Clinical Disorders of Social Cognition

Clinical Disorders of Social Cognition provides contemporary neuroscientific theories of social cognition in a wide range of conditions across the lifespan. Taking a trans-diagnostic approach to understanding these disorders, it discusses how they present in different conditions, ranging from brain injury to neurodevelopmental disorders, psychiatric conditions and dementia.

Social cognitive disorders directly impact upon individuals' work, leisure and social functioning. This book also collates and critiques the best and most useful assessment tools across the different disorders and coalesces research into intervention strategies across disorders to provide practical information about how such disorders can be assessed and treated so individuals can have meaningful, effective and satisfying social interactions.

This book is essential reading for clinicians who work with people with clinical disorders and who are looking for new knowledge to understand, assess and treat their clients with social cognitive impairment. It will also appeal to students and professionals in clinical neuropsychology, speech and language pathology and researchers who are interested in learning more about the social brain and understanding how evidence from clinical conditions can inform this.

Skye McDonald is a world leader in understanding social cognitive disorders after brain injury and has published 200 peer-reviewed journal articles on this topic. Her interests span theory development, the development of ecologically valid assessments and the development of remediation and intervention programs.

Clinical Disorders of Social Cognition

Edited by Skye McDonald

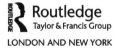

Routledge
Taylor & Francis Group

LONDON AND NEW YORK

First published 2022
by Routledge
2 Park Square, Milton Park, Abingdon, Oxon OX14 4RN

and by Routledge
605 Third Avenue, New York, NY 10158

Routledge is an imprint of the Taylor & Francis Group, an informa business

© 2022 selection and editorial matter, Skye McDonald; individual chapters, the contributors

The right of Skye McDonald to be identified as the author of the editorial material, and of the authors for their individual chapters, has been asserted in accordance with sections 77 and 78 of the Copyright, Designs and Patents Act 1988.

British Library Cataloguing-in-Publication Data
A catalogue record for this book is available from the British Library

Library of Congress Cataloging-in-Publication Data
A catalog record for this book has been requested

ISBN: 978-0-367-46120-1 (hbk)
ISBN: 978-0-367-46119-5 (pbk)
ISBN: 978-1-003-02703-4 (ebk)

DOI: 10.4324/9781003027034

Typeset in Bembo
by Apex CoVantage, LLC

Contents

Figures

Boxes: Case studies

Tables

Contributors

Vicki Anderson, Murdoch Children's Research Institute, Royal Children's Hospital, University of Melbourne, Melbourne, Australia

Miriam Beauchamp, University of Montreal, Montreal, Canada, Sainte-Justine Hospital Research Center, Montreal, Canada

Anneli Cassel, School of Psychology, UNSW, Sydney, Australia

Anita Chisholm, Murdoch Children's Research Institute, Department of Paediatrics, Faculty of Medicine, Dentistry and Health Sciences, University of Melbourne, Parkville, Victoria, Australia

Jennifer Chow, Murdoch Children's Research Institute, Melbourne, Victoria, Australia

Louise Crowe, Murdoch Children's Research Institute and Psychological Sciences & Paediatrics, University of Melbourne, Melbourne, Australia

Simone Darling, Murdoch Children's Research Institute and Psychological Sciences & Paediatrics, University of Melbourne, Melbourne, Australia

Helen Genova, Center for Neuropsychology and Neuroscience Research, Kessler Foundation, East Hanover, New Jersey, USA

Mardee Greenham, Murdoch Children's Research Institute, Melbourne, Australia

Cynthia Honan, School of Psychological Sciences, University of Tasmania, Hobart, Australia

Michelle Kelly, School of Psychology, University of Newcastle, Newcastle, NSW Australia

Fiona Kumfor, Department of Psychology, University of Sydney, Sydney, Australia

Alice Maier, Murdoch Children's Research Institute, The Royal Children's Hospital, Parkville, Victoria, Australia

Skye McDonald, School of Psychology, UNSW, Sydney, Australia

Katherine Osborne-Crowley, University of NSW, Sydney, Australia

Jonathan Payne, Murdoch Children's Research Institute, Department of Paediatrics, Faculty of Medicine, Dentistry and Health Sciences, University of Melbourne, Parkville, Victoria, Australia

Amy Pinkham, School of Behavioral and Brain Sciences, University of Texas at Dallas, Texas, USA

Nicholas P. Ryan, Murdoch Children's Research Institute, Melbourne, Australia, School of Psychology, Deakin University

Jacoba M. Spikman, Faculty of Behavioural and Social Sciences, University of Gronigen, Netherlands

Travis Wearne, School of Psychology, University of NSW, Sydney, Australia

Herma J. Westerhof-Evers, Faculty of Behavioural and Social Sciences, University of Gronigen, Netherlands

Stephanie Wong, Department of Psychology, University of Sydney, Sydney, Australia

Acknowledgements

We would like to acknowledge the kind provision of brain templates used in Chapters 1 and 5, provided by Professor George Paxinos and Professor Juergen K. Mai, NeuRA, Sydney, Australia.

Chapter 1

Introduction to social cognition

Skye McDonald and Fiona Kumfor

Social cognition refers to our ability to attend to, process and interpret social signals so as to understand other people. This is the most fundamental of human abilities. As we are essentially social animals, we need to get on with others. We need to understand whether we are welcome or not, whether our behaviour is acceptable or not, whether others intend us harm or kindness. We need to be able to determine if others are interested, enthralled, bored or outraged by what we say and do, and we need to be able to modify our behaviour based on these cues so as to achieve our own social goals.

Many clinical conditions arising from developmental, psychiatric and acquired brain disorders are associated with impaired social cognition. Indeed, a systematic review of meta-analyses concluded that a wide variety of neurological disorders produced significant impairments in social cognition with moderate to large effects sizes (d = 0.41 to 1.81) that were comparable to impairments in general cognition and in some conditions, e.g. frontotemporal dementia, exceeded them. Similar, although more variable deficits, were seen in psychiatric disorders (Cotter et al., 2018). These impairments have the potential to significantly curtail psychosocial function and, therefore, are of major clinical concern. It is only relatively recently, however, that social cognition has been considered to be a cognitive domain that is distinct from non-social abilities. There are a number of sources of evidence that speak to its functional independence.

Firstly, as social animals, it is an evolutionary imperative that humans are able to interact successfully with each other. Arguably, this is more important than possessing good intellectual ability to understand the physical environment, learn and problem solve. Provided individuals are well integrated in their community, they can rely on and benefit from the group's collective skills. This suggests that evolutionary pressures exerted on the development of social cognition are separate and possibly pre-date general cognitive abilities.

Secondly, functional neuroimaging suggests that distinct areas of the brain are activated when individuals are engaged in social compared to non-social tasks. So, for example, when thinking about oneself, thinking about psychological attributes of other people, watching emotional events or judging what

DOI: 10.4324/9781003027034-1

kind of emotions others are experiencing, constellations of neural systems in the frontal and temporal lobes are reliably implicated.

Thirdly, there are many clinical disorders in which social and non-social abilities dissociate, that is, individuals can have profound difficulties in one realm but not the other. Autism spectrum disorders (ASD) refer to a spectrum of developmental disorders that are characterised by specific impairment in social function. Individuals with ASD can have intellectual abilities that span the normal range, including those with above average or even superior intellectual skills. Despite this, they suffer from a limited capacity to understand and interact with their social world. The converse can also be found. Williams syndrome is a rare genetic disorder that leads to profound, developmental intellectual disability. Despite this, children with Williams syndrome are highly social. They seek out the company of others and display affectionate, prosocial behaviour.

Brain damage can also selectively impair social abilities. One of the most well known cases is EVR (Eslinger & Damasio, 1985). This man was a successful businessman who underwent surgical resection of a meningioma in his frontal lobe. Following this surgery, his general intellectual abilities were assessed as intact, in the superior range. Despite this, his social abilities deteriorated, and his business eventually disintegrated. In another example, AS suffered a severe brain injury in a motor bike accident. Prior to the injury, he had been a popular member of his motorbike gang and was a well-regarded fitter and turner at the local government bus depot. Following the injury, his cognitive abilities returned to premorbid (high average) levels. However, his interpersonal skills deteriorated. He was overly talkative, egocentric and did not pick up social cues. Years after the injury, he still worked in his former position but was shunned by his work mates. He had no friends and no romantic relationships. He continued to live with his parents where he would embarrass them regularly in front of their friends with tales of buying illegal drugs and engaging sex-workers. AS participated in a number of research studies where he demonstrated that, despite good neuropsychological function, he could not understand sarcasm (McDonald, 1992) and was unable to consider the listener's perspective when explaining a procedure (McDonald, 1993).

In dementia also, social abilities can be differentially impaired. Thus, for example, people with Alzheimer's disease experience loss of cognitive skills such as memory and problem-solving skills early in the disease but retain social skills until the disease advances. In contrast, people who develop the behavioural variant of frontotemporal dementia show early decline of social skills, loss of emotional understanding and empathy. Meta-analytic reviews confirm that social cognitive deficits characterise people with FTD rather than AD and are independent of impairments in cognitive function (Bora, Velakoulis, & Walterfang, 2016a).

The field of social cognition is rapidly evolving and the description of its components and processes is expanding. Essentially, however, there is agreement that social cognition provides us with the ability to use social cues to represent the mental states, i.e. beliefs, feelings, experiences and intentions, of other people, as well as the ability to understand these in relation to our own mental states and to use this information to regulate our social behavior (Adolphs, 2001; Amodio & Frith, 2006). A schematic view of the stages in social cognition, i.e. perception, evaluation and regulation, is detailed in Figure 1.1.

In terms of perceptual processes, most social cognition research has been limited to the processing of visual and auditory cues (e.g. facial expressions, voice). However, it is important to appreciate that, while less studied, other sensory cues such as touch and pheromones may also play a role. Once perceptual cues have been identified, the viewer must use these and the context to infer and evaluate the mental states they represent.

In Figure 1.1, such evaluative processes include those involved in experiencing and understanding emotions as well as social cognitive ability to understand thoughts based on the behaviour and communication of others. In reality, these are probably all entwined. Finally, in order to understand others, it is critical that we are self-aware and able to understand ourselves in relation to them. We also need to be able to regulate our own reactions and emotions. For example, when we empathise, it is useful to understand how another person feels and that may involve a degree of emotional sharing or resonance. But we must also be able to step back and understand that the emotion is not ours, so as to engage in a constructive manner. Thus, we need to be self-aware, be able to differentiate between self and other, to contextualise the events that are occurring (i.e. access language, memory, executive control, etc.) and we need to be able to self-regulate our responses.

There are a number of different aspects to social cognition that have been researched extensively in clinical populations and others that are, as yet, less well delineated and understood. In the following sections, we will focus on the better-known facets of social cognition including face identity, theory of

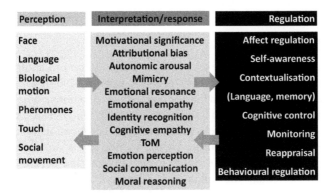

Figure 1.1 Processes involved in social cognition

mind, emotion perception, emotional empathy, self-awareness, attributional bias, moral reasoning and social behaviour.

Identity recognition

Syndromes whereby people cannot recognise the identity of other people have had a long history in neuropsychology (e.g. Bodamer, 1947) and, indeed, are among the more commonly known neuropsychological disorders in the non-scientific press thanks to popular accounts such as Oliver Sacks' book *The man who mistook his wife for a hat* (Sacks, 1985). Disorders of face recognition have not typically been included in discussions of social cognition disorders with some notable exceptions (Hutchings, Palermo, Piguet, & Kumfor, 2017; Kumfor, Hazelton, De Winter, de Langavant, & Van den Stock, 2017). Being able to discriminate between strangers on the basis of face and body characteristics is fundamental to social competence and can be selectively impaired with brain lesions (De Renzi, Scotti, & Spinnler, 1969). Equally disabling is a disorder which impairs the ability to recognise the identity of familiar people, a disorder known as prosopagnosia (Bate, Bennetts, Tree, Adams, & Murray, 2019). Such face processing disorders reflect damage to the *fusiform gyri*, especially on the right (Watson, Huis in 't Veld, & de Gelder, 2016). In a particular variant of this, the patient may recognise the face but believe it is an imposter, otherwise known as Capgras syndrome. Theories regarding Capgras syndrome suggest that it arises from the normal processing of the face but a loss of attendant arousal with an associated loss of a sense of familiarity (Ellis & Young, 1990), combined with an impaired capacity to evaluate one's own, mistaken beliefs (Coltheart, 2010). The *retrosplenial cortex* has been implicated in the reduction of familiarity detection in Capgras while the *right ventral frontal cortex* has been implicated in the impairment of the detection of expectancy violation (Darby, Laganiere, Pascual-Leone, Prasad, & Fox, 2017). Brain regions associated with face identity disorders are highlighted in Figure 1.2 and the main features of the disorders summarised in Table 1.1.

Empathy

Empathy refers to the capacity to understand and respond to another person's experience in a prosocial manner (Decety & Jackson, 2004). Empathy has a cognitive and affective component (see Figure 1.3). Cognitive empathy entails theory of mind (ToM), i.e. the ability to consider things from another persons' point of view. This can be cognitive (understanding thoughts and beliefs) or affective (understanding another person's emotional state). Affective ToM entails emotion perception, the ability to identify another person's emotional expression. It also entails the ability to deduce what kind of emotions another may be experiencing based on context. On the other hand, emotional empathy refers to the observer experiencing an emotional response that resonates with the feelings of the other. This resonance is considered to be a 'pro-social'

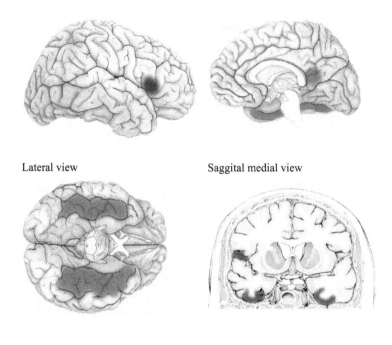

Lateral view

Saggital medial view

Ventral view

Coronal section

Lateral view: right frontal cortex implicated in Capgras; Sagittal, fusiform gyrus and retrosplenial cortex; Ventral view: fusiform gyrus; Coronal section: fusiform gyrus and right ventral frontal cortex.

Figure 1.2 Neural structures engaged in face perception

Table 1.1 Summary of disorders of face perception

	Type of task requirement	*Type of task*	*Implicated brain regions*	*Type of disorders*	*Variants*
Face perception	Match these faces	Photos	Fusiform gyrus, V5, Retrosplenial cortex, right frontal cortex	Failure to identify face across different angles, lighting, expressions	
Face recognition	Identify this face	Photos		Failure to recognise familiar faces	❖Failure to recognise the person ❖Belief the person is an imposter (Capgras)

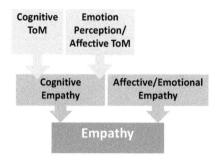

Figure 1.3 Components of empathy

process, more regulated than simple emotional contagion, which is a basic phenomenon shared across species (e.g. fear spreading through a flock). As we will discuss further, because affective ToM and emotion perception involve the processing of emotion, they are sometimes considered part of emotional empathy. Either way, both cognitive and emotional empathy work in concert. Self-awareness and self-regulation are also essential elements of empathy, enabling the observer to understand that the experiences of the other person are not their own and to control their own responses appropriately (Decety & Meyer, 2008).

Many clinical disorders are associated with deficits in empathy, including developmental disorders such as ASD (Baron-Cohen & Wheelwright, 2004), neuropsychiatric disorders such as schizophrenia (Bonfils, Lysaker, Minor, & Salyers, 2017), neurodegenerative diseases such as frontotemporal dementia (Dermody et al., 2016), non-progressive brain pathology such as traumatic brain injury (TBI) (de Sousa et al., 2010; Neumann, Zupan, Malec, & Hammond, 2013; Wood & Williams, 2008) and stroke (Adams, Schweitzer, Molenberghs, & Henry, 2019; Nijsse, Spikman, Visser-Meily, de Kort, & van Heugten, 2019) as well as mood disorders (Cusi, MacQueen, Spreng, & McKinnon, 2011).

While empathy deficits may be common across such disorders, there is variety in the way in which they manifest. For example, psychopathy and narcissistic personality disorder are characterised by normal cognitive empathy, but a lack of emotional empathy (Ritter et al., 2011; Shamay-Tsoory, Harari, Aharon-Peretz, & Levkovitz, 2010). In contrast, people with ASD tend to have low cognitive empathy and normal emotional empathy (Dziobek et al., 2008; Jones, Happé, Gilbert, Burnett, & Viding, 2010). It is also possible to have enhanced emotion perception yet poor cognitive ToM, as is seen in people with borderline personality disorders (Harari, Shamay-Tsoory, Ravid, & Levkovitz, 2010).

In neurodegenerative brain disorders, other profiles of empathy disturbance are seen. While frontotemporal disorder tends to impair both cognitive and emotional empathy, Alzheimer's disease impairs cognitive but not emotional empathy (Dermody et al., 2016). Natural ageing is associated with either stable or increasing affective empathy with age and stable or slightly lower cognitive empathy (Beadle & De La Vega, 2019). Within any clinical condition, the extent to which empathy is affected, and the kind of empathic process that is impaired, will depend on the neural structures implicated, the manner in which it is assessed and other features of the disorder. In the following sections, we will consider major components that make up the construct of empathy.

Cognitive empathy

Theory of mind

Theory of mind (ToM) refers to the ability to understand what another person may think, believe or feel, and to understand that another's thoughts are distinct from one's own (Amodio & Frith, 2006). By having a ToM, we are able to predict what others are thinking and therefore what they might do (Premack & Woodruff, 1978). ToM is pivotal to understand not simply the purpose of others' actions, but the intent behind what they say. Many of our verbal utterances are indirect, in order to hint, skirt around delicate subjects, abrade, make fun of and so on (Gibbs & Mueller, 1988). Therefore, we need to gauge what is on another's mind to understand their meaning and this requires ToM. ToM develops incrementally from the age of four years when children can understand that another person may hold a different belief to themselves (first order ToM) (Wimmer & Perner, 1983), with more sophisticated understanding about what one person believes another person believes (second order ToM) developing by the age of six or seven (Perner & Wimmer, 1985). The ability to correctly interpret indirect, ironic remarks relies upon this second order ability (Demorest, Meyer, Phelps, Gardner, & Winner, 1984). ToM may refer specifically to the ability to understand another person's thoughts and beliefs, i.e. cognitive ToM, but also extends to understanding their emotional state, i.e. affective ToM. This aspect of ToM ability overlaps with emotion perception.

Children with ASD appear to lack a ToM, regardless of level of intellectual ability (Baron-Cohen, Leslie, & Frith, 1985). Differentially poor ToM abilities, not explained by cognitive impairment, can also be seen following acquired brain injuries, neurodegenerative conditions, e.g. frontotemporal dementia, and subgroups within neuropsychiatric conditions, e.g. schizophrenia (Bora, Yucel, & Pantelis, 2009; Fanning, Bell, & Fiszdon, 2012; Martin-Rodriguez & Leon-Carrion, 2010). Thus, impaired ToM can represent a specific, discrete impairment. This is not to say, however, that poor cognitive function does not affect ToM performance. Situations in which ToM abilities are needed are usually multi-modal and interactive. The person making the ToM judgement needs to understand the other person's facial and body signals, language and context in order to appreciate what they are thinking. Tasks that are used to test ToM are often in the form of short narratives, where one story character knows something the other does not, or makes a non-literal comment such as a lie or sarcasm, or unintentionally makes a faux pas. It is common to use written stories, pictures, photos or videos to present material that requires a ToM judgement. Understanding of ToM and emotions is usually measured by asking the participant to answer questions or choose between verbal labels. Because of these cognitive demands, people who have poor working memory, language ability, new learning and/or executive abilities will have trouble with ToM tasks, with more complex ToM judgements placing greater demand on such skills. In some populations (e.g. Huntington's disease, multiple sclerosis, schizophrenia), there is a clear link between poor ToM performance and the degree of cognitive impairment (Bora, 2017; Bora, Ozakbas, Velakoulis, & Walterfang, 2016; Bora & Pantelis, 2016; Bora, Walterfang, & Velakoulis, 2015). Nevertheless, the fact that individuals or subgroups can present with poor ToM despite good cognitive skills, attests to the likelihood that ToM ability also relies upon specific, discrete, mentalising abilities.

Specific neural structures engaged in ToM

Functional magnetic resonance imaging (fMRI) in healthy adults has pointed to a specific neural network underpinning mental state judgements (Amodio & Frith, 2006). fMRI scans provide a snapshot of what brain structures are activated when performing a specific social cognitive task compared to a control task. There have been hundreds of such studies enabling meta-analytic reviews. Specifically, across the wide range of tasks used to tap ToM, there is bilateral activation along the medial aspect of the brain, in the *anterior dorsal medial prefrontal cortex* extending into the *orbitofrontal cortex* and *cingulate* as well as the *precuneus*. On the lateral surface, bilateral activation is seen in the *bilateral temporo-parietal junctions*, extending along the *superior temporal gyrus* into the *temporal poles* and into the *inferior frontal gyrus* (Molenberghs, Johnson, Henry, & Mattingley, 2016). Variation in activation and lateralisation reflects the nature of the task (verbal vs non-verbal, explicit vs implicit, etc.).

Each of the neural areas highlighted in meta-analyses have also been associated with different types of ToM reasoning. The *dorsal medial prefrontal cortex* has been shown to be activated in tasks where the participant is asked to think about themselves (Northoff et al., 2006) or about psychological attributes of others (D'Argembeau et al., 2007). Activation of the *medial prefrontal cortex* increases with the number of perspectives the participant is asked to consider (Meyer & Collier, 2020). The *anterior cingulate gyrus* plays a role in conflict monitoring (Barch et al., 2001) and activates when considering concepts related to self

(Murray, Schaer, & Debbané, 2012). The *posterior cingulate/precuneus* has been attributed a role in many high-level integrative tasks including visuospatial judgements and assuming the self and other perspective (Cavanna & Trimble, 2006; Murray et al., 2012). *Inferior dorsolateral (BA 9 and 10)* and *orbitofrontal (BA 45/47)* regions are also involved when considering another person's perspective (D'Argembeau et al., 2007). The same region *(BA 45/47)* has been theorised to form part of the human mirror neuron system, i.e. a neural system that is activated not only when planning purposeful movement, but observing it in others (Rizzolatti & Sinigaglia, 2010), discussed later in more detail.

Lesion studies suggest that *ventromedial (especially right)* lesions are associated with impaired ToM judgements, such as understanding irony and faux pas (Shamay-Tsoory, Tomer, & Aharon-Peretz, 2005). The *temporo-parietal junction* has been attributed a specific role in understanding biological movement and agency (Castelli, Frith, Happe, & Frith, 2002) while the *anterior temporal lobe* is activated for tasks requiring conceptual or semantic social knowledge (Pobric, Lambon Ralph, & Zahn, 2016).

Finally, it is important to appreciate that ToM tasks in the real world are multimodal. To understand another's mental state may require watching them, listening to their words, understanding the context they are referring to, etc. Thus, efficient ToM requires the coordinated processing of multiple channels of information and stored representations. People with congenital or acquired damage to the *corpus callosum* and other *white matter fibre tracts* have impaired naturalistic ToM judgements (McDonald, Dalton, Rushby, & Landin-Romero, 2019; McDonald, Rushby, Dalton, Allen, & Parks, 2018; Symington, Paul, Symington, Ono, & Brown, 2010).

Affective ToM

Affective ToM refers to the capacity to attribute emotional mental states to others. Affective ToM, like cognitive ToM, can range from first order judgements (gauging how another person feels) to second order judgements (gauging what one person wants another person to feel). Second order affective ToM overlaps considerably with second order cognitive ToM, as both reflect abstract judgements which could arise from a range of contextual cues, such as visual displays and verbal narratives. First order affective ToM, on the other hand, overlaps with emotion perception discussed below. A summary of the kinds of disorders of ToM is provided in Table 1.2.

Emotion perception

Emotion perception refers to the ability to attend to, process and identify the physically expressed emotional state of others and has long been considered a critical human ability.

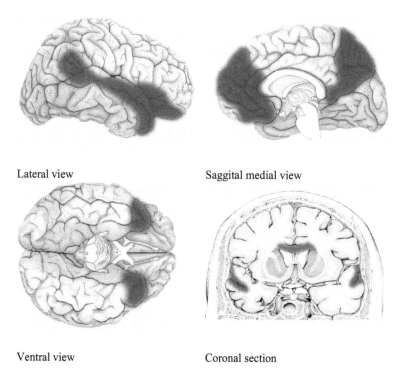

Lateral view   Saggital medial view

Ventral view   Coronal section

Lateral view: temporoparietal junction, superior temporal sulcus, temporal pole, inferior frontal gyrus, orbitofrontal cortex; Sagittal, medial view: dorsal medial prefrontal cortex, orbitofrontal cortex, anterior cingulate cortex, precuneus; Ventral view: temporal poles. Coronal view: superior temporal sulcus.

Figure 1.4 Neural structures engaged in ToM

The role of the right hemisphere in emotion perception

Initial research suggested a fundamental role for the right hemisphere in the mediation of emotions. The first report of a patient who had lost his ability to understand emotion in voice was attributed to a stroke in the right hemisphere (Heilman, Scholes, & Watson, 1975). Not long after, patients with right hemisphere lesions were reported who lost their ability to express emotion in voice (Ross & Mesulam, 1979). This was taken to suggest that the right hemisphere may mediate a parallel role to the left hemisphere's role in the production and comprehension of language, i.e. right frontal and right posterior regions might mediate the production and comprehension of affective speech respectively.

Table 1.2 Summary of disorders of ToM

	Type of knowledge	Type of tasks	Implicated brain regions	Type of disorders	Variants
Cognitive: First order	What does Sally think...	Cartoons, texts, videos	DMPFC, OFC, CG, PC, TPJ, STS, TP, IFG, CC and other white matter tracts	Impaired understanding of self-other distinction (often preserved in adults)	❖ Primary loss of mental reasoning, e.g. lack of use of mental state terms ❖ May have particular difficulty moving from own perspective to another's (problem of inhibition) ❖ Problems primarily arise due to cognitive demands of the task ❖ Problems to do with connections between multiple brain areas required to process multi-modal information
Cognitive: Second order	What does Sally think that John thinks...			Impaired judgements regarding complex perspectives or knowledge states	
Affective: First order (emotion perception)	What does Sally feel...	Cartoons, texts, videos	OFC, Insula, STS, CG, SS and MG, amygdala, BG	Impaired emotion recognition	See Table 3 for further detail
Affective: Second order	What does Sally want John to feel...		DMPFC, OFC, CG, PC, TPJ, STS, TP, IFG, CC and other white matter tracts	Impaired understanding of other people's desires and intentions, use of indirect language, faux pas	Similar to those seen in cognitive ToM

DMPFC = dorsomedial prefrontal cortex, OFC = orbitofrontal prefrontal cortex, CG = cingulate gyrus, PC = precuneus, TPJ = temporoparietal junction, STS = superior temporal sulcus, TP = temporal pole, IFG = inferior frontal gyrus, SS = somatosensory strip, MG = motor gyrus, BG = basal ganglia, CC = corpus callosum

Later reports followed that patients with right hemisphere lesions had difficulty recognising emotions in faces (Borod, Koff, Lorch, & Nicholas, 1986) as well as extracting emotional information from pictures and narratives (Brownell, Powelson, & Gardner, 1983; Cicone, Wapner, & Gardner, 1980).

This notion that the right hemisphere may be dominant for all emotions has since been challenged. An alternative point of view is that the right hemisphere may be dominant for processing negative or 'withdrawal' emotions and the left hemisphere dominant for positive and 'approach' emotions. One strand of evidence for this was the general finding that patients with right hemisphere lesions were often unrealistically euphoric or indifferent, suggesting they were no longer able to process negative emotions. Conversely, patients with left hemisphere stroke were prone to depression suggesting a loss of positive emotions (Gainotti, 1972; Sackeim et al., 1982). It is also possible that the right hemisphere is dominant for the processing of negative emotions while positive emotions are processed bilaterally (Adolphs, Jansari, & Tranel, 2001). Consistent with this view, meta-analyses of studies of emotion perception following right versus left hemisphere stroke reveals a pattern of large deficits in people with right hemisphere stroke when identifying and labelling (d = -3.02, -1.51) negative emotions with still large but relatively smaller effects for positive emotions (d = -1.33, -0.84). Left hemisphere stroke also impacted the identification and labelling of negative (d = -1.12, -0.26) and positive (d = -0.41, -0.38) emotions with smaller effect sizes that did not always reach significance. Right hemisphere stroke caused greater impairment than left hemisphere on emotion perception and this was particularly noticeable for negative emotions (d = -1.02, -1.42) (Abbott, Cumming, Fidler, & Lindell, 2013).

Specific neural structures underpinning emotion perception

Neuroimaging research suggests that the neural system underpinning emotion perception is likely to be distributed and bilateral, although the right hemisphere does appear to play a more dominant role. Computerised tomography (CT) and magnetic resonance imaging (MRI) scans of structural lesions in patients with brain damage have clearly implicated the *amygdala* in emotion processing. The *amygdala* forms part of a network connecting the *neocortex, hypothalamus, thalamus, basal forebrain* and *brainstem*, providing a mechanism for reciprocal interaction between the cortex and the autonomic nervous system (Emery & Amaral, 2000). Specific damage to the *amygdala* has been associated with loss of an autonomic fear response to aversive events (Bechara et al., 1995) and the loss of recognition of fear and other negative emotions in face (Adolphs, Tranel, Damasio, & Damasio, 1994; Kumfor, Irish, Hodges, & Piguet, 2013) and voice (Scott et al., 1997). Mostly, studies have suggested that bilateral *amygdala* damage underpins such emotional loss, but some studies have, again, suggested that right hemisphere *amygdala* lesions produce more severe deficits (Adolphs & Tranel, 2004; Adolphs, Tranel, & Damasio, 2001).

In addition to the *amygdala*, it has long been known that lesions to the *orbital/medial prefrontal cortex* and *ventral, anterior cingulate cortex* lead to personality change including disinhibition, lability, aggression and apathy (Barrash, Tranel, & Anderson, 2000; Grafman et al., 1996) and also to impairments in emotion perception and self-reported emotional experience, especially for negative emotions (Hornak, Rolls, & Wade, 1996). This constellation has lead theorists to suggest the *prefrontal cortex* (especially the right) may specifically mediate anger (Adolphs, 2002). Damage to the *anterior insula cortex* especially in the left hemisphere, along with the *basal ganglia*, have also been associated with a loss of perception of disgust in patients with focal brain lesions (Calder, Keane, Manes, Antoun, & Young, 2000) and Huntington's disease (Sprengelmeyer et al., 1996).

Interestingly, lesions to the *somatosensory cortex* and *motor cortex*, once again especially on the right, have also been linked to poor emotion perception.

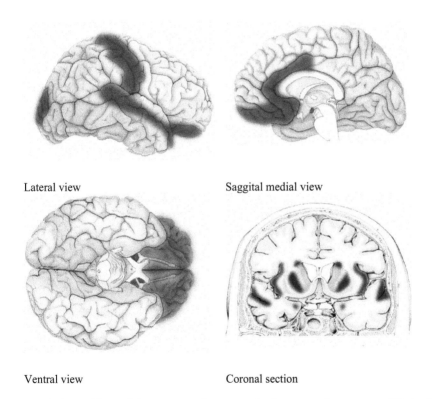

Lateral view   Saggital medial view

Ventral view   Coronal section

Lateral view: orbitomedial cortex, superior temporal sulcus, sensorimotor areas, V5 visual area (latter three regions implicated in dynamic expressions). Sagittal view: orbitomedial prefrontal cortex, anterior cingulate gyrus, amygdala; Ventral view: orbitofrontal cortex; Coronal section: insular, superior temporal sulcus, basal ganglia.

Figure 1.5 Neural structures associated with emotion perception

This finding fits in with the notion that people understand emotions in others through the process of simulation, that is, their somatosensory and motor cortex activate "as if" they were experiencing the emotion directly (Adolphs, Damasio, & Tranel, 2002; Adolphs, Damasio, Tranel, & Damasio, 1996).

Different categories of emotion

As may be apparent from the previous overview, researchers have attributed different structures to different emotions, the *amygdala* for processing fear, the *insula* for processing disgust and the *prefrontal cortex* for processing anger and high arousal emotions (as an aside, no specific structures have ever been associated with positive emotions!). However, whether there is such specialisation of brain systems to mediate different types of emotions is controversial. Once again, meta-analytic reviews of neuroimaging studies of normal healthy adults have provided some insight into this. Overall, it appears that specific structures may play a role in attributes that are important to particular emotions, rather than the emotions themselves. Thus, (Lindquist, Wager, Kober, Bliss-Moreau, & Barrett, 2012) concluded from their review that the *amygdala* may not be specific to the perception of fear, but rather, may have an important role in triggering the orienting response to novel, potentially arousing, events. Consistent with this, the *amygdala* is active even when processing masked emotional stimuli, an activation that rapidly dissipates (Costafreda, Brammer, David, & Fu, 2008; Sergerie, Chochol, & Armony, 2008). It would also appear that left versus right amygdala activation is influenced by task requirements, e.g. the *left amygdala* is more activated in tasks requiring language and the *right amygdala* more activated when processing covert emotional material (Costafreda et al., 2008; Sergerie et al., 2008). In a similar fashion, Lindquist et al argued that, rather than disgust, the *insula* may play a specific role in the integration of self-awareness and bodily states, while the *prefrontal* cortex may be critical for regulating high arousal sensations.

The special status of negative emotions

Whether or not there are discrete neural systems underpinning the processing of specific emotions, the general findings from research into many different clinical disorders is that perception of negative emotions is differentially affected relative to positive emotions (Bora, Ozakbas et al., 2016; Bora & Pantelis, 2013; Bora, Velakoulis et al., 2016a; Bora & Yener, 2017; Cotter et al., 2016; Lozier, Vanmeter, & Marsh, 2014). Even when poor performance on both positive and negative emotions has been reported, positive emotions, especially happiness, are usually affected to a lesser extent (Abbott et al., 2013; Bora & Meletti, 2016; Bora, Velakoulis, & Walterfang, 2016b; Coundouris, Adams, & Henry, 2020). There are two important possible explanations for this.

Asymmetry of representation of negative versus positive emotional categories

The first reflects a potential artefact arising from the conventional approach to assessing emotion perception. Most test batteries sample the six 'basic' emotions using actors posing an intense portrayal of the emotion. Of these six emotions, four are negative and only two positive. The negative emotions (sadness, fear, anger and disgust) require relatively subtle discrimination compared to the two positive (happy and surprised). 'Happy', in particular, is associated with the characteristic wide mouth and is, by far, the most easily recognised of all emotions with normal adults often performing at ceiling (Rosenberg, McDonald, Dethier, Kessels, & Westbrook, 2014). So a relative drop in performance for negative emotions may reflect this asymmetry in difficulty.

There is evidence for this explanation. Using the Emotion Recognition Test (Kessels, Montagne, Hendriks, Perrett, & de Haan, 2014) to assess people with TBI, the usual differentially poor performance on negative emotions was found when the participants viewed each emotion at 100% intensity (Rosenberg, Dethier, Kessels, Westbrook, & McDonald, 2015). This effect disappeared, however, when the task was modified so that each expression was displayed at a different intensity to yield roughly the same accuracy across emotions for normal healthy adults (happiness was displayed at 20%, anger at 20%, disgust at 30%, fear at 100%, sadness at 70% and surprise at 70%). In another modification, Rosenberg and colleagues developed a task with 22 emotions, 11 positive and 11 negative. This yielded not only an equal number of positive versus negative emotions but also an equal number of distractors of the same valence to choose between. Using this method, the differentially poor performance on negative emotions usually seen in people with brain injury was, again, no longer there. (Rosenberg, McDonald, Rosenberg, & Westbrook, 2016).

Engagement of automatic emotional responses to emotional stimuli

Despite problems with the arbitrary design of emotion perception tasks, there is no doubt that in other circumstances, people with brain lesions can show aberrant responses to negative emotions. There is another explanation for this, which is based on a theoretical understanding of how emotions are processed in the human brain. Based upon reviews of animal, neuroimaging and clinical studies, Phillips, Drevets, Rauch, and Lane (2003) and many others have proposed that emotion perception involves not only the identification of the emotional significance of an event, but the production of an affective state of physiological arousal in response to that stimulus and its regulation. Animal research has identified the presence of short, subcortical routes that provide rapid coarse processing of danger signals in the environment enabling the 'fight or flight' response (LeDoux, 1995), i.e. a state of physiological readiness and autonomic regulation. For humans, these pathways appear to converge on the *ventromedial prefrontal cortex* and *anterior cingulate*, the *insula, ventral striatum and amygdala* (Phillips et al., 2003). This ventral system is considered to be rapid and mainly automatic (Lieberman, 2007). For example, people can demonstrate an orientation reflex and rapid autonomic changes in arousal (measured as a change in skin conductance) to fearful materials even when they are not consciously aware of having seen them (Esteves, Dimberg, & Ohman, 1994; Ohman & Soares, 1994).

Heavily interacting with this automatic ventral route is a neural system that enables the slow detailed processing of the emotional signal, its contextualisation in memory and the regulation of the affective response as situationally appropriate. This neural system appears to entail the *dorsolateral* and *medial prefrontal cortex, dorsal anterior cingulate, hippocampus* and *temporoparietal cortex* (Lieberman, 2007; Phillips et al., 2003). These two systems work in concert. For example, emotion tasks that require verbal processing such as labeling, increase activation of the *dorsolateral prefrontal cortex* and decrease activation of the *amygdalae* (Hariri, Bookheiner, & Mazziotta, 2000; Keightly et al., 2003). Figure 1.6 provides a schematic overview of these two systems.

As the automatic network most likely evolved to help us deal with fear and danger, it stands to reason that this network may be especially tuned to exemplars of such negative emotional events; an angry face represents threat, a fearful face indicates danger in the immediate vicinity. Damage to this network has been shown to have a differential impact upon the processing of negative emotions relative to others.

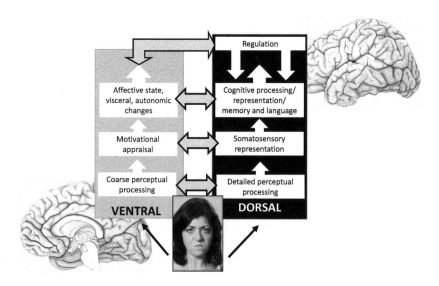

Figure 1.6 Overview of the ventral and dorsal routes to emotion processing

People with specific lesions to the *ventromedial frontal lobes* do not show a normal physiological response to negative emotionally charged pictures (Damasio, Tranel, & Damasio, 1990). Nor do patients with specific *amygdala* lesions show the usual enhancement of the 'startle' response when viewing negative images (Angrilli et al., 1996; Buchanan, Tranel, & Adolphs, 2004; Funayama, Grillon, Davis, & Phelps, 2001). Similar findings have been reported in people with TBI who frequently have damage to the *ventromedial frontal* and *temporal lobes*. People with TBI habituate unusually rapidly to angry faces (McDonald, Rushby et al., 2011). They also fail to show the normal, enhanced startle to negative images but have a normal (reduced) startle reflex when viewing positive images (Saunders, McDonald, & Richardson, 2006; Williams & Wood, 2012). Furthermore, when explicitly asked, they rated the valence of images (positive and negative) the same as did people without injuries. However, they rated the negative images as not being particularly arousing, in contrast to healthy control participants (Saunders et al., 2006). These physiological correlates of emotion perception suggest that emotion perception is not simply a cognitive task, but that emotion perception is also partially reflective of emotional resonance and empathy as we discuss further below.

Interestingly, this reciprocal relationship between ventral (automatic, autonomic) and dorsal (controlled cognitive) processes can be manipulated to ameliorate low arousal. Specifically, it has been shown that an absence of arousal (skin conductance) when viewing emotional evocative scenes in people with *ventromedial lesions* could be normalized when the patients were asked to describe the scenes, engaging cognitive and language processes (Damasio et al., 1990). A similar increased physiological response was reported when people with TBI were asked to verbally identify specific information in emotional material versus viewing this passively (McDonald, Rushby et al., 2011).

Auditory versus visual modalities

Different neural structures are also engaged depending on the mode of stimulus presentation. Partly overlapping and partly dissociable neural systems process facial versus vocal affective stimuli leading to dissociations whereby patients with brain lesions may have greater problems recognising emotions in voice versus faces and vice versa (Adolphs et al., 2002).

Static versus dynamic displays

There also appears to be a dissociation in the processing of static visual images (such as photographs) and moving images such as occur in everyday life and also captured via video. While the processing of static images appears to depend on the *amygdala, orbitofrontal cortex* and *insula* network (Adolphs, Tranel, & Damasio, 2003), dynamic visual emotional movement additionally relies upon the *superior temporal sulcus* and the *visual area V5*, regions known to be involved in the detection of biological motion (Allison, Puce, & McCarthy, 2000; Rees, Friston, & Koch, 2000), along with *parietal* and *frontal* areas (Kessler et al., 2011; Sato, Kochiyama, Yoshikawa, Naito, & Matsumura, 2004; Trautmann, Fehr, & Herrmann, 2009). Dynamic images also appear to enhance activation bilaterally in the *fusiform* (face) area and the *inferior occipital gyrus*, areas that are considered more engaged in face invariant features rather than emotion per se (Kessler et al., 2011). Other more traditional emotion perception areas including the *orbitofrontal cortex* and *amygdala* are also more activated by dynamic than static faces (Schultz & Pilz, 2009; Trautmann et al., 2009) This possibly reflects that fact that dynamic facial expressions are more familiar, socially relevant and engaging than static images. These differential systems can lead to dissociations, such as the case of B, with bilateral brain lesions, who could not recognise static emotional displays but was able to recognise dynamic (Adolphs et al., 2003).

Posed versus spontaneous emotion

A final important variation in the manner in which emotion perception tasks are designed reflects whether the images are of posed emotional displays or genuine displays. Posed emotions differ from spontaneous emotions in non-trivial ways. They are normally full intensity, with muscles pulled in line with instructions. Spontaneous emotions, on the other hand, can be subtle through to intense and are often a mixture of emotions. People rarely simply express a single emotion in an undiluted fashion. They may temper the emotion or even play against it (e.g. laughing when crying) in order to manage societal expectations. Most emotion perception tasks rely upon posed emotions, either static (Bowers, Blonder, Feinberg, & Heilman, 1991; Ekman & Freisen, 1976; Kohler et al., 2003; Matsumoto et al., 2000) or dynamic (Bryson, Bell, & Lysaker, 1997; Kessels et al., 2014). A few, however, do use actors trained to induce natural emotions (McDonald, Flanagan, Rollins, & Kinch, 2003) or untrained adults who are induced into particular emotional states (Richter & Kunzmann, 2011; Wilhelm, Hildebrandt, Manske, Schacht, & Sommer, 2014).

There is no specific research that examines whether posed versus spontaneous emotions elicit different neural systems for processing. However, natural spontaneous emotions that evolve rapidly over time will place specific processing demands on the viewer, give limited time to understand the emotional display, require an appreciation of how the social context might temper how the emotion is displayed and provide additional facial movement cues. Consequently, spontaneous emotional displays place additional cognitive demands on the viewer, such as good processing speed, working memory and memory (McDonald et al., 2006), and also provide some additional cues not available in posed displays and have been shown to ameleriate deficits in some circumstances (Davis & Gibson, 2000). For these reasons, when assessing emotion perception in clinical disorders, it is important to consider how close the assessment task is to normal social demands. For a summary of the kinds of emotion perception disorders seen, see Table 1.3.

Table 1.3 Summary of disorders of emotion perception

	Type of knowledge probed	Type of task	Implicated brain regions	Type of disorders	Variants
Faces	Which label/ face matches?	Photos, videos	OFC, STS, SS and MG, V5, CG, amygdala, insula, BG	Failure to label, match or group emotional stimuli	Dissociations can occur: ❖ Face vs voice ❖ Dynamic vs static faces ❖ Natural expressions vs posed. ❖ Negative emotions but not positive. ❖ Primary failure to understand emotion in self, e.g. lack of self awareness, alexithymia
Voices		Audio recordings, videos			
Body language		Photos, videos			

OFC = orbitofrontal prefrontal cortex, CG = cingulate gyrus, PC = precuneus, TPJ = temporoparietal junction, STS = superior temporal sulcus, V5 = visual cortex, SS = somatosensory strip, MG = motor gyrus, BG = basal ganglia

Emotional empathy

Emotional empathy is the emotional resonance that we feel when interacting with another person who is displaying emotion, relating an emotional personal experience or in an emotionally evocative situation. In order for emotional resonance to be constructively empathic, rather than simply emotional contagion, we need to regulate our emotional response and understand the difference between our self and the other, i.e. we need self awareness, ToM and self-regulation. As such, emotional empathy can be understood as an interaction between rapid, automatic responses and autonomic changes to an emotional situation (mediated by ventral frontal circuits of the brain) and cognitive processing, such as ToM and self regulation (mediated by dorsolateral frontal systems) (see Figure 1.6).

Given these different processes, emotional empathy may be disrupted in different ways. One disruption may arise due to a loss of emotional responsivity. As discussed, damage to the ventral system can lead to a diminution of physiological responses, not just to facial emotional expressions, but to any kind of emotionally evocative materials. People with *ventromedial frontal/amygdala* system damage from focal lesions or from trauma do not show a normal physiological response to faces, distressing images and films (Buchanan et al., 2004; Damasio et al., 1990; de Sousa, McDonald, & Rushby, 2012; de Sousa et al., 2010; Saunders et al., 2006; Williams & Wood, 2012). Hypoarousal is also a characteristic of individuals within clinical populations who have low empathy including psychopathy (Raine, Lencz, Bihrle, LaCasse, & Colletti, 2000; Raine, Venables, & Williams, 1995), schizophrenia (Gruzelier & Venables, 1973), attention deficit disorder (Lawrence et al., 2005) and ASD (Mathersul, McDonald, & Rushby, 2013a).

Despite this, there is little clear evidence for a relationship between hypoarousal and self-reported emotional empathy where this has been examined, for example in ASD (Mathersul et al., 2013a) and both normal adults and people with TBI (de Sousa et al., 2012; de Sousa et al., 2011; Osborne-Crowley et al., 2019a, 2019c) (although see de Sousa et al., 2010; Rushby et al., 2013). Partly, the failure to see a relationship between these constructs may reflect the way they are measured. Arousal is often measured using skin conductance, either resting state or in response to evocative materials in a laboratory setting. Empathy, on the other hand, is commonly assessed by asking the informant to reflect on their general empathic tendencies. It may be that more concordance between these constructs will be seen with different types of measurement that hone in on specific instances of empathic behaviour.

A second disruption to emotional empathy might arise from a failure to regulate one's emotional response leading to heightened emotional contagion. Cognitive strategies provide top-down processes necessary to regulate emotional distress when observing emotional events (Eippert et al., 2007). Further, impaired cognitive control in people with TBI has been associated with dysregulated emotion (McDonald, Hunt, Henry, Dimoska, & Bornhofen, 2010; Tate, 1999). Despite this, there has been no consistent evidence linking poor cognitive executive control and emotional empathy, in this population at least (Spikman, Timmerman, Milders, Veenstra, & van der Naalt, 2012; Wood & Williams, 2008). Once again, this lack of relationship may reflect reliance on measures such as standardised neuropsychological tests versus informant or self-reported empathy. Better, more specifically calibrated instruments or experimental manipulations may be necessary to uncover these theoretical relationships. A summary of disorders of emotional empathy is detailed in Table 1.4.

The role of simulation in empathy

There has been a great deal of interest in the extent to which we understand others by emulating their experiences. Simulation has been conceptualised from several theoretical view points, some from very early work in the 20th century and others more recent. These theories are helpful in understanding how empathy works and how, or why, it might break down in clinical conditions. Four main theories are (1) the facial feedback hypothesis (2) the perception-action model, (3) the mirror neuron system and (4) the default mode network.

Table 1.4 Summary of disorders of emotion empathy

	Type of task requirement	Type of task	Implicated brain regions	Type of disorders	Variants
Mimicry/ expres- sivity	Watch this face/ emotional scene/ emotional video	Photos, videos	VMPFC, ACG insula, VS, amygdala	Failure to mimic, show expressions	❖ General hypo-arousal
Arousal				Lack of arousal	❖ Lack of response to negative emotions ❖ No arousal despite mimicry
Subjective emotional changes				Lack of self-reported emotional response to emotional stimuli	❖ Deficits in arousal overcome by verbal/ cognitive mediation ❖ Heightened arousal, increased, distorted empathy ❖ Primary failure to understand emotion in self, e.g. lack of self awareness, alexithymia

VMPFC = ventromedial prefrontal cortex, ACG = anterior cingulate gyrus, VS = ventral striatum

The facial feedback hypothesis

As noted above, watching emotional faces can evoke increased arousal in the viewer. Viewers also tend to mimic the facial expressions of the person they are watching. Even if not visible, activation of the zygomaticus (cheek) muscle occurs when someone sees a happy face and, likewise, they show activation of the corrugator (brow) muscle when observing an angry facial expression (McHugo & Smith, 1996). Even their pupil size may alter to match that of the face they are observing (Harrison, Singer, Rotshtein, Dolan, & Critchley, 2006). These changes can occur even when the viewer is unaware they have seen an emotional expression (Dimberg & Ohman, 1996; Tamietto et al., 2009). So why do observers show these rapid, automatic, synchronous emotional responses when watching someone else?

This question has been one that has spurred speculation for many years. Indeed, William James (James, 1884) suggested that such physiological responses occur prior to an explicit understanding of the associated emotional state. Thus, such bodily sensations provide informational cues as to what emotion is being experienced. Lipps in 1907 (Hoffman, 1984) made a more explicit prediction. His facial feedback hypothesis stated that facial mimicry of another person was the mechanism by which the emotional state of another was processed by the viewer, i.e. the viewer mimicked the facial expression, and this mimicry subsequently engendered an emotion congruent change that facilitated understanding of the other's emotional state.

Clinical implications

In line with Lipps' theory, many studies have reported that people subjectively report emotional changes consistent with the facial expression or body posture they adopt (Flack, Laird, & Cavallaro, 1999; Laird, 1974; Soussignan, 2002; Strack, Martin, & Stepper, 1988). While a meta-analysis of a specific demonstration of this effect has cast doubt on this relationship (Wagenmakers et al., 2016) other kinds of manipulations suggest that mimicry and subjective experience are linked (Dethier, Blairy, Rosenberg, & McDonald, 2013; Osborne-Crowley et al., 2019c). People with *ventromedial frontal* pathology have reduced spontaneous facial mimicry (Angrilli, Palomba, Cantagallo, Maietti, & Stegagno, 1999; McDonald, Li et al., 2011) especially to negative facial expressions. As detailed above, they also have reduced autonomic arousal to negative facial expressions (Blair & Cipolotti, 2000; de Sousa et al., 2011; Hopkins, Dywan, & Segalowitz, 2002) further implicating a functional relationship between these processes. Interestingly, however, the association between mimicry and subjective experience can also be disrupted by brain lesions. For example, in two studies of people with TBI, it was found that when participants were asked to assume a facial expression and posture associated with a specific (negative) emotion, they either did not report emotion congruent changes in arousal (unlike their non-injured counterparts) (Dethier et al., 2013) or did not demonstrate normal changes in physiological measures of arousal (Osborne-Crowley et al., 2019c). Thus, even when mimicry was present, it did not necessarily trigger subjective or autonomic changes in people with brain lesions.

While the presence of automatic mimicry in normal healthy adults is well accepted, its role in facilitating emotion perception is mixed. Supportive evidence includes studies that have found that if the *(left) premotor cortex* is transiently disabled using transient magnetic stimulation, thus impeding mimicry, emotion recognition accuracy and reaction time are both affected deleteriously (Balconi & Bortolotti, 2013). Similarly botulinum toxin injected into facial muscles reduces both emotional experience and emotion recognition (Davis, Senghas, Brandt, & Ochsner, 2010). If normal adults are prevented from mimicry, they are also less able to recognise emotions (Niedenthal, Brauer, Halberstadt, & Innes-Ker, 2001). So too, people with locked-in syndrome and facial paralysis are less efficient when recognizing (negative) emotions than normal controls (Pistoia et al., 2010). Despite these findings, other research has not found evidence supporting a link between mimicry and emotion perception. Blairy and colleagues, for example, found mimicry and emotion recognition were not related in normal adults (Blairy, Herrera, & Hess, 1999; Hess & Blairy, 2001). While individual patients have been shown to have both poor emotion recognition and a loss of psychophysiological changes (Blair & Cipolotti, 2000), there is no evidence that the two clinical symptoms are associated in people with brain injury (McDonald, Li et al., 2011; McDonald, Rushby et al., 2011) or in a disorder of peripheral autonomic function (Heims, Critchley, Dolan, Mathias, & Cipolotti, 2004). Thus, while mimicry may facilitate emotion perception, there is insufficient evidence to conclude that it is essential.

The perception-action model

More contemporary models of emotion recognition also contest the central role of mimicry in emotion perception. The perception-action model (Preston et al., 2007) suggests that when we observe someone else's emotion, it automatically triggers a rich network of conceptual associations (e.g. associated words, situations typically associated with that type of emotion, personally relevant memories). The strength of network activation depends upon the perceived similarity (e.g. gender, age, cultural background) between ourselves and the person we observe (Preston et al., 2007). It is this network of simultaneous conceptual associations that engender understanding rather than reflexive mimicry. Indeed, according to this model, mimicry and physiological arousal may be triggered by these associations, rather than vice versa (Hofelich & Preston, 2012). Evidence for this model comes from the finding that when people are asked to categorise emotional words superimposed on an emotional face, they are slower to do so if the background face is incongruent (e.g. a happy face behind the word 'disgusted') than if the word and face are consistent (e.g. a happy face behind 'joyful') (Preston & Stansfield, 2008). This suggests that they are processing the conceptual aspects of the face automatically, even though it is irrelevant for the task at hand.

Clinical implications

The extent to which this model helps understand clinical disorders of emotion perception is, as yet, uncertain. Such automatic processing of faces has been confirmed in people with TBI but they were, otherwise, impaired on emotion recognition tasks (Osborne-Crowley et al., 2019b). So other processes must be involved. Overall, it remains unclear whether mimicry is simply a byproduct of emotion perception as suggested by the perception-action model or an integral process as suggested by the facial feedback theory. What is the case, is that clinical conditions can disrupt emotion perception and mute the extent to which mimicry occurs. It is important to consider that mimicry may serve other functions in interpersonal encounters, for example, to communicate empathic understanding (Bavelas, Black, Chovil, Lemery, & Mullett, 1988).

The mirror neuron system

In 1992 an extremely influential study was published that reported the presence of 'mirror' neurons in the F5 area of the macaque monkey's brain. These neurons fired not only when the monkey initiated a purposeful action, but also when it observed someone else performing that action (di Pellegrino, Fadiga, Fogassi, Gallese, & Rizzolatti, 1992). Further, mirror neurons were later reported in the parietal lobe (the PF/PFG complex) (Gallese, Fogassi, Fadiga, & Rizzolatti, 2002). The discovery of these mirror neurons prompted speculation that there is a neural system underlying social cognition, one that enables us to simulate the actions of others and, in doing so, understand them. Human neuroimaging and electrophysiological studies have pointed to the *ventral premotor cortex (BA 6)* and *inferior frontal gyrus (BA 44/45/47)*, along with the *inferior parietal lobe (BA 40)*, as the human equivalent of the mirror neuron system (MNS) (Rizzolatti & Sinigaglia, 2010).

However, the role of the MNS in social cognition remains controversial. Human studies are mainly limited to imaging and other indirect measures of neural activity unlike the within cell recordings that occurred in the original macaque studies. Compounding this problem, the vast majority of studies (70%) providing evidence for the human MNS have only examined observation of movement, whereas the MNS is defined as a system that is activated by both observation and execution (Molenberghs, Cunnington, & Mattingley, 2012). Further, when both observing and executing tasks have been used within a study, a wide range of neural structures are activated, including the putative MNS but extending to adjacent neural regions and well beyond that, depending on the sensory motor requirements of the task – encroaching on up to 34 Brodmann areas (Molenberghs et al., 2012). Such an extensive network calls into question the specificity of the MNS. A further problem for the MNS is the finding described above, that people with clinical disorders can have specific problems understanding negative emotions (affective ToM) but not positive. The MNS is unable to account for valence specific deficits in emotion perception.

Other accounts of simulation: the default mode network

Despite the limitations of the MNS model for explaining social cognition, the idea that there is overlap in neural activation for both one's own experience and the observation of another's emerges consistently in the cognitive neuroscience literature. For example, there is considerable (but not complete) overlap in activation of the *insula* and *anterior cingulate* when people both experience pain and when they observe someone else's pain (Jackson, Rainville, & Decety,

2006). The theorised role of the *somatosensory cortex* in emotional perception providing activation "as if" the expression were one's own is another example (Adolphs et al., 2002; Adolphs et al., 1996).

With respect to ToM reasoning, this kind of co-activation also occurs in a number of neural systems that overlap with those in what is known as the default mode network (Buckner, Andrews-Hanna, & Schacter, 2008). The default mode network was originally conceptualised as a neural system that is activated during rest but is now known to be active during internal mental activity such as thinking of the past and the future, self-reflection and daydreaming. There are at least two subsystems, a core midline system that includes the *medial prefrontal cortex* and *posterior cingulate gyrus (BA23/24)* and another encompassing the *inferior parietal lobe (temporoparietal junction and angular gyrus)*, *medial temporal lobe* and the *lateral temporal cortex* (Kim, 2012). As we discussed above, the *medial prefrontal cortex*, along with the *posterior cingulate/precuneus* is heavily engaged with self-referential thought (Northoff et al., 2006) as well as thinking about the psychological attributes of others, especially others who are similar to oneself (D'Argembeau et al., 2007). This suggests that one way we understand others is by using our own perspective as a starting point. This theoretical position is consistent with the perception-action model discussed earlier, i.e. thinking about others triggers a rich array of associations including personally relevant associations that are stronger the closer we feel we resemble the person we are thinking about (Preston et al., 2007). Of course, an important component of successful ToM reasoning is to understand that another's thoughts are actually separate to our own. To successfully move between perspectives, we need to have self-awareness and regulation in order to inhibit our own perspective for another's and vice versa. The *inferior dorsolateral* and *orbitofrontal* regions, implicated in ToM tasks, also mediate cognitive inhibition (Collette et al., 2001). Therefore, the role of these regions in ToM may be to facilitate changing perspectives between oneself and others and to inhibit one's own perspective in order to do so (Ruby & Decety, 2004).

Clinical implications

These different facets of simulation and mentalising in ToM suggest a number of ways in which ToM abilities could be affected by brain damage and clinical disorders. Certainly, evidence suggests there are differing kinds of impairment. For example, damage to the *medial prefrontal cortex* could impair the ability to think about mental states *per se*. The finding that people with TBI, often associated with medial frontal pathology, have a reduced use of mental state terms in narratives relative to non-injured control participants (Byom & Turkstra, 2012; Stronach & Turkstra, 2008) fits with this. In addition, adults with TBI report high levels of acquired alexithymia (lack of self-awareness of internal states) (Williams & Wood, 2010; Wood & Williams, 2007). Further, alexithymic symptoms, especially externally (rather than internally) oriented thinking, have been found to significantly predict poor emotion perception (Neumann et al., 2013). People with ASD also have high levels of alexithymia, and this is also related to their empathic understanding of others (Bird et al., 2010). Adults with alexithymia without brain lesions also have reduced mentalising associated with reduced medial prefrontal activation (Moriguchi et al., 2006).

ToM may also be impaired due to a failure to move from the self-perspective to another due to *orbitofrontal* damage and a loss of inhibitory control. For example, in one study, we found that people with TBI were relatively good at considering the perspectives of others; for example, choosing a holiday destination for a family with children when they, themselves were single (McDonald et al., 2014). However, they were much less able to do this if they were first asked to describe their own ideal holiday. Once their egocentric perspective had been activated, they could not consider another's point of view. Thus, loss of inhibition may impair the capacity for a detached, third-person perspective to take place.

Social (verbal) communication

Social communication is often considered a distinct facet of social cognition. While all manner of social cues may be used to communicate, language, in particular, can be used flexibly, to infer rather that state outright. Thus, social communication alludes to the capacity that we have to understand indirect, pragmatic meanings in conversation, such as understanding sarcastic comments whereby the speaker means the opposite to what they literally assert. Hints, metaphors, lies, jokes, hyperbole, understatement and polite deference are all examples of how language is used indirectly and there are many more. In fact, humans are far more likely to use language indirectly than directly, as they negotiate social relationships (Brown & Levinson, 1978). In terms of conversations and other extended verbal interactions, speakers also need social cognition so as to know how to cooperate with each other, take turns appropriately, start and end conversations effectively, probe for and give information that addresses the other party's needs and otherwise oil the wheels of social discourse.

It has long been recognised that patients can retain basic language ability following a brain insult but lose the ability to use language effectively to communicate. Thus, acquired brain damage can lead to patients becoming literal in their understanding of language, clumsy and ineffective in their expression and insensitive to the needs of their conversational partner. Arguably, description of the communicative difficulties in patients, such as those with right hemisphere stroke in the 1980s, provided the first real insight into the unique role played by social cognition in everyday function. Such difficulties have been variously described as pragmatic language disorders, higher language disorders and cognitive-communication disorders. It is probable that many such social communicative deficits overlap with, or are in fact synonymous with, aspects of social cognition already discussed, in particular ToM. Indeed, renowned pragmatic linguistic theorists, such as Grice (1975) and later Sperber and Wilson (1986), argued that the way in which listeners understand the meaning of language in context is by searching for its relevance. This requires an appraisal of the intentions of the speaker, and that is ToM. Many ToM tasks use narratives and conversations in which indirect language such as sarcasm, lies and jokes are embedded. Thus, social communication and ToM are closely entwined. In addition, aspects of social behaviour, such as initiation, regulation and inhibition, as discussed further below, are integral to dynamic, effective social interaction and communication.

Self-awareness

Critical to social cognition in general and empathy in particular, is self-awareness. We need to be self-aware to know that our emotional reaction when observing another person's distress is separate to their distress and to regulate this accordingly. We also need self-awareness to move flexibly from our viewpoint to another's and to understand the difference. Insight and self-awareness are commonly disrupted in many clinical conditions including severe TBI (Levin, Goldstein, Williams, & Eisenberg, 1991), stroke (Spalletta et al., 2007) and dementia (Bozeat, Gregory, Ralph, & Hodges, 2000). Loss of self-awareness can range from a lack of awareness of physical impairments, or anosognosia (Vuilleumier, 2004), to an absence of awareness of emotion and internal states, i.e. alexithymia (Larsen, Brand, Bermond, & Hijman, 2003), to an absence of meta-cognition, i.e. failure to reflect on and appraise one's own mental abilities and processes (Boake, Freelands, Ringholz, Nance, & Edwards, 1995; Godfrey, Partridge, Knight, & Bishara, 1993). Such impairments can also manifest as a failure to self-monitor 'on-line' when performing specific tasks, leading to a failure to detect and correct errors when they occur (Ham et al., 2014; O'Keeffe, Dockree, Moloney, Carton, & Robertson, 2007).

In general, loss of awareness has been associated with more severe and widespread brain damage (Prigatano & Altman, 1990; Sherer, Hart, Whyte, Nick, & Yablon, 2005). However, specific neural systems have also been implicated. For example, anosognosia is commonly associated with *right hemisphere* lesions (Marcel, Tegnér, & Nimmo-Smith, 2004) while deficits in meta-cognition and on-line awareness are associated with lesions in the *frontal lobes* (Alexander, Benson, & Stuss, 1989; Hoerold, Pender, & Robertson, 2013; Stuss & Benson, 1986), the *dorsal anterior cingulate*, and *the insula* (Ham et al., 2014).

Despite the obvious theoretical relationship between self-awareness and empathy, there has been very little research in this field, most of which points to a relationship. For example, people with high alexithymia made fewer ToM judgements and self-reported less cognitive and affective empathy than those with low levels of alexithymia (Moriguchi et al., 2006). Similarly, lack of clinical insight and awareness has been associated with poor ToM in people with schizophrenia (Zhang et al., 2016) and TBI (Bivona et al., 2014).

Table 1.5 Summary of impairments in self-awareness

	Type of knowledge probed	Type of tasks	Implicated brain regions	Type of disorders	Variants
Self-awareness	How have you changed?	Interview with self versus other	Widespread brain damage	Lack of insight	
Anosognosia	What are your physical limitations?		Right hemisphere lesions	Denial of impairment	Specific to particular impairments
Alexithymia	What are you feeling?	Questionnaires	Frontal lobes and range of clinical conditions	Lack of understanding of internal states	❖ Externally oriented thinking ❖ Absence of arousal changes ❖ Intact arousal changes but absence of awareness
Meta-cognition	Do you have any problems thinking?	Interview, evaluation of performance on cognitive tasks	Frontal lobes, ACG, insula	Impaired understanding of one's own performance and abilities	❖ Overestimate abilities ❖ Underestimate abilities (often due to psychogenic rather than neurogenic reasons) ❖ Poor on-line monitoring of errors

ACG = anterior cingulate gyrus

Moral reasoning

Moral reasoning refers to our capacity to make judgements concerning the 'rightness' of particular actions according to our internal moral and social code. On the one hand, it has been common to see moral judgements as a rationale process of weighing up various factors requiring abstraction and perspective taking (Kohlberg, Levine, & Hewer, 1983). On the other hand, moral reasoning is increasingly seen to involve automatic, emotional responses (Greene & Haidt, 2002). These two sides of moral reasoning map fairly clearly onto ToM reasoning – the ability to see the perspectives and intentions of agents in a given situation – and emotional empathy – the empathic concern we hold for people who may be adversely affected by the actions of others. For example, the extent to which a harmful act is seen as morally wrong is directly influenced by the degree to which it is seen as intentional versus accidental. Furthermore, when viewing such acts, people are far more likely to attend to, and be aroused by, the victim rather than the perpetrator and to view the perpetrator's intentions more harshly if the harm is to another person rather than an object (Decety, Michalska, & Kinzler, 2012). In general, the *medial prefrontal cortex, middle temporal gyrus* and *temporoparietal junction* appear to be commonly activated by tasks requiring ToM, empathy and moral reasoning (Bzdok et al., 2012). Observing intentional harm also triggers early activation of the *amygdala* (Hesse et al., 2016) which, in concert with the *orbitofrontal cortex*, is activated when evaluating potential sources of threat.

The engagement of these processes has also been used to explain the seemingly illogical disparity in people's choices when faced with superficially similar moral dilemmas: the trolley versus the footbridge. In the trolley scenario, a runaway trolley is about to hit five people, but this can be diverted on to another track where it will hit only one person by you flicking a switch. In the footbridge version, you are standing on a bridge over the tracks beside a large stranger as the trolley speeds towards the five people and you can avert disaster to them by pushing one large man off the bridge in front of the trolley. Most people tend to believe the first action is acceptable but not the second despite both resulting in the sacrifice of one person to save five. One way of explaining this disparity is to consider the footbridge situation as demanding personal (emotional) ownership of an intention to harm, whereas the trolley scenario does not require the same intention. Consistent with this, relative to the trolley scenario, the footbridge scenario is associated with greater activation of both ToM and emotion related neural networks (Greene, Nystrom, Engell, Darley, & Cohen, 2004).

Loss of moral reasoning can be seen in people with acquired brain lesions (Anderson, Bechara, Damasio, Tranel, & Damasio, 1999). For example, patients with *ventromedial prefrontal lesions* tend to have a more 'utilitarian' approach to dilemmas like the trolley dilemma relative to healthy control participants while their approach to less personal moral dilemmas was similar (Koenigs et al., 2007). People with behavioural-variant frontotemporal dementia, a condition that selectively damages the *fronto-temporal* system, also show a similar utilitarian view of the trolley task (Mendez, Anderson, & Shapira, 2005) and, in general, do not see moral transgressions as more reprehensible than other social misdemeanours, unlike controls (Lough et al., 2006). They also have difficulty differentiating between situations on the basis of whether intentional harm is present and show lower empathic concern when it is (Baez et al., 2016). Consistent with a general loss of their moral compass, antisocial behaviours are relatively common in this population, including unsolicited sexual approaches and indecent exposure, stealing food and shoplifting, urinating in public places, traffic violations and hit and run accidents. While expressing remorse when asked, these patients may not act in a way that suggests genuine contrition or concern for the consequences (Mendez, Chen, Shapira, & Miller, 2005).

Table 1.6 Summary of disorders of moral reasoning

	Type of knowledge probed	Type of tasks	Implicated brain regions	Type of disorders	Variants
Loss of moral judgement	Is this morally right?	Moral dilemmas, images of harm, everyday observation	MPFC, MTG, TPJ, amygdala, OFC	Lack of 'moral compass'	❖ Failure to grasp other's perspectives when weighing moral decisions ❖ Utilitarian approach to moral dilemmas ❖ Sociopathic behaviours ❖ Lack of contrition ❖ Insensitivity to impact of intentional harm

MPFC = medial prefrontal cortex, MTG= medial temporal gyrus, TPJ = temporoparietal junction, OFC = orbitofrontal cortex

Attributional bias

Everyone tends to have a filter through which they view the world and this filter influences the attributions they make regarding why particular events occur, the intent of others and their own experiences. These belief systems strongly influence social judgements and behavioural choices (Moore & Stambrook, 1995). While everyone has an 'attributional style', distorted attributional biases characterise many clinical disorders. These biases influence the extent to which individuals attribute events to external agents, due to situations or other people, or internally, due to themselves. One kind of bias relates to the trustworthiness of a stranger's face. It transpires that trustworthiness is fairly reliably rated across normal healthy individuals. However, people with specific *amygdala* damage can have abnormally high ratings of approachability and trustworthiness of faces that normal healthy adults view as very untrustworthy (Adolphs, Tranel, & Damasio, 1998). A similar pattern has been reported in some adults with ASD (Adolphs, Sears, & Piven, 2001) but not all (Mathersul, McDonald, & Rushby, 2013b). However, this bias can also go in the other direction. Increased perception of untrustworthiness has been associated with increasing levels of trait paranoia and hostility in people with psychosis (Buck, Pinkham, Harvey, & Penn, 2016).

Other attributional biases have also been commonly attributed to various forms of psychosis. For example, people who experience persecutory delusions and paranoid thinking tend to have a personalising bias that attributes negative events to external agents rather than situations (Bentall, Corcoran, Howard, Blackwood, & Kinderman, 2001). Paranoid thinking is also associated with the

Table 1.7 Summary of disorders of attributional bias

	Type of knowledge probed	Type of tasks	Implicated brain regions	Type of disorders	Variants
Trustworthy biases	Is this person trustworthy?	Photos	Amygdala	Misjudge trust	❖ Over-trusting (brain damage, some devlopmental disorders) ❖ Under-trusting (paranoia, hostility)
Personalising biases	What is the cause for this event?	Texts	Damage to frontal brain systems	Misplace attributions	❖ Over-attribute negative events to external agents rather than situations (psychosis, brain damage) ❖ Over-attribute negative events to self rather than situations (depression) ❖ Over-attribute negative events externally rather than self (brain damage) ❖ Hasty decisions and jumping to conclusions (psychosis, brain damage)
Negative attribution biases	What is the cause of this event?	Texts, photos	Unknown	Negativity bias	❖ Negative recall of memories (depression) ❖ Negative interpretation of interpersonal cues (depression) ❖ Hostile intention inferred in ambiguous events (paranoid psychosis)

attribution of hostile intention in ambiguous events (Combs, Penn, Wicher, & Waldheter, 2007). The tendency to make such judgements hastily and on little information is also characteristic of psychosis in general (So, Siu, Wong, Chan, & Garety, 2016). Likewise, other disorders are associated with specific biases. Depression, for example is associated with a tendency to attribute negative events to the self (Sweeney, Anderson, & Bailey, 1986) and to cause a bias in recall of negative memories (Lloyd & Lishman, 1975).

Such attributional biases directly impact upon social cognition. A tendency to blame others has been associated with poorer ToM in normal adults (Rowland et al., 2013). People with depression are impaired when recognising both positive and negative emotional expressions (George et al., 1998; Montagne et al., 2007; Zwick & Wolkenstein, 2016) and also making ToM judgements (Bora & Berk, 2016). Psychosis in general, and delusions in particular, are associated with impaired ToM reasoning (Bora & Pantelis, 2013; Corcoran, Mercer, & Frith, 1995) even more so in individuals with schizophrenia who have committed homicidal acts (Engelstad et al., 2019). Distorted thinking about the intentions of others may interfere with accurate ToM reasoning and, equally, impaired ToM reasoning may contribute to delusional systems (Bentall et al., 2001).

Disorders of social behaviour

While we have mainly concerned ourselves with social cognition in this chapter, it is important to briefly consider social behaviour. Disorders of social cognition will disrupt social behaviour, as seen in people with FTD who, with a loss of moral judgement, behave in an antisocial manner, or people with TBI who lack ToM and empathy and are, therefore, egocentric and insensitive in their conversation. But, additionally, brain damage, often in similar regions to those associated with social cognition, leads to disorders in the regulation of behaviour itself.

Apathy

Apathy is a diminished motivation for goal directed activity that is independent of impaired consciousness, severe cognitive disturbance and/or emotional distress (Marin, 1991, 1996). Apathy can manifest as a cognitive loss of higher-level executive abilities leading to impaired goal setting, loss of initiative, rigidity and poor planning, usually reflected in damage to the *dorsolateral prefrontal cortex* and related *dorsal basal ganglia* (Johnson & Kumfor, 2018; Kumfor, Zhen, Hodges, Piguet, & Irish, 2018). High cognitive apathy correlates with executive impairments (Andersson & Bergedalen, 2002; Njomboro & Deb, 2014). Alternatively, apathy can manifest as emotional blunting, with a loss of interest or concern for others due to damage in the *orbito-frontal cortex* and *ventral basal ganglia* structures. A third kind of apathy appears to be essentially behavioral, reflected in a loss of initiation of behavior due to lesions bilaterally in the associative and limbic territories of *the globas pallidas* (Levy & Dubois, 2006). People high in apathy demonstrate reduced overall activity and more frequent daytime naps, which may reflect the more behavioral dimension of apathy (Muller, Czymmek, Thone-Otto, & Von Cramon, 2006)

High apathy has been associated with disorders of social cognition. For example, high emotional apathy is correlated with blunted physiological and subjective responses to novel events, emotional memories and stressful tasks (Andersson & Finset, 1999; Andersson, Gundersen, & Finset, 1999; Andersson, Krogstad, & Finset, 1999). Further, in adults with acquired brain injuries, those with high apathy scores have a higher tolerance for the personal moral dilemma (trolley scenario) and are less able to recognise when behaviour is unacceptable relative to people with brain injury who do not experience apathy and normal healthy adults. This is despite having similar ToM and emotion perception scores and similar performance on impersonal moral dilemmas (Njomboro & Deb, 2014). Thus, *orbitomedial* lesions result in the disruption of emotional processes that underpin both initiation and maintenance of behaviour and the processing of incoming social information (Levy & Dubois, 2006). Consequently, apathy and social cognitive impairments may be expected to co-occur.

Disinhibition

People with *ventromedial* lesions show many characteristics of apathy such as lack of initiative and persistence and blunted affect. Simultaneously, they can show symptoms of disinhibition such as poor frustration tolerance, irritability and social inappropriateness (Barrash et al., 2000). At a physiological and behavioural level, there is evidence that damage to the *prefrontal lobes* can be reflected in both a loss of arousal, as we have previously discussed, and increased reactivity as reflected in the behaviours described by Barrash et al. (2000). Such lability can also be captured in a heightened arousal response (skin conductance) to self-relevant anger inductions (Aboulafia-Brakha, Allain, & Ptak, 2016). According to the model described in Figure 1.4, this may be explained as a loss of the automatic capacity to regulate subcortical structures (e.g. *the amygdala*) that mediate autonomic excitation (e.g. the flight or fight response) (Thayer, Hansen, Saus-Rose, & Johnsen, 2009).

Cognitive inhibition and cognitive control are also often impaired with *orbitofrontal* lesions (Collette et al., 2001). For example, people with TBI often demonstrate an impairment in the capacity to inhibit prepotent responses during neuropsychological tests (Dimoska-Di Marco, McDonald, Kelly, Tate, & Johnstone, 2011). Furthermore, poor response inhibition predicts disinhibited behavior as reported by informants (Lipszyc et al., 2014; Osborne-Crowley, McDonald, & Francis, 2016; Tate, 1999). Relatedly, people with damage to the *orbitofrontal cortex* have difficulties changing their behaviour when it is no longer rewarded, i.e. they show a deficit in reversal learning (Fellows & Farah, 2003; Hornak et al., 2004; Rolls, Hornak, Wade, & McGrath, 1994). Interestingly, these kinds of reversal learning impairments are heightened in specifically socio-emotional contexts (Kelly, McDonald, & Kellett, 2014), especially in people who have high observed social disinhibition (Osborne-Crowley, McDonald, & Rushby, 2016). Like apathy, disinhibited behaviour can co-exist with impairments in social cognition arising from similar regions

Table 1.8 Summary of disorders of social behaviour

	Type of tasks	*Implicated brain regions*	*Type of disorders*	*Variants*
Cognitive Apathy	Cognitive tasks, behavioural observation	DLPFC, dBG	Loss of executive function	❖Poor goal setting ❖Poor planning ❖Rigidity
Emotional Apathy	Behavioural observation	OFC, vBG	Emotional blunting	❖Lack of arousal ❖Loss of interest in others ❖Loss of concern
Behavioural Apathy	Behavioural observation, actigraphy	GP	Loss of activity	❖Loss of initiative ❖Lack of self initiation ❖Lack of activity ❖Excessive naps
Cognitive Disinhibition	Cognitive tasks	OFC	Loss of cognitive control	❖Poor inhibition of prepotent response ❖Poor reversal learning
Social Disinhibition	Physiological tasks, behavioural observation, questionnaires	VMPFC	Loss of regulation of emotion and behaviour	❖Heightened arousal response ❖Socially inappropriate behaviours ❖Poor reversal learning (social stimuli) ❖Poor frustration tolerance ❖Irritability ❖Anger ❖Mood swings

DLPFC = dorsolateral prefrontal cortex, dBG = dorsal basal ganglia, OFC = orbitofrontal cortex, vBG = ventral basal ganglia, GP = globas pallidus

of neuropathology (Lough & Hodges, 2002). There may also be a functional relationship as we described when discussing ToM, i.e. loss of inhibition may make it more difficult to supress the prepotent focus on self in order to consider the perspective of another (McDonald et al., 2014). Certainly, problems with social behaviour regulation need to be considered alongside deficits in social cognition, as they are likely to co-occur, are likely to be functionally entwined and will exacerbate problems in social cognition with respect to poor social functioning.

A bioneuropsychosocial perspective on social cognition

In this chapter we have considered a range of areas of impairments in social cognition and social behaviour arising from brain lesions and/or clinical disorders of a developmental or neuropsychiatric nature. In the following chapters of this book, we will look at some of the more common clinical disorders in further detail. We will also consider how to both assess and treat social cognitive disorders. It is important, however, to also place social cognitive disorders in a broader neuropsychological and psychosocial context. In Figure 1.7 we have adapted a model of social cognition from that described by Cassel and colleagues (Cassel, McDonald, Kelly, & Togher, 2019), which highlights the important role of neuropsychological, psychological and environmental factors in social cognition.

Social cognition will be impacted to varying degrees by other cognitive abilities such as memory, attention and information processing. When we assess and think about social cognitive impairments, we need to be aware of these interactions.

Perhaps even more importantly, people who develop clinical disorders will come from a wide variety of social and cultural backgrounds and with enormous individual differences in personality characteristics and mental dispositions (e.g. denial, anger, defensiveness, resilience and so on). These differences will not only colour the way in which they process social information (e.g. their attributional style), but may have fundamental impacts upon how they read social information and also the relevance of particular social assessment tools. We consider cross-cultural factors in social cognition in the next chapter.

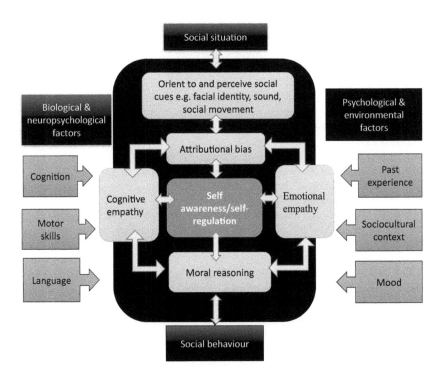

Figure 1.7 A bioneuropsychosocial model of social cognition

Finally, the environment in which the person functions can both limit and extend their abilities and opportunities to function. When we consider children with clinical disorders, the interaction becomes even more complex as we need to factor in maturation of skills and how and when disruption might affect this (Beauchamp & Anderson, 2010). These matters are always important when working with people with clinical disorders. However, they are fundamentally important when we discuss social information processing.

To conclude, social cognition represents a fundamental neuropsychological domain that, when impaired, is likely to have serious consequences for the most fundamental of human abilities, the ability to interact and get on with others. We have come a long way in understanding some of the basic features of social cognition, as touched on in this chapter. The unique aspects of social cognition, especially its reliance on other cognitive skills, its multi-modal nature and its interaction with culture, present special challenges in our efforts to develop sensitive assessment measures and treatment paradigms. The following chapters address these concerns.

References

Abbott, J. D., Cumming, G., Fidler, F., & Lindell, A. K. (2013). The perception of positive and negative facial expressions in unilateral brain-damaged patients: A meta-analysis. *Laterality: Asymmetries of Body, Brain and Cognition*, 18(4), 437–459.

Aboulafia-Brakha, T., Allain, P., & Ptak, R. (2016). Emotion regulation after traumatic brain injury: Distinct patterns of sympathetic activity during anger expression and recognition. *The Journal of Head Trauma Rehabilitation*, 31(3), E21–E31.

Adams, A. G., Schweitzer, D., Molenberghs, P., & Henry, J. D. (2019). A meta-analytic review of social cognitive function following stroke. *Neuroscience and Biobehavioral Reviews*, 102, 400–416.

Adolphs, R. (2001). The neurobiology of social cognition. *Current Opinion in Neurobiology*, 11, 231–239.

Adolphs, R. (2002). Recognizing emotion from facial expressions: Psychological and neurological mechanisms. *Behavioral & Cognitive Neuroscience Reviews*, 1(1), 21–62.

Adolphs, R., Damasio, H., & Tranel, D. (2002). Neural systems for recognition of emotional prosody: A 3-D lesion study. *Emotion*, 2(1), 23–51.

Adolphs, R., Damasio, H., Tranel, D., & Damasio, A. R. (1996). Cortical systems for the recognition of emotion in facial expressions. *Journal of Neuroscience*, 16(23), 7678–7687.

Adolphs, R., Jansari, A., & Tranel, D. (2001). Hemispheric perception of emotional valence from facial expressions. *Neuropsychology*, 15(4), 516–524.

Adolphs, R., Sears, L., & Piven, J. (2001). Abnormal processing of social information from faces in autism. *Journal of Cognitive Neuroscience*, 13(2), 232–240.

Adolphs, R., & Tranel, D. (2004). Impaired judgments of sadness but not happiness following bilateral amygdala damage. *Journal of Cognitive Neuroscience*, 16(3), 453–462.

Adolphs, R., Tranel, D., & Damasio, A. R. (1998). The human amygdala in social judgment. *Nature*, 393(6684), 470–474.

Adolphs, R., Tranel, D., & Damasio, A. R. (2003). Dissociable neural systems for recognizing emotions. *Brain & Cognition*, 52(1), 61–69.

Adolphs, R., Tranel, D., & Damasio, H. (2001). Emotion recognition from faces and prosody following temporal lobectomy. *Neuropsychology, 15*(3), 396–404.

Adolphs, R., Tranel, D., Damasio, H., & Damasio, A. R. (1994). Impaired recognition of emotion in facial expressions following bilateral damage to the human amygdala. *Nature, 372*(6507), 669–672.

Alexander, M. P., Benson, D. F., & Stuss, D. T. (1989). Frontal lobes and language. *Brain and Language, 37*, 656–691.

Allison, T., Puce, A., & McCarthy, G. (2000). Social perception from visual cues: Role of the STS region. *Trends in Cognitive Sciences, 4*(7), 267–278.

Amodio, D. M., & Frith, C. D. (2006). Meeting of minds: The medial frontal cortex and social cognition. *Nature Reviews Neuroscience, 7*(4), 268–277. doi:10.1038/nrn1884

Anderson, S. W., Bechara, A., Damasio, H., Tranel, D., & Damasio, A. R. (1999). Impairment of social and moral behavior related to early damage in human prefrontal cortex. *Nature Neuroscience, 2*(11), 1032–1037.

Andersson, S. W., & Bergedalen, A. M. (2002). Cognitive correlates of apathy in traumatic brain injury. *Neuropsychiatry, Neuropsychology, & Behavioral Neurology, 15*(3), 184–191.

Andersson, S. W., & Finset, A. (1999). Electrodermal responsiveness and negative symptoms in brain injured patients. *Journal of Psychophysiology, 13*(2), 109–116.

Andersson, S. W., Gundersen, P. M., & Finset, A. (1999). Emotional activation during therapeutic interaction in traumatic brain injury: Effect of apathy, self-awareness and implications for rehabilitation. *Brain Injury, 13*(6), 393–404.

Andersson, S. W., Krogstad, J. M., & Finset, A. (1999). Apathy and depressed mood in acquired brain damage: Relationship to lesion localization and psychophysiological reactivity. *Psychological Medicine, 29*(2), 447–456.

Angrilli, A., Mauri, A., Palomba, D., Flor, H., Birbaumer, N., Sartori, G., & di Paola, F. (1996). Startle reflex and emotion modulation impairment after a right amygdala lesion. *Brain, 119*(Pt 6), 1991–2000.

Angrilli, A., Palomba, D., Cantagallo, A., Maietti, A., & Stegagno, L. (1999). Emotional impairment after right orbitofrontal lesion in a patient without cognitive deficits. *NeuroReport, 10*(8), 1741–1746.

Baez, S., Morales, J. P., Slachevsky, A., Torralva, T., Matus, C., Manes, F., & Ibanez, A. (2016). Orbitofrontal and limbic signatures of empathic concern and intentional harm in the behavioral variant frontotemporal dementia. *Cortex, 75*, 20–32.

Balconi, M., & Bortolotti, A. (2013). The "simulation" of the facial expression of emotions in case of short and long stimulus duration. The effect of pre-motor cortex inhibition by rTMS. *Brain and Cognition, 83*, 114–120.

Barch, D. M., Braver, T. S., Akbudak, E., Conturo, T., Ollinger, J., & Snyder, A. (2001). Anterior cingulate cortex and response conflict: Effects of response modality and processing domain. *Cereb Cortex, 11*(9), 837–848.

Baron-Cohen, S., Leslie, A. M., & Frith, U. (1985). Does the autistic child have a "theory of mind"? *Cognition, 21*, 37–46.

Baron-Cohen, S., & Wheelwright, S. (2004). The empathy quotient: An investigation of adults with Asperger syndrome or high functioning autism, and normal sex differences. *Journal of Autism and Developmental Disorders, 34*(2), 163–175.

Barrash, J., Tranel, D., & Anderson, S. W. (2000). Acquired personality disturbances associated with bilateral damage to the ventromedial prefrontal region. *Developmental Neuropsychology, 18*(3), 355–381.

Bate, S., Bennetts, R. J., Tree, J. J., Adams, A., & Murray, E. (2019). The domain-specificity of face matching impairments in 40 cases of developmental prosopagnosia. *Cognition, 192*, ArtID 104031.

Bavelas, J. B., Black, A., Chovil, N., Lemery, C. R., & Mullett, J. (1988). Form and function in motor mimicry topographic evidence that the primary function is communicative. *Human Communication Research, 14*(3), 275–299.

Beadle, J. N., & De La Vega, C. E. (2019, June). Impact of aging on empathy: Review of psychological and neural mechanisms. *Frontiers in Psychiatry, 10*. doi:10.3389/fpsyt.2019.00331

Beauchamp, M. H., & Anderson, V. A. (2010). SOCIAL: An integrative framework for the development of social skills. *Psychological Bulletin, 136*(1), 39–64.

Bechara, A., Tranel, D., Damasio, H., Adolphs, R., Rockland, C., & Damasio, A. R. (1995). Double dissociation of conditioning and declarative knowledge relative to the amygdala and hippocampus in humans. *Science, 269*, 1115–1118.

Bentall, R. P., Corcoran, R., Howard, R., Blackwood, N., & Kinderman, P. (2001). Persecutory delusions: A review and theoretical integration. *Clinical Psychology Review, 21*(8), 1143–1192.

Bird, G., Silani, G., Brindley, R., White, S., Frith, U., & Singer, T. (2010). Empathic brain responses in insula are modulated by levels of alexithymia but not autism. *Brain: A Journal of Neurology, 133*(5), 1515–1525.

Bivona, U., Riccio, A., Ciurli, P., Carlesimo, G. A., Delle Donne, V., Pizzonia, E., . . . Costa, A. (2014). Low self-awareness of individuals with severe traumatic brain injury can lead to reduced ability to take another person's perspective. *Journal of Head Trauma Rehabilitation, 29*(2), 157–171.

Blair, R. J. R., & Cipolotti, L. (2000). Impaired social response reversal: A case of "acquired sociopathy". *Brain, 123*, 1122–1141.

Blairy, S., Herrera, P., & Hess, U. (1999). Mimicry and the judgment of emotional facial expressions. *Journal of Nonverbal Behavior, 23*(1), 5–41.

Boake, C., Freelands, J. C., Ringholz, G. M., Nance, M. L., & Edwards, K. E. (1995). Awareness of memory loss after severe close head injury. *Brain Injury, 9*(3), 273–283.

Bodamer, J. (1947). Die prosopagnosie. *Archiv fur Psychiatrie und Zeitschift fur Neuroologie, 179*, 6–54.

Bonfils, K. A., Lysaker, P. H., Minor, K. S., & Salyers, M. P. (2017). Empathy in schizophrenia: A meta-analysis of the interpersonal reactivity index. *Psychiatry Research, 249*, 293–303.

Bora, E. (2017). Meta-analysis of social cognition in amyotrophic lateral sclerosis. *Cortex: A Journal Devoted to the Study of the Nervous System and Behavior, 88*, 1–7.

Bora, E., & Berk, M. (2016). Theory of mind in major depressive disorder: A meta-analysis. *Journal of Affective Disorders, 191*, 49–55.

Bora, E., & Meletti, S. (2016). Social cognition in temporal lobe epilepsy: A systematic review and meta-analysis. *Epilepsy & Behavior, 60*, 50–57.

Bora, E., Ozakbas, S., Velakoulis, D., & Walterfang, M. (2016). Social cognition in multiple sclerosis: A meta-analysis. *Neuropsychology Review, 26*(2), 160–172.

Bora, E., & Pantelis, C. (2013). Theory of mind impairments in first-episode psychosis, individuals at ultra-high risk for psychosis and in first-degree relatives of schizophrenia: Systematic review and meta-analysis. *Schizophrenia Research, 144*(1), 31–36.

Bora, E., & Pantelis, C. (2016). Social cognition in schizophrenia in comparison to bipolar disorder: A meta-analysis. *Schizophrenia Research, 175*(1–3), 72–78.

Bora, E., Velakoulis, D., & Walterfang, M. (2016a). Meta-analysis of facial emotion recognition in behavioral variant frontotemporal dementia: Comparison with Alzheimer disease and healthy controls. *Journal of Geriatric Psychiatry and Neurology*, *29*(4), 205–211.

Bora, E., Velakoulis, D., & Walterfang, M. (2016b). Social cognition in Huntington's disease: A meta-analysis. *Behavioural Brain Research*, *297*, 131–140.

Bora, E., Walterfang, M., & Velakoulis, D. (2015). Theory of mind in Parkinson's disease: A meta-analysis. *Behavioural Brain Research*, *292*, 515–520. doi:10.1016/j.bbr.2015.07.012

Bora, E., & Yener, G. G. (2017). Meta-analysis of social cognition in mild cognitive impairment. *Journal of Geriatric Psychiatry and Neurology*, *30*(4), 206–213.

Bora, E., Yucel, M., & Pantelis, C. (2009). Theory of mind impairment in schizophrenia: Meta-analysis. *Schizophrenia Research*, *109*(1–3), 1–9.

Borod, J. C., Koff, E., Lorch, M. P., & Nicholas, M. (1986). The expression and perception of facial emotion in brain-damaged patients. *Neuropsychologia*, *24*(2), 169–180.

Bowers, D., Blonder, L. X., Feinberg, T., & Heilman, K. M. (1991). Differential impact of right and left hemisphere lesions on facial emotion and object imagery. *Brain*, *114*, 2593–2609.

Bozeat, S., Gregory, C. A., Ralph, M. A., & Hodges, J. R. (2000). Which neuropsychiatric and behavioural features distinguish frontal and temporal variants of frontotemporal dementia from Alzheimer's disease? *Journal of Neurology, Neurosurgery & Psychiatry*, *69*(2), 178–186.

Brown, P., & Levinson, S. (1978). Universals in language usage: Politeness phenomena. In E. N. Goody (Ed.), *Questions and Politeness: Strategies in Social Interaction*. Melbourne: Cambridge University Press.

Brownell, H. H., D., M., Powelson, J., & Gardner, H. (1983). Surprise but not sensitivity to verbal humour in right hemisphere patients. *Brain and Language*, *18*, 20–27.

Bryson, G., Bell, M., & Lysaker, P. (1997). Affect recognition in schizophrenia: A function of global impairment or a specific cognitive deficit. *Psychiatry Research*, *71*(2), 105–113.

Buchanan, T. W., Tranel, D., & Adolphs, R. (2004). Anteromedial temporal lobe damage blocks startle modulation by fear and disgust. *Behavioral Neuroscience*, *118*(2), 429–437.

Buck, B. E., Pinkham, A. E., Harvey, P. D., & Penn, D. L. (2016). Revisiting the validity of measures of social cognitive bias in schizophrenia: Additional results from the social cognition psychometric evaluation (SCOPE) study. *British Journal of Clinical Psychology*, *55*(4), 441–454.

Buckner, R. L., Andrews-Hanna, J. R., & Schacter, D. L. (2008). The brain's default network: Anatomy, function, and relevance to disease. *Annals of the New York Academy of Sciences*, *1124*, 1–38. doi:10.1196/annals.1440.011

Byom, L. J., & Turkstra, L. (2012). Effects of social cognitive demand on theory of mind in conversations of adults with traumatic brain injury. *International Journal of Language and Communication Disorders*, *47*(3), 310–321.

Bzdok, D., Schilbach, L., Vogeley, K., Schneider, K., Laird, A. R., Langner, R., & Eickhoff, S. B. (2012). Parsing the neural correlates of moral cognition: ALE meta-analysis on morality, theory of mind, and empathy. *Brain Structure and Function*, *217*(4), 783–796.

Calder, A. J., Keane, J., Manes, F., Antoun, N., & Young, A. W. (2000). Impaired recognition and experience of disgust following brain injury. *Nature Neuroscience*, *3*(11), 1077–1078.

Cassel, A., McDonald, S., Kelly, M., & Togher, L. (2019). Learning from the minds of others: A review of social cognition treatments and their relevance to traumatic brain injury. *Neuropsychological Rehabilitation*, *29*(1), 22–55.

Castelli, F., Frith, C., Happe, F., & Frith, U. (2002). Autism, Asperger syndrome and brain mechanisms for the attribution of mental states to animated shapes. *Brain, 125*, 1839–1849.

Cavanna, A. E., & Trimble, M. R. (2006). The precuneus: A review of its functional anatomy and behavioural correlates. *Brain, 129*(3), 564–583.

Cicone, M., Wapner, W., & Gardner, H. (1980). Sensitivity to emotional expressions and situations in organic patients. *Cortex, 16*(1), 145–158.

Collette, F., Van der Linden, M., Delfiore, G., Degueldre, C., Luxen, A., & Salmon, E. (2001). The functional anatomy of inhibition processes investigated with the Hayling task. *Neuroimage, 14*(2), 258–267.

Coltheart, M. (2010). The neuropsychology of delusions. *Annals of the New York Academy of Sciences, 1191*, 16–26.

Combs, D. R., Penn, D. L., Wicher, M., & Waldheter, E. (2007). The ambiguous intentions hostility questionnaire (AIHQ): A new measure for evaluating hostile social-cognitive biases in paranoia. *Cognitive Neuropsychiatry, 12*(2), 128–143.

Corcoran, R., Mercer, G., & Frith, C. D. (1995). Schizophrenia, symptomology and social inference: Investigating "theory of mind" in people with schizophrenia. *Schizophrenia Research, 17*, 5–13.

Costafreda, S. G., Brammer, M. J., David, A. S., & Fu, C. H. (2008). Predictors of amygdala activation during the processing of emotional stimuli: A meta-analysis of 385 PET and fMRI studies. *Brain Research Reviews, 58*(1), 57–70.

Cotter, J., Firth, J., Enzinger, C., Kontopantelis, E., Yung, A. R., Elliott, R., & Drake, R. J. (2016). Social cognition in multiple sclerosis: A systematic review and meta-analysis. *Neurology, 87*(16), 1727–1736.

Cotter, J., Granger, K., Backx, R., Hobbs, M., Looi, C. Y., & Barnett, J. H. (2018). Social cognitive dysfunction as a clinical marker: A systematic review of meta-analyses across 30 clinical conditions. *Neuroscience and Biobehavioral Reviews, 84*, 92–99.

Coundouris, S. P., Adams, A. G., & Henry, J. D. (2020). Empathy and theory of mind in Parkinson's disease: A meta-analysis. *Neuroscience and Biobehavioral Reviews, 109*, 92–102.

Cusi, A. M., MacQueen, G. M., Spreng, R., & McKinnon, M. C. (2011). Altered empathic responding in major depressive disorder: Relation to symptom severity, illness burden, and psychosocial outcome. *Psychiatry Research, 188*(2), 231–236.

Damasio, A. R., Tranel, D., & Damasio, H. (1990). Individuals with sociopathic behavior caused by frontal damage fail to respond autonomically to social stimuli. *Behavioural Brain Research, 41*(2), 81–94.

Darby, R., Laganiere, S., Pascual-Leone, A., Prasad, S., & Fox, M. D. (2017). Finding the imposter: Brain connectivity of lesions causing delusional misidentifications. *Brain: A Journal of Neurology, 140*(2), 497–507.

D'Argembeau, A., Ruby, P., Collette, F., Degueldre, C., Balteau, E., Luxen, A., . . . Salmon, E. (2007). Distinct regions of the medial prefrontal cortex are associated with self-referential processing and perspective taking. *Journal of Cognitive Neuroscience, 19*(6), 935–944.

Davis, J. I., Senghas, A., Brandt, F., & Ochsner, K. N. (2010). The effects of BOTOX injections on emotional experience. *Emotion, 10*(3), 433–440.

Davis, P. J., & Gibson, M. G. (2000). Recognition of posed and genuine facial expressions of emotion in paranoid and nonparanoid schizophrenia *Journal of Abnormal Psychology, 109*(3), 445–450.

Decety, J., & Jackson, P. L. (2004). The functional architecture of human empathy. *Behavioral and Cognitive Neuroscience Reviews, 3*(2), 71–100.

Decety, J., & Meyer, M. (2008). From emotion resonance to empathic understanding: A social developmental neuroscience account. *Development and Psychopathology, 20*(4), 1053–1080.

Decety, J., Michalska, K. J., & Kinzler, K. D. (2012). The contribution of emotion and cognition to moral sensitivity: A neurodevelopmental study. *Cerebral Cortex, 22*(1), 209–220.

Demorest, A., Meyer, C., Phelps, E., Gardner, H., & Winner, E. (1984). Words speak louder than actions: Understanding deliberately false remarks. *Child Development, 55*(4), 1527–1534.

De Renzi, E., Scotti, G., & Spinnler, H. (1969). Perceptual and associative disorders of visual recognition: Relationship to the site of lesion. *Neurology, 19*, 634–642.

Dermody, N., Wong, S., Ahmed, R., Piguet, O., Hodges, J. R., & Irish, M. (2016). Uncovering the neural bases of cognitive and affective empathy deficits in Alzheimer's disease and the behavioral-variant of frontotemporal dementia. *Journal of Alzheimer's Disease, 53*(3), 801–806.

de Sousa, A., McDonald, S., & Rushby, J. (2012). Changes in emotional empathy, affective responsivity and behaviour following severe traumatic brain injury. *Journal of Clinical and Experimental Neuropsychology, 34*(6), 606–623.

de Sousa, A., McDonald, S., Rushby, J., Li, S., Dimoska, A., & James, C. (2010). Why don't you feel how I feel? Insight into the absence of empathy after severe traumatic brain injury. *Neuropsychologia, 48*, 3585–3595.

de Sousa, A., McDonald, S., Rushby, J., Li, S., Dimoska, A., & James, C. (2011). Understanding deficits in empathy after traumatic brain injury: The role of affective responsivity. *Cortex, 47*(5), 526–535. doi:10.1016/j.cortex.2010.02.004

Dethier, M., Blairy, S., Rosenberg, H., & McDonald, S. (2013). Deficits in processing feedback from emotional behaviours following severe TBI. *Journal of the International Neuropsychological Society, 19*(4), 367–379.

Dimberg, U., & Ohman, A. (1996). Behold the wrath: Psychophysiological responses to facial stimuli. *Motivation and Emotion, 20*, 149–182.

Dimoska-Di Marco, A., McDonald, S., Kelly, M., Tate, R. L., & Johnstone, S. (2011). A meta-analysis of response inhibition and Stroop interference control deficits in adults with traumatic brain injury (TBI). *Journal of Clinical and Experimental Neuropsychology, 33*(4), 471–485.

di Pellegrino, G., Fadiga, L., Fogassi, L., Gallese, V., & Rizzolatti, G. (1992). Understanding motor events: A neurophysiological study. *Experimental Brain Research, 91*(1), 176–180.

Dziobek, I., Rogers, K., Fleck, S., Bahnemann, M., Heekeren, H. R., Wolf, O. T., & Convit, A. (2008). Dissociation of cognitive and emotional empathy in adults with Asperger syndrome using the multifaceted empathy test (MET). *Journal of Autism & Developmental Disorders, 38*(3), 464–473.

Eippert, F., Veit, R., Weiskopf, N., Erb, M., Birbaumer, N., & Anders, S. (2007). Regulation of emotional responses elicited by threat-related stimuli. *Human Brain Mapping, 28*(5), 409–423.

Ekman, P., & Freisen, W. V. (1976). *Pictures of Facial Affect*. Palo Alto, CA: Consulting Psychological Press.

Ellis, H. D., & Young, A. W. (1990). Accounting for delusional misidentifications. *British Journal of Psychiatry, 157*, 239–248.

Emery, N. A., & Amaral, D. G. (2000). The role of the amygdala in primate social cognition. In R. D. Lane & L. Nadel (Eds.), *Cognitive Neuroscience of Emotion*. Oxford: Oxford University Press.

Engelstad, K. N., Rund, B. R., Torgalsboen, A. K., Lau, B., Ueland, T., & Vaskinn, A. (2019). Large social cognitive impairments characterize homicide offenders with schizophrenia. *Psychiatry Research, 272*, 209–215.

Eslinger, P. J., & Damasio, A. R. (1985). Severe disturbance of higher cognitive function after bilateral frontal ablation: Patient EVR. *Neurology, 35*, 1731–1741.

Esteves, F., Dimberg, U., & Ohman, A. (1994). Automatically elicited fear: Conditioned skin conductance responses to masked facial expressions. *Cognition & Emotion, 8*(5), 393–413.

Fanning, J. R., Bell, M. D., & Fiszdon, J. M. (2012). Is it possible to have impaired neurocognition but good social cognition in schizophrenia? *Schizophrenia Research, 135*(1), 68–71.

Fellows, L. K., & Farah, M. J. (2003). Ventromedial frontal cortex mediates affective shifting in humans: Evidence from a reversal learning paradigm. *Brain, 126*(Pt 8), 1830–1837.

Flack, W. F., Laird, J. D., & Cavallaro, L. A. (1999). Separate and combined effects of facial expressions and bodily postures on emotional feelings. *European Journal of Social Psychology, 29*(2–3), 203–217.

Funayama, E. S., Grillon, C., Davis, M., & Phelps, E. A. (2001). A double dissociation in the affective modulation of startle in humans: Effects of unilateral temporal lobectomy. *Journal of Cognitive Neuroscience, 13*(6), 721–729.

Gainotti, G. (1972). Emotional behavior and hemispheric side of the lesion. *Cortex, 8*, 41–55.

Gallese, V., Fogassi, L., Fadiga, L., & Rizzolatti, G. (2002). Action representation and the inferior parietal lobule. In W. Prinz & B. Hommel (Eds.), *Common Mechanisms in Perception and Action: Attention and Performance* (Vol. XIX, pp. 247–226). New York: Oxford University Press.

George, M. S., Huggins, T., McDermut, W., Parekh, P. I., Rubinow, D., & Post, R. M. (1998). Abnormal facial emotion recognition in depression: Serial testing in an ultra-rapid-cycling patient. *Behavior Modification, 22*(2), 192–204.

Gibbs, R. W., & Mueller, R. A. (1988). Conversational sequences and preferences for indirect speech acts. *Discourse Processes, 11*(1), 101–116.

Godfrey, H. P., Partridge, F. M., Knight, R. G., & Bishara, S. N. (1993). Course of insight disorder and emotional dysfunction following closed head injury: A controlled cross-sectional follow-up study. *Journal of Clinical and Experimental Neuropsychology, 15*(4), 503–515.

Grafman, J., Schwab, K., Warden, D., Pridgen, A., Brown, H. R., & Salazar, A. M. (1996). Frontal lobe injuries, violence, and aggression: A report of the Vietnam Head Injury Study. *Neurology, 46*(5), 1231–1238.

Greene, J. D., & Haidt, J. (2002). How (and where) does moral judgment work? *Trends in Cognitive Sciences, 6*(12), 517–523.

Greene, J. D., Nystrom, L. E., Engell, A. D., Darley, J. M., & Cohen, J. D. (2004). The neural bases of cognitive conflict and control in moral judgment. *Neuron, 44*(2), 389–400.

Grice, H. P. (1975). Logic and conversation. In P. Cole & J. Morgan (Eds.), *Syntax and Semantics: Speech Acts* (Vol. 3). New York: Academic Press.

Gruzelier, J. H., & Venables, P. H. (1973). Skin conductance responses to tones with and without attentional significance in schizophrenic and nonschizophrenic psychiatric patients. *Neuropsychologia, 11*(2), 221–230.

Ham, T. E., Bonnelle, V., Hellyer, P., Jilka, S., Robertson, I. H., Leech, R., & Sharp, D. J. (2014). The neural basis of impaired self-awareness after traumatic brain injury. *Brain, 137*(Pt 2), 586–597.

Harari, H., Shamay-Tsoory, S. G., Ravid, M., & Levkovitz, Y. (2010). Double dissociation between cognitive and affective empathy in borderline personality disorder. *Psychiatry Research, 175*(3), 277–279.

Hariri, A. R., Bookheiner, S. Y., & Mazziotta, J. C. (2000). Modulating emotional responses: Effects of a neocortical network on the limbic system. *NeuroReport, 11*, 43–48.

Harrison, N. A., Singer, T., Rotshtein, P., Dolan, R. J., & Critchley, H. D. (2006). Pupillary contagion: Central mechanisms engaged in sadness processing. *Social Cognitive and Affective Neuroscience, 1*(1), 5–17.

Heilman, K. M., Scholes, R., & Watson, R. (1975). Auditory affective agnosia: Disturbed comprehension of affective speech. *Journal of Neurology, Neurosurgery & Psychiatry, 38*, 69–72.

Heims, H., Critchley, H., Dolan, R., Mathias, C., & Cipolotti, L. (2004). Social and motivational functioning is not critically dependent on feedback of autonomic responses: Neuropsychological evidence from patients with pure autonomic failure. *Neuropsychologia, 42*(14), 1979–1988.

Hess, U., & Blairy, S. (2001). Facial mimicry and emotional contagion to dynamic emotional facial expressions and their influence on decoding accuracy. *International Journal of Psychophysiology, 40*(2), 129–141.

Hesse, E., Mikulan, E., Decety, J., Sigman, M., del Carmen Garcia, M., Silva, W., . . . Ibanez1, A. (2016). Early detection of intentional harm in the human amygdala. *Brain, 139*(Pt 1), 54–61.

Hoerold, D., Pender, N. P., & Robertson, I. H. (2013). Metacognitive and online error awareness deficits after prefrontal cortex lesions. *Neuropsychologia, 51*(3), 385–391.

Hofelich, A. J., & Preston, S. D. (2012). The meaning in empathy: Distinguishing conceptual encoding from facial mimicry, trait empathy, and attention to emotion. *Cognition & Emotion, 26*(1), 119–128.

Hoffman, M. L. (1984). Interaction of affect and cognition on empathy. In P. Phillippot, R. Feldman, & E. Coats (Eds.), *The Social Context of Nonverbal Behaviour* (pp. 103–131). Cambridge: Cambridge University Press.

Hopkins, M. J., Dywan, J., & Segalowitz, S. J. (2002). Altered electrodermal response to facial expression after closed head injury. *Brain Injury, 16*, 245–257.

Hornak, J., O'Doherty, J., Bramham, J., Rolls, E., Morris, R., Bullock, P., & Polkey, C. (2004). Reward-related reversal learning after surgical excisions in orbito-frontal or dorsolateral prefrontal cortex in humans. *Journal of Cognitive Neuroscience, 16*(3), 463–478.

Hornak, J., Rolls, E. T., & Wade, D. (1996). Face and voice expression identification in patients with emotional and behavioural changes following ventral frontal lobe damage. *Neuropsychologia, 34*(4), 247–261.

Hutchings, R., Palermo, R., Piguet, O., & Kumfor, F. (2017). Disrupted Face processing in frontotemporal dementia: A review of the clinical and neuroanatomical evidence. *Neuropsychology Review, 27*(1), 18–30.

Jackson, P. L., Rainville, P., & Decety, J. (2006). To what extent do we share the pain of others? Insight from the neural bases of pain empathy. *Pain, 125*(1–2), 5–9.

James, W. (1884). What is an emotion. *Mind, 9*, 188–205.

Johnson, E., & Kumfor, F. (2018). Overcoming apathy in frontotemporal dementia: Challenges and future directions. *Current Opinion in Behavioral Sciences, 22*. doi:10.1016/j.cobeha.2018.01.022

Jones, A. P., Happé, F., Gilbert, F., Burnett, S., & Viding, E. (2010). Feeling, caring, knowing: Different types of empathy deficit in boys with psychopathic tendencies and autism spectrum disorder. *Journal of Child Psychology and Psychiatry, 51*(11), 1188–1197.

Keightly, M. L., Winocur, G., Graham, S. J., Matyberg, H. S., Hevenor, S. J., & Grady, C. L. (2003). An fMRI study investigating cognitive modulation of brain regions associated with emotional processing of visual stimuli. *Neuropsychologia, 41*, 585–596.

Kelly, M., McDonald, S., & Kellett, D. (2014). Development of a novel task for investigating decision making in a social context following traumatic brain injury. *Journal of Clinical and Experimental Neuropsychology*, *36*(9), 897–913.

Kessels, R. P. C., Montagne, B., Hendriks, A. W., Perrett, D. I., & de Haan, E. H. F. (2014). Assessment of perception of morphed facial expressions using the emotion recognition task: Normative data from healthy participants aged 8–75. *Journal of Neuropsychology*, *8*(1), 75–93.

Kessler, H., Doyen-Waldecker, C., Hofer, C., Hoffmann, H., Traue, H. C., & Abler, B. (2011). Neural correlates of the perception of dynamic versus static facial expressions of emotion. *Psycho-Social-Medicine*, *8*, Doc03. doi:10.3205/psm000072

Kim, H. (2012). A dual-subsystem model of the brain's default network: Self-referential processing, memory retrieval processes, and autobiographical memory retrieval. *Neuroimage*, *61*(4), 966–977.

Koenigs, M., Young, L., Adolphs, R., Tranel, D., Cushman, F., Hauser, M., & Damasio, A. (2007). Damage to the prefrontal cortex increases utilitarian moral judgements. *Nature*, *446*(7138), 908–911.

Kohlberg, L., Levine, C., & Hewer, A. (1983). *Moral Stages: A Current Formulation and a Response to Critics*. New York: Karger.

Kohler, C. G., Turner, T. H., Bilker, W. B., Brensinger, C. M., Siegel, S. J., Kanes, S. J., . . . Gur, R. C. (2003). Facial emotion recognition in schizophrenia: Intensity effects and error pattern. *American Journal of Psychiatry*, *160*(10), 1768–1774.

Kumfor, F., Hazelton, J., De Winter, F.-L., de Langavant, L. C., & Van den Stock, J. (2017). Clinical studies of social neuroscience: A lesion model approach. In A. Ibanez, L. Sedeno, & A. M. Garcia (Eds.), *Neuroscience and Social Science: The Missing Link*. New York: Springer.

Kumfor, F., Irish, M., Hodges, J. R., & Piguet, O. (2013). Discrete neural correlates for the recognition of negative emotions: Insights from frontotemporal dementia. *PLoS ONE*, *8*(6), e67457.

Kumfor, F., Zhen, A., Hodges, J. R., Piguet, O., & Irish, M. (2018). Apathy in Alzheimer's disease and frontotemporal dementia: Distinct clinical profiles and neural correlates. *Cortex*, *103*, 350–359.

Laird, J. D. (1974). Self-attribution of emotion: The effects of expressive behavior on the quality of emotional experience. *Journal of Personality and Social Psychology*, *29*(4), 475–486.

Larsen, J. K., Brand, N., Bermond, B., & Hijman, R. (2003). Cognitive and emotional characteristics of alexithymia: A review of neurobiological studies. *Journal of Psychosomatic Research*, *54*(6), 533–541.

Lawrence, C. A., Barry, R. J., Clarke, A. R., Johnstone, S. J., McCarthy, R., Selikowitz, M., & Broyd, S. J. (2005). Methylphenidate effects in attention deficit/hyperactivity disorder: Electrodermal and ERP measures during a continuous performance task. *Psychopharmacology*, *183*(1), 81–91.

LeDoux, J. (1995). Emotions: Clues from the brain. *Annual Reviews: Psychology*, *46*, 209–235.

Levin, H. S., Goldstein, F. C., Williams, D. H., & Eisenberg, H. M. (1991). The contribution of frontal lobe lesions to the neurobehavioral outcome of closed head injury. In H. S. Levin & H. M. Eisenberg (Eds.), *Frontal Lobe Function and Dysfunction* (pp. 318–338). London: Oxford University Press.

Levy, R., & Dubois, B. (2006). Apathy and the functional anatomy of the prefrontal cortex-basal ganglia circuits. *Cerebral Cortex*, *16*(7), 916–928.

Lieberman, M. D. (2007). Social cognitive neuroscience: A review of core processes. *Annual Review of Psychology, 58,* 259–289.

Lindquist, K. A., Wager, T. D., Kober, H., Bliss-Moreau, E., & Barrett, L. F. (2012). The brain basis of emotion: A meta-analytic review. *Behavioral and Brain Sciences, 35*(3), 121–143.

Lipszyc, J., Levin, H., Hanten, G., Hunter, J., Dennis, M., & Schachar, R. (2014). Frontal white matter damage impairs response inhibition in children following traumatic brain injury. *Archives of Clinical Neuropsychology, 29*(3), 289–299.

Lloyd, G. G., & Lishman, W. A. (1975). Effect of depression on the speed of recall of pleasant and unpleasant experiences. *Psychological Medicine, 5*(2), 173–180.

Lough, S., & Hodges, J. R. (2002). Measuring and modifying abnormal social cognition in frontal variant frontotemporal dementia. *Journal of Psychosomatic Research, 53*(2), 639–646.

Lough, S., Kipps, C. M., Treise, C., Watson, P., Blair, J. R., & Hodges, J. R. (2006). Social reasoning, emotion and empathy in frontotemporal dementia. *Neuropsychologia, 44*(6), 950–958.

Lozier, L. M., Vanmeter, J. W., & Marsh, A. A. (2014). Impairments in facial affect recognition associated with autism spectrum disorders: A meta-analysis. *Development and Psychopathology, 26*(4), 933–945.

Marcel, A. J., Tegnér, R., & Nimmo-Smith, I. (2004). Anosognosia for plegia: Specificity, extension, partiality and disunity of bodily unawareness. *Cortex, 40*(1), 19–40.

Marin, R. S. (1991). Apathy: A neuropsychiatric syndrome. *The Journal of Neuropsychiatry and Clinical Neurosciences, 3*(3), 243–254. doi:10.1176/jnp.3.3.243

Marin, R. S. (1996). Apathy: Concept, syndrome, neural mechanisms, and treatment. *Seminars in Clinical Neuropsychiatry, 1*(4), 304–314.

Martin-Rodriguez, J. F., & Leon-Carrion, J. (2010). Theory of mind deficits in patients with acquired brain injury: A quantitative review. *Neuropsychologia, 48,* 1181–1191.

Mathersul, D., McDonald, S., & Rushby, J. A. (2013a). Autonomic arousal explains social cognitive abilities in high-functioning adults with autism spectrum disorder. *International Journal of Psychophysiology, 89*(3), 475–482.

Mathersul, D., McDonald, S., & Rushby, J. A. (2013b). Psychophysiological correlates of social judgement in high-functioning adults with autism spectrum disorder. *International Journal of Psychophysiology, 87*(1), 88–94.

Matsumoto, D., LeRoux, J., Wilson-Cohn, C., Raroque, J., Kooken, K., Ekman, P., . . . Goh, A. (2000). A new test to measure emotion recognition ability: Matsumoto and Ekman's Japanese and Caucasian brief affect recognition test (JACBERT). *Journal of Nonverbal Behavior, 24*(3), 179–209.

McDonald, S. (1992). Differential pragmatic language loss after closed head injury: Ability to comprehend conversational implicature. *Applied Psycholinguistics, 13*(3), 295–312.

McDonald, S. (1993). Pragmatic language skills after closed head injury: Ability to meet the informational needs of the listener. *Brain and Language, 44*(1), 28–46.

McDonald, S., Bornhofen, C., Shum, D., Long, E., Saunders, C. J., & Neulinger, K. (2006). Reliability and validity of the awareness of social inference test (TASIT): A clinical test of social perception. *Disability and Rehabilitation: An International, Multidisciplinary Journal, 28*(24), 1529–1542.

McDonald, S., Dalton, K. I., Rushby, J. A., & Landin-Romero, R. (2019). Loss of white matter connections after severe traumatic brain injury (TBI) and its relationship to social cognition. *Brain Imaging and Behavior, 13*(3), 819–829.

McDonald, S., Flanagan, S., Rollins, J., & Kinch, J. (2003). TASIT: A new clinical tool for assessing social perception after traumatic brain injury. *The Journal of Head Trauma Rehabilitation, 18*(3), 219–238.

McDonald, S., Gowland, A., Randall, R., Fisher, A., Osborne-Crowley, K., & Honan, C. (2014). Cognitive factors underpinning poor expressive communication skills after traumatic brain injury: Theory of mind or executive function? *Neuropsychology, 28*(5), 801–811.

McDonald, S., Hunt, C., Henry, J. D., Dimoska, A., & Bornhofen, C. (2010). Angry responses to emotional events: The role of impaired control and drive in people with severe traumatic brain injury. *Journal of Clinical and Experimental Neuropsychology, 32*(8), 855–864.

McDonald, S., Li, S., De Sousa, A., Rushby, J., Dimoska, A., James, C., & Tate, R. L. (2011). Impaired mimicry response to angry faces following severe traumatic brain injury. *Journal of Clinical and Experimental Neuropsychology, 33*(1), 17–29.

McDonald, S., Rushby, J. A., Dalton, K. I., Allen, S. K., & Parks, N. (2018). The role of abnormalities in the corpus callosum in social cognition deficits after traumatic brain injury. *Social Neuroscience, 13*(4), 471–479.

McDonald, S., Rushby, J., Li, S., de Sousa, A., Dimoska, A., James, C., . . . Togher, L. (2011). The influence of attention and arousal on emotion perception in adults with severe traumatic brain injury. *International Journal of Psychophysiology, 82*(1), 124–131.

McHugo, G. J., & Smith, C. A. (1996). The power of faces: A review of John Lanzetta's research on facial expression and emotion. *Motivation and Emotion, 20*, 85–120.

Mendez, M. F., Anderson, E., & Shapira, J. S. (2005). An investigation of moral judgement in frontotemporal dementia. *Cognitive and Behavioral Neurology, 18*, 193–197.

Mendez, M. F., Chen, A. K., Shapira, J. S., & Miller, B. L. (2005). Acquired sociopathy and frontotemporal dementia. *Dementia and Geriatric Cognitive Disorders, 20*(2–3), 99–104.

Meyer, M. L., & Collier, E. (2020). Theory of minds: Managing mental state inferences in working memory is associated with the dorsomedial subsystem of the default network and social integration. *Social Cognitive and Affective Neuroscience, 15*(1), 63–73.

Molenberghs, P., Cunnington, R., & Mattingley, J. B. (2012). Brain regions with mirror properties: A meta-analysis of 125 human fMRI studies. *Neuroscience and Biobehavioral Reviews, 36*(1), 341–349.

Molenberghs, P., Johnson, H., Henry, J. D., & Mattingley, J. B. (2016). Understanding the minds of others: A neuroimaging meta-analysis. *Neuroscience and Biobehavioral Reviews, 65*, 276–291.

Montagne, B., Nys, G. M. S., Van Zandvoort, M. J. E., Kappelle, L. J., de Haan, E. H. F., & Kessels, R. P. C. (2007). The perception of emotional facial expressions in stroke patients with and without depression. *Acta Neuropsychiatrica, 19*(5), 279–283.

Moore, A. D., & Stambrook, M. (1995). Cognitive moderators of outcome following traumatic brain injury: A conceptual model and implications for rehabilitation. *Brain Injury, 9*(2), 109–130.

Moriguchi, Y., Ohnishi, T., Lane, R. D., Maeda, M., Mori, T., Nemoto, K., . . . Komaki, G. (2006). Impaired self-awareness and theory of mind: An fMRI study of mentalizing in alexithymia. *Neuroimage, 32*(3), 1472–1482.

Muller, U., Czymmek, J., Thone-Otto, A., & Von Cramon, D. Y. (2006). Reduced daytime activity in patients with acquired brain damage and apathy: A study with ambulatory actigraphy. *Brain Injury, 20*(2), 157–160.

Murray, R. J., Schaer, M., & Debbané, M. (2012). Degrees of separation: A quantitative neu-roimaging meta-analysis investigating self-specificity and shared neural activation between self- and other-reflection. *Neuroscience & Biobehavioral Reviews, 36*(3), 1043–1059.

Neumann, D., Zupan, B., Malec, J. F., & Hammond, F. (2013). Relationships between alexithymia, affect recognition, and empathy after traumatic brain injury. *Journal of Head Trauma Rehabilitation, 29*(1), E18–E27.

Niedenthal, P. M., Brauer, M., Halberstadt, J. B., & Innes-Ker, Å. H. (2001). When did her smile drop? Facial mimicry and the influences of emotional state on the detection of change in emotional expression. *Cognition & Emotion, 15*(6), 853–864.

Nijsse, B., Spikman, J. M., Visser-Meily, J. M., de Kort, P. L., & van Heugten, C. M. (2019). Social cognition impairments are associated with behavioural changes in the long term after stroke. *PLoS One, 14*(3), ArtID e0213725.

Njomboro, P., & Deb, S. (2014). Distinct neuropsychological correlates of cognitive, behavio-ral, and affective apathy sub-domains in acquired brain injury. *Frontiers in Neurology, 5*, 73.

Northoff, G., Heinzel, A., de Greck, M., Bermpohl, F., Dobrowolny, H., & Panksepp, J. (2006). Self-referential processing in our brain – a meta-analysis of imaging studies on the self. *Neuroimage, 31*(1), 440–457.

Ohman, A., & Soares, J. J. F. (1994). "Unconscious anxiety": Phobic responses to masked stimuli. *Journal of Abnormal Psychology, 103*(2), 231–240.

O'Keeffe, F., Dockree, P., Moloney, P., Carton, S., & Robertson, I. (2007). Characterising error-awareness of attentional lapses and inhibitory control failures in patients with trau-matic brain injury. *Experimental Brain Research, 180*(1), 59–67.

Osborne-Crowley, K., McDonald, S., & Francis, H. (2016). Development of an observa-tional measure of social disinhibition after traumatic brain injury. *Journal of Clinical and Experimental Neuropsychology, 38*(3), 341–353.

Osborne-Crowley, K., McDonald, S., & Rushby, J. A. (2016). Role of reversal learning impairment in social disinhibition following severe traumatic brain injury. *Journal of the International Neuropsychological Society, 22*(3), 303–313.

Osborne-Crowley, K., Wilson, E., De Blasio, F., Wearne, T., Rushby, J., & McDonald, S. (2019a). Empathy for people with similar experiences: Can the perception-action model explain empathy impairments after traumatic brain injury? *Journal of Clinical and Experi-mental Neuropsychology*, 1–14.

Osborne-Crowley, K., Wilson, E., De Blasio, F., Wearne, T., Rushby, J., & McDonald, S. (2019b). Preserved rapid conceptual processing of emotional expressions despite reduced neuropsychological performance following traumatic brain injury. *Neuropsychology, 33*(6), 872–882.

Osborne-Crowley, K., Wilson, E., De Blasio, F., Wearne, T., Rushby, J., & McDonald, S. (2019c). Subjective emotional experience and physiological responsivity to posed emo-tions in people with traumatic brain injury. *Neuropsychology, 33*(8), 1151–1162.

Perner, J., & Wimmer, H. (1985). "John thinks that Mary thinks that . . .": Attribution of second-order beliefs by 5- to 10-year-old children. *Journal of Experimental Child Psychol-ogy, 39*(3), 437–471.

Phillips, M. L., Drevets, W. C., Rauch, S. L., & Lane, R. (2003). Neurobiology of emotion perception I: The neural basis of normal emotion perception. *Biological Psychiatry, 54*(5), 504–514.

Pistoia, F., Conson, M., Trojano, L., Grossi, D., Ponari, M., Colonnese, C., . . . Sara, M. (2010). Impaired conscious recognition of negative facial expressions in patients with locked-in syndrome. *The Journal of Neuroscience, 30*(23), 7838–7844.

Pobric, G., Lambon Ralph, M. A., & Zahn, R. (2016). Hemispheric specialization within the superior anterior temporal cortex for social and nonsocial concepts. *Journal of Cognitive Neuroscience, 28*(3), 351–360.

Premack, D., & Woodruff, G. (1978). Does the chimpanzee have a theory of mind? *Behavioral and Brain Sciences, 1*(4), 515–526.

Preston, S. D., Bechara, A., Damasio, H., Grabowski, T. J., Stansfield, R., Mehta, S., & Damasio, A. R. (2007). The neural substrates of cognitive empathy. *Social Neuroscience, 2*(3–4), 254–275.

Preston, S. D., & Stansfield, R. B. (2008). I know how you feel: Task-irrelevant facial expressions are spontaneously processed at a semantic level. *Cognitive, Affective and Behavioral Neuroscience, 8*(1), 54–64.

Prigatano, G. P., & Altman, I. W. (1990). Impaired awareness of behavioural limitations after traumatic brain injury. *Archives of Physical Medication and Rehabilitation, 71*, 1058–1064.

Raine, A., Lencz, T., Bihrle, S., LaCasse, L., & Colletti, P. (2000). Reduced prefrontal gray matter volume and reduced autonomic activity in antisocial personality disorder. *Archives of General Psychiatry, 57*(2), 119–127.

Raine, A., Venables, P. H., & Williams, M. (1995). High autonomic arousal and electrodermal orienting at age 15 years as protective factors against criminal behavior at age 29 years. *American Journal of Psychiatry, 152*(11), 1595–1600.

Rees, G., Friston, K., & Koch, C. (2000). A direct quantitative relationship between the functional properties of human and macaque V5. *Nature Neuroscience, 3*(7), 716–723.

Richter, D., & Kunzmann, U. (2011). Age differences in three facets of empathy: Performance-based evidence. *Psychology and Aging, 26*(1), 60–70.

Ritter, K., Dziobek, I., Preißler, S., Rüter, A., Vater, A., Fydrich, T., . . . Roepke, S. (2011). Lack of empathy in patients with narcissistic personality disorder. *Psychiatry Research, 187*(1), 241–247.

Rizzolatti, G., & Sinigaglia, C. (2010). The functional role of the parieto-frontal mirror circuit: Interpretations and misinterpretations. *Nature Reviews Neuroscience, 11*(4), 264–274.

Rolls, E. T., Hornak, J., Wade, D., & McGrath, J. (1994). Emotion-related learning in patients with social and emotional changes associated with frontal lobe damage. *Journal of Neurology, Neurosurgery & Psychiatry, 57*(12), 1518–1524.

Rosenberg, H., Dethier, M., Kessels, R. P. C., Westbrook, R. F., & McDonald, S. (2015). Emotion perception after moderate-severe traumatic brain injury: The valence effect and the role of working memory, processing speed, and nonverbal reasoning. *Neuropsychology, 29*(4), 509–521.

Rosenberg, H., McDonald, S., Dethier, M., Kessels, R. P. C., & Westbrook, R. F. (2014). Facial emotion recognition deficits following moderate-severe traumatic brain injury (TBI): Re-examining the valence effect and the role of emotion intensity. *Journal of the International Neuropsychological Society, 20*(10), 994–1003.

Rosenberg, H., McDonald, S., Rosenberg, J., & Westbrook, R. F. (2016). Amused, flirting or simply baffled? Is recognition of all emotions affected by traumatic brain injury? *Journal of Neuropsychology, 12*(2), 145–164.

Ross, E. D., & Mesulam, M.-M. (1979). Dominant language functions of the right hemisphere? Prosody and emotional gesturing. *Archives of Neurology, 36*(3), 144–148.

Rowland, J. E., Hamilton, M. K., Vella, N., Lino, B. J., Mitchell, P. B., & Green, M. J. (2013, January). Adaptive associations between social cognition and emotion regulation are absent in schizophrenia and bipolar disorder. *Frontiers in Psychology, 3*. doi:10.3389/fpsyg.2012.00607

Ruby, P., & Decety, J. (2004). How would you feel versus how do you think she would feel? A neuroimaging study of perspective-taking with social emotions. *Journal of Cognitive Neuroscience, 16*(6), 988–999.

Rushby, J. A., McDonald, S., Randall, R., de Sousa, A., Trimmer, E., & Fisher, A. (2013). Impaired emotional contagion following severe traumatic brain injury. *International Journal of Psychophysiology, 89*(3), 466–474.

Sackeim, H. A., Greenberg, M. S., Weiman, A. L., Gur, R. C., Hungerbuhler, J. P., & Geschwind, N. (1982). Hemispheric asymmetry in the expression of positive and negative emotions. *Archives of Neurology, 39*, 210–218.

Sacks, O. (1985). *The Man Who Mistook His Wife for a Hat.* New York: Summit Books.

Sato, W., Kochiyama, T., Yoshikawa, S., Naito, E., & Matsumura, M. (2004). Enhanced neural activity in response to dynamic facial expressions of emotion: An fMRI study. *Cognitive Brain Research, 20*(1), 81–91.

Saunders, J. C., McDonald, S., & Richardson, R. (2006). Loss of emotional experience after traumatic brain injury: Findings with the startle probe procedure. *Neuropsychology, 20*(2), 224–231.

Schultz, J., & Pilz, K. S. (2009). Natural facial motion enhances cortical responses to faces. *Experimental Brain Research, 194*(3), 465–475.

Scott, S. K., Young, A. W., Calder, A. J., Hellawell, D. J., Aggleton, J. P., & Johnsons, M. (1997). Impaired auditory recognition of fear and anger following bilateral amygdala lesions. *Nature, 385*(6613), 254–257.

Sergerie, K., Chochol, C., & Armony, J. L. (2008). The role of the amygdala in emotional processing: A quantitative meta-analysis of functional neuroimaging studies. *Neuroscience & Biobehavioral Reviews, 32*(4), 811–830.

Shamay-Tsoory, S. G., Harari, H., Aharon-Peretz, J., & Levkovitz, Y. (2010). The role of the orbitofrontal cortex in affective theory of mind deficits in criminal offenders with psychopathic tendencies. *Cortex, 46*(5), 668–677.

Shamay-Tsoory, S. G., Tomer, R., & Aharon-Peretz, J. (2005). The neuroanatomical basis of understanding sarcasm and its relationship to social cognition. *Neuropsychology, 19*, 288–300.

Sherer, M., Hart, T., Whyte, J., Nick, T. G., & Yablon, S. A. (2005). Neuroanatomic basis of impaired self-awareness after traumatic brain injury: Findings from early computed tomography. *The Journal of Head Trauma Rehabilitation, 20*(4), 287–300.

So, S. H., Siu, N. Y., Wong, H. L., Chan, W., & Garety, P. A. (2016). 'Jumping to conclusions' data-gathering bias in psychosis and other psychiatric disorders – two meta-analyses of comparisons between patients and healthy individuals. *Clinical Psychology Review, 46*, 151–167.

Soussignan, R. (2002). Duchenne smile, emotional experience, and autonomic reactivity: A test of the facial feedback hypothesis. *Emotion, 2*(1), 52–74.

Spalletta, G., Serra, L., Fadda, L., Ripa, A., Bria, P., & Caltagirone, C. (2007). Unawareness of motor impairment and emotions in right hemispheric stroke: A preliminary investigation. *International Journal of Geriatric Medicine, 22*, 1241–1246.

Sperber, D., & Wilson, D. (1986). *Relevance: Communication and Cognition.* Oxford: Basil Blackwell.

Spikman, J. M., Timmerman, M. E., Milders, M. V., Veenstra, V. S., & van der Naalt, J. (2012). Social cognition impairments in relation to general cognitive deficits, injury severity, and prefrontal lesions in traumatic brain injury patients. *Journal of Neurotrauma, 29*(1), 101–111.

Sprengelmeyer, R., Young, A. W., Calder, A. J., Karnat, A., Lange, H., Homber, G. V., . . . Rowland, D. (1996). Loss of disgust: Perception of faces and emotion in Huntingdon's disease. *Brain, 119,* 1647–1665.

Strack, F., Martin, L. L., & Stepper, S. (1988). Inhibiting and facilitating conditions of the human smile: A nonobtrusive test of the facial feedback hypothesis. *Journal of Personality and Social Psychology, 54*(5), 768–777.

Stronach, S. T., & Turkstra, L. S. (2008). Theory of mind and use of cognitive state terms by adolescents with traumatic brain injury. *Aphasiology, 22*(10), 1054–1070.

Stuss, D. T., & Benson, D. F. (1986). *The Frontal Lobes.* New York: Raven Press.

Sweeney, P. D., Anderson, K., & Bailey, S. (1986). Attributional style in depression: A meta-analytic review. *Journal of Personality and Social Psychology, 50*(5), 974–991.

Symington, S. H., Paul, L. K., Symington, M. F., Ono, M., & Brown, W. S. (2010). Social cognition in individuals with agenesis of the corpus callosum. *Social Neuroscience, 5*(3), 296–308.

Tamietto, M., Castelli, L., Vighetti, S., Perozzo, P., Geminiani, G., Weiskrantz, L., & de Gelder, B. (2009). Unseen facial and bodily expressions trigger fast emotional reactions. *PNAS Proceedings of the National Academy of Sciences of the United States of America, 106*(42), 17662–17666.

Tate, R. L. (1999). Executive dysfunction and characterological changes after traumatic brain injury: Two sides of the same coin? *Cortex, 35*(1), 39–55.

Thayer, J. F., Hansen, A. L., Saus-Rose, E., & Johnsen, B. H. (2009). Heart rate variability, prefrontal neural function, and cognitive performance: The neurovisceral integration perspective on self-regulation, adaptation, and health. *Annals of Behavioral Medicine, 37*(2), 141–153.

Trautmann, S. A., Fehr, T., & Herrmann, M. (2009). Emotions in motion: Dynamic compared to static facial expressions of disgust and happiness reveal more widespread emotion-specific activations. *Brain Research, 1284,* 100–115.

Vuilleumier, P. (2004). Anosognosia: The neurology of beliefs and uncertainties. *Cortex, 40*(1), 9–17.

Wagenmakers, E.-J., Beek, T., Dijkhoff, L., Gronau, Q. F., Acosta, A., Adams, R. B., . . . Zwaan, R. A. (2016). Registered replication report: Strack, Martin, & Stepper (1988). *Perspectives on Psychological Science, 11*(6), 917–928.

Watson, R., Huis in 't Veld, E. M., & de Gelder, B. (2016). The neural basis of individual face and object perception. *Frontiers in Human Neuroscience, 10,* ArtID 066.

Wilhelm, O., Hildebrandt, A., Manske, K., Schacht, A., & Sommer, W. (2014). Test battery for measuring the perception and recognition of facial expressions of emotion. *Frontiers in Psychology, 5,* 404.

Williams, C., & Wood, R. L. (2010). Alexithymia and emotional empathy following traumatic brain injury. *Journal of Clinical and Experimental Neuropsychology, 32*(3), 259–267.

Williams, C., & Wood, R. L. (2012). Affective modulation of the startle reflex following traumatic brain injury. *Journal of Clinical and Experimental Neuropsychology, 34*(9), 948–961.

Wimmer, H., & Perner, J. (1983). Beliefs about beliefs: Representation and constraining function of wrong beliefs in young children's understanding of deception. *Cognition, 13*(1), 103–128.

Wood, R. L., & Williams, C. (2007). Neuropsychological correlates of organic alexithymia. *Journal of the International Neuropsychological Society, 13,* 471–479.

Wood, R. L., & Williams, C. (2008). Inability to empathize following traumatic brain injury. *Journal of the International Neuropsychological Society, 14*, 289–296.

Zhang, Q., Li, X., Parker, G. J., Hong, X.-h., Wang, Y., Lui, S. S., . . . Chan, R. C. (2016). Theory of mind correlates with clinical insight but not cognitive insight in patients with schizophrenia. *Psychiatry Research, 237*, 188–195.

Zwick, J., & Wolkenstein, L. (2016). Facial emotion recognition, theory of mind and the role of facial mimicry in depression. *Journal of Affective Disorders, 210*. doi:10.1016/j.jad.2016.12.022

Chapter 2

Research methodologies, brain correlates, cross-cultural perspectives

Fiona Kumfor and Skye McDonald

Social cognition is complex and multifactorial. While the concept that abilities that support social interactions are unique has historical roots (Cannon, 1927; Darwin, 1872; James, 1884), research investigating social cognition has mostly lagged behind other traditional cognition domains, such as language and memory. As outlined in Chapter 1, social cognition is usually defined as those abilities which enable perception, judgement and action in social situations. This chapter considers the most common research techniques employed when investigating social cognition in clinical syndromes. We consider some of the limitations of existing tasks and study designs and highlight emerging paradigms which aim to address some of these criticisms. Next, we discuss the considerable impact neuroimaging has had on the field. We outline the most common techniques used and their pros and cons, and also explain how case studies are complementary to more advanced neuroimaging approaches. Finally, we contemplate how culture impacts on social cognition performance, with a particular emphasis on the need to account for cultural differences in the research setting. This chapter aims to provide clinicians and researchers with a snapshot of some of the key current themes in the research domain and considers the next steps for this rapidly developing field.

Common research methodologies

Clinical research has largely focused on assessment of emotion perception and theory of mind (Baron-Cohen, Wheelwright, Hill, Raste, & Plumb, 2001; Ekman, 1976; Kumfor, Hazelton, De Winter, Cleret de Langavant, & Van den Stock, 2017). Emotion perception tasks tend to use still photographs of posed facial expressions (Calder, Rowland, Young, Nimmo-Smith, Keane, & Perrett, 2000; Calder, Young, Perrett, Etcoff, & Rowland, 1996; Calder, Young, Rowland, & Perrett, 1997; Ekman, 1976; Matsumoto & Ekman, 1988; Tottenham et al., 2009). Several stimulus sets have been developed, which typically include exemplars of the six basic emotions (happiness, sadness, disgust, anger, fear, surprise) as well as neutral expressions. Task requirements vary, but may include (1) selecting the written label that matches the facial expression, (2) deciding

DOI: 10.4324/9781003027034-2

whether two expressions are the same or different, or (3) selecting an expression from an array of faces to match a verbally presented label (Kumfor, Hazelton et al., 2017; Kumfor et al., 2014). These tasks have the benefit of being easy to score, with answers clearly correct or not. Furthermore, they are relatively quick to administer and typically have a similar format to other neuropsychological tests of cognition. Tests that assess emotion perception through other domains have also been developed. For example, a test for emotion expressed via vocal prosody (Buchanan et al., 2000; Grandjean et al., 2005; Perry et al., 2001; Rohrer, Sauter, Scott, Rossor, & Warren, 2010; Ross, Thompson, & Yenkosky, 1997; Sander et al., 2005). Notably, recognition of emotion from facial expressions and vocal prosody are at least partially dissociable (Adolphs, Damasio, & Tranel, 2002).

However, such tests are poor at approximating performance that is required in real world social situations. Firstly, the stimuli are static and from a single modality. Secondly, the stimuli tend to be context-free. In social situations, determining the emotional expression of another person's face is usually informed by the context the face is presented in. Seminal work by Aviezer, Trope, and Todorov (2012) demonstrated how the same facial expression can be interpreted differently depending on contextual cues provided. In this case, participants were presented with faces showing high intensity facial expressions and body expressions (winning or losing). The results showed that participants could reliably discriminate between body expressions but not facial expressions (Aviezer et al., 2012; Hassin, Aviezer, & Bentin, 2013). Follow-up studies have confirmed that when faces attached to bodies are presented, their interpretation changes (Aviezer et al., 2008). Importantly, the degree of influence appears to change in clinical syndromes where frontal and/or temporal brain regions are affected (Kumfor et al., 2018). Hence, facial expressions in isolation may be inadequate to provide a full picture of an individual's capacity to understand emotion.

The other large field of research has focused on theory of mind (Premack & Woodruff, 1978). A number of tasks have been developed and widely used to assess an individual's ability to infer what another person is thinking, believing or feeling, with Simon Baron-Cohen a leader in this field. Arguably the first test of theory of mind was the Sally-Anne test (Baron-Cohen, Leslie, & Frith, 1985). Participants are introduced to two characters – Sally and Anne – and watch a short skit, where Sally hides a marble and then leaves the room. While she is absent, Anne moves the marble to a new location. The participant is then asked, "Where will Sally look for her marble?" In order to demonstrate theory of mind, the participant should respond with Location 1, which is consistent with Sally's knowledge, but differs from the participant's own knowledge/mental state. This classic false belief task has had multiple iterations to assess first-second- and third-order false beliefs (Frith & Frith, 2005; Kumfor, Hazelton et al., 2017). However, one of the drawbacks of this task is that it has considerable working memory and language demands.

Another common theory of mind test is the Reading the Mind in the Eyes test. Here, individuals are shown cropped images of the eye region of the face and asked to select what the person is thinking or feeling from four verbally presented options (e.g., irritated, thoughtful, encouraging, sympathetic) (Baron-Cohen et al., 2001). While widely used, it has been criticised for its high language demands as well as considerable demands on emotion recognition (Oakley, Brewer, Bird, & Catmur, 2016; Olderbak et al., 2015). Furthermore, because the stimuli were of actors and actresses gathered from magazines, the actual person's mental state at the time of the expression was not known. Rather, responses were considered "correct" if at least five of eight judges agreed (Baron-Cohen et al., 2001). Thus, while the Reading the Mind in the Eyes test has been widely used and appears sensitive to autism spectrum disorder, it has a number of theoretical, methodological and psychometric limitations (Olderbak et al., 2015). Subsequent tests, such as the Animated Shapes task (Abell, Happé, & Frith, 2000), and Faux Pas cartoons (Baron-Cohen, O'Riordan, Stone, Jones, & Plaisted, 1999) have been developed in an attempt to minimise cognitive and language demands when assessing theory of mind.

In addition, many studies employ self- or informant-report. For example, the Socioemotional Questionnaire was initially developed to assess aspects of social cognition in individuals with prefrontal cortex lesions (Bramham, Morris, Hornak, Bullock, & Polkey, 2009). Consistent with what would be expected based on their pattern of lesions, patients with unilateral orbitofrontal lesions reported more antisocial behaviour, and individuals with bilateral orbitofrontal lesions showed even greater social and emotional functioning impairment than those with unilateral lesions (Bramham et al., 2009). While these techniques have the advantage of being cheap, fast and easy to use, they are also subjective and therefore potentially less reliable and/or valid.

Although these common research tools have been indispensable for advancing our knowledge of social cognition impairment in clinical disorders, as outlined above, they do suffer from a number of critical limitations. Subjective measures may be unsuitable in cases where the participants have impaired insight. On the other hand, objective measures tend to have a high level of cognitive demand. This means it is possible to perform poorly due to working memory impairment, episodic memory impairment and/or language impairment. This makes it difficult to isolate social cognition impairment. See Chapter 9 for a full discussion of the reliability, validity and sensitivity of current measures used to assess social cognition.

Emerging trends

In the past couple of decades, research studies have started to move away from the relatively simplistic approach of using static stimuli to develop new tasks and approaches that better reflect the demands of day-to-day social interactions.

Where possible, newer approaches also attempt to parse out, or account for, the potential influence of cognitive impairment.

Accounting for cognitive demands

One way to address the potential influence of cognitive impairment is for tasks to have a control condition, which is as similar as possible to the experimental condition and only differs with respect to the demand on social cognition. A good example of this is The Awareness of Social Inference Test (TASIT) Part 2 (McDonald, Bornhofen, Shum, Long, & Neulinger, 2006; McDonald, Flanagan, Martin, & Saunders, 2004; McDonald, Flanagan, Rollins, & Kinch, 2003). On this task, participants watch a short video vignette and are asked questions about what the characters are thinking or feeling. On half the items, the exchanges are sincere, whereas for the remaining items the exchange is sarcastic. In order to answer the questions correctly, the person must be able to decode the sarcasm of the exchange. Importantly, if a person performs poorly on both the sincere and sarcasm items, this may indicate that cognition impairment is impacting on their performance. TASIT has been used in a number of clinical populations, where it has been demonstrated that differential performance on the sarcasm compared to the sincere items is associated with atrophy of regions in the social brain (Kumfor, Honan et al., 2017).

For emotion recognition, finding an equivalent "non-social" task is somewhat more challenging. Use of "neutral" facial expressions is tempting; however, research has found that people tend to interpret neutral expressions as somewhat negative. Indeed, neutral expressions may be more difficult to recognise than emotional expressions (Honan et al., 2016). In some cases, use of non-social stimuli has been employed. For example, tasks of face recognition often use car recognition as a comparison task (Dennett et al., 2012).

An alternative is to use tasks which are "implicit" and hence have minimal cognitive demands (Nosek et al., 2011). An advantage of implicit social cognition tasks is that they better approximate real-world conditions. If you consider everyday social interactions, it is quite rare that someone will directly ask you how another person is feeling (and even rarer for them to give you options to choose between!). Rather, processing of social information tends to happen automatically, and with minimal cognitive effort. Implicit tasks exploit this automaticity to study responses to social stimuli. The advantage of implicit tasks is that they assess mental content indirectly. Hence, different information is gleaned than from explicit tasks or self-report (Nosek et al., 2011). Two of the most common types of implicit tasks of social cognition are the implicit association test and priming tasks, such as the sequential evaluative priming task. While these tasks are increasingly employed in healthy participants, and particularly in studies interested in individual differences, they have only occasionally been used in clinical research (e.g., (McDonald et al., 2011) and are arguably yet to reach their full potential.

In comparison to behavioural measures of social cognition or questionnaires, psychophysiological markers provide a direct measure of socioemotional function. In healthy adults, negative facial expressions elicit increased skin conductance, increased corrugator response and decelerated heart rate, than happy faces, but these responses are compromised in clinical populations (e.g., de Sousa et al., 2012; de Sousa et al., 2011; Kumfor et al., 2019). Psychophysiological measures are advantageous in that they are relatively non-invasive and tend to be well tolerated in clinical populations. Furthermore, they are less susceptible to floor and ceiling effects than performance-based tasks. This means that psychophysiological measures can be suitable for use across different disorders and levels of severity. Moreover, psychophysiological measures may be more suitable for clinical trials where repeat measures across various disease stages are required. The downside of psychophysiological measurement is the inherent variability of the measures that make it difficult to obtain reliable, intra-participant measures. Nonetheless, these different techniques therefore provide a complementary approach to more traditional facial emotion recognition and performance-based theory of mind tasks. Physiological measures are discussed further in Chapter 9.

Ecological validity and truly social tasks

As mentioned above, an important distinction between existing tests of social cognition and real-world demands is that most stimuli are single modality and static in nature (with the notable exception of TASIT). While this is helpful from a mechanistic point of view (i.e., to determine whether perception of facial expression is dissociable from prosody), it means that performance may not necessarily reflect behaviour under real-world conditions. Pioneering neurologists addressed this lack of ecological validity by placing their patients in situations that better approximate reality. For example, Lhermitte (1983, 1986) examined utilisation behaviour in patients with frontal lobe lesions. When presented with an orange, plate and knife the patient would cut the orange and begin to eat; when presented with a packet of cigarettes and a lighter the patient would smoke the cigarette (and on occasion offer one to the examiner). Lhermitte noted that on only one occasion did the patient use the urinal in the room (Lhermitte, 1983). Lhermitte also set up more complex situations to assess social behaviours. He reported that one patient "behaved like a guest at a buffet; after receiving a decoration, he wanted to express his thanks by making a speech". In another, a patient was offered a revolver and pistol, and the patient selected the pistol that matched the cartridges on the table. In a third situation, the patient gave the examiner an intramuscular injection when presented with a syringe (Lhermitte, 1986). These remarkable examples of disordered social behaviour in clinical patients, however, are unsuitable for broader application due to their inherent ethical issues, as well as lack of control.

Increasingly, there are also calls for social cognition research to take a second-person approach (Redcay et al., 2019; Schilbach et al., 2013). Proponents of the second-person approach point out that while the majority of our social lives are spent in reciprocal interactions, the study of social cognition has largely been conducted using tasks that do not require interaction (Redcay et al., 2019; Schilbach et al., 2013). Crucially, the neural and cognitive processes that are engaged in second-person tasks (i.e., studies in which individuals are participants in a social interaction and/or otherwise feel engaged with a social partner) appear to differ at least somewhat from those during traditional third-person contexts, which only require observation of social stimuli. Second-person tasks may involve interaction with another real person; but may also include interactions with an avatar or may give the impression of interaction via deception. Examples of second-person tasks include mutual gaze and joint attention tasks (Caruana et al., 2015; Caruana et al., 2018), "cyberball" (Williams et al., 2006), the trust game (Bellucci et al., 2017) and some behavioural mimicry tasks (Yun et al., 2012).

New technologies present a unique opportunity for examining behaviour in complex situations while minimising potential risk to the patient and examiner and enabling replicability across participants and trials. Virtual reality is growing as a potential tool to assess social cognition, as it addresses some of these calls for improved ecological validity and social interaction while maintaining experimental control. In healthy adults, physiological reactions while participating in virtual reality scenarios are similar to those elicited in real-life situations (Parsons, Gaggioli, & Riva, 2017). Moreover, the use of virtual reality in clinical populations, such as dementia, has been shown to be tolerable and feasible (Mendez, Joshi, & Jimenez, 2015). In virtual reality, the measurement of physiological processes responding to environmental demands can occur simultaneously during situations aimed at increasing autonomic arousal.

Virtual reality also provides an opportunity for interventions using social cognition training. In people with autism spectrum disorder, virtual reality has been used as an opportunity to practice dynamic and real-life social interactions (Didehbani et al., 2016; Kandalaft et al., 2013). Here, participants enter a virtual world which includes locations where typical social interactions take place, such as an office building, fast food restaurant, café, school or park. Participants enter the virtual world with their clinician and are prompted to interact with another person in a specific social situation (e.g., meeting new people, conflict with a roommate, interviewing for a job). Typical social cognition measures are also collected pre- and post-intervention. In the study by Kandalaft et al. following 10 sessions of the intervention, participants showed improved social and occupational functioning, as well as improved emotion recognition and theory of mind test performance (Kandalaft et al., 2013). While these results are only preliminary, they demonstrate the potential utility of virtual reality for providing realistic social interactions under highly controlled environments, which poses substantial advantages from a clinical, methodological and ethical standpoint.

Neuroimaging – from research to the clinic

The other major advancement in studies of social cognition is its integration with neuroscience (Kumfor et al., in press). The growth of the field of social cognition occurred alongside the development of neuroimaging techniques. At the research level, most neuroimaging studies have focused on developing and testing neurobiological models of social cognition. However, it was not until the last decade or so that the "social brain" was eponymized (Adolphs, 1999, 2009) see also (Dunbar, 1998). Most research studies use either structural or functional brain imaging to identify brain regions which are correlated with the specific social cognition domain of interest (see Chapter 1 for a comprehensive review of these brain structures).

Neuroimaging techniques can be roughly divided into structural and functional imaging. Computerized tomography (CT) scans are useful for identifying large structural changes, such as a stroke or tumour. While they are cheap and widely available, they are mostly used in clinical rather than research settings, because their spatial resolution is fairly limited. In contrast, structural magnetic resonance imaging (MRI), scans have much greater spatial resolution and can be used to identify atrophy, vascular changes, white matter lesions etc. MRI scans can also be combined with analytic tools such as voxel-based morphometry (VBM) and cortical thickness to assess grey matter integrity, and diffusion tensor imaging (DTI) to measure white matter integrity. VBM detects differences in the regional grey matter density by measuring the intensity of individual voxels (i.e., three dimensional pixels) while accounting for global brain shape differences (Ashburner et al., 2000; Mechelli et al., 2005). In contrast, cortical thickness analyses, such as Freesurfer, segment the grey matter cortical ribbon from white matter and measure the thickness of the cortical ribbon across the surface of the brain (Fischl, 2012). Finally, diffusion tensor imaging (DTI) is an MRI technique that allows mapping of the diffusion of water in brain tissue to provide measures of fractional anisotropy and mean diffusivity, which are used to determine the structural integrity of white matter tracts. Together, these analytic tools can be used to examine differences in brain integrity between groups (i.e., patients vs. controls) and measure correlations between the integrity of brain structures and performance on a behavioural task of interest. These analyses can either take a region of interest approach, where hypothesis-driven analyses are confined to specific brain regions based or they can be conducted at the whole-brain level.

Positron emission tomography (PET) and single photon emission computed tomography (SPECT) are useful in assessing metabolic changes of brain function. Both PET and SPECT can be useful in identifying regions of hypometabolism (i.e., reduced functioning) in the brain. These scans are mostly useful clinically, because they may be sensitive to brain changes before struc-tural abnormalities are able to be detected. However, they are less useful for understanding brain-behaviour relationships, because of their poor spatial and temporal resolution as well as their relative cost and the need for intrusive injections of radioactive glucose.

Electroencephalography (EEG) and magnetoencephalography (MEG) have much better temporal resolution than PET or SPECT. EEG records electrical fields which are emitted by the brain, whereas MEG records magnetic fields emitted from the brain from ionic currents which are biochemically generated at the cellular level (Lopes da Silva, 2013). These techniques are exquisitely suited to paradigms where processing occurs very quickly. One of the best examples is the N/M170 response, which is greater when viewing upright faces than inverted faces or other objects (Bentin et al., 1996; Rossion et al., 2000). The drawback of EEG and MEG is that spatial resolution is poor.

In contrast, functional MRI (fMRI) has excellent spatial resolution. Here, participants engage in a task while changes in blood-oxygen-level-dependent contrast are measured. fMRI is arguably the most common functional brain imaging technique, because it is non-invasive and well tolerated, even in many clinical disorders. Commonly, participants view and make judgements on socially salient stimuli. Designing tasks which involve social interaction can be challenging. Typically, deception is used so that the participant is under the impression they are interacting with another person located in a remote loca-tion. Less commonly, studies have used hyperscanning, where two individuals are scanned and can communicate via videolink (Montague et al., 2002). In some studies, a second person may also be present during the fMRI scan, to assess the influence of another person's presence on brain activity (Coan et al., 2006).

fMRI has also been used to examine the functional connectivity between different neural systems thought to underpin social cognition. This is achieved by examining the synchrony in activation/deactivation across brain regions either when the research participant is at rest, i.e., not engaging in a particular task (resting state functional connectivity, e.g., Fareri et al., 2017; Fox et al., 2017) or during performance of a task (to identify what brain regions are engaged at the same time). For example, an inverse relation between *amygdala* and *prefrontal* activation when exposed to negative emotional events has been thought to reflect the regulatory nature of prefrontal systems on amygdala activity (Lee et al., 2012).

Because MRI machines are large, and the magnetic shielding required is considerable, the practicalities of social interactions during fMRI present a considerable challenge. Functional near infrared spectroscopy (fNIRS) offers an alternative method to measure functional brain changes while interacting with others. fNIRS uses infrared light to measure changes in haemoglobin, reflecting brain activity. While fNIRS is best suited to measuring surface-level brain activity, it is relatively small and portable and therefore can be suitable for studying real-time interactions between people in a more realistic setting (Holper et al., 2012; Nozawa et al., 2016; Quaresima et al., 2019).

While the use of these different imaging techniques is increasingly widespread and has undoubtedly informed neurobiological models of social cognition, they do have limitations. First, the information that can be gleaned from neuroimaging studies is dependent on the strength of the experimental design. For functional neuroimaging studies, brain activity is compared between two tasks, and the difference in activity is indicative of brain regions that are specific to the task of interest. For example, if a study is interested in brain regions that respond to angry faces, they could compare brain activity when viewing neutral faces. But an equally valid design would be to compare activity when viewing sad or happy faces. While the experimental condition may remain consistent, differences in the control condition directly influence the overall results. Hence, experimental designs that have appropriate and adequate control conditions are essential. Even then, it is impossible to demonstrate that the difference in neural activation triggered by the experimental task relative to its control task is unique to the specific demands of the experimental task. It is very difficult to control what research participants are doing in scanners and the extent to which stimuli may trigger other processes (e.g., semantic associations, emotion) when this was not the intent. Additionally, the dynamics of neural activation are affected in fundamental ways by a change in task requirements. For example, greater *visual cortex* activation is observed when a participant is asked to read words out loud than when silent reading even though the visual demands are identical. (Price et al., 1997). This effect is exaggerated when the stimuli have emotional significance (Padmala et al., 2008).

Second, the statistical analysis of neuroimaging data is complex. Often, the number of comparisons are far beyond what would be conducted for behavioural studies. For example, a standard fMRI analysis involves thousands of simultaneous significance tests (Lieberman et al., 2009). There is, therefore, a need to control for family wise error in order to minimise the risk of Type I error. Traditionally in behavioural studies, a Bonferroni-type approach might be taken, where the significance level (e.g., 0.05) is divided by the number of statistical tests being conducted. In neuroimaging literature, this is known as a "corrected" *p* value. While this addresses the issue of Type I error, it is increasingly recognised that the effect of this conservative approach is an increased risk of Type II error (Lieberman et al., 2009; Noble et al., 2020). The analogy of an iceberg can be useful when interpreting MRI findings. If a conservative statistical threshold is used, then few very small peaks will be identified; however, this effect is likely to be very strong. Conversely, if a more liberal threshold is used, more peaks will be observed; however, the effect may be weaker (and may represent false positives). This statistical conundrum is an ongoing issue for the field. Careful consideration of the statistical thresholds employed is important when interpreting the robustness of reported findings.

Third, as with any correlative technique, causation cannot be inferred. For the most part, functional studies that identify brain activity or structural studies that report brain-behaviour relationships can only make claims about how a brain region is correlated with task performance. However, these studies are inadequate to determine whether brain regions are necessary or sufficient. For these reasons, lesion studies still play an important complementary role, particularly when inferring causation. Indeed, understanding of brain behaviour relationships initially had its roots in lesion model approaches. For example, pioneers such as Broca provided unparalleled insights into the function of limbic brain regions (Broca, 1878), classic case studies such as Phineas Gage revealed the role of the *prefrontal* cortex in personality and social behaviour (Damasio et al., 1994), patient SM highlighted the importance of the *amygdala* in emotion perception (Adolphs et al., 1994, 1995) and work by Kluver and Bucy illustrated the role of *temporal pole* in fear (Kluver et al., 1937). While historically, case studies were important, they are still an important complement to newer neuroimaging technology. For example, Feinstein et al. (2016) reported a patient "Roger" with widespread damage to the *insula, anterior cingulate* and *amygdala*. While fMRI studies have implicated these regions in the experience of pain, interestingly Roger's expression and experience of pain was intact, based on a comprehensive assessment which included self-report, facial expression, vocalisation, behaviour and autonomic physiological responses. Such case studies demonstrate how regions which are active during fMRI tasks are not necessarily sufficient for task performance.

As the neuroimaging field grows, it is now possible to use meta-analytic techniques to identify common neural regions which are active across tasks. This approach is useful as it helps to control for some differences in methodological design and power. One of the first such studies was a meta-analysis of PET and fMRI studies of emotion (Phan et al., 2002). The analysis included 55 studies which reported 761 individual peaks. This meta-analysis found both emotion general and emotion-specific brain regions. Specifically, the *medial prefrontal cortex* was active in response to emotion processing generally. In contrast, fear specifically engaged the *amygdala*, whereas sadness engaged the *subcallosal cingulate*. Cognitively demanding tasks or those where an emotional state was induced through emotional recall or imagery were associated with greater activation of the *anterior cingulate* and *insula*. This study has undoubtedly been influential in assimilating information across studies; however, given this study was published almost two decades ago, an update of this meta-analysis is clearly warranted. Indeed, we found that since 2001, more than 55,000 papers have been published in the field of social and affective neuroscience (Kumfor et al., in press) and numerous meta-analyses have also been reported (Costafreda et al., 2008; Kober et al., 2008; Lindquist et al., 2012; Vytal et al., 2010).

More recently, a meta-analysis of fMRI studies investigating theory of mind was published (Molenberghs et al., 2016). This study included 144 studies which had employed various theory of mind tasks including stories, cartoons, photographs, Reading the Mind in the Eyes test, videos, animations and interactive games. A brain network was identified that was activated across studies, which included the *medial prefrontal cortex* and *bilateral temporoparietal junction*. Importantly, however, the specific brain regions varied across task type. This type of research demonstrates how methodological differences can directly influence study results; but importantly, it also confirms that across studies, common brain regions associated with social cognition ability can be revealed.

Cross-cultural assessment

As outlined above, a growing body of work has focused on developing tools to assess aspects of social cognition and demonstrate their utility in a clinical setting. However, whether these tests are appropriate in culturally and linguistically diverse (CALD) populations is unclear.

Like research on cognition more broadly, the vast majority of research on social cognition has been conducted in Western, Industrialised and Democratic countries and their norms based on well-Educated and Rich people; sometimes referred to as "W.E.I.R.D" people (Gurven, 2018). Indeed, most tests of social cognition have been developed in Western countries, particularly from the U.S. and Europe. For example, both the Reading the Mind in the Eyes Test and the Facial Expressions of Emotion were developed and published in England (Baron-Cohen et al., 2001; Young et al., 2002).

In neuropsychology, the limitations of applying tests in culturally diverse populations has been recognised for at least several decades (e.g., Levinson, 1959; Wysocki et al., 1969). The impact can range from obvious – for example – a verbal memory test will be more difficult for someone whose first language is Japanese if the test is conducted in English. Or the effect can be more subtle – for example an Australian may be less likely to recognise a "beaver", whereas an American may have more difficulty recognising an "echidna".

For verbal tests, the most common approach to enable neuropsychological tests to be used across cultures is through translation and back translation. Here, the test is translated by a native speaker (e.g., from English to Spanish). Then, a second independent expert translates the test back to the original language (i.e., from Spanish to English). This process helps to identify any potential ambiguity or confusion, and discrepancies can be resolved between the experts. Thus, back translation is helpful to ensure that items are equivalent across versions. Normative data is also necessary to determine expected performance in the population of interest. For questionnaires assessing social cognition, this straightforward approach can be employed. For example, the Neuropsychiatric Inventory, which assesses disorders of social behaviour such as apathy and disinhibition (Cummings et al., 1994), is available in Korean (Choi et al., 2000), Portuguese (Camozzato et al., 2008), Chinese (Leung et al., 2001), Japanese (Hirono et al., 1997) and Dutch (Kat et al., 2002). Translated versions are also available for questionnaires assessing empathy such as the Interpersonal Reactivity Index (De Corte et al., 2007; Gilet et al., 2013; Kang et al., 2009; Zhang et al., 2010) and the Basic Empathy Scale (Albiero et al., 2009; Anastácio et al., 2016; Bensalah et al., 2016; Heynen et al., 2016).

For non-verbal tests, the suitability of tests across cultures may be more variable. As Charles Darwin stated, *"it seemed to me highly important to ascertain whether the same expressions and gestures prevail, as has often been asserted without much evidence, with all the races of mankind, especially those who have associated but little with Europeans."* (Darwin, 1872). To explore this, Darwin sent a series of queries to missionaries, fellow scientists and members of the public across the world living and working in non-European cultures (see Table 2.1).

The descriptions received by Darwin largely confirmed his observations, with reports about Aboriginal Australians, Maoris from New Zealand, the Dyaks of Borneo, indigenous people from Malacca, Chinese immigrants in

Table 2.1 Darwin's descriptions of emotional expressions and social norms. From (Darwin, 1872, p. 16)

1. Is astonishment expressed by the eyes and mouth being opened wide, and by the eyebrows being raised?
2. Does shame excite a blush when the colour of the skin allows it to be visible? And especially how low down the body does the blush extend?
3. When a man is indignant or defiant, does he frown, hold his body and head erect, square his shoulders and clench his fists?
4. When considering deeply on any subject, or trying to understand any puzzle, does he frown, or wrinkle the skin beneath the lower eyelids?
5. When in low spirits, are the corners of the mouth depressed, and the inner corner of the eyebrows raised by the muscle which the French call the "Grief muscle"? The eyebrow in this state becomes slightly oblique, with a little swelling at the inner end; and the forehead is transversely wrinkled in the middle part, but not across the whole breadth, as when the eyebrows are raised in surprise.
6. When in good spirits, do the eyes sparkle, with the skin a little wrinkled round and under them, and with the mouth a little drawn back at the corners?
7. When a man sneers or snarls at another, is the corner of the upper lip over the canine or eye tooth raised on the side facing the man who he addresses?
8. Can a dogged or obstinate expression be recognised, which is chiefly shown by the mouth being firmly closed, a lowering brow and a slight frown?
9. Is contempt expressed by a slight protrusion of the lips and by turning up the nose with a slight expiration?
10. Is disgust shown by the lower lip being turned down, the upper lip slightly raised, with a sudden expiration, something like incipient vomiting, or like something spit out of the mouth?

(Continued)

Table 2.1 (Continued)

11. Is extreme fear expressed in the same general manner as with Europeans?
12. Is laughter ever carried to such an extreme as to bring tears to the eyes?
13. When a man wishes to show that he cannot prevent something being done, or cannot himself do something, does he shrug his shoulders, turn inwards his elbows, extend outwards his hands and open the palms; with the eyebrows raised?
14. Do the children when sulky, pout or greatly protrude the lips?
15. Can guilty, or sly or jealous expressions be recognized? Though as I know not how these can be defined.
16. Is the head nodded vertically in affirmation, and shrunken laterally in negation?

the Malay archipelago, people living across India, Africa and Native American Indians, reporting remarkable similarities across cultures (Darwin, 1872). These keen observations and careful description, which are detailed in full by Darwin, highlight the remarkable commonalities across different nationalities and formed the basis of claims that basic emotions are innate and universal (Darwin, 1872).

Assessment methods

How might such observations influence the current widespread use of tests of emotion recognition? Is the simple translation of verbal labels adequate? Or does expression and recognition of non-verbal facial emotional expressions vary across cultures?

Emotion perception

Subsequent research, including seminal research by Paul Ekman (Ekman, 1973; Ekman et al., 1971b, 1986) largely confirmed the existence of emotions that are preserved across cultures. Evidence for the universality of emotional expressions in humans subsequently arose from seminal work (Ekman et al., 1971a; Izard, 1971) on cross–cultural comparisons of emotional expressions. The conclusion was that across cultures, including pre-literate cultures, people were consistent in the manner in which they expressed basic emotions of anger, fear, disgust, sadness, happiness and surprise. This cross–cultural consistency is taken as evidence for the "hard-wired" nature of emotional expression. Based on this assumption, many facial emotion perception tests have disregarded the potential influence of race, with Caucasian stimuli widely used across countries.

However, the existence of prototypical expressions which are maintained across cultures does not adequately convey the full story. Using computer simulations, Jack and colleagues (Jack et al., 2012) demonstrated that Eastern Asian individuals do not produce these emotion categories as discretely as do Western Caucasians and that the eye region conveys greater information than the mouth (vice versa for Western Caucasians). There is also, obviously, a great variety of emotions beyond the basic six that are expressed and observed in human inter-actions. These too differ in terms of salience across cultures, e.g., shame, pride and guilt may play a particular role in Eastern cultures (Bedford et al., 2003; Li et al., 2004; Tracy et al., 2004). Other social emotions can be reliably identified (Rosenberg et al., 2016) although the cultural variation of these is probably much greater than for the basic six.

Indeed, studies have demonstrated that the race and/or ethnicity of the stim-uli can influence both behavioural performance as well as the results of neuro-imaging studies (Elfenbein et al., 2002; Lieberman et al., 2005; Phelps et al., 2000; Tottenham et al., 2009). A meta-analysis was conducted that included 97 separate studies of more than 22,000 participants and examined emotion recog-nition across cultures (Elfenbein et al., 2002). The most common study design was where the same stimulus set was presented to participants from the same or different culture and performance was compared across groups. A smaller num-ber of studies used a balanced design where both groups responded to stimuli from both cultural backgrounds. For the vast majority of studies, decoding of prototypical emotional expressions (e.g., happiness, anger) was above chance (Elfenbein et al., 2002). Importantly, however, recognition of expressions from one's own national, ethnic or regional group was higher than expression from another cultural background, demonstrating an in-group advantage (Elfenbein et al., 2002). Not only that, but brain activation in response to emotional faces differs with respect to the viewer's cultural background and that of the target face (Brooks et al., 2019; Lieberman et al., 2005). This variability suggests that neural processes underpinning emotion processing are not innately assigned. Rather, top-down, learned conceptual knowledge about emotions guides and influences bottom-up perceptual processing (Lindquist et al., 2012). Such cul-tural differences call into question the use of standardised tests adapted from one culture for use in another to identify neural substrates of social cognition.

For this reason, stimulus sets which have adequate race representation are important. The most commonly employed facial emotion perception test in research publications is the Ekman and Friesen stimuli (Ekman & Freisen, 1976; Young et al., 2002). These include 10 models (six female and four male) displaying the six basic emotions as well as a neutral expression. Of relevance here, all the models have a Caucasian appearance. Some attempts have been made to redress this lack of race representation in facial emotional stimuli. For example, the Japanese and Caucasian Facial Expressions of Emotion (JACFEE) (Matsumoto et al., 1988) were developed to examine cultural differences in emotion recognition. The JACFEE consists of 56 colour photographs of 56 different individuals, with each portraying one of seven emotions (the six basic emotions plus contempt). It includes 28 male and 28 female models, with equal numbers of Caucasian and Japanese individuals. Another widely used stimulus set is the NimStim (Tottenham et al., 2009). The NimStim Set of Facial Expressions includes 672 images of naturally posed photographs by 43 professional actors. The models are racially diverse and include 10 African, 6 Asian, 25 European and 2 Latino-American models. The expressions include happy, sad, angry, fearful, surprised, disgusted, neutral and calm with either an open or closed mouth. Notably, the stimuli are freely available. However, while widely used, validity data are lacking.

Other stimulus sets which have non-Caucasian models include Mandal's set, which includes Indian models (Mandal, 1987), the Montreal Set of Facial Displays of Emotion, which includes black and white photos of Chinese, French-Canadian White and sub-Saharan African models portraying anger, disgust, fear, happiness, sadness and shame (Beaupré et al., 2000), and Wang and Markham's Chinese facial expressions of emotion (Wang et al., 1999). The Emotion Recognition Test by Kessels and colleagues (Kessels et al., 2014; Montagne et al., 2007) includes Caucasian models, but the response labels are available in Dutch, German, French, English, Spanish, Finnish, Italian, Russian, Greek, Portuguese, Lithuanian and Turkish. Thus, while the availability of some stimuli with improved race representation is encouraging, information about psychometric properties and normative data are mostly lacking. Additional research is needed in order to develop stimulus sets that are suitable for clinical settings in CALD populations.

Theory of mind

As outlined above, tasks to assess theory of mind are diverse. Some of the most commonly used tasks include the Reading the Mind in the Eyes Test, cartoons, faux pas detection and classic false-belief tasks. Unsurprisingly, culture appears to have a substantial impact on various tests of theory of mind, at both the behavioural and neural levels. This is clearly seen in a study of decoding mental states on the Reading the Mind in the Eyes test. A small fMRI study including 14 white American young healthy participants and 14 Japanese young healthy participants completed the original and a Japanese version of the Reading the Mind in the Eyes test (Adams Jr et al., 2010). To develop the test, the verbal labels were back-translated from English to Japanese. Then, images of "Asian eyes" were gathered from internet and magazine sources. A pilot study was conducted to identify stimuli that were reliably selected to match the target label by at least 5/9 Japanese students. The behavioural results confirmed an interaction between task and cultural background, with Japanese participants performing better on the Japanese task and vice versa, although both groups exceeded 60% accuracy on both tests (chance = 25%). The fMRI results found common brain regions, including the *bilateral superior temporal sulcus, fusiform, middle* and *inferior frontal gyrus* and *the temporal pole*, were activated in both groups. Notably, however, greater activation was observed in the *bilateral superior temporal sulcus* in the same culture condition than in the other culture condition. What does this mean clinically? While it is reassuring that tasks that have been adapted to use different stimuli activate similar brain regions, there are clear differences both at the behavioural and neural level when completing tasks using stimuli from one's own culture compared to another culture. This likely also extends to performance in the real world.

Another approach is to use cartoons to assess understanding of others' mental states. One popular example of this is the use of cartoons that dissociate between physical (slapstick) and theory of mind (mentalising) jokes (Corcoran et al., 1997; Happé et al., 1999). Individuals with impairments in theory of mind find the physical jokes funny, but do not understand the items which require understanding of another person's mental state. This raises the issue of whether humour is consistent across cultures. While review of this issue is beyond the scope of this chapter, anecdotal reports suggest that despite being largely non-verbal stimuli, the use of cartoons may be unsuitable in some cultures. Thus, validation of the stimuli in the cultural group of interest is needed before abnormal performance on such tasks can be considered indicative of impairment in clinical populations.

False belief tasks have also been used to assess theory of mind. One of the most common examples is the "unexpected transfer" test; a variation on the Sally-Ann test. Here, a short scenario is shown during which an object is moved from one location to another while the protagonist is out of the room. In order to successfully demonstrate theory of mind on the test, the individual must inhibit their knowledge about the new location of the object and indicate that the protagonist will expect the object to remain in the original location. Cross-cultural studies using these tasks in clinical populations are scant. But evidence from developmental psychology suggests that interpretation of these scenarios across cultures may differ (Kobayashi Frank et al., 2009). For example, Japanese children appear to show differences in reasoning about others, with explanations tending to be attributed to behavioural or situational cues rather than mental states. Specifically, whereas Western children tend to use personal justifications e.g., "he wanted the toy", Japanese children tended to refer to social rules e.g., "he said to wait there". While these studies were conducted with children, it suggests there may be qualitative differences in how individuals perform false-belief tasks across cultures.

Attempts have also been made to translate dynamic test stimuli, such as TASIT (Westerhof-Evers et al., 2014). This is obviously more resource heavy as it requires verbal content to be translated, new video stimuli to be developed, as well as ensuring that the stimuli hold their intended meaning once translated. The Dutch version of TASIT has successfully been developed, suggesting that this is feasible, at least for other Western cultures. Whether complex social interactions such as sarcasm are suitable to be applied in other cultural groups (e.g., Asian cultures) is an important avenue for future research.

Clinical presentation – variation across cultures?

A second important question is whether clinical disorders manifest in a qualitatively different way across cultures. Impaired social cognition leads to inability in the perception of others' emotions, understanding others' mental states and behaving accordingly with these judgements. We have already discussed how social perception may vary across cultures. In addition, knowledge of appropriate social behaviour, referred to as social norms, is highly context and culture-dependent. For example, while some cultures tolerate swearing during an interview or entering a bank barefoot, in other cultures such behaviours represent a clear break of social rules. Differences in socially appropriate behaviour can also be extended to the assessment setting. Is it appropriate to greet the clinician by their first name, or should they be greeted as "Doctor" or "Professor"? Should one wear a suit to the appointment, or are shorts and a T-shirt appropriate? In the clinical setting, social norms are often assessed through clinical observation during the initial interview. If in the dominant culture, the use of formal titles and attire is considered appropriate, then a client who arrives in casual wear and uses the clinician's first name might be seen as an indicator of socially inappropriate behaviour, despite this behaviour being entirely appropriate in a different cultural context

In an attempt to formalise the assessment of social norms, tests have been developed where the client is asked to detect whether the behaviour is appropriate or not. For example, the Social Norms Questionnaire (Kramer et al., 2014; Possin et al., 2013) asks people to determine whether it is appropriate to "cry during a movie in a theatre" or "talk out loud during a movie in a theatre". However, while cross-cultural studies are lacking, even demographics appear to influence performance. For example, fewer men than women recognised that it is inappropriate to ask a co-worker their age, while women, on the whole, scored higher than men, suggesting that some social norms do not apply equally across genders (Ganguli et al., 2018). Older adults were also less likely to report items as inappropriate than younger adults, although the authors speculated this may be due to cohort effects rather than age-related decline (Ganguli et al., 2018). From these findings, it is plausible to assume that people from different cultural backgrounds would also perform differently on this questionnaire. More conservative cultures may identify more behaviours as inappropriate than more liberal countries. Some items may also be culturally specific (e.g., "Is it appropriate to blow your nose in public?"). For both clinical observation and formal assessment of social norms, it is important that clinicians are aware of the potential influence of the dominant culture when interpreting clients' behaviour. Clinicians should be aware of these cultural issues and consider how behavioural features and/or scores may be influenced by the individual's cultural background before ascribing abnormal performance to impaired social cognition.

In the research setting, exclusion criteria often include insufficient fluency in the dominant (testing) language. While most cross-cultural studies have employed a design where performance is compared across groups of people from different countries (usually recruited at the same site), these types of designs are susceptible to confounds. For example, how much exposure the groups have had to the dominant culture and how long they have been living in the study country. Recent calls have identified the need for a more nuanced approach, which is both inclusive and representative (Barrett, 2020). This requires studies to be conducted on a larger scale and with more sophisticated study designs.

One such example is an unpublished multisite study that included 587 healthy adult participants from 12 countries (Quesque et al., preprint doi:10.31234/ osf.io/tg2ay). All participants completed the Ekman faces test from the Facial Expressions of Emotion: Stimulus Test (FEEST) (Young et al., 2002) and the Faux Pas test (Baron-Cohen et al., 1999). They found that 20% of the variation in emotion recognition performance could be attributed to the effect of country. This variance was observed after controlling for the influence of sex, age and education. For emotion recognition, while the overall pattern of responses was largely similar across countries, there were some notable exceptions. For example, fear was misclassified as surprise 25% of the time in Germany but 50% of the time in Canada, while for neutral, Italians misclassified this expression as sadness 21% of the time, but this error was never observed in the Chinese participants. For the Faux Pas test, 24% of performance could be accounted for by country. Notably, this effect appeared to be independent of the language the test was conducted in. Studies such as this highlight the considerable potential influence of culture on test performance.

The influence of these cultural variations in the clinic is likely to be important, particularly in situations where international diagnostic criteria are used as well as for multisite clinical trials. For example, the diagnostic criteria for behavioural-variant frontotemporal dementia include behavioural disinhibition, apathy, loss of sympathy or empathy, perseverative or stereotyped behaviour, dietary changes, and/or executive dysfunction (Rascovsky et al., 2011). While the sensitivity of these criteria is high (0.85) in Westernised countries (USA, Australia, Europe), a landmark study indicated that these criteria have much lower sensitivity in the early disease stage in an Indian population (Ghosh et al., 2013). These findings suggest that the manifestation of frontotemporal dementia may differ across cultures, which is further compounded by potential variation in sensitivity and specificity of tests across cultures. It can be thus extrapolated that other syndromes with hallmark social cognition impairment may also have variable sensitivity and specificity across cultures.

Comments on cross-cultural research in a multicultural society – cultural and linguistic diversity (CALD) in the clinical setting

In the clinical setting, people from CALD backgrounds may perform differently from non-CALD individuals because of a lack of in-group advantage. The effect of this is two-fold. Firstly, it is possible that this absence of in-group advantage may mean these tests are more sensitive to subtle declines in CALD individuals.

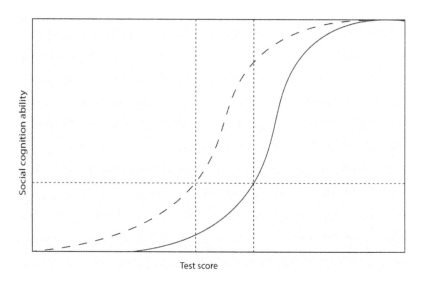

Figure 2.1 Performance on social cognition tests according to cultural background

For example, a person with mild social cognition impairment from a cultur-ally different background may perform worse than a person with a culturally similar background when tested on a task with Western stimuli. However, this increase in sensitivity has the trade-off of a reduction in specificity, whereby peo-ple with CALD backgrounds may perform below expectations, due to differ-ences in cultural background despite not having any social cognition impairment (see Box 2.1: Case and Figure 2.1). Importantly, the overall profile on tests, i.e., the relative scores across emotions, is likely to be the same. That is, an individual incorrectly perceiving happy faces as angry, is unlikely to be due to cultural effects.

Box 2.1   Case 1: Mr E: Influence of cultural and linguistic diversity (CALD) on social cognitive test performance

History:

Mr E was born in Egypt in 1950. He emigrated to Australia aged 39 years and worked as a banker. He held a bachelor of commerce and a bachelor of economics, both attained in Egypt. Me E self-reported irritability, low mood and a feeling he was underperforming at work, leading to him leaving the workforce and applying for a disability pension.

Presentation:

He was polite and cooperative and showed good effort during the assessment, part of which was conducted with the aid of an Arabic translator. His premorbid intelligence was estimated to be high average to superior. On cognitive testing, he performed below expectations in mental arithmetic, working memory, fluency, naming, general knowledge and processing speed. Comprehension and word-finding were impaired, and he showed a degree of surface dyslexia. Widening of the interhemispheric fissure between the frontal lobes was seen on MRI. On Ekman's faces, he scored 45/60 (z = -1.17); on TASIT Part 1 he scored 19/24 (z = -2.75) and on TASIT Part 2 he scored 47/60 (z = -1.63). A self-report version of the Cambridge Behavioural Inventory suggested difficulty with social interactions (frequent tactless or suggestive remarks and impulsive behaviour) as well as apathy and rigid thinking; however, his wife's reports did not concur.

Opinion:

An initial review of this case would appear to be consistent with frontotemporal dementia. There is evidence of impaired working memory, fluency and surface dyslexia, borderline to impaired social cognition, changes in social behaviour and apparent frontal lobe atrophy on MRI. However, a number of caveats should be noted. Most of the cognitive impairment was present on language-based tests. While an interpreter assisted with some testing, scores are not directly comparable to normative data from a non-CALD population. Furthermore, the reductions on social cognition tests may reflect the absence of an in-group advantage. This fits with his wife's report of no change in social behaviour. While the MRI findings are unusual, in the absence of a repeat scan, this may simply reflect individual variability.

Summary:

This high-functioning man self-reported concerns in his ability to perform at work and with his behaviour. His performance on formal testing was below expectations based on his estimated premorbid functioning. However, his CALD background likely accounts for this reduced performance. His intact insight and his wife's report that his behaviour has not changed, suggest that impaired social cognition is unlikely. Repeat testing 12 months later showed no decline in performance on testing.

Table 2.2 Recommendations for clinical assessment of culturally and linguistically diverse individuals

Test type	Recommendation
Emotion Perception	❖ Select non-verbal over verbal stimuli ❖ Check understanding of response terms if the client speaks a language different from the test materials; offer translated response options ❖ Where available, select stimuli from the clients' cultural background or with culturally diverse stimuli e.g., JACFEE; NimStim ❖ Where possible, use normative data that reflect the client's cultural background
Theory of Mind	❖ Select non-verbal tasks or tasks with minimal language requirements ❖ Preference tasks that have a "non-social" control task ❖ Where possible, use normative data that reflect the client's cultural background
Questionnaires	❖ Where possible, employ both self- and informant-reported versions ❖ Focus on change from premorbid behaviour rather than comparison with "typical" behaviour

In the research setting, people who are not fluent in English, or who have grown up in the non-dominant culture, are typically excluded from participation in studies. While this approach has benefits methodologically as it enables researchers to parse out how performance is affected by the neurological disorder from the influence of culture, it leaves clinicians in a relatively uninformed position when faced with a CALD client. In the case of assessment of social cognition, some tests are arguably more appropriate than others. As is true for other cognitive domains, non-verbal tests are less susceptible to cultural influence than verbal tests. Hence, tests such as facial emotion recognition, where the clinician can confirm the client understands the meaning of basic emotion labels, may be less influenced by culture than more complex multimodal stimuli. Involving family members or a knowledgeable informant is also essential to determine whether behaviours are out of character and represent a change from what is typical for the individual.

Conclusions

The abilities which make up social cognition are remarkably complex and interact with other cognitive abilities such as language, memory, attention and processing speed. Hence, tests that can parse out specific components of social cognition are challenging to develop. Clinical research in this field has made considerable headway in developing and modifying tasks from developmental psychology and social psychology, and employing techniques from neuroscience and computer science to improve our understanding of these complex behaviours. Tasks that take into account cognitive requirements and maximise ecological validity will help to further advance our knowledge in this domain. In particular, implicit tasks, tasks employing a second-person approach and tasks using virtual reality appear promising in offering new insights into social cognition. Neuroimaging has undoubtedly been essential in developing understanding of the neurobiological basis of social cognition. Savvy task design and selection of appropriate neuroimaging techniques and analyses are essential in order for results to be meaningful. Finally, recognition that social cognition varies across cultures is important. While assessing social cognition in CALD groups is challenging, it is an important issue both clinically and theoretically. Examination of differences and commonalities across cultures is a rich field of research, with exciting new findings undoubtedly likely to emerge. As this chapter demonstrates, social cognition is an active and rich field, with many important questions still to be explored.

References

Abell, F., Happé, F., & Frith, U. (2000). Do triangles play tricks? Attribution of mental states to animated shapes in normal and abnormal development. *Cognitive Development, 15*(1), 1–16.

Adams Jr, R., Rule, N., Franklin Jr, R., Wang, E., Stevenson, M., Yoshikawa, S., . . . Ambady, N. (2010). Cross-cultural reading the mind in the eyes: An fMRI investigation. *Journal of Cognitive Neuroscience, 22*(1), 97–108.

Adolphs, R., Damasio, & Tranel. (2002). Neural systems for recognition of emotional prosody: A 3-D lesion study. *Emotion, 2*(1), 23.

Adolphs, R., Tranel, D., Damasio, H., & Damasio, A. (1994). Impaired recognition of emotion in facial expressions following bilateral damage to the human amygdala. *Nature, 372*(6507), 669–672.

Adolphs, R., Tranel, D., Damasio, H., & Damasio, A. (1995). Fear and the human amygdala. *The Journal of Neuroscience, 15*(9), 5879–5891.

Adolphs, R. (1999). Social cognition and the human brain. *Trends in Cognitive Sciences, 3*(12), 469–479.

Adolphs, R. (2009). The social brain: Neural basis of social knowledge. *Annual Review of Psychology, 60*, 693–716.

Albiero, P., Matricardi, G., Speltri, D., & Toso, D. (2009). The assessment of empathy in adolescence: A contribution to the Italian validation of the "Basic Empathy Scale". *Journal of Adolescence, 32*(2), 393–408.

Anastácio, S., Vagos, P., Nobre-Lima, L., Rijo, D., & Jolliffe, D. (2016). The Portuguese version of the basic empathy scale (BES): Dimensionality and measurement invariance in a community adolescent sample. *European Journal of Developmental Psychology, 13*(5), 614–623.

Ashburner, J., & Friston, K. (2000). Voxel-based morphometry – the methods. *Neuroimage, 11*, 805–821.

Aviezer, H., Hassin, R. R., Ryan, J., Grady, C., Susskind, J., Anderson, A., . . . Bentin, S. (2008). Angry, disgusted, or afraid?: Studies on the malleability of emotion perception. *Psychological Science, 19*(7), 724–732.

Aviezer, H., Trope, Y., & Todorov, A. (2012). Body cues, not facial expressions, discriminate between intense positive and negative emotions. *Science, 338*(6111), 1225–1229.

Baron-Cohen, S., Leslie, A. M., & Frith, U. (1985). Does the autistic child have a "theory of mind"? *Cognition, 21*(1), 37–46.

Baron-Cohen, S., O'Riordan, M., Stone, V., Jones, R., & Plaisted, K. (1999). Recognition of Faux Pas by normally developing children and children with Asperger syndrome or high-functioning autism. *Journal of Autism and Developmental Disorders, 29*(5), 407–418.

Baron-Cohen, S., Wheelwright, S., Hill, J., Raste, Y., & Plumb, I. (2001). The "reading the mind in the eyes" test revised version: A study with normal adults, and adults with Asperger syndrome or high-functioning autism. *The Journal of Child Psychology and Psychiatry and Allied Disciplines, 42*(2), 241–251.

Barrett, H. (2020). Towards a cognitive science of the human: Cross-cultural approaches and their urgency. *Trends in Cognitive Sciences, 24*(8), 620–638.

Beaupré, Cheung, & Hess. (2000). *The Montreal set of Facial Displays of Emotion.* Montreal, Quebec, Canada. http://www.psychophysiolab.com/msfde/terms.php

Bedford, O., & Hwang, K. (2003). Guilt and shame in Chinese culture: A cross-cultural framework from the perspective of morality and identity. *Journal for the Theory of Social Behaviour, 33,* 127–144.

Bellucci, G., Chernyak, S. V., Goodyear, K., Eickhoff, S. B., & Krueger, F. (2017). Neural signatures of trust in reciprocity: A coordinate-based meta-analysis. *Human Brain Mapping, 38*(3), 1233–1248.

Bensalah, L., Stefaniak, N., Carre, A., & Besche-Richard, C. (2016). The basic empathy scale adapted to French middle childhood: Structure and development of empathy. *Behavior Research Methods, 48*(4), 1410–1420.

Bentin, S., Allison, T., Puce, A., Perez, E., & McCarthy, G. (1996). Electrophysiological studies of face perception in humans. *Journal of Cognitive Neuroscience, 8*(6), 551–565.

Bramham, J., Morris, R., Hornak, J., Bullock, P., & Polkey, C. (2009). Social and emotional functioning following bilateral and unilateral neurosurgical prefrontal cortex lesions. *Journal of Neuropsychology, 3*(1), 125–143.

Broca, P. (1878). Anatomie comparée des circonvolutions cérébrales: Le grand lobe limbique et la scissure limbique dans la serie des mammifères. *Revue Anthropologique, 1,* 385–498.

Brooks, J, Chikazoe, J. Sadato, N. & Freeman, J. (2019). The neural representation of facial-emotion categories reflects conceptual structure. *PNAS Proceedings of the National Academy of Sciences of the United States of America, 116*(32), 15861–15870.

Buchanan, T., Lutz, K., Mirzazade, S., Specht, K., Jon Shah, N., Zilles, K., & Jancke, L. (2000). Recognition of emotional prosody and verbal components of spoken language: An fMRI study. *Cognitive Brain Research, 9*(3), 227–238.

Calder, A., Rowland, D., Young, A., Nimmo-Smith, I., Keane, J., & Perrett, D. (2000). Caricaturing facial expressions. *Cognition, 76*(2), 105–146.

Calder, A., Young, A., Perrett, D., Etcoff, N., & Rowland, D. (1996). Categorical perception of morphed facial expressions. *Visual Cognition, 3*(2), 81–117.

Calder, A., Young, A., Rowland, D., & Perrett, D. (1997). (1997). Computer-enhanced emotion in facial expressions. *Proceedings of the Royal Society London B, 264,* 919–925.

Camozzato, A., Kochhann, R., Simeoni, C., Konrath, C., Franz, A., Carvalho, A., & Chaves, M. L. (2008). Reliability of the Brazilian Portuguese version of the neuropsychiatric inventory (NPI) for patients with Alzheimer's disease and their caregivers. *International Psychogeriatrics, 20*(2), 383–393.

Cannon, W. (1927). The James-Lange theory of emotions: A critical examination and an alternative theory. *The American Journal of Psychology, 39*(1/4), 106–124.

Caruana, N., Brock, J., & Woolgar, A. (2015). A frontotemporoparietal network common to initiating and responding to joint attention bids. *Neuroimage, 108*, 34–46.

Caruana, N., Stieglitz Ham, H., Brock, J., Woolgar, A., Kloth, N., Palermo, R., & McArthur, G. (2018). Joint attention difficulties in autistic adults: An interactive eye-tracking study. *Autism, 22*(4), 502–512.

Choi, S., Na, D., Kwon, H., Yoon, S., Jeong, J., & Ha, C. (2000). The Korean version of the neuropsychiatric inventory: A scoring tool for neuropsychiatric disturbance in dementia patients. *Journal of Korean Medical Science, 15*(6), 609–615.

Coan, J., Schaefer, H., & Davidson, R. (2006). Lending a hand: Social regulation of the neural response to threat. *Psychological Science, 17*(12), 1032–1039.

Corcoran, R., Cahill, C., & Frith, C. (1997). The appreciation of visual jokes in people with schizophrenia: A study of 'mentalizing' ability. *Schizophrenia Research, 24*(3), 319–327.

Costafreda, S., Brammer, M., David, A., & Fu, C. (2008). Predictors of amygdala activation during the processing of emotional stimuli: A meta-analysis of 385 PET and fMRI studies. *Brain Research Reviews, 58*(1), 57–70.

Cummings, J., Mega, M., Gray, K., Rosenberg-Thompson, S., Carusi, D., & Gornbein, J. (1994). The neuropsychiatric inventory comprehensive assessment of psychopathology in dementia. *Neurology, 44*(12), 2308–2308.

Damasio, H., Grabowski, T., Frank, R., Galaburda, A., & Damasio, A. (1994). The return of Phineas Gage: Clues about the brain from the skull of a famous patient. *Science, 264*(5162), 1102.

Darwin, C. (1872). *The Expression of the Emotions in Man and Animals.* London: John Murray.

De Corte, K., Buysse, A., Verhofstadt, L., Roeyers, H., Ponnet, K., & Davis, M. (2007). Measuring empathic tendencies: Reliability and validity of the Dutch version of the interpersonal reactivity index. *Psychologica Belgica, 47*(4), 235–260.

Dennett, H., McKone, E., Tavashmi, R., Hall, A., Pidcock, M., Edwards, M., & Duchaine, B. (2012). The Cambridge car memory test: A task matched in format to the Cambridge face memory test, with norms, reliability, sex differences, dissociations from face memory, and expertise effects. *Behavior Research Methods, 44*(2), 587–605.

de Sousa, A., McDonald, S., & Rushby, J. (2012). Changes in emotional empathy, affective responsivity, and behavior following severe traumatic brain injury. *Journal of Clinical and Experimental Neuropsychology, 34*(6), 606–623.

de Sousa, A., McDonald, S., Rushby, J., Li, S., Dimoska, A., & James, C. (2011). Understanding deficits in empathy after traumatic brain injury: The role of affective responsivity. *Cortex, 47*(5), 526–535.

Didehbani, N., Allen, T., Kandalaft, M., Krawczyk, D., & Chapman, S. (2016). Virtual reality social cognition training for children with high functioning autism. *Computers in Human Behavior, 62*, 703–711.

Dunbar, R. (1998). The social brain hypothesis. *Brain, 9*(10), 178–190.

Ekman, P., & Friesen, W. (1971a). Constants across culture in the face and emotion. *Journal of Personality and Social Psychology, 17*, 124–129.

Ekman, P. & Friesen, W. (1971b). Constants across cultures in the face and emotion. *Journal of Personality and Social Psychology, 17*(2), 124.

Ekman, P., & Friesen, W. (1986). A new pancultural facial expression of emotion. *Motivation Emotion, 10*, 159–168.

Ekman, P. (1973). Cross-cultural studies of facial expression. *Darwin and Facial Expression: A Century of Research in Review, 169222*, 1.

Ekman, P., & Friesen, W. (1976). *Pictures of Facial Affect*. Palo Alto, CA: Consulting Psychologists Press.

Elfenbein, H., & Ambady, N. (2002). On the universality and cultural specificity of emotion recognition: A meta-analysis. *Psychological Bulletin, 128*(2), 203.

Fareri, D., Gabard-Durnam, L., Goff, B., Flannery, F., Gee, D., Lumian, D., . . . Tottenham, N. (2017). Altered ventral striatal-medial prefrontal cortex resting-state connectivity mediates adolescent social problems after early institutional care. *Development and Psychopathology, 29*(5), 1865–1876.

Feinstein, J., Khalsa, S., Salomons, T., Prkachin, K., Frey-Law, L., Lee, J., . . . Rudrauf, D. (2016). Preserved emotional awareness of pain in a patient with extensive bilateral damage to the insula, anterior cingulate, and amygdala. *Brain Structure and Function, 221*(3), 1499–1511.

Fischl, B. (2012). FreeSurfer. *Neuroimage, 62*(2), 774–781.

Fox, J., Abram, S., Reilly, J., Eack, S., Goldman, M., Csernansky, J., . . . Smith, M. (2017). Default mode functional connectivity is associated with social functioning in schizophrenia. *Journal of Abnormal Psychology, 126*(4), 392–405.

Frith, C., & Frith, U. (2005). Theory of mind. *Current Biology, 15*(17), R644–R646.

Ganguli, M., Sun, Z., McDade, E., Snitz, B., Hughes, T., Jacobsen, E., & Chang, C.-C. (2018). That's inappropriate! Social norms in an older population-based cohort. *Alzheimer Disease and Associated Disorders, 32*(2), 150.

Ghosh, A., Dutt, A., Ghosh, M., Bhargava, P., & Rao, S. (2013). Using the revised diagnostic criteria for frontotemporal dementia in India: Evidence of an advanced and florid disease. *PloS One, 8*(4), e60999.

Gilet, A.-L., Mella, N., Studer, J., Grühn, D., & Labouvie-Vief, G. (2013). Assessing dispositional empathy in adults: A French validation of the interpersonal reactivity index (IRI). *Canadian Journal of Behavioural Science/Revue canadienne des sciences du comportement, 45*(1), 42.

Grandjean, D., Sander, D., Pourtois, G., Schwartz, S., Seghier, M., Scherer, K., & Vuilleumier, P. (2005). The voices of wrath: Brain responses to angry prosody in meaningless speech. *Nature Neuroscience, 8*(2), 145–146.

Gurven, M. (2018). Broadening horizons: Sample diversity and socioecological theory are essential to the future of psychological science. *Proceedings of the National Academy of Sciences, 115*(45), 11420–11427.

Happé, F., Brownell, H., & Winner, E. (1999). Acquired 'theory of mind' impairments following stroke. *Cognition, 70*(3), 211–240.

Hassin, R., Aviezer, H., & Bentin, S. (2013). Inherently ambiguous: Facial expressions of emotions, in context. *Emotion Review, 5*(1), 60–65.

Heynen, E., Van der Helm, G., Stams, G., & Korebrits, A. (2016). Measuring empathy in a German youth prison: A validation of the German version of the basic empathy scale (BES) in a sample of incarcerated juvenile offenders. *Journal of Forensic Psychology Practice, 16*(5), 336–346.

Hirono, N., Mori, E., Ikejiri, Y., Imamura, T., Shimomura, T., Hashimoto, M., . . . Ikeda, M. (1997). Japanese version of the neuropsychiatric inventory – a scoring system for neuropsychiatric disturbance in dementia patients. *No to Shinkei= Brain and Nerve, 49*(3), 266–271.

Holper, L., Scholkmann, F., & Wolf, M. (2012). Between-brain connectivity during imitation measured by fNIRS. *Neuroimage, 63*(1), 212–222.

Honan, C., McDonald, S., Sufani, C., Hine, D., & Kumfor, F. (2016). The awareness of social inference test: Development of a shortened version for use in adults with acquired brain injury. *The Clinical Neuropsychologist, 30*(2), 243–264.

Izard, C. (1971). *The Face of Emotion* (Vol. xii). New York: Appleton-Century-Crofts.

Jack, R., Garrod, O., Yu, H., Caldara, R., & Schyns, P. (2012). Facial expressions of emotion are not culturally universal. *Proceedings of the National Academy of Sciences, 109*(19), 7241–7244.

James, H. (1884). What is an emotion? *Mind, 9*(34), 188–205.

Kandalaft, M., Didehbani, N., Krawczyk, D., Allen, T., & Chapman, S. (2013). Virtual reality social cognition training for young adults with high-functioning autism. *Journal of Autism and Developmental Disorders, 43*(1), 34–44.

Kang, I., Kee, S.-W., Kim, S.-E., Jeong, B.-S., Hwang, J.-H., Song, J.-E., & Kim, J.-W. (2009). Reliability and validity of the Korean-version of interpersonal reactivity index. *Journal of Korean Neuropsychiatric Association, 48*(5), 352–358.

Kat, M., De Jonghe, J., Aalten, P., Kalisvaart, C., Dröes, R.-M., & Verhey, F. (2002). Neuropsychiatric symptoms of dementia: Psychometric aspects of the Dutch version of the neuropsychiatric inventory (NPI). *Tijdschift voor Gerontologie en Geriatrie, 33*(4), 150–155.

Kessels, R., Montagne, B., Hendriks, A., Perrett, D., & de Haan, E. (2014). Assessment of perception of morphed facial expressions using the emotion recognition task: Normative data from healthy participants aged 8–75. *Journal of Neuropsychology, 8*(1), 75–93.

Kluver, H., & Bucy, P. (1937). "Psychic blindness" and other symptoms following temporal lobectomy. *American Journal of Physiology, 119*, 254–284.

Kobayashi Frank, C., & Temple, E. (2009). Cultural effects on the neural basis of theory of mind. *Progress in Brain Research, 178*, 213–223

Kober, H., Feldman, L., Joseph, J., Bliss-Moreau, E., Lindquist, K., & Wagera, T. (2008). Functional grouping and cortical – subcortical interactions in emotion: A meta-analysis of neuroimaging studies. *NeuroImage, 42*, 998–1031.

Kramer, J., Mungas, D., Possin, K., Rankin, K., Boxer, A., Rosen, H., . . . Widmeyer, M. (2014). NIH EXAMINER: Conceptualization and development of an executive function battery. *Journal of the International Neuropsychological Society: JINS, 20*(1), 11.

Kumfor, F., Hazelton, J., De Winter, F., Cleret de Langavant, L., & Van den Stock, J. (2017). Clinical studies of social neuroscience: A lesion model approach. In A. Ibanez, L. Sedeno, & A. M. Garcia (Eds.), *Neuroscience and Social Science: The Missing Link*. New York: Springer.

Kumfor, F., Hazelton, J., Rushby, J., Hodges, J., & Piguet, O. (2019). Facial expressiveness and physiological arousal in frontotemporal dementia: Phenotypic clinical profiles and neural correlates. *Cognitive, Affective, & Behavioral Neuroscience, 19*(1), 197–210.

Kumfor, F., Honan, C., McDonald, S., Hazelton, J., Hodges, J., & Piguet, O. (2017). Assessing the "social brain" in dementia: Applying TASIT-S. *Cortex, 93*, 166–177.

Kumfor, F., Ibanez, A., Hutchings, R., Hazelton, J., Hodges, J., & Piguet, O. (2018). Beyond the face: How context modulates emotion processing in frontotemporal dementia subtypes. *Brain*, doi:10.1093/brain/awy1002.

Kumfor, F., Sapey-Triomphe, L., Leyton, C., Burrell, J., Hodges, J., & Piguet, O. (2014). Degradation of emotion processing ability in corticobasal syndrome and Alzheimer's disease. *Brain, 137*(Pt 11), 3061–3072.

Kumfor, F., Tracy, L., Wei, G., Chen, Y., Dominguez, J., Whittle, S., . . . Kelly, M. (in press). Social and affective neuroscience: An Australian perspective. *Social Cognitive and Affective Neuroscience*.

Lee, H., Heller, A., van Reekum, C., Nelson, B., & Davidson, R. (2012). Amygdala – prefrontal coupling underlies individual differences in emotion regulation. *NeuroImage*, *62*(3), 1575–1581.

Leung, V., Lam, L., Chiu, H., Cummings, J., & Chen, Q. (2001). Validation study of the Chinese version of the neuropsychiatric inventory (CNPI). *International Journal of Geriatric Psychiatry*, *16*(8), 789–793.

Levinson, B. (1959). Traditional Jewish cultural values and performance on the Wechsler tests. *Journal of Educational Psychology*, *50*(4), 177.

Lhermitte, F. (1983). 'Utilization behaviour'and its relation to lesions of the frontal lobes. *Brain*, *106*(2), 237–255.

Lhermitte, F. (1986). Human autonomy and the frontal lobes. Part II: Patient behavior in complex and social situations: The "environmental dependency syndrome". *Annals of Neurology*, *19*(4), 335–343.

Li, J., Wang, L., & Fischer, K. (2004). The organisation of Chinese shame concepts? *Cognition and Emotion*, *18*(6), 767–797.

Lieberman, M., & Cunningham, W. (2009). Type I and Type II error concerns in fMRI research: Re-balancing the scale. *Social Cognitive and Affective Neuroscience*, *4*(4), 423–428.

Lieberman, M., Hariri, A., Jarcho, J., Eisenberger, N., & Bookheimer, S. (2005). An fMRI investigation of race-related amygdala activity in African-American and Caucasian-American individuals. *Nature Neuroscience*, *8*(6), 720–722.

Lindquist, K., Wager, T., Kober, H., Bliss-Moreau, E., & Barrett, L. (2012). The brain basis of emotion: A meta-analytic review. *Behavioral and Brain Sciences*, *35*(3), 121–143.

Lopes da Silva, F. (2013). EEG and MEG: Relevance to neuroscience. *Neuron*, *80*(5), 1112–1128.

Mandal, M. (1987). Decoding of facial emotions, in terms of expressiveness, by schizophrenics and depressives. *Psychiatry*, *50*(4), 371–376.

Matsumoto, D., & Ekman, P. (1988). *Japanese and Caucasian Facial Expressions of Emotion (JACFEE) and Neutral Faces (JACNeuF)*. San Francisco: San Francisco State University.

McDonald, S., Bornhofen, C., Shum, D., Long, E., Saunders, C., & Neulinger, K. (2006). Reliability and validity of the awareness of social inference test (TASIT): A clinical test of social perception. *Disability and Rehabilitation*, *28*(24), 1529–1542.

McDonald, S., Flanagan, S., Martin, I., & Saunders, C. (2004). The ecological validity of TASIT: A test of social perception. *Neuropsychological Rehabilitation*, *14*(3), 285–302.

McDonald, S., Flanagan, S., Rollins, J., & Kinch, J. (2003). TASIT: A new clinical tool for assessing social perception after traumatic brain injury. *The Journal of Head Trauma Rehabilitation*, *18*(3), 219.

McDonald, S., Saad, A., & James, C. (2011). Social dysdecorum following severe traumatic brain injury: Loss of implicit social knowledge or loss of control? *Journal of Clinical and Experimental Neuropsychology*, *33*(6), 619–630.

Mechelli, A., Price, C., Friston, C., & Ashburner, J. (2005). Voxel-based morphometry of the human brain: Methods and applications. *Current Medical Imaging Reviews 1*(2), 105–113.

Mendez, M., Joshi, A., & Jimenez, E. (2015). Virtual reality for the assessment of frontotemporal dementia, a feasibility study. *Disability and Rehabilation: Assistive Technology, 10*, 160–164.

Molenberghs, P., Johnson, H., Henry, J., & Mattingley, J. (2016). Understanding the minds of others: A neuroimaging meta-analysis. *Neuroscience and Biobehavioral Reviews*, *65*, 276–291.

Montagne, B., Kessels, R., De Haan, E., & Perrett, D. (2007). The emotion recognition task: A paradigm to measure the perception of facial emotional expressions at different intensities. *Perceptual and Motor Skills*, *104*(2), 589–598.

Montague, P. Berns, G., Cohen, J., McClure, S., Pagnoni, G., Dhamala, M., . . . Fisher, R. (2002). Hyperscanning: Simultaneous fMRI during linked social interactions. *Neurimage*, *16*(4), 1159–1164.

Noble, S., Scheinost, D., & Constable, R. (2020). Cluster failure or power failure? Evaluating sensitivity in cluster-level inference. *Neuroimage*, *209*, 116468.

Nosek, B., Hawkins, C., & Frazier, R. (2011). Implicit social cognition: From measures to mechanisms. *Trends in Cognitive Sciences*, *15*(4), 152–159.

Nozawa, T., Sasaki, Y., Sakaki, K., Yokoyama, R., & Kawashima, R. (2016). Interpersonal frontopolar neural synchronization in group communication: An exploration toward fNIRS hyperscanning of natural interactions. *Neuroimage*, *133*, 484–497.

Oakley, B., Brewer, R., Bird, G., & Catmur, C. (2016). Theory of mind is not theory of emotion: A cautionary note on the reading the mind in the eyes test. *Journal of Abnormal Psychology*, *125*(6), 818–823.

Olderbak, S., Wilhelm, O., Olaru, G., Geiger, M., Brenneman, M., & Roberts, R. (2015). A psychometric analysis of the reading the mind in the eyes test: Toward a brief form for research and applied settings. *Frontiers in Psychology*, *6*, 1503–1503.

Padmala, S., & Pessoa, L. (2008). Affective learning enhances visual detection and responses in primary visual cortex. *The Journal of Neuroscience*, *28*(24), 6202–6210.

Parsons, T., Gaggioli, A., & Riva, G. (2017). Virtual reality for research in social neuroscience. *Brain Science*, *7*(4), 42. doi:10.3390/brainsci7040042

Perry, R., Rosen, H., Kramer, J., Beer, J., Levenson, R., & Miller, B. (2001). Hemispheric dominance for emotions, empathy and social behaviour: Evidence from right and left handers with frontotemporal dementia. *Neurocase*, *7*(2), 145–160.

Phan, K., Wager, T., Taylor, S., & Liberzon, I. (2002). Functional neuroanatomy of emotion: A meta-analysis of emotion activation studies in PET and fMRI. *Neuroimage*, *16*(2), 331–348.

Phelps, E., O'Connor, K., Cunningham, W., Funayama, E., Gatenby, J., Gore, J., & Banaji, M. (2000). Performance on indirect measures of race evaluation predicts amygdala activation. *Journal of Cognitive Neuroscience*, *12*(5), 729–738.

Possin, K., Feigenbaum, D., Rankin, K., Smith, G., Boxer, A., Wood, K., . . . Kramer, J. (2013). Dissociable executive functions in behavioral variant frontotemporal and Alzheimer dementias. *Neurology*, *80*(24), 2180–2185.

Premack, D., & Woodruff, G. (1978). Does the chimpanzee have a theory of mind? *Behavioral and Brain Sciences*, *1*, 515–526.

Price, C., & Friston, K. (1997). The temporal dynamics of reading: A PET study. *Proceedings. Biological sciences*, *264*(1389), 1785–1791.

Quaresima, V., & Ferrari, M. (2019). Functional near-infrared spectroscopy (fNIRS) for assessing cerebral cortex function during human behavior in natural/social situations: A concise review. *Organizational Research Methods*, *22*(1), 46–68.

Quesque, F., Coutrot, A., Cox, S., Baez, S., Felipe, C., Hannah, M.-P., . . . Luciana, C. (preprint doi:10.31234/osf.io/tg2ay). Culture shapes our understanding of others' thoughts and emotions: An investigation across 12 countries. *PsyArXiv*. doi:10.31234/osf.io/tg2ay

Rascovsky, K., Hodges, J., Knopman, D., Mendez, M., Kramer, J., Neuhaus, J., . . . Miller, B. (2011). Sensitivity of revised diagnostic criteria for the behavioural variant of fronto-temporal dementia. *Brain, 134*(9), 2456–2477.

Redcay, E., & Schilbach, L. (2019). Using second-person neuroscience to elucidate the mechanisms of social interaction. *Nature Reviews Neuroscience, 20*(8), 495–505.

Rohrer, J., Sauter, D., Scott, S., Rossor, M., & Warren, J. (2010). Receptive prosody in nonfluent primary progressive aphasias. *Cortex, 48*(3), 308–316.

Rosenberg, H., McDonald, S., Rosenberg, J., & Westbrook, F. (2016). Amused, flirting or simply baffled? Is recognition of all emotions affected by traumatic brain injury? *Journal of Neuropsychology, 12*(2), 145–164.

Ross, E., Thompson, R., & Yenkosky, J. (1997). Lateralisation of affective prosody in brain and the callosal integration of hemispheric language functions. *Brain and Language, 56*(1), 27–54.

Rossion, B., Gauthier, I., Tarr, M., Despland, P., Bruyer, R., Linotte, S., & Crommelinck, M. (2000). The N170 occipito-temporal component is delayed and enhanced to inverted faces but not to inverted objects: An electrophysiological account of face-specific processes in the human brain. *Neuroreport, 11*(1), 69–72.

Sander, D., Grandjean, D., Pourtois, G., Schwartz, S., Seghier, M., Scherer, K., & Vuilleumier, P. (2005). Emotion and attention interactions in social cognition: Brain regions involved in processing anger prosody. *Neuroimage, 28*(4), 848–858.

Schilbach, L., Timmermans, B., Reddy, V., Costall, A., Bente, G., Schlicht, T., & Vogeley, K. (2013). A second-person neuroscience in interaction. *Behavioral and Brain Sciences, 36*(4), 441–462.

Tottenham, N., Tanaka, J., Leon, A., McCarry, T., Nurse, M., Hare, T., . . . Nelson, C. (2009). The NimStim set of facial expressions: Judgments from untrained research participants. *Psychiatry Research, 168*(3), 242–249.

Tracy, J., & Robins, R. (2004). Show your pride: Evidence for a discrete emotion expression. *Psychological Science, 15*(3), 194–197.

Vytal, K., & Hamann, S. (2010). Neuroimaging support for discrete neural correlates of basic emotions: A voxel-based meta-analysis. *Journal of Cognitive Neuroscience, 22*(12), 2864–2885.

Wang, L., & Markham, R. (1999). The development of a series of photographs of Chinese facial expressions of emotion. *Journal of Cross-Cultural Psychology, 30*(4), 397–410.

Westerhof-Evers, H., Visser-Keizer, A., McDonald, S., & Spikman, J. (2014). Performance of healthy subjects on an ecologically valid test for social cognition: The short, Dutch version of the awareness of social inference test (TASIT). *Journal of Clinical and Experimental Neuropsychology, 36*(10), 1031–1041.

Williams, K., & Jarvis, B. (2006). Cyberball: A program for use in research on interpersonal ostracism and acceptance. *Behavior Research Methods, 38*(1), 174–180.

Wysocki, B., & Wysocki, A. (1969). Cultural differences as reflected in Wechsler-Bellevue intelligence (WBII) test. *Psychological Reports, 25*(1), 95–101.

Young, A., Perrett, D., Calder, A., Sprengelmeyer, R., & Ekman, P. (2002). *Facial Expressions of Emotion – Stimuli and Tests (FEEST)*. Bury St Edmunds, England: Thames Valley Test Company.

Yun, K., Watanabe, K., & Shimojo, S. (2012). Interpersonal body and neural synchronization as a marker of implicit social interaction. *Scientific Reports, 2*(1), 959.

Zhang, F.-f., Dong, Y., & Wang, K. (2010). Reliability and validity of the Chinese version of the interpersonal reactivity index-C. *Chinese Journal of Clinical Psychology, 18*(2), 155–157.

Chapter 3

Impact of early brain insult on the development of social competence

Vicki Anderson, Mardee Greenham, Nicholas P Ryan and Miriam Beauchamp

Childhood acquired brain injury (ABI) is among the most frequent causes of death and lifelong disability in children and adolescents. It results in disruptions to normal development and, depending on its severity, may lead to residual impairments across a wide range of domains: physical, cognitive, behavioural, memory and social. Long-term follow-up studies have demonstrated that, even with access to rehabilitation, problems often persist. These deficits impact on the child's capacity to interact with the environment effectively, leading to lags in skill acquisition and increasing gaps between injured children and their typically developing peers. Predicting outcome from childhood ABI is challenging, and the long-term consequences depend on a complex interaction of numerous factors, including premorbid child abilities and socio-emotional function, injury characteristics, environmental context, developmental stage and access to rehabilitation.

This chapter reviews the current literature examining social outcomes from childhood ABI, focusing on traumatic brain injury (TBI), paediatric stroke and childhood cancers, recognising that social impairment has been identified as among the most frequent and debilitating consequences of ABI, with reports that up to 50% of childhood ABI survivors (Anderson et al., 2013, 2014; McCarthy et al., 2010; Rosema, Crowe, & Anderson, 2012) experience difficulties in the social domain. Despite this, post-childhood ABI social outcomes, especially in the social cognitive domain, are poorly documented, largely due to the lack of definitional clarity and scarcity of appropriate, ecologically valid and psychometrically robust measurement tools.

Childhood acquired brain insult

The term ABI refers to damage to the brain that occurs after birth and which is not related to congenital disorders, developmental disabilities or processes that progressively damage the brain. Underlying injury mechanisms vary but can generally be classified into one of the following: traumatic, vascular, developmental, infective or neuroplastic. Location and extent of resultant damage can also vary, ranging from unilateral or bilateral, focal or diffuse, and frontal

DOI: 10.4324/9781003027034-3

or extra-frontal. The unifying factor for childhood ABIs is that they occur in the context of a rapidly developing brain where: (1) cerebral organisation is incomplete; (2) serious damage has the potential to derail the genetic blueprint for normal brain development; (3) neurobehavioural skills are immature and (4) environmental factors, such as injury, parent influences or family functioning, may significantly influence development.

Traumatic brain injury (TBI) is by far the most common form of ABI, with incidence ranging from 47 to 280 per 100,000 children (Dewan et al., 2016). Rates of other forms of childhood ABI fall between 1.3–13.0 per 100,000 for stroke (Greenham et al., 2016), 1.12–5.14 per 100,000 for brain tumours (Johnson et al., 2014), 36.3–688 per 100,000 for viral and bacterial infections (Rantakallio, Leskinen, & von Wendt, 1986) and 18 per 100,000 for encephalitis (Bale, 2009).

Consequences of childhood ABI depend on a complex interaction of factors including aetiology, insult characteristics, premorbid child abilities and socio-emotional function, environmental context, developmental stage and access to resources. As a result, predicting outcomes from childhood ABI is challenging. Accumulating evidence indicates that, for most domains (e.g., motor, cognitive, language), injury severity is by far the best-established index for child outcome (Taylor et al., 1999; Anderson, Catroppa, Morse, Haritou, & Rosenfeld, 2005). Age, or developmental level, at the time of injury, is a further critical factor for recovery. Though some have argued that younger children recover better than adolescents and adults because their brains are more adaptable (or 'plastic'), studies now show that the developing brain may, in fact, be more vulnerable to early injury because of the potential for such insults to disrupt neural and cognitive maturation (Anderson, Spencer-Smith, & Wood, 2011). Pre-injury and environmental risks (pre-injury learning and behaviour problems, adjustment difficulties, family burden and stress, social disadvantage) are also significant contributing factors (Anderson et al., 2006, 2014; Gerring & Wade, 2012; Yeates et al., 2004).

Social development

The development of intact social skills is fundamental to human existence and to quality of life. The manner in which a child operates within a social environment, by relying on social skills and interacting with others, is critical for developing and forming lasting relationships and participating and functioning within the community (Beauchamp & Anderson, 2010; Blakemore, 2010; Cacioppo, 2002). What appears to happen so naturally is, in fact, a highly complex process involving the adequate development and activation of distributed neural networks, acquisition of multiple socio-cognitive and affective abilities and the culmination of the individual's life experiences and social knowledge.

Social skills emerge gradually through infancy and childhood, consolidating during adolescence, with this progression reflecting a dynamic interplay between the individual and their environment. In the first few months of life, the infant begins to smile and engage with others and imitate the actions of those around them in an interactive manner. By 5–8 months, infants display evidence of goal-directed social behaviour. At 3–4 years, children can describe the mental states or beliefs of others, distinct from their own (Beaudoin & Beauchamp, 2020; Saxe, Carey, & Kanwisher, 2004), and by 7–8 years they can begin to predict the behaviour of others based on past experiences (Rholes, Ruble, & Newman, 1990). Social decision-making and judgement mature later, in early adolescence (Van Overwalle, 2009; Beauchamp, Dooley, & Anderson, 2013; Beauchamp et al., 2019). During this protracted developmental process, any disruption that impacts on normal neural or cognitive maturation processes could impair future social and behavioural progress.

Disruption to social function at any stage across the lifespan may have nega-tive implications for a range of domains including mental health, academic success, career achievement and quality of life. Failure to acquire and consoli-date social skills in early life may interfere with the child's capacity to develop complex social skills required to function appropriately in society. ABI is an example of such disruption in childhood. It is well established that brain insult occurring during childhood can result in physical dysfunction, cognitive and communication deficits, behavioral problems and poor academic performance (Anderson, Catroppa, Morse, Haritou, & Rosenfeld, 2009a). Less research has examined social function in children with paediatric brain insult; however, given that many social skills are rapidly emerging through childhood, it is highly likely that victims of such insults will have a compromised social development.

Mechanisms underpinning the development of social skills

Social skills and the social brain network

Advances in the social neurosciences demonstrate that social skills are inti-mately linked with neurological and cognitive functions (Adolphs, 2001, 2009). For example, to be socially competent, an individual must attend to others and inhibit inappropriate behaviours (executive functions), communi-cate effectively (language skills) and interpret other's social cues and behaviours (social cognition). These skills have been linked to the structure and function of specific brain regions (e.g., theory of mind to prefrontal cortices), with the end product, the social functions we observe in daily behaviour, represented by an integrative, distributed neural network, coined the social brain network. Brain regions identified as contributing to this social brain network include, among others, the *prefrontal cortex, temporo-parietal junction, temporal poles, superior temporal sulcus, insula* and *amygdala* (Adolphs, 2001) (see also Chapter 1). As has been demonstrated for cognitive functions, it is likely that this network devel-ops and becomes refined through childhood and adolescence (Beauchamp &

Anderson, 2010; Burnett, Sebastian, Cohen, Kadosh, & Blakemore, 2011; Tousignant, Eugène, & Jackson, 2017). An injury to the brain, particularly during the formative childhood years, has the potential to disrupt this network and result in social dysfunction (Yeates et al., 2007), with recent work from our group identifying associations between social cognition (e.g., theory of mind) and brain correlates using various methods assessing brain volumes (Ryan et al., 2016, 2017), white matter microstructure (Ryan et al., 2018) and microhemorrhagic brain lesions (Ryan et al., 2015a, 2015b, 2016).

Social skills: environmental influences

The importance of the child's environment has been well established in the developmental psychology literature, with distal factors, such as socio-economic status, and more proximal influences (e.g., parent mental health, family environment) each implicated in the development of intact social functions (Ackerman & Brown, 2006; Belsky & de Haan, 2011; Bowlby, 1962; Bulotsky, Fantuzzo, & McDermott, 2008; Guralink, 1999; Masten et al., 1999). These links are also supported by studies of children raised in abnormal environments. For example, there is a wealth of research describing Romanian children raised in conditions of severe environmental deprivation which illustrate the potential for environment to negatively impact on social development (Belsky & de Haan, 2011; Bos, Fox, Zeanah, & Nelson, 2009; Raizada & Kishiyama, 2010). These have also illustrated the close association between environment factors, brain development and these social skills (Adolphs, 2009; Kolb et al., 1998; Ryan et al., 2017; Van Overwalle, 2009).

In the context of childhood ABI, parents and family can either support or undermine a child's social development (Gerring & Wade, 2012). Not surprisingly, in the wake of ABI, family routine can be disrupted. Parents may need to attend hospital and outpatient appointments, and some families may experience financial hardship associated with caring for their child. The associated burden may increase stress and family dysfunction. A secondary impact of early brain insult is the elevated risk of clinically significant mental health problems for parents (McCarthy et al., 2010), with up to one third of parents presenting with such symptoms even six months after diagnosis. Such parent psychopathology has been shown to impact negatively on the quality of the family environment and on the child's well-being, with research identifying a clear link between such factors and children's social and behavioral adjustment (Anderson et al., 2006; Yeates, Taylor, Walz, Stancin, & Wade, 2010).

Functional impairment

Medical factors may also restrict opportunities for social development, in particular, social participation. For example, a hemiplegia will reduce the child's mobility and thus their capacity to independently interact with peers during informal play and sporting activities. Speech difficulties may lead to reduced expressive language fluency and thus impact on opportunities for communication with peers. Seizures may cause those around the child to feel wary or anxious about the child's well-being and thus influence social interactions. Further, many instances of TBI can be conceptualized as chronic illness, involving ongoing medical care, health concerns and frequent absences from school, thus limiting normal exposure to social interactions.

Child status

The child's cognitive status, temperament and adjustment to their condition will contribute to their social function (Lo et al., 2014: Greenham et al., 2018; Séguin et al., 2020). It is not uncommon for children experiencing an ABI to experience post-traumatic stress symptoms, in response to the initial insult and hospitalization, reduced self-esteem and/or 'feeling different' from their peers for the medical reasons noted above, which can commonly translate into social anxiety and withdrawal. An additional symptom, common to early stages of recovery from brain injury, is excessive fatigue (Crichton et al., 2018, Greenham et al., 2018), which can severely impair the child's motivation and endurance of social interactions, further reducing social exposure. In response to these medical problems, some parents will be over-protective of their vulnerable child, potentially further restricting their child's opportunities for engaging independently with peers.

Social function and childhood ABI: What are the challenges?

A review of the literature investigating social outcomes following ABI reveals a dearth of evidence. Various factors may contribute to this current situation. First, until recently, health professionals working with children with ABI have often failed to recognise the significance of social competence for recovery and reintegration, concentrating primarily on physical and cognitive domains. This is well illustrated in a seminal study of child TBI conducted by Bonhert and colleagues (Bohnert, Parker, & Warschausky, 1997). These authors report that, when asked to rank the relative importance of health, education and friendships for the child with ABI, both parents and health professionals agreed that friendships were of least importance. In contrast, children ranked friendships as their top priority.

Additional challenges exist in accurately defining, labelling and measuring components of social skills. Within the social domain, there are few developmentally driven and appropriately age-normed social assessment measures. Most available standardized options are either rating scales or questionnaires, and these commonly canvas only parent or teacher perceptions. Many of these are global measures of adaptive ability, behaviour or quality of life, which mostly include only a small subset of items relevant to day-to-day social skills and social cognition. There exists a small group of measures specific to social skills such as relationships, social interaction, social participation and loneliness (Crowe, Beauchamp, Catroppa, & Anderson, 2011). An even smaller selection of more empirical measures is available, mostly tapping aspects of social cognition, including empathy, perspective taking and intent attribution. While many possess good face validity, few have normative data or robust psychometric properties. Pediatric assessment issues are discussed further in Chapter 10.

Social function and childhood ABI: a theoretical framework

In response to a largely atheoretical approach to the investigation of social consequences of child brain insult in the literature to date, two complementary neuropsychological models of social function in the context of childhood ABI have been described (Beauchamp & Anderson, 2010; Yeates et al., 2007). Both propose that disruption to development, via an injury or insult to the child's brain, can have significant consequences for the acquisition of intact everyday social skills and social cognition.

Yeates et al. (2007) present a heuristic describing social outcomes (social information processing, social interaction and social adjustment) within a developmental psychology framework and with a focus on outcomes from TBI. Social outcomes are conceptualised as susceptible to insult-related risk factors, such as type and severity of insult and nature and extent of brain pathology, as well as non-insult factors including parenting style, family function and socio-economic status.

Beauchamp and Anderson (2010) offer a similar framework (Figure 3.1), placing their emphasis on the mediating role of brain (development and integrity) and environment (family, temperament) on neurobehavioural skills (attention/executive function, communication and social cognition) and, consequently,

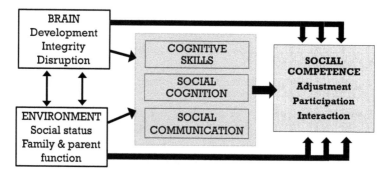

Figure 3.1 Social skills in children: A biopsychosocial model

Source: Adapted from Beauchamp & Anderson (2010)

Table 3.1 Definitions of commonly used terms in social cognitive neuroscience

Term	Definition	Reference
Social Skills/ Social Competence	". . . include the abilities to (a) accurately select relevant and useful information from an interpersonal context, (b) use that information to determine appropriate goal-directed behavior and (c) execute verbal and nonverbal behaviors that maximize the likelihood of goal attainment and the maintenance of good relations with others."	Bedell & Lennox, 1997
Social Adjustment	"The degree to which children get along with their peers; the degree to which they engage in adaptive, competent social behavior; and the extent to which they inhibit aversive, incompetent behavior."	Crick & Dodge, 1994
Social Interaction	". . . is a dynamic, changing sequence of social actions between individuals (or groups) who modify their actions and reactions according to the actions by their interaction partner(s). In other words they are events in which people attach meaning to a situation, interpret what others are meaning, and respond accordingly."	http://en. wikipedia. org/wiki/ social_ interaction
Social Partici-pation	" engagement in socially interactive play, activities and situations"	Muscara & Crowe, 2012
Social Cognition	"(. . .) those aspects of higher cognitive function which underlie smooth social interactions by understanding and processing interpersonal cues and planning appropriate responses."	Scourfield et al., 1999
Social Information Processing Theory	". . . social information processing theory is more broadly concerned with all of the mental operations that are deployed to generate a behavioral response during one's own social interaction."	Dodge & Rabiner, 2004

on social competence. The following review of the research examining the social consequences of ABI will draw on the models described by Yeates et al. and Beauchamp and Anderson, as a framework to structure available findings, with definitions for aspects of social skills provided in Table 3.1.

Social function and ABI: What do we know?

Over the past few years, in keeping with the recognition of their debilitating and persisting impact, research has begun to describe the social deficits associated with childhood ABI. The limited research available has demonstrated deficits in the cognitive skills central to social function (e.g., executive function and communication skills) (Anderson et al., 2009b; Catroppa & Anderson, 2005; Didus, Anderson, & Catroppa, 1999; Hanten et al., 2008; Janusz, Kirkwood, Yeates, & Taylor, 2002; Long et al., 2011a), providing a platform for conceptualizing the presence of social dysfunction. Only a very small number of studies have attempted to examine possible links between specific cognitive domains implicated in social function and social outcomes (Ganesalingham, Sanson, Anderson, & Yeates, 2007a; Ganesalingham, Yeates, Sanson, & Anderson, 2007b, Greenham, Spencer-Smith, Anderson, Coleman, & Anderson, 2010; Muscara, Catroppa, & Anderson, 2008), with early cross-sectional findings supporting the presence of such relationships.

Social outcomes from traumatic brain injury (TBI)

TBI is the most common cause of ABI. It occurs as a result of a blow to the head and, for more serious injuries, this characteristically leads to both localized brain damage at the site of impact and the 'contrecoup site', and more diffuse axonal injury. Due to the shape of the skull, and the effect of injury forces, some brain regions are more vulnerable to damage than others. These include the *frontal* and *temporal* regions of the brain and white matter. Several additional subcortical structures are also impacted in the context of child TBI, including the *hippocampus, corpus callosum* and *amygdala* (Beauchamp et al., 2011). Of note, many of these regions contribute to the 'social brain', suggesting that children with TBI are likely to be particularly vulnerable to social difficulties of an organic basis.

By far, the majority of research into social development after ABI has focused on TBI. Early research showed that children with TBI had lower levels of self-esteem and adaptive behaviour, higher levels of loneliness and behaviour problems (Andrews, Rose, & Johnson, 1998) and more difficulties in peer relationships (Bohnert et al., 1997) than typically developing controls. Further, prospective, longitudinal studies (e.g., Yeates and colleagues, 2004; Anderson, Brown, & Newitt, 2010; Rosema et al., 2012) have highlighted the persistence of social problems post-TBI, reporting no substantial recovery in social function, and in some cases worsening levels of social function, up to 10 years post-injury. In support of these findings, long-term outcome studies identify links between poor social function following child TBI and persisting social maladjustment and reduced quality of life in adulthood (Anderson, Godfrey, Rosenfeld, & Catroppa, 2012; Cattelani, Lombardi, Brianti, & Mazzucchi, 1998).

Social adjustment

The majority of studies examining social adjustment have done so by administering broad-band parent questionnaires. Overall, findings are inconsistent, with some studies reporting social impairment post child TBI (Fletcher et al., 1990; Levin, Hanten, & Li, 2009; Poggi et al., 2005) and others identifying

intact social skills (Anderson et al., 2001; Hanten et al., 2008; Papero, Prigatano, Snyder, & Johnson, 1993; Poggi et al., 2005). A smaller number of studies have incorporated findings from multiple respondents to investigate social
adjustment. Ganesalingam and colleagues (Ganesalingham, Sanson, Anderson, & Yeates; Ganesalingham et al., 2006, 2007a, 2007b) used both parent
ratings and direct child measures with consistent evidence of social impairment
for children with moderate and severe TBI. Whether greater injury severity
leads to poorer social adjustment is also unclear (Asarnow et al., 1991; Fletcher
et al., 1990; Max et al., 1998; Yeates et al., 2004), with studies failing to detect
consistent dose-response relationships (Papero et al., 1993).

Social interaction

While there are variations in research findings in this domain, the bulk of
work supports reductions in friendship networks, less close relationships (Prigatano & Gupta, 2006) and higher levels of loneliness (Andrews et al., 1998) in
children post-TBI. A higher likelihood of aggressive or antisocial behaviours
compared with controls was identified as a potential determinant (Andrews
et al., 1998; Dooley, Anderson, Hemphill, & Ohan, 2008). Further, in a retrospective study of 160 young adults with a history of child TBI, we found
that survivors of severe child TBI reported significant problems with relationships, with few of these young people having a stable friendship or life partners
and minimal engagement in leisure activities. In contrast, young adults with a
history of mild-moderate child TBI were less likely to report long-term challenges with relationships (Anderson et al., 2010). The impact of such socio-
emotional problems following child TBI and stroke is illustrated by two case
studies, Jessica and Tim, outlined in Boxes 3.1 and 3.2.

Box 3.1   Case 1: Jessica: Young person with severe TBI impacting the social brain network

History:

Jessica is a young person who had normal development prior to being
hit by a car at age 11 years. She suffered a severe traumatic brain injury,
with brain contusions in the left frontal area, linked to the social brain
network, and neurological signs consistent with cerebellar involvement.
She was hospitalized for one week, received some inpatient and outpatient rehabilitation for balance problems and returned to school gradually
over a six-month period.

Presentation:

Jessica and her mother describe persisting socio-emotional and behavioural problems (e.g., violent, disruptive outbursts) as the most concerning consequences of her injuries. Jessica reports that she struggles to participate in social interactions and often misses the emotional cues of those around her. Her volatile, aggressive outburst are triggered by Jessica's feeling that she has lost friendships and that her peers are judging her as being 'different'. These behaviours were so disruptive that they have resulted in Jessica being excluded from school and required to participate in a home school program.

Assessment:

On assessment, self-confidence was low and Jessica demonstrated poor emotional control and low frustration tolerance, and parent ratings indicated clinically significant problems for externalizing behaviours, anxiety and adaptive abilities. In contrast, attention, task persistence and functional language skills were intact, and Jessica demonstrated good insight.

Intervention strategy:

Jessica's intact cognitive skills have been important in supporting Jessica's involvement in a peer relationships intervention program, which has enabled her to understand her weaknesses (emotion recognition and perception, social information processing, impulse control) and develop compensatory strategies to manage them. At a broader level, she has been able to establish and maintain new friendships, resulting in improved self-esteem and reductions in anxiety symptoms.

Box 3.2   Case 2: Tim: Young person receiving intervention for social anxiety

History:

Tim is a 15-year old boy, previously healthy and well-functioning, who suffered a stroke at age 10, which was associated with right frontal pathology. Of note, he and his parents report no pre-insult anxiety or social difficulties.

Presentation:

Post-stroke, Tim experienced persistent excessive fatigue, which led to a reduction in participation in out-of-school activities and a major focus on his academic studies. Several years on, in mid-adolescence, Tim was referred for treatment of newly developed social anxiety. At the time of referral, Tim reported that he is doing well academically and had no behaviour problems. Assessment also revealed intact social cognition, both basic and complex. However, he had become increasingly unable to participate in school sports or go to crowded places, such as shopping centres or cinemas, because of high levels of anxiety in these contexts.

Intervention goals:

Tim identified his goal for intervention was to reduce his anxiety in social situations, so that he could be more involved in sports and join his friends when they went to the local shopping centre or the movies.

Intervention outcomes:

Tim completed the Cool Kids Adolescent Anxiety program via Skype, as he lived several hours from the city centre. Formal ratings on pre- and post-treatment questionnaires showed reductions in social anxiety, social avoidance and fear of negative peer evaluation. There was also a small decrease in depressive symptoms. Tim also described everyday benefits not tapped by formal questionnaires including being proud that he had been able to meet the goals that he had set for himself and feeling more confident. In particular, he reported feeling subjectively less anxious and better able to participate in school sports and spend time with his friends in his local shopping centre.

Tim's experience of emerging social anxiety in the context of significant fatigue is not uncommon following childhood ABI and highlights the importance of taking a broad view of the causes of social problems post brain injury.

Social participation

A recent systematic review (Greenham et al., 2020) indicates that social participation following childhood TBI has received limited attention in the scientific literature. However, available results consistently identify reduced levels of participation, lowest for children and adolescents with more severe TBI (Beddell & Dumas, 2004), ongoing medical problems and lower levels of education.

In addition to time since injury, the importance of the family environment has also been documented, such that the poorest social participation outcomes are linked to greater parent mental health problems at two years post-injury (Anderson et al., 2017).

Social cognition

Social cognition refers to the mental processes used to perceive and process social cues, stimuli and environments (Beauchamp & Anderson, 2010). In contrast to social adjustment and social interaction, measurement within this domain is largely based on direct child assessments, although these are currently restricted to mostly experimental tools. Social cognition has attracted recent attention, with a growing number of publications investigating outcomes in this area following child TBI. A recent systematic review and meta-analysis from our group (Zhi et al., in press) provide a comprehensive overview of the state of the art in social cognition following childhood TBI.

Emotion recognition

Zhi et al. (in press), conclude that lower-order aspects of social cognition, such as emotion perception/recognition, which develop early in life are relatively preserved following child TBI (Lawrence, Campbell, & Skuse, 2015; Schmidt et al., 2010). Integration of findings in this area suggested some inconsistencies across different modalities (McDonald & Pierce, 1996), with children with TBI having problems recognising emotions expressed in the eyes, but intact skills where more context was provided (e.g., facial expressions; Tonks et al., 2007). Interestingly, similar findings have been reported for basic ToM, on first-order belief tasks (Turkstra et al., 2008), supporting the view that lower-order social cognitive skills may be relatively intact after child TBI.

Theory of mind (ToM)

In child TBI research, ToM is typically examined as a single construct tapped using basic false belief type tasks. One such study reported largely intact performances for children injured in the preschool years, but significant deficits in children with TBI incurred at an older age (5–7 years), raising the possibility that ToM impairment may only be detectable later in childhood. Supporting this proposition, Turkstra et al. (2004) have reported that, relative to healthy controls, adolescents with TBI show deficiencies in judging whether a speaker is talking at the listener's level and recognising an individual monopolising a conversation.

Recently, a more comprehensive 'tripartite' model of ToM has been employed in child TBI research. The model incorporates multiple elements: cognitive ToM, which develops in infancy and early childhood, and complex aspects of ToM, which show protracted development through mid-to-late adolescence (Dennis et al., 2013). Complex aspects of ToM can be partitioned into *conative*, defined as the ability to understand how indirect speech acts involving irony and empathy are used to influence the mental or affective state of the listener; and *affective*, concerned with understanding that facial expressions are often used for social purposes to convey emotions that we want people to think we feel. Comparing these aspects of ToM in a school-aged sample, Ryan et al. (2017) found that conative and affective ToM were most vulnerable to the effects of TBI, with cognitive ToM relatively spared. A newly published large-scale, multisite study of school-aged children (n=218) (Ryan et al., 2020) confirms the elevated risk of impaired ToM following child TBI and documents links between ToM and injury severity, as well as parent ratings of social adjustment, behaviour and social communication.

Taken together, the current literature suggests that the differential impact of child TBI on various aspects of ToM is likely explained by a combination of injury and developmental factors. Skills that are better established at the time of injury (e.g., cognitive ToM) are less vulnerable than those skills that are emerging or not yet developed (e.g., conative and affective ToM).

Social problem solving

Several recent studies have investigated social problem-solving in children and adolescents post TBI. Hanten et al. (2008) and Janusz et al. (2002) both used the Interpersonal Negotiation Strategies task, derived from the Crick and Dodge (1994) social information processing paradigm, which consists of hypothetical interpersonal dilemmas involving four steps: defining the problem, generating alternative strategies, selecting and implementing a specific strategy and evaluating outcomes. Both studies found that children with TBI demonstrated significantly poorer social problem-solving skills, with the greatest problems selecting the optimal solution. Taking a similar approach, Warschausky et al. (1997) examined children (TBI and healthy controls) aged 7 and 13 years, demonstrating that children with TBI generated fewer peer entry solutions in social engagement situations. Some recent work from our team has employed a novel task of socio-moral reasoning (So Moral: Beauchamp et al., 2013, 2019; Dooley, Beauchamp, & Anderson, 2010), which assesses specific aspects of social information processing, in children and adolescents post-TBI. Supporting many findings in the socio-cognitive domain, we found that a history of TBI was associated with poorer moral choices and lower levels of moral maturity. Similarly, recent meta-analytic findings (Wardlaw et al., in submission) show that children with moderate-severe TBI have significantly poorer social problem-solving skills, characterised by impulsive rather than collaborative strategies.

Exploring the underlying mechanisms for these social problem-solving difficulties, Muscara et al. (2008) examined the relationship between executive function and social function 10 years post-child TBI and found that greater executive dysfunction was associated with less sophisticated social problem-solving skills and poorer social outcomes. Further, the maturity of social problem-solving skills mediated the relationship between executive function and social outcomes. These findings provide empirical evidence for a link between executive and social skills in the context of childhood ABI, due to the mediating link of social problem-solving, consistent with the Yeates et al. (2007) and Beauchamp and Anderson (2010) frameworks.

In summary, the weight of evidence indicates that children sustaining TBI are at elevated risk of experiencing social deficits, including social adjustment, social interaction and social cognition. These problems persist long-term post-insult and are not able to be fully explained by injury severity. However, the developmental stage does appear to play a role. Fewer problems are identified in younger children, where only basic social adjustment, social interaction and socio-cognitive abilities are established, with greater difficulties emerging in older children and adolescents where socio-cognitive demands are more complex (Ryan et al., 2015b). However, further work is needed to describe the potential impact of injury-related factors (e.g., severity, age at insult) and environmental influences on these social consequences, particularly in very young children in whom there is a dearth of studies specifically assessing social-cognitive outcomes after ABI (Beauchamp et al., 2020).

Social outcomes from pediatric stroke

Pediatric stroke (PS) is an acute cerebrovascular event that can occur at any stage during childhood, affecting 1.3–13.0 per 100,000 children and 1 per 1,200 live births in neonates. (Mallick et al., 2010; Dunbar et al., 2020). There are two forms of PS: arterial ischemic stroke and hemorrhagic stroke. Arterial stroke occurs due to a blockage or obstruction of an artery due to a clot, resulting in disrupted blood flow, and causes relatively focal damage. Hemorrhagic stroke, in contrast, involves the rupture of an artery, often leading to more diffuse brain damage. Depending on the type of stroke and the artery affected, brain lesions caused by PS will vary in size, extent and location (Greenham, Gordon, Anderson, & Mackay, 2016). Infarcts impacting the middle cerebral artery will affect *dorsolateral frontal cortex, basal ganglia* and *white matter*, while anterior cerebral artery stroke leads to bilateral lesions in *orbito-frontal, temporal* and *parietal cortices*. Given the distributed nature of the social brain network, it is not surprising that damage from PS may contribute to social problems.

Children recovering from stroke often have unique social challenges due to the high risk of functional and physical impairments affecting 60–85% of cases (Brower, Rollins, & Roach, 1996; Ganesan et al., 2000; Gordon, Ganesan, Towell, & Kirkham, 2002; Sofranas et al., 2006). In contrast to the large body of research documenting social dysfunction in the context of child TBI, relatively little evidence exists regarding social outcomes of PS. There is, however, evidence of disruption to cognitive skills underpinning social competence, with studies reporting post-stroke deficits in executive skills, attention (Long et al., 2011b) and communication (Bates et al., 2001).

Two general reviews, primarily of cross-sectional studies with small samples, and standard measurement tools have provided some insights into social outcomes following PS. Goodman and Graham (1996) highlighted that children with stroke require additional assistance for optimal school and home participation, and Ganesan et al. (2000) reported that 37% of parents of children with stroke were "concerned" about their child's socio-emotional function. In contrast, findings from recent studies are more specific, identifying social deficits emerging 6- and 12-months post-stroke (Greenham et al., 2017, 2018).

Social interaction

A handful of studies have commented on this area of social function in the context of PS, using specific measures to characterise the quality of social interactions. Everts et al. (2008) examined children who suffered stroke from birth to 18 years and provided qualitative reports of low peer acceptance, mood instability and decreased social support from peers for many participants. Using parent-report data, De Schryver et al. (2000) described changes in children's social behaviour and companionship post-stroke, while Steinlin, Roellin, and Schroth (2004) detected changes in social interactions, including a qualitative difference in friendships with peers. Findings underscored children's difficulties in implementing social skills in real-life situations, linking these problems to the impact of cognitive deficits, (e.g., processing speed), though this relationship was not statistically tested. More recently, Lo and colleagues (2014) and Greenham et al. (2017) have reported quantitative data supporting reduced social interactions in children post-stroke compared to typically developing children.

Social participation

To date, patterns of social participation following PS remain relatively unknown. In one study of 29 adult survivors of PS, Hurvitz and colleagues found that daily living skills, communication and socialization were in the moderately low range (Hurvitz, Warschausky, Berg, & Tsai, 2004). Tonks et al. (2011) have also studied social participation in children with stroke, and other acquired brain insults (n=135). They found that, compared to healthy controls, children with stroke demonstrated a restricted level of diversity and intensity across a range of activities: recreational, social and self-improvement. These authors highlighted the key role of intact social participation for children's general health and quality of life. Our group has also explored social participation in children with PS and found significant reductions compared to both typically developing children and those with chronic illness (Anderson et al., 2014). Social participation was also linked to self-esteem and parent-reported social cognition.

Social cognition

Very little attention has been directed to social cognition following PS to date. One study, authored by Greenham and colleagues (2018), reported no differences between children with PS and normative expectations for measures of pragmatic language and emotion recognition. However, when age at stroke was examined, children sustaining childhood stroke had a four-fold risk of deficits in pragmatic language. Lo et al. (2020) have also reported on social cognition post-PS, reporting poorer results on tasks tapping conative ToM for children with PS compared to healthy controls.

Social outcome from PS: potential contributors

Brain-related predictors of social outcomes

Following childhood stroke, severity, often indexed by lesion size, may be a useful predictor of outcome. However, to date, relationships between social outcomes and infarct volume have not been found (Everts et al., 2008; Nass & Trauner, 2004). A small body of research has demonstrated that localisation of infarction is predictive of functional outcome (Long et al., 2011a; Roach, 2000), but others have failed to replicate these findings (Anderson et al., 2019). Overall, however, studies investigating the general impact of lesion size and location have been inconclusive due to small sample size and limited socially-oriented outcome measures.

Age at stroke onset

In keeping with findings of cognitive domains, age at stroke onset may impact social outcomes. Research in this area has been limited to a single study by Greenham et al. (2018) who found poorer social adjustment and social cognition associated with childhood-onset PS, compared to neonatal stroke.

Environment

Follow-up studies of children with PS from our group have linked environmental factors with social outcomes in the chronic stages of recovery. In particular, family function and parent mental health have been consistent predictors of social outcomes across multiple cohorts, and, as for child TBI, these influences increase with time post-stroke (Anderson et al., 2020; Greenham et al., 2017, 2015).

Social outcomes from brain tumour

Childhood cancers, and in particular brain tumours, have been related to higher levels of stress and trauma than most other brain-related conditions (McCarthy et al., 2010). While relatively uncommon, treatment advances in childhood cancers have led to improved survival rates and an increasing focus on quality of life outcomes. Psychosocial consequences have received considerable attention, although little research to date has focused on the brain bases of these problems. Rather, the emphasis has been on adjustment to life-threatening disease, extended treatment and their impact on self-concept and quality of life. However, regardless of the assessment approach employed, or the social domain under study, findings consistently document long-term social problems in these children (Schulte & Barrera, 2010; Desjardins et al., 2020a, 2020b).

Social adjustment

As with studies of children with TBI and PS, research with this group has mainly employed broad-band measurement tools. Using parent and teacher-based ratings, numerous studies have reported poor social adjustment after diagnosis and treatment of a brain tumour (Aarsen et al., 2006; Bhat et al., 2005; Poretti et al., 2004; Sands et al., 2005; Upton & Eiser, 2006; Varni, Seid, & Rode, 1999), with Mabbott et al. (2005) noting that, while social adjustment may appear intact acutely, problems increase with time since diagnosis.

Social interaction

Survivors of childhood brain tumours are also reported to struggle with peer interaction and social participation more generally. Studies describe these children as having fewer friends (Barrera, Schule, & Spiegler, 2008) as well as experiencing limited social opportunities, social isolation, peer exclusion and bullying (Boydell et al., 2008; Upton & Eiser, 2006; Vance, Eiser, & Home, 2004).

Social cognition

Bonner et al. (2008) have conducted one of the few studies evaluating social cognition in children with brain tumours. They examined facial expression recognition and found that these children made greater errors than expected when interpreting facial expressions.

Predictors of social problems post-tumour

Brain factors

Several risk and resilience factors have been investigated in the context of childhood tumours. Somewhat surprisingly, treatment factors have been shown to have little impact on social outcomes (Schulte et al., 2010). In contrast, there is evidence that the developmental stage is relevant, with the greatest social consequences identified in association with both early childhood diagnosis (social adjustment, social cognition: Bonner et al., 2008; Foley, Barakat, Herman-Liu, Radcliffe, & Molloy, 2000) and diagnosis during adolescence (reduced quality of life: Aarsen et al., 2006), perhaps suggesting that disturbances in social competence are most likely during 'critical periods' of social development. As noted above, and in keeping with observations of increasing brain pathology and neurocognitive impairment with greater time from diagnosis, social competence also appears to deteriorate over time with most problems emerging between 7–11 years post-illness (Aarsen et al., 2006; Kullgren, 2003; Mabbott et al., 2005; Poretti et al., 2004).

Internal and environmental factors

In the brain tumour population, several studies have addressed child-related contributors to social outcomes. For example, a number of studies have identified poorer social competence in survivors with lower levels of intelligence (Carey et al., 2001; Holmquist & Scott, 2003; Poggi et al., 2005). Interestingly, these studies have reported greater links between non-verbal skills and social skills, with less evidence of a relationship between verbal skills and the social domain. Poorer social adjustment and social participation have also been associated with lower body mass index (Schulte et al., 2010). Perhaps contrary to expectations, to date, links with social and family factors have been less compelling. In a review of this literature, Schulte and Barrera (2010) advise caution in interpreting these findings, noting the heterogeneous nature of brain tumour samples in terms of age at injury, time since diagnosis, retrospective design and inadequate assessment tools.

Conclusions

There is growing interest in the social consequences of paediatric brain insult; however, evidence to date is relatively scarce. Not surprisingly, the available literature does indicate that the presence of a brain injury in early life is associated with an elevated risk of social dysfunction across a range of dimensions – social adjustment, social interaction and participation, and social cognition. The ways in which these domains interact with one another, and with the child's other skills, remain unclear, and the measures generally employed in such studies are not intended for the assessment of social skills specifically. In addition, it appears that the injury-related risk factors established as predictors of cognitive and physical outcomes from early brain insult (injury severity, lesion location, age at insult) are unable to predict social outcomes in isolation. Rather, findings suggest that environmental factors play a key role. Social context, family function, child temperament and adjustment to brain insult are all important in determining the child's social outcome. Recent theoretical models of social function and early brain insult, integrating social neuroscience, developmental and developmental psychopathology literatures, and findings emerging from longitudinal studies of childhood ABI show great promise and will facilitate future research and the design of evidence-based interventions in this field.

References

Aarsen, F., Paquier, P., Reddingius, R., Streng, I., Arts, W., Evera-Preesman, M., & Catsman-Berrevoets, C. (2006). Functional outcome after low grade astrocytoma treatment in childhood. *Cancer, 106*, 396–402.

Ackerman, B. P., & Brown, E. D. (2006). Income poverty, poverty co-factors, and the adjustment of children in elementary school. *Advances in Child Development and Behavior, 34*, 91–129.

Adolphs, R. (2001). The neurobiology of social cognition. *Current Opinion in Neurobiology, 11*, 231–239.

Adolphs, R. (2009). The social brain: Neural basis of social knowledge. *Annual Review of Psychology, 60*, 693–716.

Anderson, V., Beauchamp, M. H., Yeates, K. O., Crossley, L., Hearps, S. J. C., & Catroppa, C. (2013). Social competence at 6 months following childhood traumatic brain injury. *Journal of the International Neuropsychological Society, 19*(5), 539–550.

Anderson, V., Beauchamp, M. H., Yeates, K. O., Crossley, L., Hearps, S. J. C., & Catroppa, C. (2017). Social competence at 2 years following child traumatic brain injury. *Journal of Neurotrauma, 34*(14), 2261–2271.

Anderson, V., Brown, S., & Newitt, H. (2010). What contributes to quality of life in adult survivors of childhood traumatic brain injury? *Journal of Neurotrauma, 27*(5), 863–870.

Anderson, V., Catroppa, C., Dudgeon, P., Morse, S., Haritou, F., & Rosenfeld, J. (2006). Understanding predictors of functional recovery and outcome thirty-months following early childhood head injury. *Neuropsychology, 20*, 42–57.

Anderson, V., Catroppa, C., Morse, S., Haritou, F., & Rosenfeld, J. (2001). Outcome from mild head injury in young children: A prospective study. *Journal of Clinical and Experimental Neuropsychology, 23*, 705–717.

Anderson, V., Catroppa, C., Morse, S., Haritou, F., & Rosenfeld, J. (2005). Functional plasticity or vulnerability after early brain injury? *Pediatrics, 116*(6), 1374–1382.

Anderson, V., Catroppa, C., Morse, S., Haritou, F., & Rosenfeld, J. (2009a). Intellectual outcome from preschool traumatic brain injury: A 5-year prospective, longitudinal study. *Pediatrics, 124*(6), pp. e1064–e1071.

Anderson, V., Darling, S., Mackay, M., Monagle, P., Greenham, M., Cooper, A., . . . Gordon, A. L. (2020). Cognitive resilience following paediatric stroke: Biological and environmental predictors. *European Journal of Paediatric Neurology, 25*, 52–58.

Anderson, V., Godfrey, G., Rosenfeld, J., & Catroppa. (2012). Ten-year outcome from childhood traumatic brain injury. *International Journal of Developmental Neuroscience, 30*(3), 217–224.

Anderson, V., Gomes, A., Greenham, M., Hearps, S., Gordon, A., Rinehart, N., . . . Mackay, M. (2014). Social competence following pediatric stroke: Contributions of brain insult and family environment. *Social Neuroscience, 9*(5), 471–483.

Anderson, V., Spencer-Smith, M., & Wood, A. (2011). Do children really recover better? Neurobehavioural plasticity after early brain insult. *Brain, 134*(8), 2197–2221.

Anderson, V., Spencer-Smith, M., Leventer, R., Coleman, L., Anderson, P., Williams, J., . . . Jacobs, R. (2009b). Childhood brain insult: Can age at insult help us predict outcome? *Brain, 132*(1), 45–56.

Andrews, T. K., Rose, F. D., & Johnson, D. A. (1998). Social and behavioural effects of traumatic brain injury in children. *Brain Injury, 12*, 133–138.

Asarnow, R. F., Satz, P., Light, R., Lewis, R., & Neumann, E. (1991). Behavior problems and adaptive functioning in children with mild and severe closed head injury. *Journal of Pediatric Psychology, 16*, 543–555.

Bale Jr, J. F. (2009). Encephalitis. In L. R. Squire (Ed.), *Encyclopedia of Neuroscience* (Vol. 1, pp. 953–962). USA: Elsevier.

Barrera, M., Schule, F., & Spiegler, B. (2008). Factors influencing depressive symptoms of children treated for a brain tumor. *Journal of Psychosocial Oncology, 26*, 1–16.

Bates, E., Reilly, J., Wilfeck, B., Donkers, N., Opie, M., Fenson, J., . . . Herbst, K. (2001). Differential effects of unilateral lesions on language production in children and adults. *Brain and Language, 79*, 223–265.

Beauchamp, M. H., & Anderson, V. (2010). SOCIAL: An integrative framework for the development of social skills. *Psychological Bulletin, 136*, 39–64.

Beauchamp, M. H., Degeilh, F., Yeates, K., Gagnon, I., Tang, K., . . . Deschênes, S. (2020). Kids' Outcomes and long-term abilities (KOALA): Protocol for a prospective, longitudinal cohort study of mild traumatic brain injury in children 6 months to 6 years of age. *British Medical Journal Open, 10*(10), e040603. doi:10.1136/bmjopen-2020-040603

Beauchamp, M. H., Ditchfield, M., Catroppa, C., Kean, M., Godfrey, C., Rosenfeld, J. V., & Anderson, V. (2011). Focal thinning of the posterior corpus callosum: Normal variant or post traumatic? *Brain Injury, 25*(10), 950–957.

Beauchamp, M. H., Dooley, J. J., & Anderson, V. (2013). A preliminary investigation of moral reasoning and empathy after traumatic brain injury in adolescents. *Brain Injury, 27*(7–8), 896–902.

Beauchamp, M. H., Vera-Estay, E., Forasse, F., Anderson, V., & Dooley, J. (2019) Moral reasoning and decision-making in adolescents who sustain traumatic brain injury. *Brain Injury, 33*(1), 32–39.

Beaudoin, C., & Beauchamp, M. H. (2020). Social cognition. *Handbook of Clinical Neurology, 173*, 255–264.

Bedell, G. M., & Dumas, H. M. (2004). Social participation of children and youth with acquired brain injuries discharged from inpatient rehabilitation: A follow-up study. *Brain Injury, 18*(1), 65–82.

Bedell, J., & Lennox, S. (1997). *Handbook for Communication and Problem-Solving Skills Training: A Cognitive Behavioral Approach*. New York: Wiley, 1996.

Belsky, J., & de Haan, M. (2011). Parenting and children's brain development: The end of the beginning. *Journal of Child Psychology and Psychiatry, 52*, 409–428.

Bhat, S., Goodwin, T., Burwinkle, T., Lansdale, M., Dahl, G., Huhn, S., Gibbs, I., Donaldson, S., Rosenblum, R., Varni, J., & Fisher, P. (2005). Profile of daily life in children with brain tumors: An assessment of health-related quality of life. *Journal of Clinical Oncology, 23*, 5493–5500.

Blakemore, S. (2010). The developing social brain. *Neuron, 65*, 774–777.

Bohnert, A. M., Parker, J. G., & Warschausky, S. A. (1997). Friendship and social adjustment of children following a traumatic brain injury: An exploratory investigation. *Developmental Neuropsychology, 13*, 477–486.

Bonner, M., Hardy, K., Willard, V., Anthon, K., Hood, M., & Gururangan, S. (2008). Social function and facial expression recognition in survivors of pediatric brain tumors. *Journal of Pediatric Psychology, 33*, 1142–1152.

Bos, K., Fox, N., Zeanah, C., & Nelson, C. (2009). Effects of early psychological deprivation on the development of memory and executive function. *Frontiers in Behavioural
Neuroscience.* doi:0.3389/neuro.08.016.2009

Bowlby, J. (1962). *Deprivation of Maternal Care.* Geneva: World Health Organization.

Boydell, K., Stasiulis, E., Greenberg, M., Greenberg, C., & Spiegler, B. (2008). I'll show
them: The social construction of (in)competence in survivors of childhood brain tumors.
Journal of Pediatric Oncology Nursing, 25, 164–174.

Brower, M. C., Rollins, N., & Roach, E. S. (1996). Basal ganglia and thalamic infarction in
children. *Archives of Neurology, 53,* 1252–1256.

Bulotsky, R., Fantuzzo, J., & McDermott, P. (2008). An investigation of classroom situational dimensions of emotional and behavioral adjustment and cognitive and social outcomes for Head Start children. *Developmental Psychology, 44,* 139–154.

Burnett, S., Sebastian, C., Cohen, Kadosh, K., & Blakemore, S. J. (2011). The social brain
in adolescence: Evidence from functional magnetic imaging and behavioural studies. *Neuroscience and Biobehavioural Reviews, 35,* 1654–1664.

Cacioppo, J. (2002). Social neuroscience: Understanding the pieces fosters understanding of
the whole and vice versa. *American Psychologist, 57,* 819–831.

Carey, M., Barakat, L., Foley, B., Gyato, K., & Phillips, P. (2001). Neuropsychological functioning and social functioning of survivors of pediatric brain tumors: Evidence of nonverbal learning disability. *Child Neuropsychology, 7,* 265–272.

Catroppa, C., & Anderson, V. (2005). A prospective study of the recovery of attention from
acute to 2 years post pediatric traumatic brain injury. *Journal of the International Neuropsychological Society, 11,* 84–98.

Cattelani, R., Lombardi, R., Brianti, R., & Mazzucchi, A. (1998). Traumatic brain injury
in childhood: Intellectual, behavioural and social outcome in adulthood. *Brain Injury, 12,*
283–296.

Crichton, A., Oakley, E., Babl, F. E., Greenham, M., Hearps, S., Delzoppo, C., Beauchamp,
M. H., Hutchison, J. S., Guerguerian, A. M., Boutis, K., & Anderson, V. (2018). Predicting fatigue 12 months after child traumatic brain injury: Child factors and post injury
symptoms. *Journal of the International Neuropsychological Society, 24*(3), 224–236.

Crick, N. R., & Dodge, K. A. (1994). A review and reformulation of social information
processing mechanisms in children's social adjustment. *Psychological Bulletin, 115,* 74–101.

Crowe, L. M., Beauchamp, M. H., Catroppa, C., & Anderson, V. (2011). Social function
assessment tools for children and adolescents: A systematic review from 1988 to 2010.
Clinical Psychology Review, 31, 767–785.

Dennis, M., Simic, N., Bigler, E. D., Abildskov, T., Agostino, A., Taylor, H. G., . . . Yeates,
K. O. (2013). Cognitive, affective, and conative theory of mind (ToM) in children with
traumatic brain injury. *Developmental Cognitive Neuroscience, 5,* 25–39.

De Schryver, E. L., Kappelle, L. J., Jennekens-Schinkel, A., & Boudewyn Peters, A. C.
(2000). Prognosis of ischemic stroke in childhood: A long-term follow-up study. *Developmental Medicine and Child Neurology, 42*(5), 313–318.

Desjardins, L., Rodriguez, E., Dunn, M., Bemis, H., Murphy, L., Manring, S., . . . Compas,
B. E. (2020b). Coping and social adjustment in pediatric oncology: From diagnosis to 12
months. *Journal of Pediatric Psychology, 45*(10), 1199–1207.

Desjardins, L., Solomon, A., Janzen, L., Bartels, U., Schulte, F., Chung, J., . . . Barrera, M.
(2020a). Executive functions and social skills in pediatric brain tumor survivors. *Applied
Neuropsychology Child.* 9(1), 83–91.

Dewan, M. C., Mummareddy, N., Wellons III, J. C., & Bonfield, C. M. (2016). Epidemiology of global pediatric traumatic brain injury: Qualitative review. *World Neurosurgery, 91*, 497–509. e491.

Didus, E., Anderson, V., & Catroppa, C. (1999). The development of pragmatic communication skills in head injured children. *Pediatric Rehabilitation, 3*, 177–186.

Dodge, K. A., & Rabiner, D. L. (2004). Returning to roots: On social information processing and moral development. *Child Development, 75*(4), 1003–1008.

Dooley, J. J., Anderson, V., Hemphill, S., & Ohan, J. (2008). Aggression after pediatric traumatic brain injury: A theoretical approach. *Brain Injury, 22*(11), 836–846.

Dooley, J. J., Beauchamp, M. H., & Anderson, V. A. (2010). The measurement of sociomoral reasoning in adolescents with traumatic brain injury: A pilot investigation. *Brain Impairment, 11*(2), 152–161

Dunbar, M. J., & Kirton, A. (2020). The incidence of perinatal stroke is 1: 1200 live births: A population-based study in Alberta Canada. *Stroke. 51*, A51.

Everts, R., Pavlovic, J., Kaufmann, F., Uhlenberg, B., Seidel, U., Nedeltchev, K., . . . Steinlin, M. (2008). Cognitive functioning, behavior, and quality of life after stroke in childhood. *Neuropsychology, Development, and Cognition. Section C, Child Neuropsychology, 14*(4), 323–338.

Fletcher, J. M., Ewing-Cobbs, L., Miner, M. E., Levin, H. S., & Eisenberg, H. M. (1990). Behavioral changes after closed head injury in children. *Journal of Consulting and Clinical Psychology, 58*, 93–98.

Foley, B., Barakat, L. P., Herman-Liu, A., Radcliffe, J., & Molloy, P. (2000). The impact of childhood hypothalamic/chiasmatic brain tumors on child adjustment and family function. *Child Health Care, 29*, 209–223.

Ganesalingam, K., Sanson, A., Anderson, V., & Yeates, K. O. (2006). Self-regulation and social and behavioral functioning following childhood traumatic brain injury. *Journal of the International Neuropsychological Society, 12*, 609–621.

Ganesalingam, K., Sanson, A., Anderson, V., & Yeates, K. O. (2007a). Self-regulation as a mediator of the effects of childhood traumatic brain injury on social and behavioral functioning. *Journal of the International Neuropsychological Society, 13*, 298–311.

Ganesalingam, K., Yeates, K. O., Sanson, A., & Anderson, V. (2007b). Social problem-solving skills following childhood traumatic brain injury and its association with self-regulation and social and behavioral functioning. *Journal of Neuropsychology, 1*, 149–170.

Ganesan, V., Hogan, A., Shack, N., Gordon, A., Isaacs, E., & Kirkham, F. J. (2000). Outcome after ischaemic stroke in childhood. *Developmental Child Neurology, 42*, 455–461.

Gerring, J., & Wade, S. (2012). The essential role of psychosocial risk and protective factors in pediatric traumatic brain injury resaerch. *Journal of Neurotrauma, 29*, 621–628.

Goodman, R., & Graham, P. (1996). Psychiatric problems in children with hemiplegia: Cross-sectional epidemiological survey. *British Medical Journal, 312*, 1065–1069.

Gordon, A. L., Ganesan, V., Towell, A., & Kirkham, F. J. (2002). Functional outcome following stroke in children. *Journal of Child Neurology, 17*(6), 429–434.

Greenham, M., Anderson, V., Cooper, A., Hearps, S., Ditchfield, M., Coleman, L., Hunt, R. W., Mackay, M. T., Monagle, P., & Gordon, A. L. (2017). Early predictors of psychosocial functioning 5 years after pediatric stroke. *Developmental Medicine and Child Neurology. 59*(10), 1034–1041.

Greenham, M., Botchway, E., Knight, S., Bonyhady, B., Tavender, E., Scheinberg, A., Anderson, V., & Muscara, F. (2020). Predictors of participation and quality of life following major traumatic injuries in childhood. A systematic review. *Disability and Rehabilitation.* doi:10.1080/09638288.2020.1849425

Greenham, M., Gordon, A. L., Anderson, V., & Mackay, M. T. (2016). Outcome in childhood stroke. *Stroke, 47*(4), 1159–1164.

Greenham, M., Gordon, A. L., Cooper, A., Ditchfield, M., Coleman, L., Hunt, R. W., Mackay, M. T., Monagle, P., & Anderson, V. (2018). Social functioning following pediatric stroke: Contribution of neurobehavioral impairment. *Developmental Neuropsychology, 43*(4), 312–328.

Greenham, M., Hearps, S., Gomes, A., Rinehart, N., Gonzalez, L., Gordon, A., Mackay, M., Lo, W., Yeates, K., & Anderson, V. (2015). Environmental contributions to social and mental health outcomes following pediatric stroke. *Developmental Neuropsychology, 40*(6), 348–362.

Greenham, M., Spencer-Smith, M. M., Anderson, P. J., Coleman, L., & Anderson, V. A. (2010). Social functioning in children with brain insult. *Frontiers in Human Neuroscience, 4*(22), EPub.

Guralink, M. (1999). Family and child influences on the peer-related social competence of young children with developmental delays. *Mental Retardation and Developmental Disabilities Research Reviews, 5,* 21–29.

Hanten, G., Wilde, E. A., Menefee, D. S., Li, X., Lane, S., Vasquez, C., Chu, Z., Ramos, M. A., Yallampalli, R., Swank, P., Chapman, S. B., Gamino, J., Hunter, J. V., & Levin, H. S. (2008). Correlates of social problem solving during the first year after traumatic brain injury in children. *Neuropsychology, 22,* 357–370.

Holmquist, L., & Scott, J. (2003). Treatment, age and time-related predictors of behavioral oputcome in pediatric brain tumor survivors. *Journal of Clinical Psychology and Medical Settings, 9,* 315–321.

Hurvitz, E., Warschausky, S., Berg, M., & Tsai, S. (2004). Long-term functional outcome of pediatric stroke survivors. *Topics in Stroke Rehabilitation, 11*(2), 51–59.

Janusz, J. A., Kirkwood, M. W., Yeates, K. O., & Taylor, G. (2002). Social problem-solving skills in children with traumatic brain injury: Long-term outcomes and prediction of social competence. *Child Neuropsychology, 8,* 179–194.

Johnson, K. J., Cullen, J., Barnholtz-Sloan, J. S., Ostrom, Q. T., Langer, C. E., Turner, M. C., . . . Scheurer, M. E. (2014). Childhood brain tumor epidemiology: A brain tumor epidemiology consortium review. *Cancer Epidemiology, Biomarkers & Prevention: A Publication of the American Association for Cancer Research, Cosponsored by the American Society of Preventive Oncology, 23*(12), 2716–2736. doi:10.1158/1055-9965.EPI-14-0207

Kolb, B., Forgie, M., Gibb, R., Gorny, G., & Rowntree, S. (1998). Age, experience and the changing brain. *Neuroscience and Biobehavioral Reviews, 22*(2), 143–159.

Kullgren, K., (2003). Risk factors associated with long-term social and behavioural problems among children with brain tumors. *Journal of Psychosocial Oncology, 21,* 73–87.

Lawrence, K., Campbell, R., & Skuse, D. (2015). Age, gender, and puberty influence the development of facial emotion recognition. *Frontiers in Psychology, 6,* 761.

Levin, H. S., Hanten, G., & Li, X. (2009). The relation of cognitive control to social outcome after paediatric TBI: Implications for interventions. *Developmental NeuroRehabilitation, 12,* 320–329.

Lo, W., Gordon, A., Hajek, C., Gomes, A., Greenham, M., Perkins, E., Zumberge, N., Anderson, V., Yeates, K., & Mackay, M. (2014). Social competence following neonatal and childhood stroke. *International Journal of Stroke, 9,* 1037–1044.

Lo, W., Li, X., Hoskinson, K., McNally, K., Chung, M., Lee, J., Wang, J., Lu, Z., & Yeates, K. (2020). Pediatric Stroke Impairs Theory of Mind Performance. *Journal of Child Neurology*, 35(3), 228–234.

Long, B., Anderson, V., Jacobs, R., Mackay, M., Leventer, R., Barnes, C., & Spencer-Smith, M. M., (2011a). Executive function following child stroke: The impact of lesion location. *Journal of Child Neurology*. 26(3), 279–287.

Long, B., Anderson, V., Jacobs, R., Mackay, M., Leventer, R., Barnes, C., & Spencer-Smith, M. (2011b). Executive function following child stroke: The impact of lesion location. *Developmental Neuropsychology*, 36(8), 971–987.

Mabbott, D., Spiegler, S., Greenberg, M., Rutka, J., Hyder, D., & Bouffet, E. (2005). Serial evaluation of academic and behavioral outcome after treatment with cranial radiation in childhood. *Journal of Clinical Oncology*, 23, 2256–2263.

Mallick, A. A., & O'Callaghan, F. J. (2010). The epidemiology of childhood stroke. *European Journal of Paediatric Neurology*, 3, 197–205.

Masten, A., Hubbard, J., Gest, S., Tellegen, A., Garmezy, N., & Ramirez, M. (1999). Competence in the context of adversity: Pathways to resilience and maladaptation from childhood to late adolescence. *Development and Psychopathology*, 11, 143–169.

Max, J. E., Koele, S. L., Lindgren, S. D., Robin, D. A., Smith, W. L., Sato, Y., & Arndt, S. (1998). Adaptive functioning following traumatic brain injury and orthopedic injury: A controlled study. *Archives of Physical Medicine & Rehabilitation*, 79, 893–899.

McCarthy, M. C., Clarke, N. E., Lin Ting, C., Conroy, R., Anderson, V., & Heath, J. A. (2010). Prevalence and predictors of parental grief and depression after the death of a child from cancer. *Journal of Palliative Medicine*, 13(11), 1321–1326.

McDonald, S., & Pierce, S. (1996). Clinical insights into pragmatic theory: Frontal lobe deficit and sarcasm. *Brain and Language*, 53, 81–104.

Muscara, F., Catroppa, C., & Anderson, V. (2008). Social problem-solving skills as a mediator between executive function and long-term social outcome following paediatric traumatic brain injury. *Journal of Neuropsychology*, 2, 445–461.

Muscara, F., & Crowe, L. (2012). Measuring children's social skills: Questionnaires and rating scales. In V. Anderson & M. Beauchamp (Eds.), *Developmental Social Neuroscience: Implications for Theory and Clinical Practice*. New York: Guilford.

Nass, R. D., & Trauner, D. (2004). Social and affective impairments are important recovery after acquired stroke in childhood. *CNS Spectrums*, 9(6), 420–434.

Papero, P. H., Prigatano, G. P., Snyder, H. M., & Johnson, D. L. (1993). Children's adaptive behavioural competence after head injury. *Neuropsychological Rehabilitation*, 3, 321–340.

Poggi, G., Liscio, M., Adduci, A., Galbiati, S., Massimino, M., Sommovigo, M., Zettin, M., Figini, E., & Castelli, E. (2005). Psychological and adjustment problems due to acquired brain lesions in childhood: A comparison between post-traumatic patients and brain tumor survivors. *Brain Injury*, 19, 777–785.

Poretti, A., Grotzer, M., Ribi, K., Schonle, E., & Bolthauser, E. (2004). Outcome of craniopharyngioma in children: Long-term complications and quality of life. *Developmental Medicine and Child Neurology*, 46, 220–229.

Prigatano, G. P., & Gupta, S. (2006). Friends after traumatic brain injury in children. *Journal of Head Trauma Rehabilitation*, 21, 505–513.

Raizada, R., & Kishiyama, M. (2010). Effects of socioeconomic status on brain development, and how cognitive neuroscience may contribute to levelling the playing field. *Frontiers in Human Neuroscience*, 4, 1–11. doi:10.3389/neuro 09.003.2010

Rantakallio, P., Leskinen, M., & von Wendt, L. (1986). Incidence and prognosis of central nervous system infections in a birth cohort of 12 000 children. *Scandinavian Journal of Infectious Diseases, 18*(4), 287–294.

Rholes, W., Ruble, D., & Newman, L. (1990). Children's understanding of self and other: Developmental and motivational aspects of perceiving persons in terms of invariant dispositions. In R. Sorention & E. Higgins (Eds.), *The Handbook of Motivation and Cognition: Foundations and Social Behavior* (Vol. II, pp. 369–407). Hillsdale, NJ: LEA.

Roach, E. S. (2000). Stroke in children. *Current Treatment Options in Neurology, 2*(4), 295–304.

Rosema, S., Crowe, L., & Anderson, V. (2012). Social function in children and adolescents after traumatic brain injury: A systematic review 1989–2011. *Journal of Neurotrauma, 29*(7), 1277–1291.

Ryan, N. P., Anderson, V. A., Bigler, E. D., Dennis, M., Taylor, H. G., Rubin, K. H., . . . Yeates, K. O. (2020). Delineating the nature and correlates of social dysfunction after childhood traumatic brain injury using common data elements: Evidence from an international multi-cohort study. *Journal of Neurotrauma*. doi:10.1089/neu.2020.7057.

Ryan, N. P., Catroppa, C., Beare, R., Silk, T. J., Crossley, L., Beauchamp, M. H., . . . Anderson, V. A. (2016). Theory of mind mediates the prospective relationship between abnormal social brain network morphology and chronic behavior problems after pediatric traumatic brain injury. *Social Cognitive and Affective Neuroscience, 11*(4), 683–692.

Ryan, N., Catroppa, C., Cooper, J., Beare, R., Ditchfield, M., Coleman, L., . . . Anderson, V. (2015a). Relationship between acute imaging biomarkers and theory of mind impairment in post-acute pediatric traumatic brain injury: A prospective analysis using susceptibility weighted imaging (SWI). *Neuropsychologia, 66*, 32–38.

Ryan, N., Catroppa, C., Cooper, J., Beare, R., Ditchfield, M., Coleman, L., . . . Anderson, V. (2015b). The emergence of age-dependent social cognitive deficits after generalized insult to the developing brain: A longitudinal prospective study using susceptibility-weighted imaging. *Human Brain Mapping, 36*(5), 1677–1691.

Ryan, N., Catroppa, C., Godfrey, C., Noble-Haeusslein, L., Shultz, S., O'Brien, T., . . . Semple, B. (2016). Social dysfunction after pediatric traumatic brain injury: A translational perspective. *Neuroscience & Biobehavioral Reviews, 64*, 196–214.

Ryan, N., Genc, S., Beauchamp, M., Yeates, K., Hearps, S., Catroppa, C., Anderson, V., & Silk, T. (2018). White matter microstructure predicts longitudinal social cognitive outcomes after paediatric traumatic brain injury: A diffusion tensor imaging study. *Psychological Medicine. 48*(4), 679–691.

Ryan, N. P., Catroppa, C., Beare, R., Silk, T, Hearps, S., Beauchamp, M. H., Yeates, K. O., & Anderson, V. (2017). Uncovering the neuroanatomical correlates of cognitive, affective, and conative theory of mind in pediatric traumatic brain injury: A neural systems perspective. *Social Cognitive and Affective Neuroscience, 12*(9), 1414–1427.

Sands, S., Milner, J., Goldberg, J., Mukhi, V., Moliterno, J., Maxfield, C., & Wisoff, J. (2005). Quality of life and behavioral follow-up study of pediatric survivors of craniopharyngioma. *Journal of Neurosurgery, 103*, 302–311.

Saxe, R., Carey, S., & Kanwisher, N. (2004). Understanding other minds: Linking developmental psychology and functional neuroimaging. *Annual Review of Psycholog, 55*, 87–124.

Schmidt, A. T., Hanten, G. R., Li, X., Orsten, K. D., & Levin, H. S. (2010). Emotion recognition following pediatric traumatic brain injury: Longitudinal analysis of emotional prosody and facial emotion recognition. *Neuropsychologia, 48*(10), 2869–2877.

Schulte, F., & Barrera, M. (2010). Social competence in childhood brain tumor survivors: A comprehensive review. *Support Care Cancer, 18*, 1499–1513.

Schulte, F., Bouffet, E., Janzen, L., Hamilton, J., & Barrera, M. (2010). Body weight, social competence and cognitiev functioning in survivors of childhood brain tumors. *Pediatric Blood and Cancer, 55*, 532–539.

Scourfield, J., Martin, N., Lewis, G., & McGuffin, P. (1999). Heritability of social cognitive skills in children and adolescents. *British Journal of Psychiatry, 175*, 559–564.

Séguin, M., Dégeilh, F., Bernier, A., El-Jalbout, R., & Beauchamp, M. H. (2020). It's a matter of surgency: Traumatic brain injury is associated with changes in preschoolers' temperament. *Neuropsychology, 34*(4), 375–387.

Sofranas, M., Ichord, R. N., Fullerton, H. J., Lynch, J. K., Massicotee, P., Willan, A. R., . . . deVeber, G. (2006). Pediatric stroke initiatives and preliminary studies: What is knowns and what is needed? *Pediatric Neurology, 34*(6), 439–445.

Steinlin, M., Roellin, K., & Schroth, G. (2004). Long-term follow-up after stroke in childhood. *European Journal of Pediatrics, 163*, 245–250.

Taylor, H. G., Yeates, K., Wade, S., Drotar, D., Klein, S. K., & Stancin, T. (1999). Influences on first year recovery from traumatic brain injury in children. *Neuropsychology, 13*, 76–89.

Tonks, J., Williams, W. H., Frampton, I., Yates, P., & Slater, A. (2007). Reading emotions after child brain injury: A comparison between children with brain injury and non-injured controls. *Brain Injury, 21*, 731–739.

Tonks, J., Williams, W. H., Yates, P., & Slater, A. (2011). Cognitive correlates of psychosocial outcome following traumatic brain injury in early childhood: Comparisons between groups of children aged under and over 10 years of age. *Clinical Child Psychology and Psychiatry, 16*, epub.

Tousignant, B., Eugène, F., & Jackson, P. L. (2017). A developmental perspective on the neural bases of human empathy. *Infant Behavior, 48*(Pt A), 5–12.

Turkstra, L. S., Dixon, T. M., & Baker, K. K. (2004). Theory of mind and social beliefs in adolescents with traumatic brain injury. *NeuroRehabilitation, 19*, 245–256.

Turkstra, L. S., Williams, W. H., Tonks, J., & Frampton, I. (2008). Measuring social cognition in adolescents: Implications for students with TBI returning to school. *NeuroRehabilitation, 23*, 501–509.

Upton, P., & Eiser, C. (2006). School experiences after treatment for a brain tumor. *Child Care and Healthy Development, 32*, 9–17.

Vance, Y., Eiser, C., & Home, B. (2004). Parents' views of the impact of childhood brain tumors and their treatment on young people's social and family functioning. *Clinical Child Psychology and Psychiatry, 9*, 271–288.

Van Overwalle, F. (2009). Social cognition and the brain: A meta-analysis. *Human Brain Mapping, 30*, 829–858.

Varni, J., Seid, M., & Rode, C. (1999). The PedsQL: Measurement model for pediatric quality of life inventory. *Medical Care, 37*, 126–139.

Warschausky, S., Cohen, E. H., Parker, J. G., Levendosky, A. A., & Okun, A. (1997). Social problem-solving skills of children with traumatic brain injury. *Pediatric Rehabilitation, 1*, 77–81.

Yeates, K. O., Bigler, E. D., Dennis, M., Gerhardt, C. A., Rubin, K. H., Stancin, T., Taylor, H. G., & Vannatta, K. (2007). Social outcomes in childhood brain disorder: A heuristic integration of social neuroscience and developmental psychology. *Psychological Bulletin, 133*, 535–556.

Yeates, K. O., Swift, E., Taylor, H. G., Wade, S. L., Drotar, D., Stancin, T., & Minich, N. (2004). Short- and long-term social outcomes following pediatric traumatic brain injury. *Journal of the International Neuropsychological Society, 10*, 412–426.

Yeates, K. O., Taylor, H., Walz, N., Stancin, T., & Wade, S. (2010). The family environment as a moderator of psychosocial outcome following traumatic brain injury in young children. *Neuropsychology, 24*, 345–356.

Zhi, X. O., Ryan, N. P., Konjarski, M., Catroppa, C., & Stargatt, R. (in press). Social cognition in paediatric traumatic brain injury: A systematic review and meta-analysis. *Neuropsychology Reviews*.

Chapter 4

Social cognition in autism spectrum disorder and neurogenetic syndromes

Alice Maier, Nicholas P Ryan, Anita Chisholm and Jonathan M Payne

This chapter provides an overview of social cognition in individuals with autism spectrum disorder (ASD). In many ways, the bond between social cognition and ASD is unique among the clinical conditions associated with poor social cognition, as social cognitive deficits have been postulated to be primary drivers of autism symptomatology (Baron-Cohen, 1989; Frith, Morton, & Leslie, 1991; Klin, Jones, Schultz, & Volkmar, 2003; Patriquin, DeRamus, Libero, Laird, & Kana, 2016; Schultz, 2005). Apart from social (pragmatic) communication disorder, no other clinical condition in the DSM-5 holds such a theorised link between social cognition deficits and core clinical symptoms than ASD. This chapter reviews the literature on social cognition in ASD, which shows that the causal role of social cognitive deficits in ASD remains unclear and that while social cognitive deficits are prevalent in ASD, they are neither necessary nor sufficient for diagnosis. We then discuss the heterogeneity inherent in ASD, at the symptom, cognitive and aetiological levels, and conclude by outlining the value of investigating social cognition in 'subpopulations' of ASD that are caused by single-gene syndromes. These 'genetic models' of ASD offer a unique opportunity to shed light on the neurobiological and developmental processes that underpin ASD and social cognition.

Autism spectrum disorder

ASD is a neurodevelopmental disorder diagnosed on the basis of impairing behavioural symptoms, including deficits in social communication and interaction skills together with restricted interests, repetitive behaviours and sensory abnormalities (American Psychiatric Association, 2013). Symptoms required for diagnosis as per the American Psychiatric Association *Diagnostic and Statistical Manual of Mental Disorders*, (DSM-5) are presented in Table 4.1.

(American Psychiatric Association, 2013)

Importantly, DSM-5 allows for comorbid diagnoses of common clinical conditions associated with ASD, including attention deficit hyperactivity disorder (ADHD), intellectual disability, language disorders and known genetic conditions. See Box 4.1 for a vignette describing the case of Emily, illustrating some common ASD symptoms and their functional impact.

DOI: 10.4324/9781003027034-4

Table 4.1 DSM-5 Diagnostic criteria for autism spectrum disorder

A. Persistent deficits in social communication and social interaction across multiple contexts, as manifested by the following, currently or by history:
   1. Deficits in social-emotional reciprocity ranging, for example, from abnormal social approach and failure of normal back-and-forth conversation to reduced sharing of interests, emotions or affect to failure to initiate or respond to social interactions.
   2. Deficits in nonverbal communicative behaviours used for social interaction ranging, for example, from abnormal social approach and failure of normal back-and-forth conversation to reduced sharing of interests, emotions or affect to failure to initiate or respond to social interactions.
   3. Deficits in developing, maintaining, and understanding relationships, ranging, for example, from difficulties adjusting behaviour to suit various social contexts to difficulties in sharing imaginative play or in making friends to absence of interest in peers.
B. Restricted, repetitive patterns of behaviour, interests or activities, as manifested by at least two of the following, currently or by history:
   1. Stereotyped or repetitive motor movements, use of objects or speech (e.g., simple motor stereotypies, lining up toys or flipping objects, echolalia, idiosyncratic phrases).
   2. Insistence on sameness, inflexible adherence to routines, or ritualised patterns or verbal nonverbal behaviour (e.g., extreme distress at small changes, difficulties with transitions, rigid thinking patterns, greeting rituals, need to take same route or eat same food every day).
   3. Highly restricted, fixated interests that are abnormal in intensity or focus (e.g., strong attachment to or preoccupation with unusual objects, excessively circumscribed or perseverative interest).
   4. Hyper- or hyporeactivity to sensory input or unusual interests in sensory aspects of the environment (e.g., apparent indifference to pain/temperature, adverse response to specific sounds or textures, excessive smelling or touching of objects, visual fascination with lights or movement).
C. Symptoms must be present in the early developmental period (but may not become fully manifest until social demands exceed limited capacities or may be masked by learned strategies in later life).
D. Symptoms cause clinically significant impairment in social, occupational or other important areas of current functioning.
E. These disturbances are not better explained by intellectual disability (intellectual developmental disorder) or global developmental delay. Intellectual disability and autism spectrum disorder frequently co-occur; to make comorbid diagnoses of autism spectrum disorder and intellectual disability, social communication should be below that expected for general developmental level.

(American Psychiatric Association, 2013)

Box 4.1   Case 1: Emily: Young person revealing clinical heterogeneity in autism spectrum disorder

History:

Emily is a 9-year-old girl with a history of challenging behaviour, emotional dysregulation and social difficulties. Speech and language concerns were noted from 2–3 years of age and coincided with the emergence of wide-ranging and persistent motor stereotypies, including bilateral hand flapping, body rocking and rhythmic side-to-side head movements. These behaviours continued to occur daily and usually coincided with periods of excitement or fatigue. She has longstanding sensory processing difficulties, including heightened sensitivity to textures and sounds.

Current symptoms/functional impact:

Emily is in Grade 4. Her teachers indicate that she rarely initiates social interaction with peers and prefers playing alone. She does not consistently understand social cues and tends to ignore classmates' attempts to engage her. Recently, she has become increasingly distressed in anticipation of social events involving unfamiliar children (e.g., school camps). Her anxiety often culminates in school refusal and self-harming on the day of the scheduled event (e.g., punching herself in the chest). Emily experiences marked distress when expected to wear socks and shoes and will often try on five different pairs in the morning. She often wears earmuffs at public events (e.g., school assemblies). Emily has a strong interest in collecting seashells. At the beach, she becomes highly distressed unless given the opportunity to remove every seashell from the dunes. Her bedtime routine involves repeatedly checking that her seashell collection is 'safely' stored under her bed.

Neuropsychological evaluation:

On assessment, Emily's overall intellectual functioning was average (*61st percentile*). Speech and language testing revealed age-appropriate receptive oral language skills but mild impairment in expressive oral language skills. Evaluation of social cognitive abilities revealed difficulties labelling basic facial emotions (*5th percentile*) and inferring what others' might be thinking or feeling (*10th percentile*). On the Autism Diagnostic Observation Schedule (ADOS-2), Emily displayed poorly modulated eye contact and did not direct facial expression toward the examiner. She exhibited poor insight into typical social situations, limited understanding of others' emotions. She made negligible social overtures and showed difficulty following conversational leads.

Prevalence rates of ASD are estimated at ~1–2% (M. C. Lai, Lombardo, & Baron-Cohen, 2014; Maenner, Shaw, & Baio, 2020). There is a well-established sex bias in favour of males, with estimates ranging from a 2.6:1 to a 5.2:1 male to female ratio (D. L. Christensen et al., 2019; Loomes, Hull, & Mandy, 2017).

The male predominance in ASD may be associated with sex-specific factors that confer increased genomic risk. For example, foetal testosterone is implicated in multiple stages of development and may interact with neurotransmitter, neuropeptide and immune pathways to increase male vulnerability (Ferri, Abel, & Brodkin, 2018). Non-biological factors may also contribute to the observed sex effect. For example, it has been suggested that females are better equipped to employ behavioural compensatory strategies, leading to differential expression of core ASD symptoms that go undetected in girls (Hull, Petrides, & Mandy, 2020; Van Wijngaarden-Cremers et al., 2014).

Family studies consistently provide evidence for a strong genetic basis for ASD. Heritability estimates typically range from 0.5 to 0.9, with twin studies indicating consistently increased concordance rates in monozygotic versus dizygotic twins (Garg & Green, 2018; Tick, Bolton, Happé, Rutter, & Rijsdijk, 2016). Several environmental risk factors for ASD have also been identified. These include advanced parental age (Janecka et al., 2017), birth complications (Modabbernia, Velthorst, & Reichenberg, 2017), premature birth (Williamson & Jakobson, 2014) and prenatal exposure to toxins including sodium valproate (J. Christensen et al., 2013). Notably, no environmental factors have been shown to be necessary (nor sufficient) for the development of ASD. Rather, they are considered to impart their effects in complex gene x environment interactions that subsequently result in ASD (Garg & Green, 2018; Modabbernia et al., 2017).

Psychological and social cognitive explanations of ASD

Traditional heuristics attempting to describe the neurodevelopmental mechanisms that contribute to ASD offer at least four inter-related levels of analysis (Joseph, 1999; Morton & Frith, 1995) consisting of: (1) *aetiology*, including genetic and environmental factors that underlie abnormal neurodevelopment; (2) *neurobiological processes*, which impact on normal brain development and function; (3) *social and domain-general cognitive processes*, an intermediary level of analysis that mediates the relationship between brain and behaviour; and (4) the *behaviours and symptoms* that arise from these brain abnormalities and associated cognitive deficits. From a clinical perspective, both genetic and environmental factors contribute to structural and functional brain abnormalities, which cause cognitive deficits that manifest as behavioural symptoms (see Figure 4.1).

Psychological theories traditionally stem from the assumption that cognitive abnormalities represent key mechanisms underlying the behavioural symptoms of ASD. According to these theories, abnormal cognitive processing offers a unifying explanation for the clinical presentation of ASD. In the following section, we evaluate three key psychological theories of ASD, including social cognitive theory.

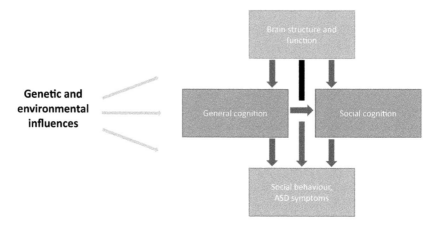

Figure 4.1 A simplified causal model

Source: Adapted from Coghill and colleagues (2005) and Morton and Frith (1995)

The executive function theory

Executive function (EF) is an umbrella term for a range of sophisticated cognitive processes that support high-level problem-solving and enable us to coordinate our thoughts, emotions and behaviour (Diamond, 2013). These skills, which include inhibitory control, planning and self-monitoring (Anderson, Jacobs, & Anderson, 2010), are essential for managing the complex dynamics of interpersonal relationships. The EF theory of ASD argues that executive dysfunction contributes to reduced initiation of social approach, poor attention and orientation to social cues, an inability to inhibit socially inappropriate behaviours and a reduced capacity to flexibly adjust behaviour. These deficits are then hypothesised to independently, or interactively, give rise to behavioural features of ASD (Brunsdon & Happé, 2014; Hill, 2004; Hughes & Russell, 1993; Ozonoff, Rogers, & Pennington, 1991). An appealing feature of this theory is that it not only provides an account for some of the social communication symptoms of ASD but an inability to shift mental set and a tendency to perseverate may also explain some of the restricted interests and repetitive behaviours associated with ASD (Lopez, Lincoln, Ozonoff, & Lai, 2005).

Group level studies suggest ASD is associated with impairments across multiple subdomains of EF. A recent meta-analysis of involving 5,991 individuals (N ASD = 2,986; N healthy controls = 3,005) found those with ASD were moderately impaired in verbal working memory (Hedges' $g = 0.67$), spatial working memory (Hedges' $g = 0.58$), flexibility (Hedges' $g = 0.59$), planning (Hedges' $g = 0.62$), and generativity (Hedges' $g = 0.60$)(C. L. E. Lai et al., 2017). After taking comorbid ADHD and general cognitive abilities into account, impairments in flexibility (Hedges' g = 0.57–0.61), generativity (Hedges' g = 0.52–0.68), and working memory (Hedges' g = 0.49–0.56) remained significant. Others have likewise reported a moderate overall effect size (Hedges' g = 0.48) for a global EF deficit in 14,081 individuals (N ASD = 6,816), with small to moderate effect sizes also apparent across separate executive subdomains (Demetriou et al., 2018). However, despite evidence that EF impairments are present at the group level, there is substantial inconsistency in these findings, with specific EF deficits noted in some studies but not others (Hill, 2004). These findings underscore significant individual variability in EF not fully accounted for in group level analyses (Geurts, Sinzig, Booth, & Happé, 2014). Studies on the association between EF and ASD symptoms also yield inconsistent findings. Although some show that executive dysfunction (e.g., poor initiation, planning, organising) explains significant variance in ASD symptoms (Leung, Vogan, Powell, Anagnostou, & Taylor, 2016; Lopez et al., 2005; Pellicano, 2013), these findings are not universal (Cantio, Jepsen, Madsen, Bilenberg, & White, 2016; Jones et al., 2018; Joseph, 1999). Indeed, recent meta-analytic evidence suggests laboratory tests of EF have limited clinical utility in differentiating between ASD and typical controls (Demetriou et al., 2018).

The central coherence theory

Another key psychological theory argues that a 'weak central coherence' contributes to the behavioural symptoms of individuals with ASD. Central coherence refers to the cognitive process of integrating pieces of information into a meaningful whole. According to this model, individuals with ASD have an information processing bias favouring detailed attention to 'local/featural' aspects of objects and situations, at the expense of integrating information into a meaningful, global gestalt (Booth & Happé, 2018; Frith, 1989; Frith & Happé, 1994; Happé & Frith, 2006). This theory has been used to explain why some individuals with ASD excel at tasks in which high attention to detail is advantageous (Happé, 1994b; Jolliffe & Baron-Cohen, 1997). The framework has also been used as an explanation for the circumscribed interests and repetitive behaviours that characterise ASD, including an increased need for sameness and the reduced ability to generalise information (Booth & Happé, 2018; Happé & Frith, 2006). A weak central coherence has also been used to account for the characteristic social difficulties of individuals with ASD. For instance, overly detailed processing of specific aspects of facial features might plausibly compromise overall recognition of a facial emotion, thereby impacting the ability to generate a meaningful understanding of social behaviour (Happé & Frith, 2006). Indeed, it has been suggested that individuals with ASD favour feature-based, as opposed to configurable processing strategies during facial recognition tasks (Dawson, Webb, & McPartland, 2005) and neutral stimuli viewing paradigms (Vlamings, Jonkman, Van Daalen, Van Der Gaag, & Kemner, 2010).

The weak central coherence theory has received mixed support (Joseph, 1999). Although there is some confirmatory evidence (Burnette et al., 2005; Neufeld et al., 2020), other research does not support the theory (Henderson, Clarke, & Snowling, 2011; López & Leekam, 2003). Furthermore, the relationship between weak central coherence and core ASD symptoms remains unclear. Although some observe no association between weak central coherence and social skills (Morgan, Maybery, & Durkin, 2003), others have documented a link between central coherence and the ability to infer the beliefs, intentions and emotional states of others; a high-level social cognitive skill termed 'theory of mind' (Skorich et al., 2016).

Social cognitive theories

Social cognitive theories differ from domain-general cognitive theories in their premise that intrinsic, domain-specific weaknesses in social cognition underpin the social interaction and communication deficits in ASD. Social cognition refers to the mental processes that enable a person to recognise, understand and behave fluidly with respect to socially relevant stimuli (Adolphs, 2001). While a widely accepted model of social cognition is not yet established, there are a growing number of heuristics incorporating lower- and higher-level social cognitive processes and their relationships to neural networks (Adolphs, 2001; Blakemore, 2008).

Lower-level social cognitive skills include the processes by which socially relevant stimuli and signals are received by an individual. These include both reflexive and intentional behaviours that involve orienting gaze to socially rich information such as faces (especially the eyes and mouth) and the physical movements of social partners (e.g., non-verbal communicative behaviours such as gestures). Higher-level social cognitive skills then enable individuals to process social information received at the 'input perception level' and use it to take the perspective of others. This process is thought to enable individuals to experience empathy, predict what others are thinking and guide future behaviour (D'Arc & Mottron, 2012). Neurobiological models of social behaviour extend these frameworks by proposing that low- and high-level social cognitive abilities are controlled by a complex 'social brain' network (see Figure 4.2) (Adolphs, 1999, 2001; Blakemore, 2008).

Both lower-level social perception and higher-level social cognitive skills are assumed to be causally linked during typical development, with the formation of basic social perceptual skills during childhood providing the necessary experiences and building blocks for higher social skill development across the lifespan (Schultz, 2005). It is intuitive that aberrant perception of social stimuli has downstream consequences for the ability to discern changes in body language and social cues, and to rapidly formulate and execute appropriate social responses. According to social cognitive theories, this process is derailed in ASD with social perception skills failing to emerge in a typical fashion during

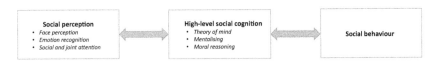

Figure 4.2 A simplified model of the key components involved in social processing. Brain regions in the temporal lobe, such as the fusiform gyrus
and superior temporal sulcus, are critical for social perception. These
regions work together with a network of interconnected structures
including the amygdala, prefrontal and orbitofrontal cortices, cingulate cortices and insula in order to process higher-level social cognitive information. This network modulates effector and emotion
output systems, which in turn enable mentalising, social and moral
reasoning and appropriate social behaviour. Abnormal brain development and/or function within the network causes social dysfunction.

Source: Adapted from Adolphs (2001, 2009)

critical developmental windows, imparting a cascade of consequences for later
social cognitive development, leading to the social communication symptoms
associated with ASD.

Low-level social cognitive skills: social perception

Substantial research indicates abnormalities in the way individuals with ASD
perceive social stimuli, including faces and emotions. Commonly described
deficits include reduced eye contact, abnormal gaze following and poor orientation to faces (Klin, Jones, Schultz, Volkmar, & Cohen, 2002; Webb et al.,
2017), together with impairments in discrimination, recognition and memory
for faces and emotions (Bi & Fang, 2017; Dawson et al., 2005; Nomi & Uddin,
2015; Vlamings et al., 2010). However, akin to EF and weak central coherence
theories, these observations are not universal. For example, there are conditions in which those with ASD may exhibit similar performances to typically
developing individuals (Jemel, Mottron, & Dawson, 2006). Moreover, while
facial processing abnormalities commonly occur across the lifespan in ASD, the
nature and extent of these deficits varies significantly between individuals and
are impacted by interrelated factors including age, overall functioning and task
demands (Webb, Neuhaus, & Faja, 2017).

Emotion recognition research in ASD has also yielded mixed results. Early
studies suggested a fundamental deficit in facial emotional processing such as
reduced accuracy and longer reaction times compared with typically developing individuals. However, these findings have been challenged by larger, better
powered, studies (Jones et al., 2011) and reviews (Harms, Martin, & Wallace,
2010). Overall, research continues to indicate a degree of emotion recognition difficulty in ASD with facial affect recognition deficits across a range of

emotions that are not better explained by deficits in domain-general intellectual abilities (Lozier, Vanmeter, & Marsh, 2014; Uljarevic & Hamilton, 2013).

Another critical social perceptual skill involves the capacity to focus attention to the movements of social partners (i.e., biological motion). Humans are highly sensitive to the movements of others, and preferential attention to biological motion is observed within the first few days of life (Simion, Regolin, & Bulf, 2008). This interest in social partners is thought to play a foundational role in the development of social communicative skills (Pavlova, 2012). Recent meta-analyses suggest a moderate deficit in the perception and interpretation of biological motion in ASD, although heterogeneity in these behaviours is also observed (Federici et al., 2020). Drawing firm conclusions regarding the role of biological motion in ASD remains difficult due to substantial differences in sample characteristics and study paradigms employed across research studies (Todorova, Hatton, & Pollick, 2019). Future work is required to establish the role of orientation to biological motion in ASD and the social cognitive and communicative deficits that characterise the disorder.

A plethora of neuroimaging studies have emerged that examine neuroanatomical markers of atypical social cognitive processes in ASD. Regions of interest include the *amygdala, fusiform gyrus* and *superior temporal gyrus*, which form part of the 'social brain' network and are hypothesised to play an important role in detecting and responding to emotional expressions (Adolphs, 2008; Basil, Westwater, Wiener, & Thompson, 2017; Hoffman & Haxby, 2000). Indeed, early studies indicated selective abnormalities in these regions in ASD individuals compared to typically developing controls (Pelphrey, Adolphs, & Morris, 2004).

Meta-analyses continue to suggest different activation patterns in neural systems implicated in social perceptive processes between ASD and typically developing individuals, including the *posterior superior temporal sulcus at the temporoparietal junction, middle frontal gyrus, fusiform face area, inferior frontal gyrus, amygdala, insula* and *cingulate cortex* (Di Martino et al., 2009; Patriquin et al., 2016). However, there is marked variability in findings between studies, and firm conclusions about specific brain-behaviour relationships in ASD remain elusive. For example, studies investigating the *amygdala* and *superior temporal sulcus* in ASD have reported both hypo- and hyper-activation in ASD individuals (D'Arc & Mottron, 2012; Di Martino et al., 2009; Jemel et al., 2006; Nomi & Uddin, 2015; Pelphrey et al., 2004). Moreover, some studies have demonstrated similar activation patterns in social brain regions in both healthy control and ASD groups on a range of tasks including passive viewing of faces (Hadjikhani et al., 2004), gender discrimination (Pierce, Haist, Sedaghat, & Courchesne, 2004) and emotion labelling (Piggot et al., 2004).

Mixed findings in this area may be explained by methodological differences, including the use of variable combinations of tasks assessing different permutations of facial expressions/emotions. A further complicating factor is that many behavioural studies rely on younger (often lower functioning) individuals, whereas neuroimaging protocols typically recruit older and higher functioning participants who can comply with the demands of neuroimaging paradigms (Nomi & Uddin, 2015). A related and plausible explanation is that the heterogeneity in neuroimaging findings is partly accounted for by between- and within-group differences in overall ASD symptom severity, as well as differences in social cognitive and domain-general abilities. For example, a recent fMRI study indicated that more severe ASD symptoms resulted in less face-related activation in the *fusiform face area* (a neural region linked to facial processing in healthy individuals) in adolescents with ASD (Scherf, Elbich, Minshew, & Behrmann, 2015). Unfortunately, many studies do not report on the clinical severity of ASD symptoms and fail to document key sample characteristics that may mediate relationships between brain and behaviour, including domain-general or social cognitive abilities (Jemel et al., 2006; Uljarevic & Hamilton, 2013).

Higher level social cognitive skills: mentalisation and theory of mind

Perhaps the most influential social cognitive theory of ASD is the theory of mind deficit model. Theory of mind (ToM) refers to the capacity to understand the mental states of others and oneself, including knowledge, beliefs, intentions and emotions (Baron-Cohen, 2001; Happé, 1994a). This sophisticated cognitive skill is thought to be responsible for the ability to comprehend and predict another person's behaviour and is often referred to as 'mentalising' (Frith et al., 1991). According to this theory, social communication deficits in ASD arise from a ToM deficit, which impedes the ability of the individual to form appropriate social responses and to successfully engage in social interactions (Baron-Cohen, 1989; Frith et al., 1991).

Classical ToM tasks involve presenting a narrative in which a character holds a belief (e.g. object location) inconsistent with reality (e.g. actual object location). Task success requires participants to draw inferences about the behaviour of the characters holding incorrect information. Early studies provided evidence that individuals with ASD typically exhibited deficits on ToM tasks, compared to age and IQ matched controls (Baron-Cohen, 1989; Baron-Cohen et al., 1985; Frith et al., 1991). More sophisticated ToM assessment tools have since been developed (see Chapter 9), due to the finding that older and higher-functioning ASD participants often demonstrate intact performances on traditional false-belief paradigms. Using these and similar tasks, many studies continue to provide evidence of ToM deficits in ASD individuals (Beaumont & Sofronoff, 2008; Senju, 2012; White, Hill, Happé, & Frith, 2009). The neuroimaging literature also supports the notion of aberrant ToM development in ASD. For example, functional neuroimaging studies have observed that adults with ASD demonstrate hypoactivation of neural regions thought to be responsible for mentalising during social tasks in typically developing individuals

(Castelli, Frith, Happé, & Frith, 2002; Di Martino et al., 2009; Molenberghs, Johnson, Henry, & Mattingley, 2016).

While many individuals with ASD experience difficulty attributing mental states to themselves or to others, this finding is not universal. In most studies at least *some* ASD participants successfully pass false belief tasks (Scheeren, De Rosnay, Koot, & Begeer, 2013; Spek, Scholte, & Van Berckelaer-Onnes, 2010; Tager-Flusberg, 2007). This raises the question of the capacity for ToM to reliably predict the social communication symptoms inherent in ASD. While substantial research has documented associations between ToM deficits and social problems (De Rosnay, Fink, Begeer, Slaughter, & Peterson, 2014; Jones et al., 2018; Mazza et al., 2017), others have failed to replicate these relationships (Bennett et al., 2013; Cantio et al., 2016; Wilson et al., 2014). A further complication is that laboratory based ToM task performances often fail to demonstrate significant correspondences with 'real world' applications of the ability (Barendse, Hendriks, Thoonen, Aldenkamp, & Kessels, 2018). As a simple illustration, while children with ASD are often rated as less empathetic than typically developing peers, this appears unrelated to their ToM development (Peterson, 2014).

Inconsistencies in research findings regarding ToM in ASD are likely due to multiple factors including diverse sample characteristics, small sample sizes, and variability in the testing paradigms employed between studies. Other explanations include the fact that higher functioning individuals with ASD may develop compensatory strategies to bolster ToM performances (Livingston, Colvert, Bolton, & Happé, 2019). Notably, successful ToM task performance hinges on skills in other general cognitive domains (e.g., attention, language). Apparent ToM task failure may therefore reflect a breakdown in any one of these domain-general cognitive abilities. For example, many ToM tasks require the inhibition of a response based on one's own belief. They therefore rely, at least partly, on intact EF skills (Brunsdon & Happé, 2014; Joseph, 1999). A further consideration is that most ToM tasks assess explicit ToM (the ability to answer direct questions about another person's belief state), which may not reflect an individual's ability to implicitly apply mentalising skills in complex social interactions or their motivation to do so (Chevallier, Kohls, Troiani, Brodkin, & Schultz, 2012; Senju, 2013). Notably, many commonly used measures exhibit weak reliability (Hayward & Homer, 2017), and relationships between measures assumed to be evaluating the same social cognitive skill are often poor (Söderstrand & Almkvist, 2012). For example, correlations between the 'eyes test' and other ToM tests (e.g., strange stories and Faux Pas task) have been shown to be low or absent (Spek et al., 2010). See Chapter 9 for further discussion of this issue.

Overall, while domain-general cognitive and specific social cognitive abnormalities are common in ASD, their prevalence, diversity and severity remain unclear, as do their relationships with primary symptoms of the disorder. Certainly, the literature does not point to simplistic causal relationships between any of these factors, central ASD symptoms and neurobiological substrates. For deficit theories to be convincing explanatory models of primary symptoms, dysfunctions must be universal features of the condition, which does not appear to be the case, and a single causal explanation for ASD seems increasingly unlikely (Happé, Ronald, & Plomin, 2006). This viewpoint aligns with research into other neurodevelopmental conditions, showing that although cognitive abnormalities often accompany clinical features of the disorders, they are neither necessary nor sufficient to cause symptoms required for diagnosis, nor are they reliable predictors of level of functional impairment (Coghill, Hayward, Rhodes, Grimmer, & Matthews, 2014; Payne et al., 2019).

Heterogeneity of ASD at symptom and aetiological levels: the challenge for research

A significant challenge for research into social cognition in ASD is the fact that most studies analyse group-level data and employ between-subject study designs. These investigations are limited in their capacity to account for the vast heterogeneity of ASD features. The primary diagnostic symptoms of ASD can manifest in a myriad of different behavioural combinations. Furthermore, there are numerous clinical comorbidities associated with the disorder including sensory sensitivities, hyperactivity and impulsivity, attention problems, mood disturbance and intellectual disability (Vannucchi et al., 2014). In addition to symptom diversity, the clinical severity of these comorbidities also varies substantially. While some individuals with ASD exhibit intellectual disability together with severe social and communication impairments, others display above average intellectual function, fluent language and only mildly compromised social skills (Charman et al., 2010; Chiang, Tsai, Cheung, Brown, & Li, 2014; Georgiades et al., 2013; Maenner et al., 2020). This variability may explain, at least in part, why the causal models discussed above are limited in their ability to reliably predict individual profiles of social cognitive abilities in ASD. While these frameworks make intuitive sense, they rest on the assumption that the behavioural features of ASD are the consequence of single underlying factors (e.g., theory of mind deficits; executive dysfunction) that are consistent across individuals with the disorder. If there is anything that the research on ASD has demonstrated conclusively, it is that the presentation of ASD is far from uniform, and that the disorder may represent not one, but many different 'spectrums' (Ure, Rose, Bernie, & Williams, 2018).

Heterogeneity in the presentation and severity of ASD symptoms is equalled by the vast polygenic and environmental risk factors that play a role in the pathogenesis of the disorder. In addition to the environmental risk factors covered earlier, hundreds of candidate genes have been identified as playing a role in the development of ASD (Betancur, 2011; O'Roak et al., 2012; Ramaswami & Geschwind, 2018). Contributions from alleles of varying frequency and type (e.g., common vs rare, large chromosomal rearrangements, copy number variations, small insertions/deletions, and single-nucleotide variants) have been implicated, although the strength of these associations vary (Masi, DeMayo, Glozier, & Guastella, 2017; Vithayathil, Pucilowska, & Landreth, 2018). This research demonstrates that the genetic architecture of ASD is undoubtedly as complex and diverse as its behavioural expression.

Importantly, while many genetic risk factors have been implicated in ASD, the exact genetic aetiology is unknown in ~85% of cases (Casanova et al., 2020). In these 'idiopathic' cases, ASD is thought to arise from a dynamic inter-action of genetic and non-genetic factors (Garg & Green, 2018). Accordingly, there are likely multiple aetiological and neurodevelopmental pathways to ASD (Toma, 2020). This aetiological complexity poses several challenges to clinical research, including the difficulties associated with stratifying samples based on common genetic/environmental factors (Garg & Green, 2018). The challenge now facing researchers is in linking the highly heterogeneous genotype of ASD with its equally striking differences in phenotype, including social cognition.

Genetic models of ASD and social cognition

To overcome the complexities and methodological challenges that arise from heterogeneous disorders like ASD, some research groups are shifting their attention to studying monogenic ('syndromic') forms of ASD. These account for ~5–10% of ASD cases (Garg & Green, 2018; Ramaswami & Geschwind, 2018; Vithayathil et al., 2018), and refer to cases of ASD that arise in the con-text of a known medical syndrome caused by genetic mutations (Abrahams & Geschwind, 2010; Fernandez & Scherer, 2017). Because the genetic 'blue-print' is identifiable in these cases, they offer the opportunity to systematically explore behavioural phenotypes that occur due to homologous aetiologies. Syndromes that have attracted significant attention to date include Williams syndrome, Fragile X, and Neurofibromatosis Type 1. These disorders and their profiles of social cognition are discussed in brief below.

Williams syndrome

Williams syndrome (WS) arises from the deletion of ~25 genes at chromo-some 7q11.23 (Dai et al., 2009) and has a prevalence of approximately 1 in 7,500 (Strømme, Bjømstad, & Ramstad, 2002). Most individuals with WS meet criteria for an intellectual disability and mean IQ typically falls around 55 (Pober, 2010). Specific cognitive deficits such as poor visuospatial ability, inattentiveness, reduced inhibitory control and increased distractibility are common (Gray & Cornish, 2012; Pober, 2010). While initial studies indicated relatively preserved language skills in WS, these views have been challenged by others showing that although vocabulary knowledge can be high in WS, it is rarely age appropriate and often characterised by shallow semantics (Karmiloff-Smith, 2007). Social problems are frequent in WS, and approximately 50%

of individuals meet criteria for ASD (Garg & Green, 2018). Interestingly, the social behaviour profile diverges substantially from idiopathic ASD. Core behavioural features of WS include *increased* social approach towards strangers, over-familiarity and social disinhibition (Pober, 2010). Despite this 'hyper-socialiabilty', WS individuals experience significant difficulties maintaining friendships and often suffer from marked anxiety in social situations (Järvinen, Korenberg, & Bellugi, 2013).

The behavioural profile in WS is thought to reflect a distinct social cognitive phenotype, characterised by social attentional and emotional processing biases. Compared to typically developing controls, individuals with WS display a greater preference for faces than non-social stimuli. This is often reflected by prolonged fixation on eye regions (Järvinen et al., 2013). Coupled with this increased attention and orientation towards faces/eyes is a distinct profile of emotion processing biases in WS. Individuals with WS consistently exhibit decreased recognition of negative social signals across visual and auditory domains, and attentional and processing biases in favour of positive social stimuli (Dodd & Porter, 2010; Plesa-Skwerer, Faja, Schofield, Verbalis, & Tager-Flusberg, 2006). Initially, the social cognitive profile of WS seems at odds with that of idiopathic ASD, which has historically been associated with *asocial* behaviour and poor orientation to facial stimuli and eyes. However, several commonalities have also been documented between idiopathic ASD and WS. For example, both share deficits in joint attention (Vivanti, Fanning, Hocking, Sievers,& Dissanayake, 2017), pragmatic language (Philofsky, Fidler, & Hepburn, 2007) and social reasoning (Porter, Coltheart, & Langdon, 2008; Tager-Flusberg & Sullivan, 2000). Social behaviours in idiopathic ASD and WS may, therefore, be viewed as both reflecting atypical social cognition together with abnormal patterns of social motivation (which are typically reduced in idiopathic ASD but enhanced in WS). While seemingly opposite, both profiles nonetheless have impairing functional social consequences (Vivanti, Hamner, & Lee, 2018).

There is ongoing debate as to whether the social problems observed in WS arise from specific social cognitive impairments or general cognitive deficits secondarily impacting on social skills. Functional neuroimaging studies suggest hypoactivation of the *amygdala* in response to threatening social stimuli in individuals with WS (Haas et al., 2009; Vivanti et al., 2018). Individuals with WS also exhibit increased autonomic arousal in response to happy faces compared to typically developing controls, suggesting that social stimuli are excessively salient and rewarding for them (Järvinen et al., 2015). One plausible inference of these studies is that individuals with WS interpret the social world as less threatening and excessively rewarding, perhaps contributing to increased and undiscerning social drive and naivety. Alternatively, their social behavioural profile may be partly explained by domain-general executive dysfunction such as poor sustained attention and inhibitory control (Rhodes, Riby, Matthews, & Coghill, 2011; Vivanti et al., 2017, 2018). While too early to establish causal relationships, existing research suggests that individuals with

WS are at increased risk of impaired social skills associated with both social cognitive and domain-general cognitive deficits.

Fragile X

Fragile X syndrome (FXS) is a monogenic disorder, with a prevalence rate of approximately 1 in 5,000 males and 1 in 4,000 to 1 in 8,000 females, caused by the silencing of the *FMR1* gene on the X chromosome at q27.3 (Hagerman et al., 2017). This genetic abnormality results in a reduction (or loss) of the protein FMRP, which is essential for synaptic growth and is therefore critical for learning and neurodevelopment. Most males with FXS display developmental delay and an IQ within the mild to severe range of intellectual disability (Gray & Cornish, 2012; Niu et al., 2017). Girls with FXS demonstrate a more variable clinical presentation due to having an unaffected X chromosome (Hagerman et al., 2017). In both sexes, however, cognitive and behavioural profiles are marked by significant attentional impairments, language delays, executive dysfunction and anxiety (Hagerman et al., 2017; Van der Molen et al., 2010). Social impairments are well documented within the FXS population and tend to include high levels of social withdrawal, avoidance of eye gaze and social awkwardness (Cornish, Gray, & Rinehart, 2010; Hagerman et al., 2017; Morel et al., 2018; Niu et al., 2017).

FXS represents one of the few, known, single gene causes of ASD. Up to 75% of boys and 25% of girls with FXS exhibit broader ASD features (Klusek, Martin, & Losh, 2014), and 21–47% of individuals meet criteria for ASD (Garg & Green, 2018). Like WS, ASD presentation in FXS appears to differ to that seen in the idiopathic population. For instance, while children with FXS exhibit reduced social skills, they are more likely to display reciprocal relationships than idiopathic ASD counterparts (Cornish et al., 2010; Gray & Cornish, 2012). Indeed, individuals with FXS and comorbid ASD are more likely than individuals with idiopathic ASD to have at least one friend (32% vs 7% respectively; Smith, Barker, Seltzer, Abbeduto, & Greenberg, 2012). Furthermore, those with FXS and comorbid ASD may display less severe social and communication symptoms and seem more responsive to social overtures than those with idiopathic ASD. Interestingly, one research group found that boys with FXS were more likely to smile in social situations than age and symptom-severity matched boys with idiopathic ASD (McDuffie, Thurman, Hagerman, & Abbeduto, 2015). Compared to idiopathic ASD controls, children with FXS and ASD also exhibit less impairment on measures of social behaviour, including gaze integration, quality of social overtures, social smiles, facial expressions and response to joint attention (Wolff et al., 2012). Wolff and colleagues (2012) also found that children with FXS differed in the expressions of restricted interests and repetitive behaviours, with FXS individuals showing lower rates of compulsive and ritual behaviours than those with idiopathic ASD.

Regardless of the presence of a comorbid ASD diagnosis, FXS is characterised by social impairment. While it has been argued that these difficulties are associated with underlying social cognitive deficits, research in this area is limited and the findings are variable. While earlier research suggested that basic emotion identification was intact in individuals with FXS, this view has been recently challenged (Morel et al., 2018). Later studies showed that relative to mental and chronological age-matched controls, FXS groups perform more poorly on emotion recognition tasks and exhibit a bias towards processing negative emotion (Burris et al., 2017; Crawford et al., 2015; Shaw & Porter, 2013; Williams, Porter, & Langdon, 2014).

While higher-level social cognitive processes such as ToM may also be impaired in children with FXS (Gray & Cornish, 2012; Morel et al., 2018), some speculate that these deficits may be less severe than those observed in idiopathic ASD (Cornish et al., 2005) and potentially attributable to domain-general cognitive/intellectual impairments. One study compared two groups of boys with FXS (a group with few ASD features and a group with severe ASD features) to a control group of children with intellectual disability (Grant, Apperly, & Oliver, 2007). The pattern of performances in both FXS groups were suggestive of ToM deficits secondary to information processing and working memory problems. Another research group compared 20 girls with FXS to age matched typically developing peers on tasks of social cognition (Turkstra, Abbeduto, & Meulenbroek, 2014). While significant between-group differences in social cognition were observed, these effects were largely driven by differences in IQ, EF, and language, which accounted for 54–69% of variance on social cognitive test performances.

Research into social cognition in FXS and WS is challenged by the fact that most individuals with these conditions present with substantial domain-general cognitive impairments (e.g., significant intellectual disability), making it difficult to disentangle low intellectual functioning from specific social cognitive deficits. Additional considerations include comorbidities (e.g., anxiety) that likely contribute to the social difficulties observed in these syndromes (Williams et al., 2014). Unfortunately, many studies do not account for comorbidities, and often employ heterogeneous social outcome measures, making it difficult to synthesise results across studies (Morel et al., 2018).

Neurofibromatosis Type 1

With a prevalence rate of 1 in 2,700, NF1 is one of the most common genetic conditions impacting the central nervous system (Evans et al., 2010). It is caused by loss of function mutations within the *NF1* gene, which encodes the protein neurofibromin. In NF1, reduced neurofibromin expression increases rat sarcoma (RAS) activity, which positively regulates the Mitogen-Activated Protein Kinase (MAPK) signalling cascade. Hyperactivation of the

RAS-MAPK signalling cascade results in the key clinical manifestation of the condition – tumours (Gutmann et al., 2017). NF1 also affects brain development (Payne et al., 2010). While not part of the diagnostic criteria, cognitive and behavioural deficits are arguably the most common complication of NF1 in childhood. While overall IQ tends to fall in the lower bounds of the normal range, specific deficits in attention, EF, visuoperception and language impact up to 80% of NF1 children (Hyman, Shores, & North, 2005; Lehtonen Howie, Trump, & Huson, 2013; Payne et al., 2019; Plasschaert et al., 2016). These deficits contribute to elevated rates of neurodevelopmental comorbidities including ADHD (Mautner, Kluwe, Thakker, & Leark, 2002) and specific learning disorders (Arnold, Barton, McArthur, North, & Payne, 2016; Watt, Shores, & North, 2008), resulting in functional impairments and reduced quality of life (Payne et al., 2019).

Like WS and FXS, NF1 is associated with social dysfunction and elevated ASD risk. Unlike these conditions, however, IQ is usually relatively well preserved in NF1, making it easier to model relationships between cognitive factors and ASD symptoms. Indeed, there is increasing evidence to suggest that NF1 presents with a unique social phenotype, and possibly, a specific ASD symptom profile. This emerging research holds promise in terms of drawing clearer links between ASD symptoms, social and domain-general cognitive deficits and specific biological pathways affected by mutations of *NF1*. The final sections of this chapter discuss emerging research into the social phenotype of NF1 and the implications of these findings for the development of precision medicine-based therapeutics.

Social dysfunction and ASD prevalence in NF1

Poor social outcomes are well documented in NF1 literature, with recent meta-analytic evidence from Chisholm and colleagues (2018) suggesting a large effect of lower social functioning in NF1 (N=1093; 518 healthy controls; Hedges' $g = 0.79$) and ASD symptoms (N=1277; 657 healthy controls; Hedges' $g = 0.91$). Included in this meta-analysis were data from the International NF1-ASD Consortium Team (INFACT; Morris et al., 2016) who pooled autism symptom ratings from six tertiary sites (NF1 N = 531) and found that 39% of individuals scored above the clinical cut-off scores on parent-reported ASD symptom trait questionnaires (Social Responsiveness Scale; SRS-2; total T score ≥ 60). Studies investigating the prevalence of ASD in NF1 using diagnostic instruments have returned similar estimates of ASD prevalence (~11–25%) in children with NF1 (Eijk et al., 2018; Garg et al., 2013; Plasschaert et al., 2015), rates much higher than the 1–2% estimated in the general population (M. C. Lai et al., 2014).

Anecdotally, children with NF1 are commonly described as friendly and willing to engage with others. Nevertheless, they display significant difficulties maintaining friendships and are often described as social 'floaters' with problems 'picking up' social cues. On parent rated questionnaires of prosocial skills (e.g., communication skills, cooperation, empathy) children with NF1 exhibit a moderate deficit relative to population norms (Payne et al., 2020). They also tend to be rated by their parents as being less popular and less likely to have close friends (Lewis, Porter, Wiliams, North, & Payne, 2016). At least 24.7% report daily bullying at school (Holland et al., 2019). Teachers also perceive children with NF1 as having poorer leadership abilities and as being more sensitive and isolated than classmate controls (Noll et al., 2007). These difficulties persist across the lifespan with consequent impacts on adaptive functioning, quality of life and well-being (Payne et al., 2020). Compared to controls, significantly more individuals with NF1 report workplace bullying (13% versus 5%; Fjermestad, 2019) and evidence suggests poor mental health outcomes in adults with NF1 (D. L. Wang et al., 2012).

Several research groups have sought to characterise profiles of social impairment in NF1 using subscale items from parent-rated questionnaires of ASD symptoms, although findings have been variable (Chisholm et al., 2018). One possibility for the mixed findings is that screening tools designed to assess ASD behaviour may lose some of their specificity in syndromic forms of ASD, such as NF1. Indeed there is evidence that popular ASD screening instruments (including the SRS and the Social Communication Questionnaire; SCQ) lose some of their specificity in syndromic forms of ASD, including FXS (Kidd et al., 2020). Interestingly, Kidd and colleagues found that, by adjusting questionnaires to remove non-discriminating/low validity items, the psychometric properties of the tools improved for an FXS population. There is a need for similar investigative work in NF1, which may facilitate more accurate ASD phenotyping in NF1, and potentially improve the predictive power of commonly used ASD screening tools in this population. See Box 4.2 for a vignette describing the case of Tom, illustrating a case of ASD diagnosed in the context of NF1.

Box 4.2   Case 2: Tom: Young person revealing clinical heterogeneity in autism spectrum disorder

History:

Tom is a 10-year-old boy with NF1. Significant concerns were noted at childcare when Tom was aged 2. While content during solitary or parallel play, he became physically aggressive if another child tried to play with his toys. He was reluctant to join any group activities and became distressed by loud noises. Attentional and literacy difficulties became evident at school. Tom was diagnosed with ADHD at age 6 and commenced stimulant medication. However, Tom's academic progress continued to be well behind age expectations. School reports described him as easily frustrated and defiant and to have an absence of age-appropriate peer relationships.

Current symptoms/functional impact:

Tom is in Grade 5. Over the past year, he has displayed increasing school refusal and aggressive and defiant behaviours (e.g., ripping up his work, kicking classmates). His academic curriculum has been modified and an area in the classroom has been nominated for Tom to remove himself from group interactions when he is feeling frustrated or overstimulated. Tom has one friend at school who shares his current 'obsessions' in Minecraft and Roblox. If this friend is away, Tom refuses to play with other children. His family's activities are limited by Tom's need for routine and his refusal to participate in activities not related to his interests.

Neuropsychological evaluation:

On assessment, Tom's overall intellectual functioning was low average (*18th percentile*). Receptive and expressive language abilities were mildly reduced, and his speech was characterised by articulation errors. Performances on measures of attention and executive function revealed impulsivity, impaired planning and organisational skills, and poor capacity to sustain and flexibly shift attention. Tom's phonological awareness was extremely low for his age. The Autism Diagnostic Interview-Revised (ADI-R) revealed a history of limited imaginative play and engagement in reciprocal social interactions, an extreme sensitivity to noise and narrow interests that dominate his play and communication. He has always insisted on adhering to a rigid routine (e.g., refusing to eat dinner before bath time). The ADOS-2 revealed fleeting eye contact, one-sided conversations focused on his topics of interest, and an unusual degree of interest in the texture of some test stimuli. This evaluation, in conjunction with clinical judgement from a multidisciplinary team, found that Tom met criteria for previously undetected ASD. While there is considerable overlap between Tom's and Emily's ASD symptoms (see Box 4.1), like most children with NF1 and ASD, Tom does not demonstrate the motor stereotypies that are relatively common in the broader ASD population.

Social cognition in NF1

To date, little research on social cognition and its relation to ASD symptoms has been conducted in NF1. Initial studies do, however, suggest that social cognitive abilities are selectively affected in NF1. Recent meta-analytic evidence indicates individuals with NF1 exhibit significantly poorer social cognition relative to controls (N = 390, 189 healthy controls; Hedges' g = 0.65; Chisholm et al., 2018). Existing data suggests that these deficits manifest at the social perception level and are also evident in higher-level social cognitive processes that require a ToM.

Regarding lower level social perceptual abilities, children with NF1 are reported to show difficulty identifying negative emotions (e.g., fear and anger; Huijbregts, Jahja, De Sonneville, De Breij, & Swaab-Barneveld, 2010; Lewis et al., 2017) and distinguishing ambiguous facial expressions (Allen et al., 2016) compared to healthy controls. This may signify problems with key foundational aspects of social information processing. Similar deficits in emotion recognition are also documented in adults with NF1 (Pride, Crawford, Payne, & North, 2013; Pride et al., 2014). Deficits have also been reported in higher-level social cognition. For example, children with NF1 have been shown to make significantly more errors than typically developing controls on a non-verbal picture sequencing task that required them to attribute mental states to characters, while showing no deficits when sequencing control stories that did not require mentalising (Payne, Porter et al., 2016). Similarly, adults with NF1 show significantly poorer performances on sarcasm detection tasks that hinge on the capacity to pick up social cues such as facial expression and tone of voice compared to unaffected controls (Pride et al., 2014).

The role that domain-general cognitive processes (e.g., IQ, EF, attention) play in influencing social cognition in NF1 is currently unclear. However, preliminary evidence suggests social cognitive deficits persist even after controlling for these domain-general cognitive factors. For instance, the generalized ToM deficit in children with NF1 has been shown independent of general cognitive abilities, EF and ADHD symptoms (Payne, Porter et al., 2016). Others have, likewise, demonstrated that deficits in bottom-up processing of social signals and overall poor social competence remains in NF1 cohorts, even after controlling for EF, IQ and ADHD symptoms (Huijbregts et al., 2010; Lewis et al., 2016). These findings align with research into ADHD in NF1, showing that cognitive variables do not necessarily predict neurodevelopmental symptoms like ADHD or functional outcomes (Payne, Hyman, Shores, & North, 2011; Payne et al., 2019). Further, well-controlled phenotyping studies are required to explore the relationships between social and domain-general cognitive factors in NF1 and how they impact the expression of ASD symptoms.

ASD symptom profiles in NF1

Existing studies indicate several commonalities between idiopathic ASD and ASD in children with NF1. Both track alongside poor attention and hyperactive behaviour (Jang et al., 2013; Morris et al., 2016; Payne et al., 2011) and both appear related to executive dysfunction (Chisholm et al., 2018). However, there are also important differences that have been observed between idiopathic ASD and ASD comorbid with NF1. For example, the well-documented male to female bias in idiopathic ASD is attenuated in NF1, with ratio estimates ranging from between 1.6 to 2.6:1 (Chisholm et al., 2018; Garg et al., 2016; Morris et al., 2016). Furthermore, age at diagnosis of ASD tends to occur later, at approximately 10 years of age for children with NF1 (Plasschaert et al., 2015) versus four years in the idiopathic ASD population. It is possible the medical and other clinical comorbidities associated with NF1 (e.g., ADHD, tumours) 'mask' ASD features, meaning that emerging ASD behavioural symptoms are less concerning to clinicians and parents than medical complications, or may not be as immediately concerning.

Interestingly, factor analysis on SRS-2 data reveals that while ASD symptoms in NF1 conforms to the same unitary factor structure as is observed for idiopathic ASD, the highest loading items on the first principal component are less specific to ASD per se than other items, perhaps suggesting a NF1-specific ASD phenotype (Morris et al., 2016). The implication of this is that ASD symptom expression in NF1 may diverge from that observed in the idiopathic ASD population. To further investigate this observation, several studies have recently investigated ASD symptom profiles in NF1 using diagnostic instruments such as the Autism Diagnostic Observation Schedule (ADOS-2) and the Autism Diagnostic Interview – Revised (ADI-R) (Lord et al., 2000; Rutter, Le Couteur, & Lord, 2003). These suggest children with NF1 and ASD show better eye contact, fewer repetitive behaviours and better language skills than idiopathic ASD counterparts (Garg et al., 2015; Plasschaert et al., 2015). Interestingly, the social perceptual deficits observed in children with NF1 also differ from those seen in idiopathic ASD. For example, while children with NF1 spend less time attending to faces presented in social scenes than controls, they often show a pattern of initially orienting their attention to faces but then spending less time focused on faces overall (Lewis et al., 2019). This conflicts with what is typically observed in idiopathic ASD, where a weak orientation to faces is commonly observed (Kornreich, 2019). Earlier work (Lewis et al., 2017) has also demonstrated that while children with NF1 spend less time viewing faces as a whole during emotional recognition tasks, they do not appear to spend less time viewing primary facial features (e.g., eyes) compared to healthy controls. These gaze patterns also seem to deviate from those frequently observed in idiopathic ASD, where there is often particularly poor attention to eyes (Webb et al., 2017). Future studies linking atypical social cognition to ASD symptom expression in NF1 are required to extend these findings.

Some critical questions remain in terms of understanding relationships between social cognition, ASD and NF1. Existing research has been hindered by the fact that many studies do not use diagnostic tools to quantify ASD symptoms, and there is variable reporting on moderating factors such as IQ and EF. Furthermore, studies often assess social cognitive abilities in isolation without considering multiple levels of the ability (e.g., explicit but not implicit ToM). Moreover, studies typically comprise of small samples. To better understand the ASD phenotype in medically defined syndromes, including NF1, future studies will need to compare children with the genetic condition of interest to those with the genetic condition *and* comorbid ASD and to those with idiopathic ASD and healthy controls. Such analysis would preferably be complemented by the characterisation of ASD symptoms using gold standard phenotyping/diagnostic tools, together with assessment of moderating factors such as IQ and EF, and in consideration with genetic and neurobiological makers (e.g., eye tracking studies, functional neuroimaging).

Pharmaceutical rescue of social deficits in neurofibromatosis type 1

Attempts at developing pharmaceutical treatments for ASD have been frustratingly ineffective (Garg & Green, 2018; Loth, Murphy, & Spooren, 2016), likely due to treatments being applied to disorders of heterogeneous aetiologies that clinically manifest as ASD. However, the genetic specificity of many syndromic forms of ASD, such as NF1, provides a unique opportunity to develop mechanism-directed 'precision' treatments. Monogenic forms of autism are a logical entry point into systematically exploring the neurobiological mechanisms of ASD within a 'human model' because the causal gene is known. Understanding these neurobiological mechanisms has the potential to inform the development of novel therapeutics to reverse the molecular, and ultimately clinical, phenotype caused by the genetic mutation. To date, mechanistic analysis of NF1 pathophysiology has primarily been conducted in murine models. These provide evidence that abnormalities in the regulation of the RAS-MAPK pathway (Shilyansky, Lee, & Silva, 2010), and other intra- and extracellular pathways (Brown et al., 2010, 2011), are related to mutation of *NF1* and may underlie the cognitive, learning and behaviour problems in humans with the condition (Molosh & Shekhar, 2018).

One class of medication that has been investigated as a potential treatment for neurobiological deficits in NF1 is statins, which act as net inhibitors of the RAS-MAPK pathway (Li et al., 2005). Preclinical trials in mice with a heterozygous inactivating mutation in the $Nf1$ gene ($Nf1^{+/-}$) demonstrated that lovastatin negatively regulated the MAPK pathway, normalised synaptic plasticity and GABA deficits, and rescued learning and attention deficits compared to placebo (Cui et al., 2008; Li et al., 2005), providing a rationale for translational human trials. Some uncontrolled (Acosta et al., 2011) and small randomised controlled trials (RCTs) suggested positive effects of lovastatin on cognitive outcomes (Bearden et al., 2016), and a small, 12 week RCT of simvastatin versus placebo in younger children with NF1 also showed some evidence of effects in brain areas previously associated with NF1 pathophysiology (Stivaros et al., 2018). However, larger well-controlled trials conducted spanning 12 weeks to 12 months have shown no clinical benefits (Krab et al., 2008; Payne, Barton et al., 2016; van der Vaart et al., 2013).

More recently, MEK inhibitors, a cancer therapy that selectively inhibits the RAS-MAPK signalling cascade, have been shown to be successful targeted treatments for tumours in NF1, and enthusiasm has emerged about the possibility of these agents as a treatment for cognitive and behavioural manifestations of NF1 (Gross et al., 2020). Mouse studies have suggested a possible therapeutic effect on the abnormal neurobiological processes in NF1 (Kim et al., 2014; Y. Wang et al., 2012). Several clinical trials are now underway evaluating MEK inhibitors for NF1 tumours in humans, some of which include cognitive and behavioural endpoints as secondary outcomes.

Applying findings from laboratory bench to clinical practice is complex, and treatments for the social, behavioural and cognitive deficits in NF1 are no exception (Drozd et al., 2018; Payne, 2015). A challenge has been reconciling human clinical trial findings with the results from mouse models. One reason for this is that animal models may not be adequate representations of brain disorders in the human condition. While mice and humans share considerable genomic homology, and some behavioural parallels, there are important between-species differences that appear to limit the ability of genetically engineered mice to model the human condition. These include differences in the timing of key brain maturation events, the limited capacity for mice to model higher cortical abilities, and a number of divergent neurodevelopment processes; all of which significantly limit conclusions that can be readily translated from animal models to human clinical trials. Significant work validating meaningful cognitive biomarkers in humans is urgently required in this area. Identifying cognitive and behavioural biomarkers, specifically and directly regulated by neurofibromin, will enable smaller pilot studies to also demonstrate proof of principle and dose refinement by testing whether promising preclinical treatments normalize pathophysiologic processes in human patients. These approaches will better inform clinical research and optimise trial designs based on findings observed in humans. Current research, using patient-derived induced pluripotent stem cell modelling techniques, is also underway to hopefully provide a deeper understanding of the disease mechanisms in NF1 patients. These studies have the potential to provide powerful models for targeted screening of therapeutic agents for neurodevelopmental deficits such as ASD (Bozaoglu et al., 2020; Wegscheid, Anastasaki, & Gutmann, 2018).

While disappointing that no viable therapy for ASD has emerged yet, preclinical and clinical research in this area is in its infancy. Most clinical trials have been underpowered to detect true change, many have methodological weaknesses, and the majority rely on data from animal studies that may not adequately model the human condition. Large, well-controlled studies driven by second- and third-generation disease modelling, which triangulate data from animal and human models, represent the next exciting chapter of research into neurodevelopmental disorders in NF1 and other monogenetic ASD syndromes.

Concluding remarks

Ultimately, the development of a complete explanatory framework for social cognition and ASD (in idiopathic and syndromic ASD populations) requires integration of genetic, neurobiological, cognitive, and behavioural mechanisms to describe complete causal chains that occur across development (Coghill et al., 2005; Joseph, 1999). Existing research has typically relied on cross-sectional designs with diverse methodological approaches focused on singular levels of analysis. This has yielded a broad but shallow collection of findings that are difficult to synthesise and translate into meaningful clinical trial endpoints and therapeutic options. The complexity inherent in understanding social cognition and the relationship it holds to ASD necessitates collaborative research that combines specialist knowledge and skills from research groups with diverse scientific and clinical backgrounds.

References

Abrahams, B. S., & Geschwind, D. H. (2010). Genetics of Autism. In *Vogel and Motilsky's Human Genetics* (pp. 699–714). Springer. doi:10.1007/978-3-540-37654-5_29

Acosta, M. T., Kardel, P. G., Walsh, K. S., Rosenbaum, K. N., Gioia, G. A., & Packer, R. J. (2011). Lovastatin as treatment for neurocognitive deficits in neurofibromatosis type 1: Phase I study. *Pediatric Neurology, 45*(4), 241–245. doi:10.1016/j.pediatrneurol.2011.06.016

Adolphs, R. (1999). Social cognition and the human brain. *Trends in Cognitive Sciences, 3*(12), 469–479.

Adolphs, R. (2001). The neurobiology of social cognition. *Current Opinion in Neurobiology, 11*(2), 231–239.

Adolphs, R. (2008). Fear, faces, and the human amygdala. *Current Opinion in Neurobiology, 18*(2), 166–172. doi:10.1016/j.conb.2008.06.006

Adolphs, R. (2009). The social brain: Neural basis of social knowledge. *Annual Review of Psychology, 60*(1), 693–716.

Allen, T., Willard, V. W., Anderson, L. M., Hardy, K. K., & Bonner, M. J. (2016). Social functioning and facial expression recognition in children with neurofibromatosis type 1. *Journal of Intellectual Disability Research, 60*(3), 282–293. doi:10.1111/jir.12248

American Psychiatric Association. (2013). *Diagnostic and Statistical Manual of Mental Disorders (DSM-5)*. American Psychiatric Pub. doi:10.1016/B978-0-12-809324-5.05530-9

Anderson, V., Jacobs, R., & Anderson, P. J. (2010). Towards a developmental model of executive function. In *Executive Functions and the Frontal Lobes: A Lifespan Perspective* (pp. 37–56). New York: Taylor and Francis.

Arnold, S. S., Barton, B., McArthur, G., North, K. N., & Payne, J. M. (2016). Phonics training improves reading in children with neurofibromatosis type 1: A prospective intervention trial. *Journal of Pediatrics, 177,* 219–226, e2. doi:10.1016/j.jpeds.2016.06.037

Barendse, E. M., Hendriks, M. P. H., Thoonen, G., Aldenkamp, A. P., & Kessels, R. P. C. (2018). Social behaviour and social cognition in high-functioning adolescents with autism spectrum disorder (ASD): Two sides of the same coin? *Cognitive Processing, 19*(4), 545–555. doi:10.1007/s10339-018-0866-5

Baron-Cohen, S. (1989). The autistic child's theory of mind: A case of specific developmental delay. *Journal of Child Psychology and Psychiatry, 30*(2), 285–297.

Baron-Cohen, S. (2001). Theory of mind in normal development and autism. *Prisme, 34,* 174–183.

Baron-Cohen, S., Leslie, A. M., & Frith, U. (1985). Does the autistic child have a "theory of mind"? *Cognition, 21,* 37–46.

Basil, R. A., Westwater, M. L., Wiener, M., & Thompson, J. C. (2017). A causal role of the right superior temporal sulcus in emotion recognition from biological motion. *Open Mind, 2*(1), 26–36. doi:10.1162/opmi_a_00015

Bearden, C. E., Hellemann, G. S., Rosser, T., Montojo, C., Jonas, R., Enrique, N., . . . Silva, A. J. (2016). A randomized placebo-controlled lovastatin trial for neurobehavioral function in neurofibromatosis I. *Annals of Clinical and Translational Neurology, 3*(4), 266–279. doi:10.1002/acn3.288

Beaumont, R. B., & Sofronoff, K. (2008). A new computerised advanced theory of mind measure for children with Asperger syndrome: The ATOMIC. *Journal of Autism and Developmental Disorders, 38*(2), 249–260. doi:10.1007/s10803-007-0384-2

Bennett, T. A., Szatmari, P., Bryson, S., Duku, E., Liezanne, V., & Tuff, L. (2013). Theory of mind, language and adaptive functioning in ASD: A neuroconstructivist perspective. *Journal of the Canadian Academy of Child and Adolescent Psychiatry, 22*(1). www.cacap-acpea.org/uploads/documents//Theory_of_Mind_Bennett_2013_02.pdf

Betancur, C. (2011). Etiological heterogeneity in autism spectrum disorders: More than 100 genetic and genomic disorders and still counting. *Brain Research, 1380,* 42–77. doi:10.1016/j.brainres.2010.11.078

Bi, T., & Fang, F. (2017). Impaired face perception in individuals with Autism spectrum disorder: Insights on diagnosis and treatment. *Neuroscience Bulletin, 33*(6), 757–759. doi:10.1007/s12264-017-0187-1

Blakemore, S. J. (2008). The social brain in adolescence. *Nature Reviews Neuroscience, 9*(4), 267–277. doi:10.1038/nrn2353

Booth, R. D. L., & Happé, F. G. E. (2018). Evidence of reduced global processing in Autism spectrum disorder. *Journal of Autism and Developmental Disorders, 48*(4), 1397–1408. doi:10.1007/s10803-016-2724-6

Bozaoglu, K., Lee, W. S., Haebich, K. M., North, K. N., Payne, J. M., & Lockhart, P. J. (2020). Generation of four iPSC lines from neurofibromatosis type 1 patients. *Stem Cell Research,* 102013.

Brown, J. A., Emnett, R. J., White, C. R., Yuede, C. M., Conyers, S. B., O'Malley, K. L., Wozniak, D. F., & Gutmann, D. H. (2010). Reduced striatal dopamine underlies the attention system dysfunction in neurofibromatosis-1 mutant mice. *Human Molecular Genetics, 19*(22), 4515–4528. doi:10.1093/hmg/ddq382

Brown, J. A., Xu, J., Diggs-Andrews, K. A., Wozniak, D. F., Mach, R. H., & Gutmann, D. H. (2011). PET imaging for attention deficit preclinical drug testing in neurofibromatosis-1 mice. *Experimental Neurology, 232*(2), 333–338.

Brunsdon, V. E. A., & Happé, F. (2014). Exploring the "fractionation" of autism at the cognitive level. *Autism*, 18(1), 17–30. doi:10.1177/1362361313499456

Burnette, C. P., Mundy, P. C., Meyer, J. A., Sutton, S. K., Vaughan, A. E., & Charak, D. (2005). Weak central coherence and its relations to theory of mind and anxiety in autism. *Journal of Autism and Developmental Disorders*, 35(1), 63–73. doi:10.1007/s10803-004-1035-5

Burris, J. L., Barry-Anwar, R. A., Sims, R. N., Hagerman, R. J., Tassone, F., & Rivera, S. M. (2017). Children with Fragile X syndrome display threat-specific biases toward emotion. *Biological Psychiatry: Cognitive Neuroscience and Neuroimaging*, 2(6), 487–492. doi:10.1016/j.bpsc.2017.06.003

Cantio, C., Jepsen, J. R. M., Madsen, G. F., Bilenberg, N., & White, S. J. (2016). Exploring 'the Autisms' at a cognitive level. *Autism Research*, 9(12), 1328–1339. doi:10.1002/aur.1630

Casanova, M. F., Casanova, E. L., Frye, R. E., Baeza-Velasco, C., LaSalle, J. M., Hagerman, R. J., . . . Natowicz, M. R. (2020, April). Editorial: Secondary vs. idiopathic Autism. *Frontiers in Psychiatry*, 11, 10–12. doi:10.3389/fpsyt.2020.00297

Castelli, F., Frith, C., Happé, F., & Frith, U. (2002). Autism, Asperger syndrome and brain mechanisms for the attribution of mental states to animated shapes. *Brain*, 125(8), 1839–1849. doi:10.1093/brain/awf189

Charman, T., Pickles, A., Simonoff, E., Chandler, S., Loucas, T., & Baird, G. (2010). IQ in children with autism spectrum disorders: Data from the special needs and Autism project (SNAP). *Psychological Medicine*, 41(3), 619–627. doi:10.1017/S0033291710000991

Chevallier, C., Kohls, G., Troiani, V., Brodkin, E. S., & Schultz, R. T. (2012). The social motivation theory of autism. *Trends in Cognitive Sciences*, 16(4), 231–239. Elsevier Ltd. doi:10.1016/j.tics.2012.02.007

Chiang, H. M., Tsai, L. Y., Cheung, Y. K., Brown, A., & Li, H. (2014). A meta-analysis of differences in IQ profiles between individuals with Asperger's disorder and high-functioning autism. *Journal of Autism and Developmental Disorders*, 44(7), 1577–1596. doi:10.1007/s10803-013-2025-2

Chisholm, A. K., Anderson, V. A., Pride, N. A., Malarbi, S., North, K. N., & Payne, J. M. (2018). Social function and autism spectrum disorder in children and adults with neurofibromatosis type 1: A systematic review and meta-analysis. *Neuropsychology Review*, 28(3), 317–340. Springer New York LLC. doi:10.1007/s11065-018-9380-x

Christensen, D. L., Maenner, M. J., Bilder, D., Constantino, J. N., Daniels, J., Durkin, M. S., Fitzgerald, R. T., Kurzius-Spencer, M., Pettygrove, S. D., Robinson, C., Shenouda, J., White, T., Zahorodny, W., Pazol, K., & Dietz, P. (2019). United States. *MMWR Surveillance Summaries*, 68(2), 1–19.

Christensen, J., Grønborg, T. K., Merete, M., Sørensen, J., Schendel, D., Parner, E. T., Pedersen, L. H., & Vestergaard, M. (2013). Prenatal valproate exposure and risk of autism spectrum disorders and childhood autism. *Jama*, 309(16), 1696–1703. www.jama.com.

Coghill, D., Hayward, D., Rhodes, S. M., Grimmer, C., & Matthews, K. (2014). A longitudinal examination of neuropsychological and clinical functioning in boys with attention deficit hyperactivity disorder (ADHD): Improvements in executive functioning do not explain clinical improvement. *Psychological Medicine*, 44(5), 1087–1099. doi:10.1017/S0033291713001761

Coghill, D., Nigg, J., Rothenberger, A., Sonuga-Barke, E., & Tannock, R. (2005). Whither causal models in the neuroscience of ADHD? *Developmental Science*, 8(2), 105–114. doi:10.1111/j.1467-7687.2005.00397.x

Cornish, K. M., Burack, J. A., Rahman, A., Munir, F., Russo, N., & Grant, C. (2005). Theory of mind deficits in children with fragile X syndrome. *Journal of Intellectual Disability Research, 49*(5), 372–378. doi:10.1111/j.1365-2788.2005.00678.x

Cornish, K. M., Gray, K. M., & Rinehart, N. J. (2010). Fragile X syndrome and associated disorders. *Advances in Child Development and Behavior – Developmental Disorders and Interventions, 39,* 211–235.

Crawford, H., Moss, J., Anderson, G. M., Oliver, C., & McCleery, J. P. (2015). Implicit discrimination of basic facial expressions of positive/negative emotion in Fragile X syndrome and autism spectrum disorder. *American Journal on Intellectual and Developmental Disabilities, 120*(4), 328–345. doi:10.1352/1944-7558-120.4.328

Cui, Y., Costa, R. M., Murphy, G. G., Elgersma, Y., Zhu, Y., Gutmann, D. H., Parada, L. F., Mody, I., & Silva, A. J. (2008). Neurofibromin regulation of ERK signaling modulates GABA release and learning. *Cell, 135*(3), 549–560.

Dai, L., Bellugi, U., Chen, X. N., Pulst-Korenberg, A. M., Järvinen-Pasley, A., Tirosh-Wagner, T., Eis, P. S., Graham, J., Mills, D., Searcy, Y., & Korenberg, J. R. (2009). Is it Williams syndrome? GTF2IRD1 implicated in visual-spatial construction and GTF2I in sociability revealed by high resolution arrays. *American Journal of Medical Genetics, Part A, 149*(3), 302–314. doi:10.1002/ajmg.a.32652

D'Arc, B. F., & Mottron, L. (2012). Social cognition in autism. In Anderson, V. & Beauchamp, M. (Eds.), *Developmental Social Neuroscience and Childhood Brain Insult: Theory and Practice* (pp. 299–315). New York: Guilford Press.

Dawson, G., Webb, S. J., & McPartland, J. (2005). Understanding the nature of face processing impairment in autism: Insights from behavioral and electrophysiological studies. *Developmental Neuropsychology, 27*(3), 403–424. doi:10.1207/s15326942dn2703_6

Demetriou, E. A., Lampit, A., Quintana, D. S., Naismith, S. L., Song, Y. J. C., Pye, J. E., Hickie, I., & Guastella, A. J. (2018). Autism spectrum disorders: A meta-analysis of executive function. *Molecular Psychiatry, 23*(5), 1198–1204. doi:10.1038/mp.2017.75

De Rosnay, M., Fink, E., Begeer, S., Slaughter, V., & Peterson, C. (2014). Talking theory of mind talk: Young school-aged children's everyday conversation and understanding of mind and emotion. *Journal of Child Language, 41*(5), 1179–1193. doi:10.1017/S0305000913000433

Diamond, A. (2013). Executive functions. *Annual Review of Psychology, 64,* 135–168. Annual Reviews Inc. doi:10.1146/annurev-psych-113011-143750

Di Martino, A., Ross, K., Uddin, L. Q., Sklar, A. B., Castellanos, F. X., & Milham, M. P. (2009). Functional brain correlates of social and nonsocial processes in autism spectrum disorders: An activation likelihood estimation meta-analysis. *Biological Psychiatry, 65*(1), 63–74. doi:10.1016/j.biopsych.2008.09.022

Dodd, H. F., & Porter, M. A. (2010). I see happy people: Attention bias towards happy but not angry facial expressions in Williams syndrome. *Cognitive Neuropsychiatry, 15*(6), 549–567. doi:10.1080/13546801003737157

Drozd, H. P., Karathanasis, S. F., Molosh, A. I., Lukkes, J. L., Clapp, D. W., & Shekhar, A. (2018). From bedside to bench and back: Translating ASD models. *Progress in Brain Research, 241,* 113–158. Elsevier B.V. doi:10.1016/bs.pbr.2018.10.003

Eijk, S., Mous, S. E., Dieleman, G. C., Dierckx, B., Rietman, A. B., de Nijs, P. F. A., . . . Legerstee, J. S. (2018). Autism spectrum disorder in an unselected cohort of children with neurofibromatosis type 1 (NF1). *Journal of Autism and Developmental Disorders, 48*(7), 2278–2285. doi:10.1007/s10803-018-3478-0

Evans, D. G., Howard, E., Giblin, C., Clancy, T., Spencer, H., Huson, S. M., & Lalloo, F. (2010). Birth incidence and prevalence of tumor-prone syndromes: Estimates from a UK family genetic register service. *American Journal of Medical Genetics Part A, 152*(2), 327–332.

Federici, A., Parma, V., Vicovaro, M., Radassao, L., Casartelli, L., & Ronconi, L. (2020). Anomalous perception of biological motion in autism: A conceptual review and meta-analysis. *Scientific Reports, 10*(1). doi:10.1038/s41598-020-61252-3

Fernandez, B. A., & Scherer, S. W. (2017). Syndromic autism spectrum disorders: Moving from a clinically defined to a molecularly defined approach. *Dialogues in Clinical Neuroscience, 19*(4), 353–371. https://pubmed.ncbi.nlm.nih.gov/29398931

Ferri, S. L., Abel, T., & Brodkin, E. S. (2018). Sex differences in autism spectrum disorder: A review. *Current Psychiatry Reports, 20*(2). doi:10.1007/s11920-018-0874-2

Fjermestad, K. W. (2019). Health complaints and work experiences among adults with neurofibromatosis 1. *Occupational Medicine, 69*(7), 504–510. doi:10.1093/occmed/kqz134

Frith, U. (1989). *Autism: Understanding the Enigma.* Maiden, MA: Blackwell.

Frith, U., & Happé, F. (1994). Autism: Beyond "theory of mind." *Cognition, 50*(1–3), 115–132.

Frith, U., Morton, J., & Leslie, A. M. (1991). The cognitive basis of a biological disorder: Autism. *Trends in Neurosciences, 14*(10), 433–438. doi:10.1016/0166-2236(91)90041-R

Garg, S., & Green, J. (2018). Studying child development in genetic models of ASD. *Progress in Brain Research, 241*, 159–192. Elsevier B.V. doi:10.1016/bs.pbr.2018.09.009

Garg, S., Green, J., Leadbitter, K., Emsley, R., Lehtonen, A., Gareth Evans, D., & Huson, S. M. (2013). Neurofibromatosis type 1 and autism spectrum disorder. *Pediatrics, 132*. www.aappublications.org/news

Garg, S., Heuvelman, H., Huson, S., Tobin, H., Green, J., Evans, D. G., . . . Steiger, C. (2016). Sex bias in autism spectrum disorder in neurofibromatosis type 1. *Journal of Neurodevelopmental Disorders, 8*(1). doi:10.1186/s11689-016-9159-4

Garg, S., Plasschaert, E., Descheemaeker, M. J., Huson, S., Borghgraef, M., Vogels, A., Evans, D. G., Legius, E., & Green, J. (2015). Autism spectrum disorder profile in neurofibromatosis type I. *Journal of Autism and Developmental Disorders, 45*(6), 1649–1657. doi:10.1007/s10803-014-2321-5

Georgiades, S., Szatmari, P., Boyle, M., Hanna, S., Duku, E., Zwaigenbaum, L., . . . Thompson, A. (2013). Investigating phenotypic heterogeneity in children with autism spectrum disorder: A factor mixture modeling approach. *Journal of Child Psychology and Psychiatry and Allied Disciplines, 54*(2), 206–215. doi:10.1111/j.1469-7610.2012.02588.x

Geurts, H. M., Sinzig, J., Booth, R., & Happé, F. (2014). Neuropsychological heterogeneity in executive functioning in autism spectrum disorders. *International Journal of Developmental Disabilities, 60*(3), 155–162. doi:10.1179/2047387714Y.0000000047

Grant, C. M., Apperly, I., & Oliver, C. (2007). Is theory of mind understanding impaired in males with Fragile X syndrome? *Journal of Abnormal Child Psychology, 35*(1), 17–28. doi:10.1007/s10802-006-9077-0

Gray, K. M., & Cornish, K. M. (2012). Genetic disorders and social problems. *Developmental Social Neuroscience and Childhood Brain Insult: Theory and Practice*, 269.

Gross, A. M., Wolters, P. L., Dombi, E., Baldwin, A., Whitcomb, P., Fisher, M. J., Weiss, B., Kim, A. R., Bornhorst, M., Shah, A. C., Martin, S., Roderick, M. C., Pichard, D. C., Carbonell, A., Paul, S. M., Therrien, J., Kapustina, O., Heisey, K., Wade Clapp, D., . . . Widemann, B. C. (2020). Selumetinib in children with inoperable plexiform neurofibromas. *New England Journal of Medicine, 382*(15), 1430–1442. doi:10.1056/NEJMoa1912735

Gutmann, D. H., Ferner, R. E., Listernick, R. H., Korf, B. R., Wolters, P. L., & Johnson, K. J. (2017). Neurofibromatosis type 1. *Nature Reviews Disease Primers, 3*. doi:10.1038/nrdp.2017.4

Haas, B. W., Mills, D., Yam, A., Hoeft, F., Bellugi, U., & Reiss, A. (2009). Genetic influences on sociability: Heightened amygdala reactivity and event-related responses to positive social stimuli in Williams syndrome. *Journal of Neuroscience, 29*(4), 1132–1139. doi:10.1523/JNEUROSCI.5324-08.2009

Hadjikhani, N., Joseph, R. M., Snyder, J., Chabris, C. F., Clark, J., Steele, S., McGrath, L., Vangel, M., Aharon, I., Feczko, E., Harris, G. J., & Tager-Flusberg, H. (2004). Activation of the fusiform gyrus when individuals with autism spectrum disorder view faces. *Neuro-Image, 22*(3), 1141–1150. doi:10.1016/j.neuroimage.2004.03.025

Hagerman, R. J., Berry-Kravis, E., Hazlett, H. C., Bailey, D. B., Moine, H., Kooy, R. F., . . . Hagerman, P. J. (2017). Fragile X syndrome. *Nature Reviews Disease Primers, 3*, 17065. doi:10.1038/nrdp.2017.65

Happé, F. (1994a). An advanced test of theory of mind: Understanding of story characters' thoughts and feelings by able autistic, mentally handicapped, and normal children and adults. *Journal of Autism and Developmental Disorders, 24*(2), 129–154. doi:10.1007/BF02172093

Happé, F. (1994b). Wechsler IQ profile and theory of mind in autism: A research note. *Journal of Child Psychology and Psychiatry, 35*(8), 1461–1471.

Happé, F., & Frith, U. (2006). The weak coherence account: Detail-focused cognitive style in autism spectrum disorders. *Journal of Autism and Developmental Disorders, 36*(1), 5–25. doi:10.1007/s10803-005-0039-0

Happé, F., Ronald, A., & Plomin, R. (2006). Time to give up on a single explanation for autism. *Nature Neuroscience, 9*(10), 1218–1220. doi:10.1038/nn1770

Harms, M. B., Martin, A., & Wallace, G. L. (2010). Facial emotion recognition in autism spectrum disorders: A review of behavioral and neuroimaging studies. *Neuropsychology Review, 20*(3), 290–322. doi:10.1007/s11065-010-9138-6

Hayward, E. O., & Homer, B. D. (2017). Reliability and validity of advanced theory-of-mind measures in middle childhood and adolescence. *British Journal of Developmental Psychology, 35*(3), 454–462. doi:10.1111/bjdp.12186

Henderson, L. M., Clarke, P. J., & Snowling, M. J. (2011). Accessing and selecting word meaning in autism spectrum disorder. *Journal of Child Psychology and Psychiatry and Allied Disciplines, 52*(9), 964–973. doi:10.1111/j.1469-7610.2011.02393.x

Hill, E. L. (2004). Executive dysfunction in autism. *Trends in Cognitive Sciences, 8*(1), 26–32.

Hoffman, E. A., & Haxby, J. V. (2000). Distinct representations of eye gaze and identity in the distributed human neural system for face perception. *Nature Neuroscience, 3*(1), 80–84. doi:10.1038/71152

Holland, A. A., Stavinoha, P. L., Swearer, S. M., Solesbee, C., Patel, S., & Klesse, L. J. (2019). Rate and frequency of bullying victimization in school-age children with neurofibromatosis type 1 (NF1). *School Psychology, 34*(6), 687–694. doi:10.1037/spq0000333

Hughes, C., & Russell, J. (1993). Autistic children's difficulty with mental disengagement from an object: Its implications for theories of autism. *Developmental Psychology, 29*(3), 498–510. doi:10.1037//0012-1649.29.3.498

Huijbregts, S., Jahja, R., De Sonneville, L., De Breij, S., & Swaab-Barneveld, H. (2010). Social information processing in children and adolescents with neurofibromatosis type 1. *Developmental Medicine and Child Neurology, 52*(7), 620–625. doi:10.1111/j.1469-8749.2010.03639.x

Hull, L., Petrides, K. V., & Mandy, W. (2020). The female autism phenotype and camouflaging: A narrative review. *Review Journal of Autism and Developmental Disorders*. Springer. doi:10.1007/s40489-020-00197-9

Hyman, S. L., Shores, A., & North, K. N. (2005). The nature and frequency of cognitive deficits in children with neurofibromatosis type 1. *Neurology*, *65*(7), 1037–1044. doi:10.1212/01.wnl.0000179303.72345.ce

Janecka, M., Mill, J., Basson, M. A., Goriely, A., Spiers, H., Reichenberg, A., Schalkwyk, L., & Fernandes, C. (2017). Advanced paternal age effects in neurodevelopmental disorders-review of potential underlying mechanisms. *Translational Psychiatry*, *7*(1). Nature Publishing Group. doi:10.1038/tp.2016.294

Jang, J., Matson, J. L., Williams, L. W., Tureck, K., Goldin, R. L., & Cervantes, P. E. (2013). Rates of comorbid symptoms in children with ASD, ADHD, and comorbid ASD and ADHD. *Research in Developmental Disabilities*, *34*(8), 2369–2378.

Järvinen, A., Korenberg, J. R., & Bellugi, U. (2013). The social phenotype of Williams syndrome. *Current Opinion in Neurobiology*, *23*(3), 414–422. doi:10.1016/j.conb.2012.12.006

Järvinen, A., Ng, R., Crivelli, D., Neumann, D., Grichanik, M., Arnold, A. J., Lai, P., Trauner, D., & Bellugi, U. (2015). Patterns of sensitivity to emotion in children with Williams syndrome and autism: Relations between autonomic nervous system reactivity and social functioning. *Journal of Autism and Developmental Disorders*, *45*(8), 2594–2612. doi:10.1007/s10803-015-2429-2

Jemel, B., Mottron, L., & Dawson, M. (2006). Impaired face processing in autism: Fact or artifact? *Journal of Autism and Developmental Disorders*, *36*(1), 91–106. doi:10.1007/s10803-005-0050-5

Jolliffe, T., & Baron-Cohen, S. (1997). Are people with autism and Asperger syndrome faster than normal on the embedded figures test? *Journal of Child Psychology and Psychiatry and Allied Disciplines*, *38*(5), 527–534. doi:10.1111/j.1469-7610.1997.tb01539.x

Jones, C. R. G., Pickles, A., Falcaro, M., Marsden, A. J. S., Happé, F., Scott, S. K., Sauter, D., Tregay, J., Phillips, R. J., Baird, G., Simonoff, E., & Charman, T. (2011). A multimodal approach to emotion recognition ability in autism spectrum disorders. *Journal of Child Psychology and Psychiatry and Allied Disciplines*, *52*(3), 275–285. doi:10.1111/j.1469-7610.2010.02328.x

Jones, C. R. G., Simonoff, E., Baird, G., Pickles, A., Marsden, A. J. S., Tregay, J., Happé, F., & Charman, T. (2018). The association between theory of mind, executive function, and the symptoms of autism spectrum disorder. *Autism Research*, *11*(1), 95–109. doi:10.1002/aur.1873

Joseph, R. M. (1999). Neuropsychological frameworks for understanding autism. *International Review of Psychiatry*, *11*(4), 309–324. doi:10.1080/09540269974195

Karmiloff-Smith, A. (2007). Quick guides Williams syndrome. *Current Biology*, *17*(24), 1035–1036.

Kidd, S. A., Berry-Kravis, E., Choo, T. H., Chen, C., Esler, A., Hoffmann, A., Andrews, H. F., & Kaufmann, W. E. (2020). Improving the diagnosis of autism spectrum disorder in Fragile X syndrome by adapting the social communication questionnaire and the social responsiveness scale-2. *Journal of Autism and Developmental Disorders*, *50*(9), 3276–3295. doi:10.1007/s10803-019-04148-0

Kim, E., Wang, Y., Kim, S. J., Bornhorst, M., Jecrois, E. S., Anthony, T. E., Wang, C., Li, Y. E., Guan, J. L., Murphy, G. G., & Zhu, Y. (2014). Transient inhibition of the ERK pathway prevents cerebellar developmental defects and improves long-term motor functions in murine models of neurofibromatosis type 1. *ELife*, *3*, 1–27. doi:10.7554/eLife.05151

Klin, A., Jones, W., Schultz, R., & Volkmar, F. (2003). The enactive mind, or from actions to cognition: Lessons from autism. *Philosophical Transactions of the Royal Society B: Biological Sciences, 358*(1430), 345–360. doi:10.1098/rstb.2002.1202

Klin, A., Jones, W., Schultz, R., Volkmar, F., & Cohen, D. (2002). Visual fixation patterns during viewing of naturalistic social situations as predictors of social competence in individuals with autism. *Archives of General Psychiatry, 59*(9), 809–816. doi:10.1001/archpsyc.59.9.809

Klusek, J., Martin, G. E., & Losh, M. (2014). Consistency between research and clinical diagnoses of autism among boys and girls with fragile X syndrome. *Journal of Intellectual Disability Research, 58*(10), 940–952. doi:10.1111/jir.12121

Kornreich, C. (2019). Face reading difficulties in children with neurofibromatosis type 1: Towards more personalized treatments. *Developmental Medicine & Child Neurology, 61*(2), 113–114.

Krab, L. C., De Goede-Bolder, A., Aarsen, F. K., Pluijm, S. M. F., Bouman, M. J., Van Der Geest, J. N., Lequin, M., Catsman, C. E., Arts, W. F. M., Kushner, S. A., Silva, A. J., De Zeeuw, C. I., Moll, H. A., & Elgersma, Y. (2008). Effect of simvastatin on cognitive functioning in children with neurofibromatosis type 1: A randomized controlled trial. *JAMA – Journal of the American Medical Association, 300*(3), 287–294. doi:10.1001/jama.300.3.287

Lai, C. L. E., Lau, Z., Lui, S. S. Y., Lok, E., Tam, V., Chan, Q., Cheng, K. M., Lam, S. M., & Cheung, E. F. C. (2017). Meta-analysis of neuropsychological measures of executive functioning in children and adolescents with high-functioning autism spectrum disorder. *Autism Research, 10*(5), 911–939. doi:10.1002/aur.1723

Lai, M. C., Lombardo, M. V., & Baron-Cohen, S. (2014). Autism. *Lancet, 383*(9920), 896–910.

Lehtonen, A., Howie, E., Trump, D., & Huson, S. M. (2013). Behaviour in children with neurofibromatosis type 1: Cognition, executive function, attention, emotion, and social competence. *Developmental Medicine and Child Neurology, 55*(2), 111–125. doi:10.1111/j.1469-8749.2012.04399.x

Leung, R. C., Vogan, V. M., Powell, T. L., Anagnostou, E., & Taylor, M. J. (2016). The role of executive functions in social impairment in autism spectrum disorder. *Child Neuropsychology, 22*(3), 336–344. doi:10.1080/09297049.2015.1005066

Lewis, A. K., Porter, M. A., Wiliams, T. A., North, K. N., & Payne, J. M. (2016). Social competence in children with neurofibromatosis type 1: Relationships with psychopathology and cognitive ability. *Journal of Childhood and Developmental Disorders, 2,* 12.

Lewis, A. K., Porter, M. A., Williams, T. A., Bzishvili, S., North, K. N., & Payne, J. M. (2017). Facial emotion recognition, face scan paths, and face perception in children with neurofibromatosis type 1. *Neuropsychology, 31*(4), 361–370. American Psychological Association. doi:10.1037/neu0000340

Lewis, A. K., Porter, M. A., Williams, T. A., Bzishvili, S., North, K. N., & Payne, J. M. (2019). Attention to faces in social context in children with neurofibromatosis type 1. *Developmental Medicine and Child Neurology, 61*(2), 174–180. doi:10.1111/dmcn.13928

Li, W., Cui, Y., Kushner, S. A., Brown, R. A. M., Jentsch, J. D., Frankland, P. W., Cannon, T. D., & Silva, A. J. (2005). The HMG-CoA reductase inhibitor lovastatin reverses the learning and attention deficits in a mouse model of neurofibromatosis type 1. *Current Biology, 15*(21), 1961–1967. doi:10.1016/j.cub.2005.09.043

Livingston, L. A., Colvert, E., Bolton, P., & Happé, F. (2019). Good social skills despite poor theory of mind: Exploring compensation in autism spectrum disorder. *Journal of Child Psychology and Psychiatry and Allied Disciplines, 60*(1), 102–110. doi:10.1111/jcpp.12886

Loomes, R., Hull, L., & Mandy, W. P. L. (2017). What is the male-to-female ratio in autism spectrum disorder? A systematic review and meta-analysis. *Journal of the American Academy of Child & Adolescent Psychiatry, 56*(6), 466–474.

López, B. R., & Leekam, S. R. (2003). Do children with autism fail to process information in context? *Journal of Child Psychology and Psychiatry and Allied Disciplines, 44*(2), 285–300. doi:10.1111/1469-7610.00121

Lopez, B. R., Lincoln, A. J., Ozonoff, S., & Lai, Z. (2005). Examining the relationship between executive functions and restricted, repetitive symptoms of autistic disorder. *Journal of Autism and Developmental Disorders, 35*(4), 445–460. doi:10.1007/s10803-005-5035-x

Lord, C., Risi, S., Lambrecht, L., Cook, E. H., Leventhal, B. L., DiLavore, P. C., Pickles, A., & Rutter, M. (2000). The autism diagnostic observation schedule – generic: A standard measure of social and communication deficits associated with the spectrum of autism. *Journal of Autism and Developmental Disorders, 30*(3), 205–223.

Loth, E., Murphy, D. G., & Spooren, W. (2016). Defining precision medicine approaches to autism spectrum disorders: Concepts and challenges. *Frontiers in Psychiatry, 7*, 188.

Lozier, L. M., Vanmeter, J. W., & Marsh, A. A. (2014). Impairments in facial affect recognition associated with autism spectrum disorders: A meta-analysis. *Development and Psychopathology, 26*(4), 933–945. doi:10.1017/S0954579414000479

Maenner, M. J., Shaw, K. A., & Baio, J. (2020). Prevalence of autism spectrum disorder among children aged 8 years – autism and developmental disabilities monitoring network, 11 sites, United States, 2016. *MMWR Surveillance Summaries, 69*(4), 1.

Masi, A., DeMayo, M. M., Glozier, N., & Guastella, A. J. (2017). An overview of autism spectrum disorder, heterogeneity and treatment options. *Neuroscience Bulletin, 33*(2), 183–193. Science Press. doi:10.1007/s12264-017-0100-y

Mautner, V. F., Kluwe, L., Thakker, S. D., & Leark, R. A. (2002). Treatment of ADHD in neurofibromatosis type 1. *Developmental Medicine and Child Neurology, 44*(3), 164–170. doi:10.1111/j.1469-8749.2002.tb00780.x

Mazza, M., Mariano, M., Peretti, S., Masedu, F., Pino, M. C., & Valenti, M. (2017). The role of theory of mind on social information processing in children with autism spectrum disorders: A mediation analysis. *Journal of Autism and Developmental Disorders, 47*(5), 1369–1379. doi:10.1007/s10803-017-3069-5

McDuffie, A., Thurman, A. J., Hagerman, R. J., & Abbeduto, L. (2015). Symptoms of autism in males with Fragile X syndrome: A comparison to nonsyndromic ASD using current ADI-R scores. *Journal of Autism and Developmental Disorders, 45*(7), 1925–1937. doi:10.1007/s10803-013-2013-6

Modabbernia, A., Velthorst, E., & Reichenberg, A. (2017). Environmental risk factors for autism: An evidence-based review of systematic reviews and meta-analyses. *Molecular Autism, 8*(1). BioMed Central Ltd. doi:10.1186/s13229-017-0121-4

Molenberghs, P., Johnson, H., Henry, J. D., & Mattingley, J. B. (2016). Understanding the minds of others: A neuroimaging meta-analysis. *Neuroscience & Biobehavioral Reviews, 65*, 276–291. doi:10.1016/j.neubiorev.2016.03.020

Molosh, A. I., & Shekhar, A. (2018). Neurofibromatosis type 1 as a model system to study molecular mechanisms of autism spectrum disorder symptoms. *Progress in Brain Research, 241*, 37–62. Elsevier B.V. doi:10.1016/bs.pbr.2018.09.014

Morel, A., Peyroux, E., Leleu, A., Favre, E., Franck, N., & Demily, C. (2018). Overview of social cognitive dysfunctions in rare developmental syndromes with psychiatric phenotype. *Frontiers in Pediatrics, 6*. doi:10.3389/fped.2018.00102

Morgan, B., Maybery, M., & Durkin, K. (2003). Weak central coherence, poor joint attention, and low verbal ability: Independent deficits in early autism. *Developmental Psychology*, *39*(4), 646–656. doi:10.1037/0012-1649.39.4.646

Morris, S. M., Acosta, M. T., Garg, S., Green, J., Huson, S., Legius, E., . . . Constantino, J. N. (2016). Disease burden and symptom structure of autism in neurofibromatosis type 1: A study of the international NF1-ASD consortium team (INFACT). *JAMA Psychiatry*, *73*(12), 1276–1284. doi:10.1001/jamapsychiatry.2016.2600

Morton, J., & Frith, U. (1995). Causal modeling: A structural approach to developmental psychopathology. In *Developmental Psychopathology, Vol. 1: Theory and Methods* (pp. 357–390). Hoboken, NJ: John Wiley & Sons.

Neufeld, J., Hagström, A., Van't Westeinde, A., Lundin, K., Cauvet, Willfors, C., Isaksson, J., Lichtenstein, P., & Bölte, S. (2020). Global and local visual processing in autism – a co-twin-control study. *Journal of Child Psychology and Psychiatry and Allied Disciplines*, *61*(4), 470–479. doi:10.1111/jcpp.13120

Niu, M., Han, Y., Dy, A. B. C., Du, J., Jin, H., Qin, J., Zhang, J., Li, Q., & Hagerman, R. J. (2017). Autism symptoms in Fragile X syndrome. *Journal of Child Neurology*, *32*(10), 903–909. doi:10.1177/0883073817712875

Noll, R. B., Reiter-Purtill, J., Moore, B. D., Schorry, E. K., Lovell, A. M., Vannatta, K., & Gerhardt, C. A. (2007). Social, emotional, and behavioral functioning of children with NF1. *American Journal of Medical Genetics Part A*, *143*(19), 2261–2273.

Nomi, J. S., & Uddin, L. Q. (2015). Face processing in autism spectrum disorders: From brain regions to brain networks. *Neuropsychologia*, *71*, 201–216. Elsevier Ltd. doi:10.1016/j.neuropsychologia.2015.03.029

O'Roak, B. J., Vives, L., Fu, W., Egertson, J. D., Stanaway, I. B., Phelps, I. G., . . . Shendure, J. (2012). Multiplex targeted sequencing identifies recurrently mutated genes in autism spectrum disorders. *Science*, *338*(6114), 1619–1622. doi:10.1126/science.1227764

Ozonoff, S., Rogers, S. J., & Pennington, B. F. (1991). Asperger's syndrome: Evidence of an empirical distinction from high-functioning autism. *Journal of Child Psychology and Psychiatry*, *32*(7).

Patriquin, M. A., DeRamus, T., Libero, L. E., Laird, A., & Kana, R. K. (2016). Neuro-anatomical and neurofunctional markers of social cognition in autism spectrum disorder. *Human Brain Mapping*, *37*(11), 3957–3978. doi:10.1002/hbm.23288

Pavlova, M. A. (2012). Biological motion processing as a hallmark of social cognition. *Cerebral Cortex*, *22*(5), 981–995. doi:10.1093/cercor/bhr156

Payne, J. M. (2015). Bridging the gap between mouse behavior and human cognition in neurofibromatosis type 1. *EBioMedicine*, *2*(10), 1290–1291. Elsevier B.V. doi:10.1016/j.ebiom.2015.09.013

Payne, J. M., Barton, B., Ullrich, N. J., Cantor, A., Hearps, S. J. C., Cutter, G., . . . North, K. N. (2016). Randomized placebo-controlled study of lovastatin in children with neurofibromatosis type 1. *Neurology*, *87*(24), 2575–2584. doi:10.1212/WNL.0000000000003435

Payne, J. M., Haebich, K. M., MacKenzie, R., Walsh, K. S., Hearps, S. J. C., Coghill, D., . . . North, K. N. (2019). Cognition, ADHD symptoms, and functional impairment in children and adolescents with neurofibromatosis type 1. *Journal of Attention Disorders*. doi:10.1177/1087054719894384

Payne, J. M., Hyman, S. L., Shores, E. A., & North, K. N. (2011). Assessment of executive function and attention in children with neurofibromatosis type 1: Relationships between cognitive measures and real-world behavior. *Child Neuropsychology*, *17*(4), 313–329.

Payne, J. M., Moharir, M. D., Webster, R., & North, K. N. (2010). Brain structure and function in neurofibromatosis type 1: Current concepts and future directions. *Journal of Neurology, Neurosurgery and Psychiatry*, *81*(3), 304–309. doi:10.1136/jnnp.2009.179630

Payne, J. M., Porter, M., Pride, N. A., & North, K. N. (2016). Theory of mind in children with neurofibromatosis type 1. *Neuropsychology*, *30*(4), 439–448. doi:10.1037/neu0000262

Payne, J. M., Walsh, K. S., Pride, N. A., Haebich, K. M., Maier, A., Chisholm, A., Glad, D. M., Casnar, C. L., Rouel, M., Lorenzo, J., Del Castillo, A., North, K. N., & Klein-Tasman, B. (2020). Social skills and autism spectrum disorder symptoms in children with neurofibromatosis type 1: Evidence for clinical trial outcomes. *Developmental Medicine and Child Neurology*, *62*(7), 813–819. doi:10.1111/dmcn.14517

Pellicano, E. (2013, March). Testing the predictive power of cognitive atypicalities in autistic children : Evidence from a 3-year follow-up study. *Autism Research*, *6*, 258–267. doi:10.1002/aur.1286

Pelphrey, K., Adolphs, R., & Morris, J. P. (2004). Neuroanatomical substrates of social cognition dysfunction in autism. *Mental Retardation and Developmental Disabilities Research Reviews*, *10*(4), 259–271. doi:10.1002/mrdd.20040

Peterson, C. (2014). Theory of mind understanding and empathic behavior in children with autism spectrum disorders. *International Journal of Developmental Neuroscience*, *39*, 16–21. doi:10.1016/j.ijdevneu.2014.05.002

Philofsky, A., Fidler, D. J., & Hepburn, S. (2007). Pragmatic language profiles of school-age children with autism spectrum disorders and Williams Syndrome. *American Journal of Speech-Language Pathology*, *16*(4), 368–380. doi:10.1044/1058-0360(2007/040)

Pierce, K., Haist, F., Sedaghat, F., & Courchesne, E. (2004). The brain response to personally familiar faces in autism: Findings of fusiform activity and beyond. *Brain*, *127*(12), 2703–2716. doi:10.1093/brain/awh289

Piggot, J., Ch, M. B. B., Kwon, H., Blasey, C., Lotspeich, L., Menon, V., Bookheimer, S., & Reiss, A. L. (2004). Emotional attribution in high-functioning individuals with autistic spectrum disorder: A functional imaging study. *Journal of the American Academy of Child and Adolescent Psychiatry*, *43*(4), 473–480. doi:10.1097/01.chi.0000111363.94169.37

Plasschaert, E., Descheemaeker, M. J., Van Eylen, L., Noens, I., Steyaert, J., & Legius, E. (2015). Prevalence of autism spectrum disorder symptoms in children with neurofibromatosis type 1. *American Journal of Medical Genetics, Part B: Neuropsychiatric Genetics*, *168*(1), 72–80. doi:10.1002/ajmg.b.32280

Plasschaert, E., Van Eylen, L., Descheemaeker, M. J., Noens, I., Legius, E., & Steyaert, J. (2016). Executive functioning deficits in children with neurofibromatosis type 1: The influence of intellectual and social functioning. *American Journal of Medical Genetics, Part B: Neuropsychiatric Genetics*, *171*(3), 348–362. doi:10.1002/ajmg.b.32414

Plesa-Skwerer, D., Faja, S., Schofield, C., Verbalis, A., & Tager-Flusberg, H. (2006). Perceiving facial and vocal expressions of emotion in individuals with Williams syndrome. *American Association on Mental Retardation*, *15*. http://meridian.allenpress.com/ajidd/article-pdf/111/1/15/2029433/0895-8017

Pober, B. R. (2010). Medical progress: Williams-Beuren syndrome. *New England Journal of Medicine*, *362*(3), 239–252. Massachussetts Medical Society. doi:10.1056/NEJMra0903074

Porter, M. A., Coltheart, M., & Langdon, R. (2008). Theory of mind in Williams syndrome assessed using a nonverbal task. *Journal of Autism and Developmental Disorders*, *38*(5), 806–814. doi:10.1007/s10803-007-0447-4

Pride, N. A., Crawford, H., Payne, J. M., & North, K. N. (2013). Social functioning in adults with neurofibromatosis type 1. *Research in Developmental Disabilities, 34*(10), 3393–3399.

Pride, N. A., Korgaonkar, M. S., Barton, B., Payne, J. M., Vucic, S., & North, K. N. (2014). The genetic and neuroanatomical basis of social dysfunction: Lessons from neurofibromatosis type 1. *Human Brain Mapping, 35*(5), 2372–2382. doi:10.1002/hbm.22334

Ramaswami, G., & Geschwind, D. H. (2018). Genetics of autism spectrum disorder. *Handbook of Clinical Neurology, 147*, 321–329. Elsevier B.V. doi:10.1016/B978-0-444-63233-3.00021-X

Rhodes, S. M., Riby, D. M., Matthews, K., & Coghill, D. R. (2011). Attention-deficit/hyperactivity disorder and Williams syndrome: Shared behavioral and neuropsychological profiles. *Journal of Clinical and Experimental Neuropsychology, 33*(1), 147–156. doi:10.1080/13803395.2010.495057

Rosema, S., Crowe, L., & Anderson, V. (2012). Social function in children and adolescents after traumatic brain injury: A systematic review 1989–2011. *Journal of Neurotrauma, 29*(7), 1277–1291.

Rutter, M., Le Couteur, A., & Lord, C. (2003). *Autism Diagnostic Interview-Revised* (Vol. 29, p. 30). Los Angeles, CA: Western Psychological Services.

Scheeren, A. M., De Rosnay, M., Koot, H. M., & Begeer, S. (2013). Rethinking theory of mind in high-functioning autism spectrum disorder. *Journal of Child Psychology and Psychiatry and Allied Disciplines, 54*(6), 628–635. doi:10.1111/jcpp.12007

Scherf, K. S., Elbich, D., Minshew, N., & Behrmann, M. (2015). Individual differences in symptom severity and behavior predict neural activation during face processing in adolescents with autism. *NeuroImage: Clinical, 7*, 53–67. doi:10.1016/j.nicl.2014.11.003

Schultz, R. T. (2005). Developmental deficits in social perception in autism: The role of the amygdala and fusiform face area. *International Journal of Developmental Neuroscience, 23*(2–3 SPEC. ISS.), 125–141. doi:10.1016/j.ijdevneu.2004.12.012

Senju, A. (2012). Spontaneous theory of mind and its absence in autism spectrum disorders. *Neuroscientist, 18*(2), 108–113. doi:10.1177/1073858410397208

Senju, A. (2013). Atypical development of spontaneous social cognition in autism spectrum disorders. *Brain and Development, 35*(2), 96–101. doi:10.1016/j.braindev.2012.08.002

Shaw, T. A., & Porter, M. A. (2013). Emotion recognition and visual-scan paths in fragile X syndrome. *Journal of Autism and Developmental Disorders, 43*(5), 1119–1139. doi:10.1007/s10803-012-1654-1

Shilyansky, C., Lee, Y. S., & Silva, A. J. (2010). Molecular and cellular mechanisms of learning disabilities: A focus on NF1. *Annual Review of Neuroscience, 33*, 221–243. doi:10.1146/annurev-neuro-060909-153215

Simion, F., Regolin, L., & Bulf, H. (2008). A predisposition for biological motion in the newborn baby. *Proceedings of the National Academy of Sciences of the United States of America, 105*(2), 809–813. doi:10.1073/pnas.0707021105

Skorich, D. P., May, A. R., Talipski, L. A., Hall, M. H., Dolstra, A. J., Gash, T. B., & Gunningham, B. H. (2016). Is social categorization the missing link between weak central coherence and mental state inference abilities in autism? Preliminary evidence from a general population sample. *Journal of Autism and Developmental Disorders, 46*(3), 862–881. doi:10.1007/s10803-015-2623-2

Smith, L. E., Barker, E. T., Seltzer, M. M., Abbeduto, L., & Greenberg, J. S. (2012). Behavioral phenotype of Fragile X syndrome in adolescence and adulthood. *American Journal on Intellectual and Developmental Disabilities, 117*(1), 1–17. doi:10.1352/1944-7558-117.1.1

Söderstrand, P., & Almkvist, O. (2012). Psychometric data on the eyes test, the Faux pas test, and the Dewey social stories test in a population-based Swedish adult sample. *Nordic Psychology, 64*(1), 30–43. doi:10.1080/19012276.2012.693729

Spek, A. A., Scholte, E. M., & Van Berckelaer-Onnes, I. A. (2010). Theory of mind in adults with HFA and asperger syndrome. *Journal of Autism and Developmental Disorders, 40*(3), 280–289. doi:10.1007/s10803-009-0860-y

Stivaros, S., Garg, S., Tziraki, M., Cai, Y., Thomas, O., Mellor, J., . . . Steiger, C. (2018). Randomised controlled trial of simvastatin treatment for autism in young children with neurofibromatosis type 1 (SANTA). *Molecular Autism, 9*(1). doi:10.1186/s13229-018-0190-z

Strømme, P., Bjømstad, P. G., & Ramstad, K. (2002). Prevalence estimation of Williams syndrome. *Journal of Child Neurology, 17*(4), 269–271. doi:10.1177/088307380201700406

Tager-Flusberg, H. (2007). *Evaluating the theory-of-mind hypothesis of autism. Current Directions in Psychological Science, 16*(6), 311–315.

Tager-Flusberg, H., & Sullivan, K. (2000). A componential view of theory of mind: Evidence from Williams syndrome. *Cognition, 76.* www.elsevier.com/locate/cognit

Tick, B., Bolton, P., Happé, F., Rutter, M., & Rijsdijk, F. (2016). Heritability of autism spectrum disorders: A meta-analysis of twin studies. *Journal of Child Psychology and Psychiatry and Allied Disciplines, 57*(5), 585–595. doi:10.1111/jcpp.12499

Todorova, G. K., Hatton, R. E. M. B., & Pollick, F. E. (2019). Biological motion perception in autism spectrum disorder: A meta-analysis. *Molecular Autism, 10*(1). doi:10.1186/s13229-019-0299-8

Toma, C. (2020). Genetic variation across phenotypic severity of autism. *Trends in Genetics, 36*(4), 228–231. doi:10.1016/j.tig.2020.01.005

Turkstra, L. S., Abbeduto, L., & Meulenbroek, P. (2014). Social cognition in adolescent girls with Fragile X syndrome. *American Journal on Intellectual and Developmental Disabilities, 119*(4), 319–339. American Association on Mental Retardation. doi:10.1352/1944-7558-119.4.319

Uljarevic, M., & Hamilton, A. (2013). Recognition of emotions in autism: A formal meta-analysis. *Journal of Autism and Developmental Disorders, 43*(7), 1517–1526. doi:10.1007/s10803-012-1695-5

Ure, A., Rose, V., Bernie, C., & Williams, K. (2018). Autism: One or many spectrums? *Journal of Paediatrics and Child Health, 54*(10), 1068–1072. doi:10.1111/jpc.14176

Van der Molen, M. J. W., Huizinga, M., Huizenga, H. M., Ridderinkhof, K. R., Van der Molen, M. W., Hamel, B. J. C., . . . Ramakers, G. J. A. (2010). Profiling Fragile X syndrome in males: Strengths and weaknesses in cognitive abilities. *Research in Developmental Disabilities, 31*(2), 426–439. doi:10.1016/j.ridd.2009.10.013

van der Vaart, T., Plasschaert, E., Rietman, A. B., Renard, M., Oostenbrink, R., Vogels, A., de Wit, M. C. Y., Descheemaeker, M. J., Vergouwe, Y., Catsman-Berrevoets, C. E., Legius, E., Elgersma, Y., & Moll, H. A. (2013). Simvastatin for cognitive deficits and behavioural problems in patients with neurofibromatosis type 1 (NF1-SIMCODA): A randomised, placebo-controlled trial. *The Lancet Neurology, 12*(11), 1076–1083. doi:10.1016/S1474-4422(13)70227-8

Vannucchi, G., Masi, G., Toni, C., Dell'Osso, L., Marazziti, D., & Perugi, G. (2014). Clinical features, developmental course, and psychiatric comorbidity of adult autism spectrum disorders. *CNS Spectrums, 19*(2), 157–164. doi:10.1017/S1092852913000941

Van Wijngaarden-Cremers, P. J. M., Van Eeten, E., Groen, W. B., Van Deurzen, P. A., Oosterling, I. J., & Van Der Gaag, R. J. (2014). Gender and age differences in the core triad of impairments in autism spectrum disorders: A systematic review and meta-analysis. *Journal of Autism and Developmental Disorders, 44*(3), 627–635. doi:10.1007/s10803-013-1913-9

Vithayathil, J., Pucilowska, J., & Landreth, G. E. (2018). ERK/MAPK signaling and autism spectrum disorders. *Progress in Brain Research, 241*, 63–112. Elsevier B.V. doi:10.1016/bs.pbr.2018.09.008

Vivanti, G., Fanning, P. A. J., Hocking, D. R., Sievers, S., & Dissanayake, C. (2017). Social attention, joint attention and sustained attention in autism spectrum disorder and Williams syndrome: Convergences and divergences. *Journal of Autism and Developmental Disorders, 47*(6), 1866–1877. doi:10.1007/s10803-017-3106-4

Vivanti, G., Hamner, T., & Lee, N. R. (2018). Neurodevelopmental disorders affecting sociability: Recent research advances and future directions in autism spectrum disorder and Williams syndrome. *Current Neurology and Neuroscience Reports, 18*(12). Current Medicine Group LLC 1. doi:10.1007/s11910-018-0902-y

Vlamings, P. H. J. M., Jonkman, L. M., Van Daalen, E., Van Der Gaag, R. J., & Kemner, C. (2010). Basic abnormalities in visual processing affect face processing at an early age in autism spectrum disorder. *Biological Psychiatry, 68*(12), 1107–1113. doi:10.1016/j.biopsych.2010.06.024

Wang, D. L., Smith, K. B., Esparza, S., Leigh, F. A., Muzikansky, A., Park, E. R., & Plotkin, S. R. (2012). Emotional functioning of patients with neurofibromatosis tumor suppressor syndrome. *Genetics in Medicine, 14*(12), 977–982. doi:10.1038/gim.2012.85

Wang, Y., Kim, E., Wang, X., Novitch, B. G., Yoshikawa, K., Chang, L. S., & Zhu, Y. (2012). ERK inhibition rescues defects in fate specification of Nf1-deficient neural progenitors and brain abnormalities. *Cell, 150*(4), 816–830. doi:10.1016/j.cell.2012.06.034

Watt, S. E., Shores, E. A., & North, K. N. (2008). An examination of lexical and sublexical reading skills in children with neurofibromatosis type 1. *Child Neuropsychology, 14*(5), 401–418.

Webb, S. J., Neuhaus, E., & Faja, S. (2017). Face perception and learning in autism spectrum disorders. *Quarterly Journal of Experimental Psychology, 70*(5), 970–986. doi:10.1080/17470218.2016.1151059

Wegscheid, M. L., Anastasaki, C., & Gutmann, D. H. (2018). Human stem cell modeling in neurofibromatosis type 1 (NF1). *Experimental Neurology, 299*, 270–280.

White, S., Hill, E., Happé, F., & Frith, U. (2009). Revisiting the strange stories: Revealing mentalizing impairments in autism. *Child Development, 80*(4), 1097–1117. doi:10.1111/j.1467-8624.2009.01319.x

Williams, T. A., Porter, M. A., & Langdon, R. (2014). Social approach and emotion recognition in Fragile X syndrome. *American Journal on Intellectual and Developmental Disabilities, 119*(2), 133–150. doi:10.1352/1944-7558-119.2.133

Williamson, K. E., & Jakobson, L. S. (2014). Social perception in children born at very low birthweight and its relationship with social/behavioral outcomes. *Journal of Child Psychology and Psychiatry and Allied Disciplines, 55*(9), 990–998. doi:10.1111/jcpp.12210

Wilson, C. E., Happé, F., Wheelwright, S. J., Ecker, C., Lombardo, M. V., Johnston, P., Daly, E., Murphy, C. M., Spain, D., Lai, M. C., Chakrabarti, B., Sauter, D. A., Baron-Cohen, S., Murphy, D. G. M., Bailey, A. J., Bolton, P. F., Bullmore, E. T., Carrington, S., Catani, M., . . . Williams, S. C. (2014). The neuropsychology of male adults with high-functioning autism or Asperger syndrome. *Autism Research, 7*(5), 568–581. doi:10.1002/aur.1394

Wolff, J. J., Bodfish, J. W., Hazlett, H. C., Lightbody, A. A., Reiss, A. L., & Piven, J. (2012). Evidence of a distinct behavioral phenotype in young boys with Fragile X syndrome and autism. *Journal of the American Academy of Child and Adolescent Psychiatry, 51*(12), 1324–1332. doi:10.1016/j.jaac.2012.09.001

Chapter 5

Disorders of social cognition in adults with acquired brain injury

Travis Wearne, Michelle Kelly and Skye McDonald

Acquired brain injuries refer to a complex group of non-progressive conditions that result from damage to the brain occurring any time after birth. These can range from common traumatic brain injuries or strokes to rarer forms of brain damage incurred by anoxia, cancer, drugs and alcohol, or encephalitis. This chapter aims to outline the social cognitive changes that are typically identified following these conditions. The majority of this chapter is dedicated to traumatic brain injury and stroke, as these are the most prevalent forms of brain injuries and the most researched within the field of social cognitive neuroscience. An overview of the emerging research on social cognition in other acquired brain injuries is provided at the end of the chapter.

Traumatic brain injury

A traumatic brain injury (TBI) occurs when brain tissue is damaged by a penetrating instrument (e.g., sharp objects or missiles) or an external mechanical force. The latter – often referred to as a 'closed head injury' – accounts for most TBIs and commonly results from falls, vehicle (and pedestrian) accidents, assaults and sporting injuries. TBI disproportionally affects adolescents and young adults, particularly men, who are 1.5 to 3 times more likely to sustain a TBI than women (Frost, Farrer, Primosch, & Hedges, 2013). The elderly are also susceptible given the higher incidence of falls within this group. Given the declining death rates of TBI due to advances in the acute treatment of brain trauma, together with the younger age of victims, there is an increasingly growing population of TBI survivors worldwide. Indeed, TBI is the leading international cause of disability in those under the age of 45 (Werner & Engelhard, 2007). TBIs typically fall across a spectrum of severity, which is determined based on the initial loss of consciousness (assessed using the Glasgow Coma Scale) and the duration of post-traumatic amnesia (i.e., a period whereby the person is unable to form new memories after the injury). Approximately 80% of TBIs fall within the mild category while the remaining 20% of cases are moderate to extremely severe injuries (Servadei, Graham, & Merry, 2001).

DOI: 10.4324/9781003027034-5

There are primary and secondary neuropathological mechanisms of TBI. Primary injuries are due to the immediate effects of the mechanical forces on the brain tissue. These include contusions (i.e., bruising), lacerations, haematoma (localised bleeding) and diffuse axonal injury (i.e., where neurons are stretched and torn). Acceleration-deceleration forces at the time of insult displace the brain and brush the orbital surfaces of the tissue across the bony anterior and middle fossa of the skull (Bigler, 2007). The frontal and temporal lobes are particularly vulnerable to contusions due to their direct impact with the skull (i.e., the frontal and temporal bones). As a result, the neuropathology following TBI is typically concentrated towards the *ventrolateral, ventromedial* and *orbital frontal lobes* and the *ventromedial temporal lobes* (Bigler, 2007) (Figure 5.1). Additionally, diffuse axonal injury can lead to significant atrophy of major white matter tracts including the *corpus callosum* (Figure 5.2). This along with herniation and Wallarian degeneration (i.e., loss of downstream structures due to loss of input) can disrupt connections between cortical and subcortical regions. Secondary injuries are physiological changes that follow primary injuries and usually have a delayed presentation. These include increased cranial pressure and cerebral oedema, inflammation, herniation, hypoxia and tissue death, brain lesions and infection (Werner & Engelhard, 2007).

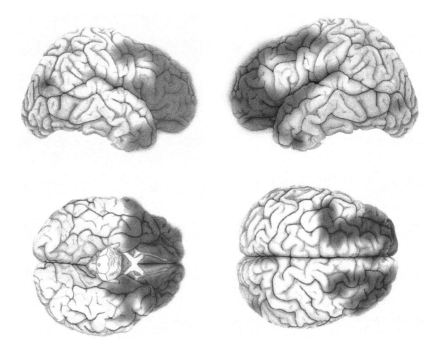

Figure 5.1 Cortical areas that are prone to pathology in TBI

Source: Based upon studies such as Courville (1945) and Yeates et al. (2007)

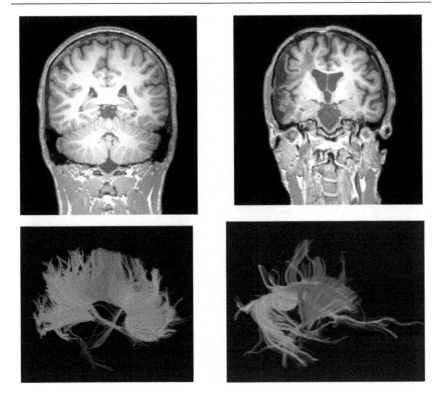

Figure 5.2 Magnetic resonance imaging (MRI), coronal section demonstrating loss of volume of corpus callosum and other white matter tracts following TBI (top frames: left, normal healthy adult; right, adult with TBI) and diffusion tensor imaging (bottom frames: left, normal healthy adult; right, adult with TBI) showing reduction of fibre tracts in corpus callosum.

Cognitively, difficulties with attention and speed of information processing are the most ubiquitous symptoms experienced following TBI, regardless of severity (Olver, Ponsford, & Curran, 1996). These difficulties typically resolve within three months for those with mild injuries while they persist for more severe TBIs (Carroll et al., 2004). Other sequelae following moderate to severe TBI include difficulties with verbal and visual learning and memory, communication (i.e., fluency, word-finding and tracking conversations) and higher-order executive skills, including problems with planning and organisation, goal-directed behaviour, problem-solving, judgement, flexibility, self-monitoring, impulsivity and insight and/or awareness (Azouvi, Arnould, Dromer, & Vallat-Azouvi, 2017). Mood (i.e., depression and anxiety) and adjustment disorders are also common (Gould, Ponsford, Johnston, & Schönberger, 2011). Overall, TBI has a profound impact on one's cognitive, emotional and physical functioning both in the acute and long-term following injury. However, an additional prominent, and often overlooked consideration, is the impact of TBI on social behaviour.

Traumatic brain injury and social outcomes

The relationship between brain injury and altered social behaviour was first reported as far back as the renowned case of Phineas Gage. In 1848, Gage sustained a penetrative brain injury after a large metal rod was driven through his head whilst working on the railroad track, extremely damaging his left frontal lobe. While his survival within of itself was remarkable, a notable repercussion of his injuries was changes to his personality, social understanding and behaviour. The descriptions of him post-injury describe him as vulgar, profane, impatient and lacking in respect for those around him, to the point whereby he was routinely described – at least in academic sources – as being "no longer Gage" (O'Driscoll & Leach, 1998). While the objectivity of such descriptions of his behaviour has been questioned (Kotowicz, 2007), the case nevertheless provided seminal evidence of the complex relationship between brain damage and the regulation and control of social functioning.

Similar descriptions are routinely reported by family members of those who have sustained a TBI. Childishness, dislike and disinterest in others, socially inappropriate behaviour, self-centredness and disputatiousness are frequently described (Brooks, Campsie, Symington, Beattie, & McKinlay, 1986; Mcdonald & Saunders, 2005; Weddell & Leggett, 2006). These personality and behavioural difficulties lead to a range of psychosocial problems, including loss and deterioration of intimate relationships (Tam, McKay, Sloan, & Ponsford, 2015), difficulty establishing and maintaining social relationships and friendships (Hoofien, Gilboa, Vakil, & Donovick, 2001), reduction or loss of job opportunities (Temkin, Corrigan, Dikmen, & Machamer, 2009), poor social integration (Winter, Moriarty, & Short, 2018), limited social participation (Cattran, Oddy, Wood, & Moir, 2011) and increased social withdrawal (Demakis et al., 2007). Such changes also cause elevated caregiver burdens for families (Katsifaraki & Wood, 2014). It has been suggested that the impact of TBI on psychosocial functioning and behaviour pose an even greater contribution to caregiver burden (Kinsella, Packer, & Olver, 1991) and distress (Kelly, Brown, Todd, & Kremer, 2008), and barriers to adjustment and rehabilitation (Yates, 2003), than the effects on physical and cognitive functioning.

Given the impact and pervasiveness of these social difficulties, research has shifted to focus on the underlying processes that subserve, maintain and predict such functional changes post TBI. Initial work suggested a role of neuropsychological components to the regulation of post-injury social behaviour (Kendall, 1996; Kendall & Terry, 2009). Some work has shown that executive ability predicts general functional outcomes following TBI post-injury (Spitz, Ponsford, Rudzki, & Maller, 2012). Others, however, have shown that the relationships between cognitive functioning and social outcomes are not so robust (Ownsworth & McKenna, 2004; Wood & Rutterford, 2006). Additionally, there can be functional dissociations between intellectual and social outcomes, such that social behaviour can be disproportionally impaired while cognitive faculties can be relatively intact (Blair & Cipolotti, 2000; Tranel, Bechara, & Denburg, 2002), raising the possibility that other factors are involved in regulating social behaviour. Indeed, research over the past three decades has witnessed a proliferation of research highlighting a clear and prominent role of social cognition in the regulation and maintenance of social outcomes following TBI.

Traumatic brain injury and social cognition

While TBI typically results in multi-focal and diffuse damage, specific brain regions associated with social cognition are particularly vulnerable to harm at the time of impact. Key regions, especially in the *ventromedial frontal* and *temporal lobes*, are implicated in the brain circuitry of 'the social brain' (Chapter 1). Furthermore, recent research has shown significant associations between the degeneration of white-matter connections (e.g., *corpus callosum* and *fornix*) and social cognitive performance following TBI (McDonald, Dalton, Rushby, & Landin-Romero, 2019). As a result, the diverse and multifocal nature of TBI pathology renders it particularly sensitive to social cognitive disturbances that may underlie deleterious social functioning following injury. Here, we describe and present evidence for changes to various components of social cognition following TBI, specifically emotion perception, empathy and theory of mind (including cognitive empathy, mentalising and pragmatics).

Emotion perception in TBI

Emotion in face

Early work on social cognitive difficulties following TBI (as far back as the early 1980s; e.g., (Prigatano & Pribram, 1982)) focussed almost exclusively on facial emotion perception, whereby participants had to recognise, match, label and/ or discriminate between still photographs (i.e., static images) of facial affect. Since this time, a large body of research has found reliable and robust difficulties in facial emotion recognition following moderate-to-severe TBI. A systematic review and meta-analysis of 13 studies published up to 2009 (Babbage et al., 2011) reported that individuals with TBI performed approximately 1.1 standard deviations below matched controls on these tasks. It was concluded that between 13% and 39% of individuals with moderate-to-severe TBI demonstrate difficulties recognising emotions via static images (compared to 7% of the comparison group). These problems are present irrespective of the age of insult (Schmidt, Hanten, Li, Orsten, & Levin, 2010), do not improve with time since injury or recovery (Ietswaart, Milders, Crawford, Currie, & Scott, 2008) and are worse with greater injury severity (Spikman, Timmerman, Milders, Veenstra, & van der Naalt, 2012). Difficulties with emotion perception are hypothesised to be due to damage sustained to the ventral fronto-temporal systems of the brain (Adolphs, Tranel, & Damasio, 2003).

There is contentious evidence that particular emotions are more susceptible to the effects of TBI than others. For example, multiple studies have found greater difficulty recognising negatively valanced emotions (e.g., sad) compared to positive emotions (Croker & McDonald, 2005; Green, Turner, & Thompson, 2004; McDonald, Flanagan, Rollins, & Kinch, 2003; Rosenberg, McDonald, Dethier, Kessels, & Westbrook, 2014; Zupan & Neumann, 2016). However, this 'valence effect' could be the result of the disproportionate representation of negative emotions on emotion perception tasks (i.e., sad, anger, disgust and fear compared to just happy and surprised). Furthermore, recent evidence suggests that the differential ease in which some emotions can be recognised is a confound in the use of static image tasks. For example, happy is an emotion that is universally recognised while fear is notoriously difficult. The differential impairment across emotions may therefore reflect the ease of identifying the emotional content rather than problems with recognising specific emotions. In support of this, when item difficulty is controlled for by implementing images of varying intensity, those with TBI demonstrate an overall emotion perception difficulty irrespective of the emotional valence of the images (Rosenberg, Dethier, Kessels, Westbrook, & McDonald, 2015; Rosenberg et al., 2014; Rosenberg, McDonald, Rosenberg, & Frederick Westbrook, 2018).

The use of static images in examining emotion perception difficulties following TBI has also sparked debate. Emotions are rarely, if ever, provided as a single static facial expression for examination by the observer. Rather, emotional displays are dynamic, fleeting and typically provided within the context of multiple, different person-centered, interpersonal, modality and environmental cues. In this vein, static images may have limited validity to assess emotions and interactions within the real world and impairments in discrete aspects of emotion recognition may not have meaningful real-life consequences. Indeed, some studies have shown that performance on static emotion perception tasks does not relate to real-world problems in interpersonal functioning for those with TBI (Milders, Fuchs, & Crawford, 2003; Milders, Ietswaart, Crawford, & Currie, 2008; Osborne-Crowley & McDonald, 2016). Hence, a number of more recent studies have shifted to assess emotion perception via alternative methods that are commensurate with displays seen in the real world, such as dynamic images. Most studies show that those with TBI have difficulty discerning dynamic emotional states compared to controls (Knox & Douglas, 2009; McDonald & Flanagan, 2004; McDonald et al., 2003; McDonald & Saunders, 2005) while some have found no difference between groups (McDonald & Saunders, 2005; Zupan & Neumann, 2014). A potential reason for the discrepant findings may relate to the dissociated brain regions involved in dynamic versus static emotion recognition. Movement cues are associated with dorsal-fronto-parietal zones that may be less implicated in the neuropathology of TBI (Adolphs et al., 2003). Additionally, enriched visual scenes provide an enhanced range of cues which may facilitate recognition but simultaneously increase the cognitive load requisite for their interpretation which may tax limited cognitive resources. Given the heterogeneity of cognitive abilities following moderate to severe TBI, dynamic scenes may either facilitate or hinder emotion perception and it may be this variability that is reflected in these studies.

There is also evidence that emotion perception difficulties may index a broader problem with emotional experience. Emotion perception deficits are related to alexithymia, an inability to identify, recognise and/or experience emotions in oneself. Alexithymia affects up to 60% of individuals with TBI (Neumann, Zupan, Malec, & Hammond, 2014; Williams & Wood, 2010). Indeed, reduced emotional experience correlates with emotion perception accuracy (Croker & McDonald, 2005), and we have recently shown that the overt subjective experience of emotion is uniquely associated with the recognition of happy, sad and angry facial expressions post TBI (Wearne, Osborne-Crowley, Rosenberg, Dethier, & McDonald, 2018). In contrast, while implicit and subconscious indices of emotional experiences, such as mimicry and physiological reactivity, can also be impaired following TBI, their relationship with emotion perception has not been substantiated (McDonald, Li et al., 2011; McDonald, Rushby et al., 2011). Therefore, difficulties with emotion perception following TBI seem to relate more specifically to poor awareness and/or the overt subjective experience of one's own emotions rather than via the unconscious mechanisms involved in simulation and/or emotion processing (discussed further below).

Emotion in voice

Vocal prosody and intonation can be used to determine a person's emotional state, particularly when facial affective cues are not available in social settings. Consequently, assessment of vocal emotion is an important aspect of the examination of emotion perception following TBI. Furthermore, there is evidence that the neural systems relating to vocal emotion are somewhat separable from those with facial emotions (Adolphs, Damasio, & Tranel, 2002), although this is sometimes debated (Drapeau, Gosselin, Peretz, & McKerral, 2017). There appears to be robust evidence that those with moderate to severe TBI demonstrate reduced vocal emotion recognition ability relative to control participants (Dimoska, McDonald, Pell, Tate, & James, 2010; Hornak, Rolls, & Wade, 1996; Zupan, Babbage, Neumann, & Willer, 2014; Zupan & Neumann, 2014, 2016). Understanding emotion in voice is a complex task, as the listener needs to process both the semantic content and voice quality, which increases demands on working memory and inhibition. Consequently, people with TBI may lose efficiency in their ability to understand vocal emotion due to the dual processing demands. Nevertheless, there is also evidence for primary problems with prosodic processing itself (Dimoska et al., 2010).

Emotion perception and social outcomes

Emotion perception difficulties relate to social functioning. For example, a recent review by Maarten Milders (2019) summarised the findings from 10 studies across 378 participants that had examined the relationship between the perception of facial and vocal social cues and post-injury behaviour (as indexed by informant based measures). He found that the average correlation between emotion perception and behaviour post-TBI was of moderate effect size ($r = 0.35$), such that those who had greater performance on tests of emotion perception showed greater social outcome and adaptive social behaviour. While it is likely that other factors are also involved, these findings suggest a critical and important relationship between emotion perception and social outcomes following TBI.

(Cognitive and affective) theory of mind in TBI

Theory of mind (ToM) is the ability to identify and understand the emotions, beliefs, thoughts and intentions of another person to appreciate their perspective (i.e., perspective taking or cognitive empathy). While ToM and cognitive empathy are often used and assessed interchangeably in the TBI space, there are distinct components of ToM, some of which do not always equate to empathy. For example, affective ToM relates to the ability to infer intentions, feelings and thoughts of another person as a means to understand their perspective (i.e., cognitive empathy). Cognitive ToM, on the other hand, involves making inferences about another's beliefs without the need or result of empathic understanding (Shamay-Tsoory, Aharon-Peretz, & Perry, 2009). Approximately 50% of individuals with TBI self-report reduced cognitive empathy on questionnaires (de Sousa et al., 2010; Grattan & Eslinger, 1989; Wells, Dywan, & Dumas, 2005).

Theory of mind difficulties are present in both the acute (Muller et al., 2010) and chronic (Bosco, Angeleri, Sacco, & Bara, 2015; Spikman et al., 2012) phases post-TBI injury. A meta-analysis of 26 studies of participants with acquired brain injury, in which 50% of the entire sample had sustained a TBI, found moderate to severe difficulties across a range of ToM tasks compared to healthy controls (Martin-Rodriguez & Leon-Carrion, 2010). They reported moderate effect sizes across first-order (ES = 0.52) and second-order (ES = 0.60) belief tasks. With regard to studies that have directly examined those with TBI, there appears to be difficulties across a range of cognitive and affective ToM components. For example, those with TBI demonstrate difficulties understanding when someone has committed a faux pas or holds a belief incongruent with fact (Bibby & McDonald, 2005; Geraci, Surian, Ferraro, & Cantagallo, 2010; Spikman et al., 2012; Turkstra, Williams, Tonks, & Frampton, 2008). They also have difficulty inferring intentions (Havet-Thomassin, Allain, Etcharry-Bouyx, & Le Gall, 2006; Muller et al., 2010), understanding jokes (Bibby &

McDonald, 2005, Spikman et al., 2012), predicting thoughts/emotions and attributing mental states of others in social situations (Allain et al., 2020; Henry, Phillips, Crawford, Ietswaart, & Summers, 2006; McDonald & Flanagan, 2004; Turkstra, Dixon, & Baker, 2004).

Disorder of pragmatic language (cognitive communication) after TBI

People with TBI are also likely to experience deficits in their communicative abilities despite good language skills. Pragmatic language disorders, otherwise known as social or cognitive communication disorders, refer to the loss of the ability to decipher pragmatic inferences that arise from the use of language in context. Such skills are central to the understanding and detection of indirect speech acts such as deceit, sarcasm, humour and irony, where the literal meaning of an utterance is not the meaning the speaker intends. Many adults with TBI demonstrate reliable difficulties not only with understanding a range of pragmatic phenomena but also in producing pragmatic inference themselves (Bosco, Gabbatore, Angeleri, Zettin, & Parola, 2018; Bosco, Parola, Sacco, Zettin, & Angeleri, 2017; Evans & Hux, 2011; Johnson & Turkstra, 2012; McDonald et al., 2003; McDonald et al., 2014; Vas, Spence, & Chapman, 2015; Yang, Fuller, Khodaparast, & Krawczyk, 2010). These difficulties have been primarily attributed to a failure of ToM, i.e., knowing what is on another person's mind, or understanding their perspective. In fact, difficulties with pragmatic interference represent the largest effect size (ES = 0.87) compared to other ToM processes (Martin-Rodriguez & Leon-Carrion, 2010), highlighting the pervasiveness of these difficulties relative to other social cognitive abilities post-injury.

ToM and social outcomes

There is also a growing number of studies demonstrating that difficulties with ToM/cognitive empathy are associated with outcomes following TBI. For example, poor ToM correlates with carer distress (Wells et al., 2005) and carer quality of life (Bivona et al., 2015) while self-reported perspective-taking is associated with interpersonal difficulties post-injury (Saxton, Younan, & Lah, 2013). Additionally, those with reduced ability to make inferences about social behaviour are more likely to have unstable employment following TBI (Meulenbroek & Turkstra, 2016). Furthermore, Milders (2019) found that across six studies and 314 participants there was an average small-to-medium effect size ($r = 0.24$) between impaired ToM and worse social behaviour following TBI. Indeed, Allain et al. (2020) recently found that mentalising abilities were associated with proxy rated dysexecutive problems. Overall, while some studies that have failed to show an association (May et al., 2017), most studies suggest that ToM is important for social and interpersonal functioning, and that difficulties within many of the various subcomponents within ToM may underlie difficulties with social behaviour and social outcome.

Emotional empathy in TBI

Emotional or affective empathy refers to the ability to share and resonate with the feelings of another. It is the ability to feel what someone else is feeling while distinguishing those feelings from one's own. Approximately 60 to 70% of those with moderate to severe TBI self-report reduced emotional empathy, almost double that of their control counterparts on questionnaire-based measures (de Sousa, McDonald, & Rushby, 2012; de Sousa et al., 2010, 2011; Eslinger, Satish, & Grattan, 1996; Wood & Williams, 2008). There is also evidence that these difficulties are independent of time since insult, injury severity (Williams & Wood, 2010) and neurocognitive difficulties (Wearne et al., 2020; Wood & Williams, 2008). Importantly, changes to empathy are associated with functional and social outcomes post-TBI (de Sousa et al. (2012) and Saxton, Younan, and Lah (2013)). However, not all studies demonstrate consistent reductions post-injury (e.g., Milders et al., 2003; Osborne-Crowley, Wilson, De Blasio, Wearne, Rushby, & McDonald, 2019a), suggesting there is heterogeneity in emotional empathy post-TBI. There has also been debate surrounding the validity of self-report measures given their reliance on insight, language and attention, all of which can be compromised post-TBI injury. Despite this, similar prevalence rates have been consistently found across studies and early work showed that the scores of those with TBI were equivalent to those completed by family members (Eslinger et al., 1996).

The mechanisms of reduced emotional empathy post-TBI have also been addressed. Similar to emotion recognition, these has been typically examined through the lens of conscious (i.e., the ability to subjectively experience emotion) and unconscious (i.e., the ability to subconsciously mimic and simulate emotion) processes. In addition to alexithymia and dulled emotional experiences (Croker & McDonald, 2005), those with TBI report reduced subjective emotion in response to emotional stimuli (de Sousa et al., 2012; de Sousa et al., 2010, 2011; Saunders, McDonald, & Richardson, 2006; Williams & Wood, 2010), have difficulty generating negative affective states deliberately or spontaneously (Dethier, Blairy, Rosenberg, & McDonald, 2012) and have reduced response to emotionally-provocative postures (Dethier, Blairy, Rosenberg, & McDonald, 2013). Despite this plethora of changes in emotional experience following TBI, the extent to which these are related to self-reported empathy is unclear. On the one hand, alexithymia has shown to be negatively associated with emotional empathy in TBI (Williams & Wood, 2010), highlighting the importance of subjective emotional experience in both emotional recognition and affective empathy. However, a study of the extent to which people with TBI responded to emotional manipulations found this had no relationship to self-reported empathy (Osborne-Crowley et al., 2019b). The difference between these studies may, to an extent, reflect the heterogeneity of TBI, not all of whom suffer deficits in empathy.

Simulation models propose that individuals subconsciously mimic emotions via pupil dilation, facial muscle contractions and/or physiology. It is proposed this implicit simulation serves as a tool to synchronise our own emotions with another's as a means to experience and understand it. This synchrony is frequently synonymous with affective empathy, and impairment has been suggested to underlie the emotional empathy difficulties experienced post-TBI. Indeed, those with TBI have lowered mimicry to facial expressions (McDonald, Li et al., 2011), reduced physiological reactivity and mimicry to negative pictures and films (de Sousa et al., 2012; de Sousa et al., 2010, 2011; Neumann, Hammond, Norton, & Blumenthal, 2011; Saunders et al., 2006; Williams & Wood, 2012) and also positive stimuli (Sanchez-Navarro, Martinez-Selva, & Roman, 2005). Importantly, and unlike research on emotion recognition, there is evidence that reduced emotional empathy is associated with impaired autonomic mimicry (de Sousa et al., 2011) and emotional physiology (Rushby et al., 2013) in those with TBI, suggesting that a range of conscious and subconscious processes are potentially involved in the breakdown of empathic experiences for those with brain injury. See Box 5.1 for a case description of a person with TBI.

Box 5.1   Case 1: DS: Young adult with severe traumatic brain injury

History:

Mr DS suffered an extremely severe TBI following a high-speed car accident at age 19. His Glasgow Coma Scale was 6/15 at the scene. A brain CT scan revealed subarachnoid haemorrhage and right frontal subdural haematoma while MRI revealed diffuse axonal injury of the left frontoparietal lobe and the body of the corpus callosum. He was estimated to be in post traumatic amnesia for 43 days, consistent with a very severe TBI.

Neuropsychological functioning:

Cognitively three years after his injury, DS demonstrated reductions in his attention, working memory, speed of information processing, visuospatial skills and higher-order executive abilities, including his planning and organization, idea generation and inhibition. His verbal skills and intake and retention of new information was preserved.

Presentation:

His mother reported DS demonstrated increased irritability, impulsivity and mood swings. He was more physically and verbally aggressive and required significant prompting to initiate tasks, which was often met with opposition and refusal. He also failed to monitor his personal hygiene and would pick up the same clothes to wear each day. He regularly "butted" into others' conversations and provide uninvited opinions on his friends' relationships. He would make inappropriate jokes to his family and friends and would make comments of a sexual nature to strangers. He also failed to pick up emotional cues (such as his mother being upset over the recent passing of her father). The general consensus was he made people feel "uncomfortable". His sister ultimately moved out of home and his friends have all pulled away, leaving his mother as his main person of support. She believes his social and behavioural difficulties are getting progressively worse.

Summary and opinion:

DS has sustained cognitive difficulties as a result of his TBI. However, his interpersonal difficulties with family and friends suggest he has broader impairments than those typically detected with conventional neuropsychological testing. The kinds of difficulties reported by his mother are consistent with acquired problems of social cognition and/or social behaviour.

Additional social cognitive abilities in TBI

Additional factors under the social cognition umbrella have recently begun to be examined in TBI. For example, some have examined interpretational biases, such as negative attribution styles, and behaviour. These findings suggest that individuals who make greater externalising-personalising judgements (e.g., hostility, blame, intentional) about people or events are more likely to react with anger and irritation (Neumann, Malec, & Hammond, 2015; Neumann et al., 2020). Consequently, behavioural output post-TBI may intricately depend on the individual's causal inferences and beliefs about themselves, others and the world. Additional abilities, such as social problem-solving (Ganesalingam, Yeates, Sanson, & Anderson, 2007), social decision-making (Kelly, McDonald, & Kellett, 2014), social disinhibition (Honan, Allen, Fisher, Osborne-Crowley, & McDonald, 2017) and moral reasoning skills (Beauchamp, Vera-Estay, Morasse, Anderson, & Dooley, 2019) have also gained traction (see Chapter 4). Conclusions regarding alterations to social knowledge have been far less conclusive compared to other social cognitive domains. For example, those with TBI still have a general fund of knowledge of socially appropriate behaviour (Kocka & Gagnon, 2014), and they show intact access to social stereotypes, as assessed by the implicit association test (McDonald, Saad, & James, 2011). Consequently, changes to social behaviour do not derive from a loss of social schemas and/or comprehension of acceptable behavioural practices.

Researchers have also delved into the mechanisms underlying social disinhibition, particularly in light of an inconclusive – or small to moderate at best – relationship between cognitive response inhibition and disinhibited behaviour (Osborne-Crowley & McDonald, 2018). Reversal learning, i.e. changing behaviour when it is no longer rewarded, has been suggested as a potential mechanism of social disinhibition given that the regulation of social behaviour is a hallmark feature of *orbitofrontal cortex* function (Osborne-Crowley & McDonald, 2018). Indeed, those with orbitofrontal cortex damage demonstrate difficulties updating stimulus-reinforcement contingencies compared to participants with damage to other brain regions (Rolls, Hornak, Wade, & McGrath, 1994), and these difficulties negatively correlate with the degree of socially disinhibited behaviour. Using a specifically designed social reward reversal learning paradigm, Osborne-Crowley, McDonald, and Rushby (2016) found that individuals with TBI had difficulty updating their responses to changing social contingencies, but interestingly, this finding only applied to those with elevated disinhibited behaviour. As such, social disinhibition may derive from an inability to update or change behaviour when presented with negative and/or altered social reward cues.

Conclusions on social cognition and TBI

Overall, TBI is associated with a range of social cognitive difficulties. Research to date has highlighted that those with TBI demonstrate reductions in emotion perception (irrespective of material and/or modality), a variety of theory of mind abilities, including cognitive empathy, pragmatics and mentalising, as well as emotional empathy, attribution style, social problem-solving, social decision-making and social disinhibition. These occur against preserved understanding and comprehension of social knowledge. Studies examining the underlying mechanisms for these problems have also begun to accrue and have proposed a range of conscious and unconscious processes. However, these difficulties are not ubiquitous post-TBI. The prevalence range across abilities is around 50%, and the effect sizes examining the relationship between social cognition and social functioning are typically around the moderate range. Thus, there is considerable heterogeneity in the profile of social cognitive difficulties and how this impacts an individual's outcomes. It should also be noted that the findings presented here are from the perspective of moderate to severe TBI. Emerging research has begun to show that even those with mild brain injury have difficulties with social inference four years after injury (Theadom et al., 2019). Consequently, our understanding of social cognition following TBI – and the mechanisms and brain structure that subserve it – are far from being fully elucidated.

Stroke

Cerebrovascular accidents, or stroke, occur when the blood supply to the brain is affected. It can affect people of all ages, although it is most prevalent in older adulthood, with those above 75 approximately five times more likely to have a stroke than those in middle age (Mohammad et al., 2011). Stroke is more likely to affect men, although women tend to be older when they experience their first stroke (Petrea et al., 2009). Statistics from the World Health Organisation (WHO) place stroke as the third leading cause of disability and second cause of death worldwide (Johnson, Onuma, Owolabi, & Sachdev, 2016). Approximately 15 million strokes occur each year, five million of which lead to permanent disability and five million result in death. However, similar to TBI, better acute management of stroke is leading to declining death rates. This, coupled with an ageing population, is leading to a larger population of stroke survivors with permanent disability or long-term care needs.

Damage to the brain follows the distribution of the affected artery. For example, the anterior cerebral arteries irrigate the medial surfaces of the *frontal* and *parietal lobes*. The posterior arteries irrigate the *occipital cortex* and *ventral temporal lobes*. The middle cerebral arteries irrigate the lateral surface of the *frontal, parietal* and *temporal lobes* (Figure 5.3) and are the most common sites of both embolic (i.e., abrupt blockage caused by solid matter) and thrombotic (i.e., blockage due to gradual narrowing of vessel) stroke (Ng, Stein, Ning, & Black-Schaffer, 2007). Damage to the anterior cerebral artery supply has the potential to lead to *ventromedial frontal* damage. Given the similar

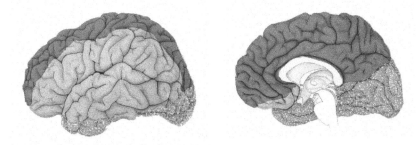

Figure 5.3 Cortical territories of the three major cerebral arteries in the lateral (left) and sagittal (right) view: light grey = middle cerebral artery, speckles = posterior cerebral artery; dark grey = anterior cerebral artery

neural systems affected, they may produce impairments in social cognition similar to those described following TBI. Damage to branches of the posterior cerebral artery has the potential to produce impairments in face recognition secondary to neuropathology affecting the *fusiform gyrus*, especially in the right hemisphere (see Chapter 1). Interestingly, damage to the middle cerebral arteries with consequential injury to regions on the lateral surfaces of either the right or left hemisphere is likely to yield impairments in social cognition that are lateralised and phenomenologically distinct to those typically seen in TBI. Here, we describe research findings that have explicitly examined the emotion perception, theory of mind and emotional empathy difficulties identified poststroke, with a unique emphasis on lateralisation between left (LH) and right (RH) hemisphere damage.

Emotion perception after stroke

As described in Chapter 1, and in our discussion of TBI, the ventral frontotemporal systems of the brain are critical to emotion perception. In addition, and of particular relevance to middle cerebral artery stroke, the *superior temporal sulcus, insula, sensorimotor* and *visual cortex* are also implicated.

Emotion in face

LH and RH stroke can result in deficits in the processing of facial emotion (Abbott, Cumming, Fidler, & Lindell, 2013; Adams et al., 2020), even when the stroke is mild (Nijsse, Spikman, Visser-Meily, de Kort, & van Heugten, 2019). This is true when stroke affects not only the cortex but also subcortical regions including the *thalamus* and *basal ganglia* (Cheung, Lee, Yip, King, & Li, 2006), which are also irrigated by the middle cerebral artery system. However, impairments are not symmetrical and tend to be more prevalent and severe when the right cortex is involved (Abbott et al., 2013; Adams, Schweitzer, Molenberghs, & Henry, 2019; Yuvaraj, Murugappan, Norlinah, Sundaraj, & Khairiyah, 2013). In RH stroke, the right frontoparietal region is particularly implicated, especially the *right somatosensory-motor cortex, anterior supramarginal gyrus,* and *insula*. The role of the somatosensory cortex is unknown but may serve to simulate the sensory experience of the perceived emotion 'as if' the viewer was experiencing it themselves as a way of facilitating conceptual understanding. Indeed, people who experience decreased sensation (touch) secondary to damage to the right somatosensory strip are more likely to experience impairment in emotion perception (Adolphs, Damasio, Tranel, Cooper, & Damasio, 2000).

People with LH stroke can also experience emotion perception deficits, particularly those specifically linked to lesions in the *left frontal operculum/insular* and/or *left supramarginal gyrus* (Adolphs et al., 2000; Corradi-Dell'Acqua et al., 2020). Using specific conceptual (e.g., sorting) versus labelling tasks,

Adolphs et al. (2000) surmised that verbal labelling of emotions may be more dependent on *supramarginal, temporal* and *opercula* lesions (in either hemisphere), whereas conceptual knowledge appears to rely upon the (right) *somatosensory cortex* and *insula.*

Emotion in voice

While damage to the LH and/or RH can interfere with the capacity to appreciate linguistic prosody (e.g., rise in pitch associated with a question), problems with affective prosody seem to be principally associated with the RH, with people with LH damage are only mildly impaired or normal relative to adults without damage (Charbonneau, Scherzer, Aspirot, & Cohen, 2003; Heilman, Bowers, Speedie, & Coslett, 1984; Kucharska-Pietura, Phillips, Gernand, & David, 2003; Pell, 2006). In an imaging study of 66 patients with focal and lateralised lesions, the majority arising from stroke, it was found that damage to the *right frontoparietal cortex* was consistently associated with affective prosody impairment (Adolphs et al., 2002).

Deficits in understanding affective prosody and facial expressions tend to co-occur, as the neural systems that mediate these abilities substantially overlap. Nonetheless, dissociations are not uncommon, where there is a deficit in one but not the other modality. Overall, people with stroke tend to have more pronounced deficits when judgements are made based upon a single modality, with voice being more difficult than face, and face more difficult than multi-modal displays (Adams et al., 2019). This possibly reflects the temporal demands of processing voice compared to face together with the facilitative context provided by multimodal displays.

Broader impairments in emotion processing post stroke

Following stroke, problems in the processing of emotion extend beyond the ability to read affect in face, body and voice. Patients with RH stroke are also often impassive with respect to emotional expressivity, more so than LH stroke (Borod, Koff, Lorch, & Nicholas, 1986; Borod, Koff, Lorch, Nicholas, & Welkowitz, 1988). Furthermore, people with RH stroke have been reported to have difficulty attributing a particular emotion to a description of nonverbal cues (e.g., "tears fell from her eyes") (Blonder, Bowers, & Heilman, 1991). Overall, this suggests that expressivity, somatosensory activation, perception and conceptual knowledge are functionally intertwined and specifically vulnerable to RH stroke. Problems may extend further into the verbal-conceptual realm. While patients with both LH and RH stroke demonstrate intact abilities in deciphering emotion from a verbal description, e.g., "it was the anniversary of the death of your child" (Blonder et al., 1991), those with damage to the RH have difficulties with more subtle aspects of emotion, such as humour in narratives and cartoons (Bowers, Bauer, & Heilman, 1993; Wapner, Hamby, & Gardner, 1981).

In summary, studies into emotion processing following stroke consistently implicate RH stroke as leading to more pervasive deficits in processing emotions than the left. There is some question as to whether this may specifically impact the experience of negatively valenced emotions. That is, patients with RH stroke can be indifferent to their impairments, while the LH patients are often depressed, suggesting a specific loss of negative emotion following RH stroke (Gainotti, 1972; Sackeim et al., 1982). This asymmetry is also seen in emotion perception where, in general, RH stroke leads to large impairments in the identification and labelling of negative emotions and relatively smaller effects for positive emotions. A similar pattern is seen for the LH but overall the effects are much smaller and sometimes not significant (Abbott et al., 2013).

Cognitive and affective theory of mind (ToM) after stroke

Theory of mind (ToM) is also frequently impaired following stroke. ToM is frequently assessed in people with stroke using written narratives, which places significant language demands on the participant, especially for those with LH lesions and compromised language processing. It has also been assessed using cartoons (Happè, Brownell, & Winner, 1999), moving shapes (Weed, McGregor, Nielsen, Roepstorff, & Frith, 2010) and videoed conversations (Honan, McDonald, Sufani, Hine, & Kumfor, 2016). Overall, people with stroke do poorly across these tasks, although deficits are generally less severe than those seen in emotion perception (Adams et al., 2019). Their performance indicates a general failure to accurately understand the mental state of others, as well as a problem inhibiting their own perspective in order to do so (Samson, Apperly, Kathirgamanathan, & Humphreys, 2005).

Once again, despite the language demands, RH stroke is more likely to produce impairments than LH (Adams et al., 2019). Although neuroimaging suggests bilateral neural structures underpin ToM processing, a preferential role for the *right temporoparietal junction* (Saxe & Wexler, 2005) and *right dorsofrontal lateral* and *medial cortex* (Corradi-Dell'Acqua et al., 2020) has been put forward, which may explain this asymmetry. Although there is strong evidence that ToM abilities are, at least partially, modular (see Chapter 1), other cognitive deficits will impact on task performance. For example, executive function has been found to have a specific relationship to ToM in stroke regardless of hemisphere (Pluta, Gawron, Sobanska, Wojcik, & Lojek, 2017).

Emotional empathy after stroke

Interestingly, there is very little evidence for emotional empathy difficulties following stroke (Adams et al., 2019). However, as discussed earlier, emotional empathy is often assessed via self-report, and this may simply reflect lack of insight, especially after RH stroke. However, when RH stroke patients were asked to rate how much they shared the feelings of a story character in a behavioural measure, they were shown to be significantly impaired, and this was correlated with the extent of damage to the *right temporal pole* and the *anterior insula*, as well as the presence of lesions in the *prefrontal cortex* and *thalamus* (Leigh et al., 2013).

Disorders of pragmatic language following right hemisphere stroke

Aphasias causing problems with language production and reception are well documented following damage to sub-branches of the left middle cerebral artery. Although patients with RH damage typically have preserved language, they tend to suffer from pragmatic language disorders. Difficulties are somewhat similar to those described post-TBI; however, the RH literature is much more extensive, where disorders are variously described as "higher order language disorders", "right hemisphere language disorders", "pragmatic language disorders" and "cognitive-communication disorders". Across these studies, people with RH stroke have been described as tangential and verbose (Mackisack, Myers, & Duffy, 1987; Roman, Brownell, Potter, & Sebold, 1987), and they have difficulty comprehending nonliteral language including metaphors (Winner & Gardner, 1977), proverbs (Hier & Kaplan, 1980), idioms (Van Lancker & Kempler, 1987), sarcasm (Kaplan, Brownell, Jacobs, & Gardner, 1990; Winner, Brownell, Happe, Blum, & Pincus, 1998) and jokes (Birhle, Brownell, Powelson, & Gardener, 1986; Gardner, Ling, Flamm, & SIlverman, 1975; Martin & McDonald, 2006). People with RH stroke also have difficulty with open-ended judgements requiring them to infer actor intentions in complex narratives (Wapner et al., 1981), are poor at making inferences about interpersonal relations or mental state so as to understand communicative intention between speakers (Kaplan et al., 1990; Winner et al., 1998) and have difficulty understanding and using indirect language that is non-conventional and therefore reliant upon understanding the speaker's intention (Stemmer, Giroux, & Joanette, 1994).

These communication disorders following RH stroke are pervasive, affecting the majority of patients with RH stroke (Fonseca & de Mattos Pimenta Parente, 2007) and strongly associated with loss in social function (Hewetson, Cornwell, & Shum, 2018). Despite this, observed impairments are variable and subtle relative to those typically seen in TBI, with ambiguous and contradictory findings across studies. This suggests that there may not be a singular clear determinant. Cluster analyses have also implicated a range of different types of RH pragmatic disorders (Parola et al., 2016). Furthermore, the neural substrate of RH pragmatic language disorders is difficult to map out. For example, while problems in speech act choice (e.g., knowing when to use a command versus question) can characterise both LH and RH stroke patients, the specific neural basis is relatively clear cut with LH lesions but not RH (Soroker et al., 2005). Neuroimaging in healthy adults paints a complex, bilateral, but not necessarily symmetrical, picture of neural activation when processing inferential language. For example, text comprehension engages the *bilateral anterior temporal lobes* and *medial prefrontal* systems with increased reliance on the right hemisphere for metaphoric and other implicit language tasks (Ferstl, Neumann, Bogler, & von Cramon, 2008; Jang et al., 2013).

Potential causes of poor pragmatic language

A number of theories have been proposed to account for at least some of these impairments. Two explanations are that these reflect the influences of impaired emotion and/or ToM. The finding that many patients with RH damage have difficulty processing emotional nuances in language, as we described earlier, fits with the first of these explanations. As regard the second, we have already discussed how the inability to attribute beliefs and intentions to others will directly interfere with the capacity to understand conversational inferences such as saying one thing and meaning another (sarcasm) or making a hint. ToM performance and pragmatic language competence have been shown to be significantly correlated in patients with both LH and RH stroke (Pluta et al., 2017).

However, there are also other theories that are RH specific. One of the earlier theories was that right hemisphere damage disrupts a general RH function that constructs mental models of the world based on synthesising incoming verbal information with context and stored knowledge (Wapner et al., 1981). As a consequence, people with RH lesions fail to appreciate language in context or make interpretations that are the most plausible given the circumstances. An alternative point of view is that many patients with RH stroke actually suffer damage to the *dorsolateral frontal lobes* due to disruption of the anterior branches of the middle cerebral artery, which leads to executive disorders reflected in concrete, stimulus bound processing and poor behaviour regulation. Where these two theories have been tested head to head (McDonald, 2000), neither were found to be a satisfactory explanation of poor performance, although there was a pattern that suggested poor pragmatic language use was more likely associated with other typical RH functions (i.e. visuospatial abilities) than executive abilities. Overall, pragmatic language impairment following RH stroke is difficult to characterise and likely to be multi-determined.

Impairments in social cognition post stroke and real-world outcomes

Deficits across the spectrum of social cognitive abilities have real world implications for people living with stroke. For example, depression in LH stroke is significantly associated with stress in the marital partner (Blonder, Langer,

Pettigrew, & Garrity, 2007), while reduced emotion perception post RH stroke is significantly associated with reduced satisfaction with relationships and social participation (Blonder, Pettigrew, & Kryscio, 2012; Cooper et al., 2014). Difficulties in social behaviour are common and represent a large effect after stroke (Adams et al., 2019). Further, poor emotion perception and poor ToM are significantly associated with behavioural difficulties as reported by relatives (Nijsse et al., 2019). Likewise, deficits in pragmatic language function are predictive of reduced social participation post discharge (Hewetson, Cornwell, & Shum, 2017). Furthermore, impairments in social cognition do not appear to resolve with time (Adams et al., 2019) and are therefore an important target for remediation. See Boxes 5.2 and 5.3 for case studies of left and right hemisphere stroke respectively.

Box 5.2   Case 2: LH: Young adult with left hemisphere stroke

History:

Ms LH is a 34-year-old young woman who suffered an embolic stroke in the anterior branches of the left middle cerebral artery secondary to a heart condition. This left her with a right hemiparesis and hesitant, faltering speech, word finding difficulties and some impairment in comprehension. She was discharged home able to walk with assistance of a stick some two months later.

Presentation:

LH was initially very frustrated and depressed about her language impairment. However, she worked hard with her speech pathologist on an outpatient basis. Gradually, her language improved and she learned compensatory strategies that increased her functional ability to interact with not only family and friends but people in the community such as bus drivers and shop keepers. Her mood also improved as she learned to compensate for her deficits.

Despite her loss of language, Ms LH remained astute in her interactions with others. She picked up quickly when someone was sad or angry and was able to communicate her own feelings effectively using verbal and non-verbal cues. With her improvement in mood, she laughed easily. She was able to follow the gist of conversations even when she had difficulty understanding or remembering the details. She maintained good relationships with her family and her immediate circle of friends.

Summary and opinion:

The kinds of strengths and weaknesses exhibited by Ms LH are instructive regarding the role of both language and social cognition in interpersonal interactions. Language impairment is clearly a major obstacle to normal everyday communication, and this was a source of frustration to LH. However, LH appears to have intact social cognitive skills, meaning she can pick up on non-verbal social cues and use these to facilitate her interactions with others.

Box 5.3   Case 3: RB: Adult with right hemisphere stroke

History:

Mr RB was a 62-year-old man working in real estate. He experienced an ischemic stroke affecting the right middle cerebral artery with subsequent pathology in the vicinity of the right parieto-frontal cortex. As a consequence, he lost function in his left arm and leg.

Neuropsychological assessment:

Cognitive testing revealed him to have slowed information processing speed, normal working memory and good vocabulary. His answers to questions concerning practical conceptual issues (e.g., what to do with an unopened letter addressed to someone else) were at times tangential and suggested a loss of understanding or regard for social conventions. His performance on visuospatial tasks, including learning tasks, suggested problems with left sided neglect. His verbal memory was good.

Presentation:

Mr RB was discharged from hospital six weeks later using a wheel chair for ambulation. At home, his wife noticed a number of changes. He demonstrated neglect of objects on his left side and had to be constantly reminded. Despite this, he minimised his impairments, was generally unconcerned and had unrealistic expectations for the future. His face became unexpressive and 'mask-like' and his voice tended to be monotonic.

He was relatively unaware of his wife's emotional state, failed to take her feelings into account when talking to others and showed little empathy.

Mr RB also tended to be very egocentric, talkative and tangential in his conversation with an odd use of words. He would elaborate minor details and sometimes frankly confabulate. He did not pick up hints and misinterpreted jokes. His wife reported his social behaviours to be very different to how he was before the stroke, and she found this quite distressing.

Summary and opinion:

Mr RB did not have any loss to basic verbal abilities although his use of language to adhere to social and conversational conventions appeared to be compromised. This could be indicative of a pragmatic language impairment. Indeed, the main features of RB's presentation, apart from his neglect, related to social cognition. These included symptoms consistent with poor emotion perception, failure to appreciate other people's perspectives (egocentricity) and lack of empathy. Aligned to these difficulties he also appeared to have poor self-awareness and disinhibition.

Other acquired brain injuries and social cognition

While this chapter has focussed exclusively on the effects of TBI and stroke in the connection between social cognition and social functioning, there is an emerging literature on the effects of various other acquired brain conditions on social cognitive abilities. For example, consistent with research on those with TBI, studies have shown that individuals with agenesis of the *corpus callosum* demonstrate difficulties with understanding social cognition in videoed conversations (Symington, Paul, Symington, Ono, & Brown, 2010). This reinforces the significance of white matter connections between brain regions in the regulation of social cognitive abilities. The utilisation of social cognitive tasks has also revealed impairments in other acquired brain conditions, such as brain tumours (Pertz, Okoniewski, Schlegel, & Thoma, 2020), Anti-N-methyl-d-aspartate (NMDA) receptor encephalitis (McKeon et al., 2016), chronic alcohol substance use disorder (Le Berre, Fama, & Sullivan, 2017) and Korsakoff's syndrome (Drost, Postma, & Oudman, 2018). These latter findings are not surprising given the pervasiveness of the various toxins and/or insults related to the conditions and the key brain regions and their connections that are affected. Research into social cognition in a diverse set of brain conditions will offer a wealth of condition-specific knowledge on the social cognitive factors underlying behavioural outcomes and social functioning.

Concluding remarks

The findings from this chapter clarify and cement the long-held belief that social cognitive difficulties are a prevalent and disabling feature of acquired brain injuries. Decades of findings from the TBI and stroke fields show that these problems appear to generalise across most areas of social cognition. Not only do these findings provide a wealth of theoretical knowledge on the intricate relationship between the brain and behaviour but also allow us to understand how such difficulties in processing social information can predict and mediate the deleterious impact brain insult has across a range of social outcomes. This illustrates the salience of social cognition within the larger umbrella of assessment and remediation. Many of these factors, however, do not have a clear or direct link with cognitive dysfunction, nor do social cognitive difficulties present in a uniform and unanimous fashion across people and conditions. It is also inappropriate to assume that difficulties in one social cognitive domain infer problems in the others. Consequently, it is pertinent for clinicians to factor social cognition (and the variety of skills that this encompasses) in their clinical assessments and treatment planning, as to provide comprehensive person-centred care when working with those with acquired brain injury.

References

Abbott, J. D., Cumming, G., Fidler, F., & Lindell, A. K. (2013). The perception of positive and negative facial expressions in unilateral brain-damaged patients: A meta-analysis. *Laterality: Asymmetries of Body, Brain and Cognition, 18*(4), 437–459.

Adams, A. G., Henry, J. D., Molenberghs, P., Robinson, G. A., Nott, Z., & von Hippel, W. (2020). The relationship between social cognitive difficulties in the acute stages of stroke and later functional outcomes. *Social Neuroscience, 15*(2), 158–169. doi:10.1080/174709 19.2019.1668845

Adams, A. G., Schweitzer, D., Molenberghs, P., & Henry, J. D. (2019). A meta-analytic review of social cognitive function following stroke. *Neuroscience and Biobehavioral Reviews, 102*, 400–416. doi:10.1016/j.neubiorev.2019.03.011

Adolphs, R., Damasio, H., & Tranel, D. (2002). Neural systems for recognition of emotional prosody: A 3-D lesion study. *Emotion, 2*(1), 23–51. doi:10.1037/1528-3542.2.1.23

Adolphs, R., Damasio, H., Tranel, D., Cooper, G., & Damasio, A. R. (2000). A role for somatosensory cortices in the visual recognition of emotion as revealed by three-dimensional lesion mapping. *Journal of Neuroscience, 20*(7), 2683–2690.

Adolphs, R., Tranel, D., & Damasio, A. R. (2003). Dissociable neural systems for recognizing emotions. *Brain and Cognition, 52*(1), 61–69.

Allain, P., Hamon, M., Saoût, V., Verny, C., Dinomais, M., & Besnard, J. (2020). Theory of mind impairments highlighted with an ecological performance-based test indicate behavioral executive deficits in traumatic brain injury. *Frontiers in Neurology, 10*(1367). doi:10.3389/fneur.2019.01367

Azouvi, P., Arnould, A., Dromer, E., & Vallat-Azouvi, C. (2017). Neuropsychology of traumatic brain injury: An expert overview. *Revue Neurologique, 173*(7), 461–472. doi:10.1016/j.neurol.2017.07.006

Babbage, D. R., Yim, J., Zupan, B., Neumann, D., Tomita, M. R., & Willer, B. (2011). Meta-analysis of facial affect recognition difficulties after traumatic brain injury. *Neuropsychology, 25*(3), 277.

Beauchamp, M. H., Vera-Estay, E., Morasse, F., Anderson, V., & Dooley, J. (2019). Moral reasoning and decision-making in adolescents who sustain traumatic brain injury. *Brain Injury, 33*(1), 32–39. doi:10.1080/02699052.2018.1531307

Bibby, H., & McDonald, S. (2005). Theory of mind after traumatic brain injury. *Neuropsychologia*, *43*(1), 99–114.

Bigler, E. D. (2007). Anterior and middle cranial fossa in traumatic brain injury: Relevant neuroanatomy and neuropathology in the study of neuropsychological outcome. *Neuropsychology*, *21*(5), 515.

Birhle, A. M., Brownell, H. H., Powelson, J. A., & Gardener, H. (1986). Comprehension of humorous and nonhumorous materials by right and left brain damaged patients. *Brain and Cognition*, *5*, 399–411.

Bivona, U., Formisano, R., De Laurentiis, S., Accetta, N., Rita Di Cosimo, M., Massicci, R., . . . Sabatini, U. (2015). Theory of mind impairment after severe traumatic brain injury and its relationship with caregivers' quality of life. *Restorative Neurology and Neuroscience*, *33*(3), 335–345.

Blair, R. J., & Cipolotti, L. (2000). Impaired social response reversal: A case ofacquired sociopathy'. *Brain*, *123*(6), 1122–1141.

Blonder, L. X., Bowers, D., & Heilman, K. M. (1991). The role of the right hemisphere in emotional communication. *Brain*, *114*, 1115–1127.

Blonder, L. X., Langer, S. L., Pettigrew, L., & Garrity, T. F. (2007). The effects of stroke disability on spousal caregivers. *NeuroRehabilitation*, *22*(2), 85–92.

Blonder, L. X., Pettigrew, L., & Kryscio, R. J. (2012). Emotion recognition and marital satisfaction in stroke. *Journal of Clinical and Experimental Neuropsychology*, *34*(6), 634–642.

Borod, J. C., Koff, E., Lorch, M. P., & Nicholas, M. (1986). The expression and perception of facial emotion in brain-damaged patients. *Neuropsychologia*, *24*(2), 169–180.

Borod, J. C., Koff, E., Lorch, M. P., Nicholas, M., & Welkowitz, J. (1988). Emotional and non-emotional facial behaviour in patients with unilateral brain damage. *Journal of Neurology, Neurosurgery and Psychiatry*, *51*(6), 826–832. doi:10.1136/jnnp.51.6.826

Bosco, F. M., Angeleri, R., Sacco, K., & Bara, B. G. (2015). Explaining pragmatic performance in traumatic brain injury: A process perspective on communicative errors. *International Journal of Language & Communication Disorders*, *50*(1), 63–83.

Bosco, F. M., Gabbatore, I., Angeleri, R., Zettin, M., & Parola, A. (2018). Do executive function and theory of mind predict pragmatic abilities following traumatic brain injury? An analysis of sincere, deceitful and ironic communicative acts. *Journal of Communication Disorders*, *75*, 102–117. doi:10.1016/j.jcomdis.2018.05.002

Bosco, F. M., Parola, A., Sacco, K., Zettin, M., & Angeleri, R. (2017). Communicative-pragmatic disorders in traumatic brain injury: The role of theory of mind and executive functions. *Brain and Language*, *168*, 73–83. doi:10.1016/j.bandl.2017.01.007

Bowers, D., Bauer, R. M., & Heilman, K. M. (1993). The nonverbal affect lexicon. Theoretical perspectives from neuropsychological studies of affect perception. *Neuropsychology*, *7*, 433–444.

Brooks, N., Campsie, L., Symington, C., Beattie, A., & McKinlay, W. (1986). The five year outcome of severe blunt head injury: A relative's view. *Journal of Neurology, Neurosurgery, and Psychiatry*, *49*(7), 764–770. doi:10.1136/jnnp.49.7.764

Carroll, L. J., Cassidy, J. D., Peloso, P. M., Borg, J., von Holst, H., Holm, L., . . . Pépin, M. (2004). Prognosis for mild traumatic brain injury: Results of the WHO Collaborating Centre Task Force on mild traumatic brain injury. *Journal of Rehabilitation Medicine*, (43 Suppl), 84–105. doi:10.1080/16501960410023859

Cattran, C. J., Oddy, M., Wood, R. L., & Moir, J. F. (2011). Post-injury personality in the prediction of outcome following severe acquired brain injury. *Brain Injury*, *25*(11), 1035–1046.

Charbonneau, S., Scherzer, B. P., Aspirot, D., & Cohen, H. (2003). Perception and production of facial prosodic emotions by chronic CVA patients. *Neuropsychologia, 41*(5), 605–613.

Cheung, C. C. Y., Lee, T. M. C., Yip, J. T. H., King, K. E., & Li, L. S. W. (2006). The differential effects of thalamus and basal ganglia on facial emotion recognition. *Brain and Cognition, 61*(3), 262–268.

Cooper, C. L., Phillips, L. H., Johnston, M., Radlak, B., Hamilton, S., & McLeod, M. J. (2014). Links between emotion perception and social participation restriction following stroke. *Brain Injury, 28*(1), 122–126.

Corradi-Dell'Acqua, C., Ronchi, R., Thomasson, M., Bernati, T., Saj, A., & Vuilleumier, P. (2020). Deficits in cognitive and affective theory of mind relate to dissociated lesion patterns in prefrontal and insular cortex. *Cortex: A Journal Devoted to the Study of the Nervous System and Behavior, 128*, 218–233.

Courville, C. B. (1945). *Pathology of the Nervous System* (2nd ed.). Mountain View, CA: California Pacific Press.

Croker, V., & McDonald, S. (2005). Recognition of emotion from facial expression following traumatic brain injury. *Brain Injury, 19*(10), 787–799.

Demakis, G. J., Hammond, F., Knotts, A., Cooper, D. B., Clement, P., Kennedy, J., & Sawyer, T. (2007). The personality assessment inventory in individuals with traumatic brain injury. *Archives of Clinical Neuropsychology, 22*(1), 123–130. doi:10.1016/j.acn.2006.09.004

de Sousa, A., McDonald, S., & Rushby, J. (2012). Changes in emotional empathy, affective responsivity, and behavior following severe traumatic brain injury. *Journal of Clinical and Experimental Neuropsychology, 34*(6), 606–623. doi:10.1080/13803395.2012.667067

de Sousa, A., McDonald, S., Rushby, J., Li, S., Dimoska, A., & James, C. (2010). Why don't you feel how I feel? Insight into the absence of empathy after severe traumatic brain injury. *Neuropsychologia, 48*(12), 3585–3595. doi:10.1016/j.neuropsychologia.2010.08.008

de Sousa, A., McDonald, S., Rushby, J., Li, S., Dimoska, A., & James, C. (2011). Understanding deficits in empathy after traumatic brain injury: The role of affective responsivity. *Cortex, 47*(5), 526–535. doi:10.1016/j.cortex.2010.02.004

Dethier, M., Blairy, S., Rosenberg, H., & McDonald, S. (2012). Spontaneous and posed emotional facial expressions following severe traumatic brain injury. *Journal of Clinical and Experimental Neuropsychology, 34*(9), 936–947. doi:10.1080/13803395.2012.702734

Dethier, M., Blairy, S., Rosenberg, H., & McDonald, S. (2013). Emotional regulation impairments following severe traumatic brain injury: An investigation of the body and facial feedback effects. *Journal of the International Neuropsychological Society: JINS, 19*(4), 367–379. doi:10.1017/S1355617712001555

Dimoska, A., McDonald, S., Pell, M. C., Tate, R. L., & James, C. M. (2010). Recognizing vocal expressions of emotion in patients with social skills deficits following traumatic brain injury. *Journal of the International Neuropsychological Society, 16*(2), 369–382. doi:10.1017/S1355617709991445

Drapeau, J., Gosselin, N., Peretz, I., & McKerral, M. (2017). Emotional recognition from dynamic facial, vocal and musical expressions following traumatic brain injury. *Brain Injury, 31*(2), 221–229. doi:10.1080/02699052.2016.1208846

Drost, R., Postma, A., & Oudman, E. (2018). Cognitive and affective theory of mind in Korsakoff's syndrome. *Acta Neuropsychiatrica, 1–7*. doi:10.1017/neu.2018.35

Eslinger, P., Satish, U., & Grattan, L. (1996). Alterations in cognitive and affectively-based empathy after cerebral damage. *Journal of the International Neuropsychological Society, 2*, 15.

Evans, K., & Hux, K. (2011). Comprehension of indirect requests by adults with severe traumatic brain injury: Contributions of gestural and verbal information. *Brain Injury*, *25*(7–8), 767–776. doi:10.3109/02699052.2011.576307

Ferstl, E. C., Neumann, J., Bogler, C., & von Cramon, D. (2008). The extended language network: A meta-analysis of neuroimaging studies on text comprehension. *Human Brain Mapping*, *29*(5), 581–593.

Fonseca, R. P., & de Mattos Pimenta Parente, M. A. (2007). Meta-analysis of communicative processing studies in right-brain-damaged patients. *Estudos de Psicologia*, *24*(4), 529–538.

Frost, R. B., Farrer, T. J., Primosch, M., & Hedges, D. W. (2013). Prevalence of traumatic brain injury in the general adult population: A meta-analysis. *Neuroepidemiology*, *40*(3), 154–159.

Gainotti, G. (1972). Emotional behavior and hemispheric side of the lesion. *Cortex*, *8*, 41–55.

Ganesalingam, K., Yeates, K. O., Sanson, A., & Anderson, V. (2007). Social problem-solving skills following childhood traumatic brain injury and its association with self-regulation and social and behavioural functioning. *Journal of Neuropsychology*, *1*(2), 149–170. doi:10.1348/174866407x185300

Gardner, H., Ling, K., Flamm, L., & SIlverman, J. (1975). Comprehension and appreciation of humor in brain damaged patients. *Brain*, *98*(399–412).

Geraci, A., Surian, L., Ferraro, M., & Cantagallo, A. (2010). Theory of mind in patients with ventromedial or dorsolateral prefrontal lesions following traumatic brain injury. *Brain Injury*, *24*(7–8), 978–987.

Gould, K. R., Ponsford, J. L., Johnston, L., & Schönberger, M. (2011). The nature, frequency and course of psychiatric disorders in the first year after traumatic brain injury: A prospective study. *Psychological Medicine*, *41*(10), 2099–2109. doi:10.1017/s003329171100033x

Grattan, L. M., & Eslinger, P. J. (1989). Higher cognition and social behavior: Changes in cognitive flexibility and empathy after cerebral lesions. *Neuropsychology*, *3*(3), 175–185. doi:10.1037/h0091764

Green, R. E., Turner, G. R., & Thompson, W. F. (2004). Deficits in facial emotion perception in adults with recent traumatic brain injury. *Neuropsychologia*, *42*(2), 133–141.

Happè, F., Brownell, H., & Winner, E. (1999). Acquired 'theory of mind' impairments following stroke. *Cognition*, *70*, 211–240.

Havet-Thomassin, V., Allain, P., Etcharry-Bouyx, F., & Le Gall, D. (2006). What about theory of mind after severe brain injury? *Brain Injury*, *20*(1), 83–91.

Heilman, K. M., Bowers, D., Speedie, L., & Coslett, H. B. (1984). Comprehension of affective and nonaffective prosody. *Neurology*, *34*(7), 917–921.

Henry, J. D., Phillips, L. H., Crawford, J. R., Ietswaart, M., & Summers, F. (2006). Theory of mind following traumatic brain injury: The role of emotion recognition and executive dysfunction. *Neuropsychologia*, *44*(10), 1623–1628.

Hewetson, R., Cornwell, P., & Shum, D. (2017). Cognitive-communication disorder following right hemisphere stroke: Exploring rehabilitation access and outcomes. *Topics in Stroke Rehabilitation*, *24*(5), 330–336. doi:10.1080/10749357.2017.1289622

Hewetson, R., Cornwell, P., & Shum, D. (2018). Social participation following right hemisphere stroke: Influence of a cognitive-communication disorder. *Aphasiology*, *32*(2), 164–182. doi:10.1080/02687038.2017.1315045

Hier, D. B., & Kaplan, J. (1980). Verbal comprehension deficits after right hemisphere damage. *Applied Psycholinguistics*, *1*, 279–294.

Honan, C. A., Allen, S. K., Fisher, A., Osborne-Crowley, K., & McDonald, S. (2017). Social disinhibition: Piloting a new clinical measure in individuals with traumatic brain injury. *Brain Impairment, 18*(1). doi:10.1017/BrImp.2016.27

Honan, C. A., McDonald, S., Sufani, C., Hine, D., & Kumfor, F. (2016). The awareness of social inference test: Development of a shortened version for use in adults with acquired brain injury. *The Clinical Neuropsychologist, 30*(2), 243–264.

Hoofien, D., Gilboa, A., Vakil, E., & Donovick, P. J. (2001). Traumatic brain injury (TBI) 10? 20 years later: A comprehensive outcome study of psychiatric symptomatology, cognitive abilities and psychosocial functioning. *Brain Injury, 15*(3), 189–209.

Hornak, J., Rolls, E. T., & Wade, D. (1996). Face and voice expression identification in patients with emotional and behavioural changes following ventral frontal lobe damage. *Neuropsychologia, 34*(4), 247–261. doi:10.0028-3932(95)00106-9 [pii]

Ietswaart, M., Milders, M., Crawford, J. R., Currie, D., & Scott, C. L. (2008). Longitudinal aspects of emotion recognition in patients with traumatic brain injury. *Neuropsychologia, 46*(1), 148–159.

Jang, G., Yoon, S.-a., Lee, S.-E., Park, H., Kim, J., Ko, J. H., & Park, H.-J. (2013). Everyday conversation requires cognitive inference: Neural bases of comprehending implicated meanings in conversations. *NeuroImage, 81*, 61–72.

Johnson, J. E., & Turkstra, L. S. (2012). Inference in conversation of adults with traumatic brain injury. *Brain Injury, 26*(9), 1118–1126.

Johnson, W., Onuma, O., Owolabi, M., & Sachdev, S. (2016). Stroke: A global response is needed. *Bulletin of the World Health Organization, 94*(9), 634–634A. doi:10.2471/BLT.16.181636

Kaplan, J. K., Brownell., H. H., Jacobs, J. R., & Gardner, H. (1990). The effects of right hemisphere damage on the pragmatic interpretation of conversational remarks. *Brain and Language, 38*, 315–333.

Katsifaraki, M., & Wood, R. L. (2014). The impact of alexithymia on burnout amongst relatives of people who suffer from traumatic brain injury. *Brain Injury, 28*(11), 1389–1395.

Kelly, G., Brown, S., Todd, J., & Kremer, P. (2008). Challenging behaviour profiles of people with acquired brain injury living in community settings. *Brain Injury, 22*(6), 457–470.

Kelly, M., McDonald, S., & Kellett, D. (2014). Development of a novel task for investigating decision making in a social context following traumatic brain injury. *Journal of Clinical and Experimental Neuropsychology, 36*(9), 897–913. doi:10.1080/13803395.2014.955784

Kendall, E. (1996). Psychosocial adjustment following closed head injury: A model for understanding individual differences and predicting outcome. *Neuropsychological Rehabilitation, 6*(2), 101–132.

Kendall, E., & Terry, D. (2009). Predicting emotional well-being following traumatic brain injury: A test of mediated and moderated models. *Social Science & Medicine, 69*(6), 947–954.

Kinsella, G., Packer, S., & Olver, J. (1991). Maternal reporting of behaviour following very severe blunt head injury. *Journal of Neurology, Neurosurgery & Psychiatry, 54*(5), 422–426.

Knox, L., & Douglas, J. (2009). Long-term ability to interpret facial expression after traumatic brain injury and its relation to social integration. *Brain and Cognition, 69*(2), 442–449. doi:10.1016/j.bandc.2008.09.009

Kocka, A., & Gagnon, J. (2014). Definition of impulsivity and related terms following traumatic brain injury: A review of the different concepts and measures used to assess impulsivity, disinhibition and other related concepts. *Behavioral Sciences, 4*(4), 352–370.

Kotowicz, Z. (2007). The strange case of Phineas Gage. *History of the Human Sciences, 20*, 115–131.

Kucharska-Pietura, K., Phillips, M. L., Gernand, W., & David, A. S. (2003). Perception of emotions from faces and voices following unilateral brain damage. *Neuropsychologia, 41*(8), 1082–1090.

Le Berre, A.-P., Fama, R., & Sullivan, E. V. (2017). Executive functions, memory, and social cognitive deficits and recovery in chronic alcoholism: A critical review to inform future research. *Alcoholism, Clinical and Experimental Research, 41*(8), 1432–1443. doi:10.1111/acer.13431

Leigh, R., Oishi, K., Hsu, J., Lindquist, M., Gottesman, R. F., Jarso, S., . . . Hillis, A. E. (2013). Acute lesions that impair affective empathy. *Brain: A Journal of Neurology, 136*, 2539–2549.

Mackisack, L. E., Myers, P. S., & Duffy, J. R. (1987). Verbosity and labelling behavious: The performance of right hemisphere and non brain damaged adults on inferential picture description task. *Clinical Aphasiology, 17*, 143–151.

Martin, I., & McDonald, S. (2006). That can't be right! What causes pragmatic language impairment following right hemisphere damage? *Brain Impairment, 7*, 202–211.

Martin-Rodriguez, J. F., & Leon-Carrion, J. (2010). Theory of mind deficits in patients with acquired brain injury: A quantitative review. *Neuropsychologia, 48*(5), 1181–1191. doi:10.1016/j.neuropsychologia.2010.02.009

May, M., Milders, M., Downey, B., Whyte, M., Higgins, V., Wojcik, Z., . . . O'Rourke, S. (2017). Social behavior and impairments in social cognition following traumatic brain injury. *Journal of the International Neuropsychological Society, 23*(5), 400–411. doi:10.1017/s1355617717000182

McDonald, S. (2000). Exploring the cognitive basis of right-hemisphere pragmatic language disorders. *Brain and Language, 75*(1), 82–107.

McDonald, S., Dalton, K. I., Rushby, J. A., & Landin-Romero, R. (2019). Loss of white matter connections after severe traumatic brain injury (TBI) and its relationship to social cognition. *Brain Imaging and Behavior, 13*(3), 819–829.

McDonald, S., & Flanagan, S. (2004). Social perception deficits after traumatic brain injury: Interaction between emotion recognition, mentalizing ability, and social communication. *Neuropsychology, 18*(3), 572–579. doi:10.1037/0894-4105.18.3.5722004-16644-018 [pii]

McDonald, S., Flanagan, S., Rollins, J., & Kinch, J. (2003). TASIT: A new clinical tool for assessing social perception after traumatic brain injury. *Journal of Head Trauma Rehabilitation, 18*(3), 219–238. doi:10.1097/00001199-200305000-00001

McDonald, S., Gowland, A., Randall, R., Fisher, A., Osborne-Crowley, K., & Honan, C. (2014). Cognitive factors underpinning poor expressive communication skills after traumatic brain injury: Theory of mind or executive function? *Neuropsychology, 28*(5), 801.

McDonald, S., Li, S., De Sousa, A., Rushby, J., Dimoska, A., James, C., & Tate, R. L. (2011). Impaired mimicry response to angry faces following severe traumatic brain injury. *Journal of Clinical and Experimental Neuropsychology, 33*(1), 17–29.

McDonald, S., Rushby, J., Li, S., de Sousa, A., Dimoska, A., James, C., . . . Togher, L. (2011). The influence of attention and arousal on emotion perception in adults with severe traumatic brain injury. *International Journal of Psychophysiology, 82*(1), 124–131. doi:10.1016/j.ijpsycho.2011.01.014

McDonald, S., Saad, A., & James, C. (2011). Social dysdecorum following severe traumatic brain injury: Loss of implicit social knowledge or loss of control? *Journal of Clinical and Experimental Neuropsychology, 33*(6), 619–630.

McDonald, S., & Saunders, J. C. (2005). Differential impairment in recognition of emotion across different media in people with severe traumatic brain injury. *Journal of the International Neuropsychological Society: JINS, 11*(4), 392.

McKeon, G. L., Scott, J. G., Spooner, D. M., Ryan, A. E., Blum, S., Gillis, D., . . . Robinson, G. A. (2016). Cognitive and social functioning deficits after anti-N-methyl-D-aspartate receptor encephalitis: An exploratory case series. *Journal of the International Neuropsychological Society, 22*(8), 828–838. doi:10.1017/s1355617716000679

Meulenbroek, P., & Turkstra, L. S. (2016). Job stability in skilled work and communication ability after moderate-severe traumatic brain injury. *Disability and Rehabilitation, 38*(5), 452–461. doi:10.3109/09638288.2015.1044621

Milders, M. (2019). Relationship between social cognition and social behaviour following traumatic brain injury. *Brain Injury, 33*(1), 62–68. doi:10.1080/02699052.2018.1531301

Milders, M., Fuchs, S., & Crawford, J. R. (2003). Neuropsychological impairments and changes in emotional and social behaviour following severe traumatic brain injury. *Journal of Clinical and Experimental Neuropsychology, 25*(2), 157–172. doi:10.1076/jcen.25.2.157.13642

Milders, M., Ietswaart, M., Crawford, J. R., & Currie, D. (2008). Social behavior following traumatic brain injury and its association with emotion recognition, understanding of intentions, and cognitive flexibility. *Journal of the International Neuropsychological Society, 14*(2), 318–326. doi:10.1017/s1355617708080351

Mohammad, Q. D., Habib, M., Hoque, A., Alam, B., Haque, B., Hossain, S., . . . Khan, S. U. (2011). Prevalence of stroke above forty years. *Mymensingh Medical Journal, 20*(4), 640–644.

Muller, F., Simion, A., Reviriego, E., Galera, C., Mazaux, J.-M., Barat, M., & Joseph, P.-A. (2010). Exploring theory of mind after severe traumatic brain injury. *Cortex, 46*(9), 1088–1099.

Neumann, D. R., Hammond, F., Norton, J., & Blumenthal, T. (2011). Using startle to objectively measure anger and other emotional responses after traumatic brain injury: A pilot study. *Journal of Head Trauma Rehabilitation, 26*(5), 375–383. doi:10.1097/HTR.0b013e3181f8d52d

Neumann, D. R., Malec, J. F., & Hammond, F. M. (2015). The association of negative attributions with irritation and anger after brain injury. *Rehabilitation Psychology, 60*(2), 155–161. doi:10.1037/rep0000036

Neumann, D. R., Sander, A. M., Perkins, S. M., Bhamidipalli, S. S., Witwer, N., Combs, D., & Hammond, F. M. (2020). Assessing negative attributions after brain injury with the ambiguous intentions hostility questionnaire. *The Journal of Head Trauma Rehabilitation, 35*(5). https://journals.lww.com/headtraumarehab/Fulltext/2020/09000/Assessing_Negative_Attributions_After_Brain_Injury.16.aspx

Neumann, D. R., Zupan, B., Malec, J. F., & Hammond, F. (2014). Relationships between alexithymia, affect recognition, and empathy after traumatic brain injury. *The Journal of Head Trauma Rehabilitation, 29*(1), E18–E27.

Ng, Y. S., Stein, J., Ning, M., & Black-Schaffer, R. M. (2007). Comparison of clinical characteristics and functional outcomes of ischemic stroke in different vascular territories. *Stroke, 38*(8), 2309–2314. doi:10.1161/STROKEAHA.106.475483

Nijsse, B., Spikman, J. M., Visser-Meily, J. M., de Kort, P. L., & van Heugten, C. M. (2019). Social cognition impairments are associated with behavioural changes in the long term after stroke. *PLoS One, 14*(3), ArtID e0213725.

O'Driscoll, K., & Leach, J. P. (1998). "No longer Gage": An iron bar through the head. Early observations of personality change after injury to the prefrontal cortex. *British Medical Journal (Clinical Research Edition), 317*(7174), 1673–1674. doi:10.1136/bmj.317.7174.1673a

Olver, J. H., Ponsford, J. L., & Curran, C. A. (1996). Outcome following traumatic brain injury: A comparison between 2 and 5 years after injury. *Brain Injury, 10*(11), 841–848. doi:10.1080/026990596123945

Osborne-Crowley, K., & McDonald, S. (2016). Hyposmia, not emotion perception, is associated with psychosocial outcome after severe traumatic brain injury. *Neuropsychology, 30*(7), 820–829. doi:10.1037/neu0000293

Osborne-Crowley, K., & McDonald, S. (2018). A review of social disinhibition after traumatic brain injury. *Journal of Neuropsychology, 12*(2), 176–199. doi:10.1111/jnp.12113

Osborne-Crowley, K., McDonald, S., & Rushby, J. A. (2016). Role of reversal learning impairment in social disinhibition following severe traumatic brain injury. *Journal of the International Neuropsychological Society, 22*(3), 303–313. doi:10.1017/S1355617715001277

Osborne-Crowley, K., Wilson, E., De Blasio, F., Wearne, T., Rushby, J., & McDonald, S. (2019a). Preserved rapid conceptual processing of emotional expressions despite reduced neuropsychological performance following traumatic brain injury. *Neuropsychology, 33*(6), 872–882. doi:10.1037/neu0000545

Osborne-Crowley, K., Wilson, E., De Blasio, F., Wearne, T., Rushby, J., & McDonald, S. (2019b). Subjective emotional experience and physiological responsivity to posed emotions in people with traumatic brain injury. *Neuropsychology, 33*(8), 1151–1162. doi:10.1037/neu0000580

Ownsworth, T., & McKenna, K. (2004). Investigation of factors related to employment outcome following traumatic brain injury: A critical review and conceptual model. *Disability and Rehabilitation, 26*(13), 765–783.

Parola, A., Gabbatore, I., Bosco, F. M., Bara, B. G., Cossa, F. M., Gindri, P., & Sacco, K. (2016). Assessment of pragmatic impairment in right hemisphere damage. *Journal of Neurolinguistics, 39*, 10–25.

Pell, M. D. (2006). Cerebral mechanisms for understanding emotional prosody in speech. *Brain and Language, 96*(2), 221–234.

Pertz, M., Okoniewski, A., Schlegel, U., & Thoma, P. (2020). Impairment of sociocognitive functions in patients with brain tumours. *Neuroscience & Biobehavioral Reviews, 108*, 370–392. doi:10.1016/j.neubiorev.2019.11.018

Petrea, R. E., Beiser, A. S., Seshadri, S., Kelly-Hayes, M., Kase, C. S., & Wolf, P. A. (2009). Gender differences in stroke incidence and poststroke disability in the Framingham heart study. *Stroke, 40*(4), 1032–1037.

Pluta, A., Gawron, N., Sobanska, M., Wojcik, A. D., & Lojek, E. (2017). The nature of the relationship between neurocognition and theory of mind impairments in stroke patients. *Neuropsychology, 31*(6), 666–681.

Prigatano, G. P., & Pribram, K. H. (1982). Perception and memory of facial affect following brain injury. *Perceptual and Motor Skills, 54*(3), 859–869.

Rolls, E. T., Hornak, J., Wade, D., & McGrath, J. (1994). Emotion-related learning in patients with social and emotional changes associated with frontal lobe damage. *Journal of Neurology, Neurosurgery & Psychiatry, 57*(12), 1518–1524.

Roman, M., Brownell, H. H., Potter, H. H., & Sebold, M. S. (1987). Script knowledge in right hemisphere damaged and in normal elderly adults. *Brain and Language, 31*, 151–170.

Rosenberg, H., Dethier, M., Kessels, R. P., Westbrook, R. F., & McDonald, S. (2015). Emotion perception after moderate-severe traumatic brain injury: The valence effect and the role of working memory, processing speed, and nonverbal reasoning. *Neuropsychology*, *29*(4), 509–521. doi:10.1037/neu0000171

Rosenberg, H., McDonald, S., Dethier, M., Kessels, R. P., & Westbrook, R. F. (2014). Facial emotion recognition deficits following moderate-severe traumatic brain injury (TBI): Re-examining the valence effect and the role of emotion intensity. *Journal of the International Neuropsychological Society*, *20*(10), 994–1003. doi:10.1017/s1355617714000940

Rosenberg, H., McDonald, S., Rosenberg, J., & Frederick Westbrook, R. (2018). Amused, flirting or simply baffled? Is recognition of all emotions affected by traumatic brain injury? *Journal of Neuropsychology*, *12*(2), 145–164. doi:10.1111/jnp.12109

Rushby, J. A., McDonald, S., Randall, R., de Sousa, A., Trimmer, E., & Fisher, A. (2013). Impaired emotional contagion following severe traumatic brain injury. *International Journal of Psychophysiology*, *89*(3), 466–474. doi:10.1016/j.ijpsycho.2013.06.013

Sackeim, H. A., Greenberg, M. S., Weiman, A. L., Gur, R. C., Hungerbuhler, J. P., & Geschwind, N. (1982). Hemispheric asymmetry in the expression of positive and negative emotions. *Archives of Neurology*, *39*, 210–218.

Samson, D., Apperly, I. A., Kathirgamanathan, U., & Humphreys, G. W. (2005). Seeing it my way: A case of a selective deficit in inhibiting self-perspective. *Brain*, *128*(Pt 5), 1102–1111. doi:10.1093/brain/awh464

Sanchez-Navarro, J., Martinez-Selva, J., & Roman, F. (2005). Emotional response in patients with frontal brain damage: Effects of affective valence and information content. *Behavioral Neuroscience*, *119*(1), 87.

Saunders, J. C., McDonald, S., & Richardson, R. (2006). Loss of emotional experience after traumatic brain injury: Findings with the startle probe procedure. *Neuropsychology*, *20*(2), 224.

Saxe, R., & Wexler, A. (2005). Making sense of another mind: The role of the right temporo-parietal junction. *Neuropsychologia*, *43*(10), 1391–1399. doi:10.1016/j.neuropsychologia.2005.02.013

Saxton, M. E., Younan, S. S., & Lah, S. (2013). Social behaviour following severe traumatic brain injury: Contribution of emotion perception deficits. *NeuroRehabilitation*, *33*(2), 263–271.

Schmidt, A. T., Hanten, G. R., Li, X., Orsten, K. D., & Levin, H. S. (2010). Emotion recognition following pediatric traumatic brain injury: Longitudinal analysis of emotional prosody and facial emotion recognition. *Neuropsychologia*, *48*(10), 2869–2877.

Servadei, F., Graham, T., & Merry, G. (2001). Defining acute mild head injury in adults: A proposal based on prognostic factors, diagnosis, and management. *Journal of Neurotrauma*, *18*(7), 657–664. doi:10.1089/089771501750357609

Shamay-Tsoory, S. G., Aharon-Peretz, J., & Perry, D. (2009). Two systems for empathy: A double dissociation between emotional and cognitive empathy in inferior frontal gyrus versus ventromedial prefrontal lesions. *Brain*, *132*(3), 617–627.

Soroker, N., Kasher, A., Giora, R., Batori, G., Corn, C., Gil, M., & Zaidel, E. (2005). Processing of basic speech acts following localized brain damage: A new light on the neuroanatomy of language. *Brain and Cognition*, *57*(2), 214–217.

Spikman, J. M., Timmerman, M. E., Milders, M. V., Veenstra, W. S., & van der Naalt, J. (2012). Social cognition impairments in relation to general cognitive deficits, injury severity, and prefrontal lesions in traumatic brain injury patients. *Journal of Neurotrauma*, *29*(1), 101–111.

Spitz, G., Ponsford, J. L., Rudzki, D., & Maller, J. J. (2012). Association between cognitive performance and functional outcome following traumatic brain injury: A longitudinal multilevel examination. *Neuropsychology*, *26*(5), 604.

Stemmer, B., Giroux, F., & Joanette, Y. (1994). Production and evaluation of requests by right hemisphere brain damaged individuals. *Brain and Language*, *47*, 1–31.

Symington, S. H., Paul, L. K., Symington, M. F., Ono, M., & Brown, W. S. (2010). Social cognition in individuals with agenesis of the corpus callosum. *Social Neuroscience*, *5*(3), 296–308. doi:10.1080/17470910903462419

Tam, S., McKay, A., Sloan, S., & Ponsford, J. (2015). The experience of challenging behaviours following severe TBI: A family perspective. *Brain Injury*, *29*(7–8), 813–821. doi:10.3109/02699052.2015.1005134

Temkin, N. R., Corrigan, J. D., Dikmen, S. S., & Machamer, J. (2009). Social functioning after traumatic brain injury. *The Journal of Head Trauma Rehabilitation*, *24*(6), 460–467.

Theadom, A., McDonald, S., Starkey, N., Barker-Collo, S., Jones, K. M., Ameratunga, S., . . . Feigin, V. L. (2019). Social cognition four years after mild-TBI: An age-matched prospective longitudinal cohort study. *Neuropsychology*, *33*(4), 560–567. doi:10.1037/neu0000516

Tranel, D., Bechara, A., & Denburg, N. L. (2002). Asymmetric functional roles of right and left ventromedial prefrontal cortices in social conduct, decision-making, and emotional processing. *Cortex*, *38*(4), 589–612.

Turkstra, L. S., Dixon, T. M., & Baker, K. K. (2004). Theory of mind and social beliefs in adolescents with traumatic brain injury. *NeuroRehabilitation*, *19*(3), 245–256.

Turkstra, L. S., Williams, W. H., Tonks, J., & Frampton, I. (2008). Measuring social cognition in adolescents: Implications for students with TBI returning to school. *NeuroRehabilitation*, *23*(6), 501–509.

Van Lancker, D. R., & Kempler, D. (1987). Comprehension of familiar phrases by left but not right hemisphere damaged patients. *Brain and Language*, *32*, 265–277.

Vas, A. K., Spence, J., & Chapman, S. B. (2015). Abstracting meaning from complex information (gist reasoning) in adult traumatic brain injury. *Journal of Clinical and Experimental Neuropsychology*, *37*(2), 152–161.

Wapner, W., Hamby, S., & Gardner, H. (1981). The role of the right hemisphere in the apprehension of complex linguistic materials. *Brain and Language*, *14*, 15–32.

Wearne, T. A., Osborne-Crowley, K., Logan, J. A., Wilson, E., Rushby, J., & McDonald, S. (2020). Understanding how others feel: Evaluating the relationship between empathy and various aspects of emotion recognition following severe traumatic brain injury. *Neuropsychology*, *34*(3), 288–297. doi:10.1037/neu0000609

Wearne, T. A., Osborne-Crowley, K., Rosenberg, H., Dethier, M., & McDonald, S. (2018). Emotion recognition depends on subjective emotional experience and not on facial expressivity: Evidence from traumatic brain injury. *Brain Injury*, 1–11. doi:10.1080/02699052.2018.1531300

Weddell, R. A., & Leggett, J. A. (2006). Factors triggering relatives' judgements of personality change after traumatic brain injury. *Brain Injury*, *20*(12), 1221–1234. doi:10.1080/02699050601049783

Weed, E., McGregor, W., Nielsen, J. F., Roepstorff, A., & Frith, U. (2010). Theory of mind in adults with right hemisphere damage: What's the story? *Brain and Language*, *113*(2), 65–72.

Wells, R., Dywan, J., & Dumas, J. (2005). Life satisfaction and distress in family caregivers as related to specific behavioural changes after traumatic brain injury. *Brain Injury*, *19*(13), 1105–1115.

Werner, C., & Engelhard, K. (2007). Pathophysiology of traumatic brain injury. *British Journal of Anaesthesia*, *99*(1), 4–9. doi:10.1093/bja/aem131

Williams, C., & Wood, R. L. (2010). Alexithymia and emotional empathy following traumatic brain injury. *Journal of Clinical and Experimental Neuropsychology, 32*(3), 259–267. doi:10.1080/13803390902976940

Williams, C., & Wood, R. L. (2012). Affective modulation of the startle reflex following traumatic brain injury. *Journal of Clinical and Experimental Neuropsychology, 34*(9), 948–961.

Winner, E., Brownell, H., Happe, F., Blum, A., & Pincus, D. (1998, March). Distinguishing lies from jokes: Theory of mind deficits and discourse interpretation in right hemisphere brain-damaged patients. *Brain and Language, 62*(1), 89–106. doi:10.1006/brln.1997.1889

Winner, E., & Gardner, H. (1977). Comprehension of metaphor in brain damaged patients. *Brain, 100*, 719–727.

Winter, L., Moriarty, H. J., & Short, T. H. (2018). Beyond anger: Emotion regulation and social connectedness in veterans with traumatic brain injury. *Brain Injury, 32*(5), 593–599. doi:10.1080/02699052.2018.1432895

Wood, R. L., & Rutterford, N. A. (2006). Demographic and cognitive predictors of long-term psychosocial outcome following traumatic brain injury. *Journal of the International Neuropsychological Society: JINS, 12*(3), 350.

Wood, R. L., & Williams, C. (2008). Inability to empathize following traumatic brain injury. *Journal of the International Neuropsychological Society: JINS, 14*(2), 289–296. doi:10.1017/S1355617708080326

Yang, F. G., Fuller, J., Khodaparast, N., & Krawczyk, D. C. (2010). Figurative language processing after traumatic brain injury in adults: A preliminary study. *Neuropsychologia, 48*(7), 1923–1929. doi:10.1016/j.neuropsychologia.2010.03.011

Yates, P. J. (2003). Psychological adjustment, social enablement and community integration following acquired brain injury. *Neuropsychological Rehabilitation, 13*(1–2), 291–306.

Yeates, K. O., Bigler, E. D., Dennis, M., Gerhardt, C. A., Rubin, K. H., Stancin, T., . . . Vannatta, K. (2007). Social outcomes in childhood brain disorder: A heuristic integration of social neuroscience and developmental psychology. *Psychological Bulletin, 133*(3), 535–556. doi:10.1037/0033-2909.133.3.535.

Yuvaraj, R., Murugappan, M., Norlinah, M. I., Sundaraj, K., & Khairiyah, M. (2013). Review of emotion recognition in stroke patients. *Dementia and Geriatric Cognitive Disorders, 36*(3–4), 179–196. doi:10.1159/000353440

Zupan, B., Babbage, D., Neumann, D., & Willer, B. (2014). Recognition of facial and vocal affect following traumatic brain injury. *Brain Injury, 28*(8), 1087–1095. doi:10.3109/02699052.2014.901560

Zupan, B., & Neumann, D. (2014). Affect recognition in traumatic brain injury: Responses to unimodal and multimodal media. *Journal of Head Trauma Rehabilitation, 29*(4), E1–e12. doi:10.1097/HTR.0b013e31829dded6

Zupan, B., & Neumann, D. (2016). Exploring the use of isolated expressions and film clips to evaluate emotion recognition by people with traumatic brain injury. *Journal of Visualized Experiments*, (111). doi:10.3791/53774

Chapter 6

Social cognition in psychiatric disorders

Amy E. Pinkham

Despite the fact that social or occupational dysfunction is required for the diagnosis of almost all psychiatric disorders, the study of social cognition in psychiatry, and how social cognition may be related to social impairment, has really only been formalized over the last 25–30 years. Social cognition initially gained traction within the fields of autism and psychosis; however, these literatures were developed largely in parallel with very little direct comparison between the two (Sasson, Pinkham, Carpenter, & Belger, 2011). This separation has led to slightly different perspectives and areas of emphasis within each class of disorders, but it has also allowed each field to grow freely and ask questions that are unconstrained by previous conceptualizations or methods. This chapter will review current knowledge of social cognition in psychiatric disorders by focusing on the psychosis literature.

Psychosis broadly refers to a loss of contact with reality and difficulty understanding what is real and what is not. It is manifest in psychiatric disorders primarily via the presence of hallucinations (without insight into their pathological nature) and/or delusions, and the primary diagnoses involving psychosis are schizophrenia and schizoaffective disorder (American Psychiatric Association, 2013; World Health Organization, 2018). Psychosis can also accompany mood disorders such as bipolar disorder and major depressive disorder. This overlap has fueled the expansion of social cognition research beyond schizophrenia spectrum illnesses to mood disorders, and social cognition is now viewed as having significant transdiagnostic value (Gur & Gur, 2016).

In this chapter, I will first review the current state of social cognitive research in psychosis by presenting how social cognition is defined within this subfield and describing the domains and topics that have received the most attention. I will then review evidence supporting impaired social cognition in psychosis and present an argument for the importance of social cognition relative to neurocognition. Next, I will provide a brief overview of the presumed neurobiological mechanisms of impaired social cognition and discuss psychosocial and pharmacological treatment approaches for improving social cognition and social functioning. I will conclude with a brief section on current challenges and areas of growth. Given that the majority of work on social cognition has

DOI: 10.4324/9781003027034-6

focused on schizophrenia and psychosis, this chapter will similarly emphasize findings from the schizophrenia literature. However, where appropriate, special mention will be made of findings that extend across diagnoses.

Definition and domains of social cognition

Definitions of social cognition vary according to sub-discipline but can broadly be summarized as perceiving, processing, and using social information. Within the psychosis area, an NIMH Workshop on Social Cognition in Schizophrenia defined social cognition as "the mental operations that underlie social interactions, including perceiving, interpreting, and generating responses to the intentions, dispositions, and behaviors of others" (Green et al., 2008, p. 1211). This definition thus encompasses a wide range of constructs spanning basic perceptual processes, such as identifying a face, to complex cognitive processes, such as trying to understand what someone else is thinking. Perhaps more importantly, however, this definition does not stop at cognition. Instead, it emphasizes the link between these diverse perceptual and cognitive processes and actual social behavior. As explained later in this chapter, the link between social cognition and real-world social functioning and behavior has been well established, and there is now consensus regarding the idea that social cognition is critical for understanding the social impairment that is seen in so many disorders.

While social cognition has traditionally been parsed into conceptual domains representing specific skills or abilities, such as emotion recognition or mental state attribution, the wide-ranging nature of its definition has led to some ambiguity about which constructs do and do not "count" as a social cognitive process. A relatively recent study attempted to provide consensus by asking experts in the fields of schizophrenia, autism, and social psychology to nominate key domains of social cognition (Pinkham, Penn et al., 2014). Nominations were compiled and presented back to the survey respondents in a second step that asked to what degree the expert thought the construct represented a valid domain of social cognition and how important they believed that construct was to their area of research. This process identified four core domains of social cognition that can be considered important for psychosis research:

1   *Emotion processing* is broadly defined as perceiving and using emotions (Green et al., 2008) and as such, represents both lower and upper level processes. At a lower perceptual level, it includes emotion perception/ recognition (i.e., identifying and recognizing emotional displays from facial expressions and/or non-face cues such as voice), and at a higher level it includes understanding emotions and managing/regulating emotions.

2   *Social perception* refers to decoding and interpreting social cues in others (Penn, Ritchie, Francis, Combs, & Martin, 2002; Sergi & Green, 2003; Toomey, Schuldberg, Corrigan, & Green, 2002). It includes social context processing and social knowledge, which can be defined as knowing

social rules and how these rules influence others' behaviors (Addington, Saeedi, & Addington, 2006; Corrigan & Green, 1993a).

3   *Mentalizing or mental state attribution* is defined as the ability to understand the mental states of others including the inference of intentions, dispositions, and/or beliefs (Frith, 1992; Penn, Addington, & Pinkham, 2006). Mentalizing is also referred to as theory of mind or cognitive empathy (Shamay-Tsoory, 2011).

4   *Attributional style/bias* describes the way in which individuals explain the causes, or make sense, of social events or interactions (Green et al., 2008; Penn et al., 2006).

It is important to point out that attributional style/bias is unique from the other domains in that it refers to tendencies to think certain ways rather than to evaluate social stimuli correctly or incorrectly. Thus, while the first three domains can be thought of as capacities or abilities that can be impaired or intact, there is no inherently correct attributional style. Instead, tendencies can be identified that may be more or less adaptive within changing social environments (Pinkham, Harvey, & Penn, 2016; Walss-Bass, Fernandes, Roberts, Service, & Velligan, 2013). Both capacities and biases are therefore likely to be involved in social functioning, and the inclusion of both within the current conceptualization of social cognition in psychosis is a notable strength.

A notable weakness of this conceptualization, however, is that the parsing of social cognition into these four domains is not empirically supported. Instead, factor analyses suggest social cognition may be best represented as a single factor (Browne et al., 2016), or if attributional style is included in the data, that a two factor solution comprising social cognitive skill and attributional style is most appropriate (Buck, Healey, Gagen, Roberts, & Penn, 2016; Etchepare & Prouteau, 2018). Other factor analyses also support the division of social cognition according to level of information processing (i.e., perception vs. inferential and regulatory processing) rather than domain of social information (i.e., emotion vs. mental state) (Lin, Wynn, Hellemann, & Green, 2012; Mancuso, Horan, Kern, & Green, 2011). It seems likely that some of the discrepancies between factor analyses are due to methodological differences (e.g., the numbers and types of tasks included; sample characteristics); however, it is clear that additional work is required before the actual factor structure is identified.

Another weakness is that these domains do not encompass the entirety of social cognition. Both metacognition, the ability to evaluate one's own thoughts and those of others (Lysaker et al., 2010), and social reciprocity, engaging in emotionally and socially appropriate turn-taking interactions with others (Constantino, Przybeck, Friesen, & Todd, 2000), were also nominated as potential domains in the expert survey but were ultimately not included due to lower ratings of validity and importance. At the time, though, these domains had received relatively little attention within the psychosis literature, and metacognition in particular has since been identified as an area of impairment in psychosis (Sellers, Varese, Wells, & Morrison, 2017) and as a domain that is amenable to treatment (Moritz & Lysaker, 2018). Empathy is another important area that is not plainly represented in the currently identified domains. While cognitive empathy overlaps with mentalizing, it is not clear where affective empathy, the relatively automatic emotional responses one has to the experiences or emotional states of others (Bonfils, Lysaker, Minor, & Salyers, 2016), fits into the identified domains. The conceptualization of social cognition will therefore need to broaden as knowledge continues to accrue. For now, though, the consensus-based domains do highlight the multidimensional nature of social cognition and provide a useful framework for reviewing social cognitive abilities in individuals with psychosis.

Social cognitive impairments in psychosis

Emotion processing

Studies addressing the lower, perceptual level of emotion processing have primarily focused on explicit recognition of emotion, typically by showing an emotional face and asking participants to select the displayed emotion from a list of choices. This work consistently demonstrates impairments in individuals with schizophrenia, and meta-analyses report large effect sizes (d = 0.91; Kohler, Walker, Martin, Healey, & Moberg, 2010 and g = 0.89; Savla, Vella, Armstrong, Penn, & Twamley, 2013) for the comparison of patients and healthy individuals. Emotion identification impairments are also present in bipolar disorder but to a lesser degree. A recent meta-analysis of comparisons between schizophrenia and bipolar disorder reported that bipolar participants outperformed schizophrenia by about a third of a standard deviation (d = 0.39; Bora & Pantelis, 2016), and the work of Ruocco and colleagues (2014) suggests that impairments are likely to exist on a continuum of increasing severity from psychotic bipolar disorder to schizoaffective disorder to schizophrenia.

Reviews of emotion recognition abilities in psychosis are numerous (Kohler et al., 2010; Pinkham, Gur, & Gur, 2007), and several points are worth emphasis here. First, recognition impairments appear to be greater for negative emotions (e.g., fear, anger) than for positive emotions (e.g., happiness), and among the negative emotions, fear appears to be the most difficult to accurately identify (Bigelow et al., 2006; Kohler et al., 2003). Individuals with schizophrenia also tend to misattribute negative emotions to neutral faces (Kohler et al., 2003), and this pattern is related to the presence of active paranoid ideation (Pinkham, Brensinger, Kohler, Gur, & Gur, 2011). Second, emotion recognition abilities are also more pronounced in individuals with more prominent negative (Sachs, Steger-Wuchse, Kryspin-Exner, Gur, & Katschnig, 2004) and disorganized symptoms (Ventura, Wood, Jimenez, & Hellemann, 2013). Specific negative symptoms may be particularly relevant as one study demonstrated that flat affect uniquely predicted emotion processing abilities (Gur et al., 2006).

Third, individuals with schizophrenia tend to show abnormal visual scanning of faces that includes reduced time looking at the most salient features of the face (e.g., eyes and mouth) (Sasson et al., 2007; Simpson, Pinkham, Kelsven, & Sasson, 2013), which may contribute to emotion recognition impairments. And finally, the debate is still open regarding whether the impairments seen in psychosis are specific to facial emotion processing or if they represent more generalized difficulties in basic perception or face perception. For example, individuals with schizophrenia also show difficulties with non-emotional face processing (e.g., identity recognition, age discrimination, etc.), and it seems likely that these impairments may feed forward to result in poorer recognition of emotions from faces (Bortolon, Capdevielle, & Raffard, 2015). However, an emerging body of work demonstrates that implicit processing of facial emotion may be intact in psychosis (Kring, Siegel, & Barrett, 2014; Shasteen et al., 2016), which suggests that emotion recognition impairments may be the result of difficulties arising during contextual appraisal and integration of information rather than the perceptual level per se (Kring et al., 2014; Sasson, Pinkham, Weittenhiller, Faso, & Simpson, 2016).

In addition to this extensive body of literature on facial emotion recognition, the ability to identify emotions from other cues, such as voice and body posture, has also been investigated. Effect size estimates for impairments in emotional prosody are comparable to those for facial affect recognition at $d = 0.92$ for recognition tasks and $d = 0.74$ for discrimination tasks (Lin, Ding, & Zhang, 2018); however, the literature is less conclusive about identifying emotions from bodies. A recent study of individuals with schizophrenia showed relatively intact performance on an explicit task of bodily emotion recognition, but with some difficulties for fearful and sad expressions (Hajdúk, Klein, Bass, Springfield, & Pinkham, 2020), and perception of emotions from bodies also appears to be intact in bipolar disorder (Lee & Van Meter, 2020). A point of focus for future work will be to replicate these initial findings, and if validated, to attempt to understand why recognition of bodily emotion would be preserved when facial emotion recognition is so clearly impaired.

As a last note on emotion processing, there have been considerably fewer studies evaluating the higher-level skills associated with this domain. Nevertheless, they also show a large effect size ($g = 0.88$) for the difference in emotion management task performance between individuals with psychosis and healthy controls (Savla et al., 2013) and reduced engagement in emotion regulation strategies, such as cognitive reappraisal or acceptance, among individuals with psychosis (Kimhy et al., 2012; Perry, Henry, & Grisham, 2011).

Social perception

Social perception has been less well investigated in psychosis, in part due to measurement issues such as poor psychometric properties of assessments (Kern et al., 2013; Pinkham, Penn, Green, & Harvey, 2016b), but perhaps also because of the wide range of skills and abilities that fall under this domain and that make it harder to succinctly measure. While social perception broadly refers to the identification and utilization of social cues, it involves multiple sub-constructs including biological motion detection, interpretation of voice and body cues to understand behavior (Rosenthal, DePaulo, & Jall, 1979), and understanding typical relationships between individuals (Bell, Fiszdon, Greig, & Wexler, 2010; Sergi et al., 2009). Social knowledge, or the awareness of the procedures and goals associated with routine social situations (Corrigan & Green, 1993b), is also included in social perception but can be viewed as a more foundational skill that aids in social perception.

Taken as a whole, the available evidence on social perception in psychosis appears to indicate that as the targeted skill increases in complexity, the level of impairment shown by patients also increases. For example, in an early series of studies, Corrigan et al. reported that individuals with schizophrenia were better able to recognize concrete social cues (e.g., "what is she doing?") as compared to abstract cues (e.g., "what are her goals?") (Corrigan, Garman, & Nelson, 1996; Corrigan & Green, 1993b; Corrigan & Nelson, 1998). Examination of effect sizes for impairments in the various skills and abilities included in social perception also follow this general pattern. Specifically, individuals with psychosis perform approximately half a standard deviation below healthy individuals on tasks of social knowledge (g = 0.54) (Savla et al., 2013) and biological motion detection (SMD = 0.66) (Okruszek & Pilecka, 2017), but about one full standard deviation below on tasks requiring the use of verbal and nonverbal cues to understand social situations (g = 1.04) (Savla et al., 2013).

Mentalizing

The ability to infer the mental states of another individual, known as mentalizing or theory of mind, has been studied extensively in psychosis. Early studies reported impairments across a broad range of mentalizing skills including understanding false beliefs (Brune, Abdel-Hamid, Lehmkamper, & Sonntag, 2007; Corcoran & Frith, 2003; Pickup & Frith, 2001), deciphering hints (Marjoram et al., 2005; Pinkham & Penn, 2006), identifying the intentions of another individual (Brunet, Sarfati, & Hardy-Bayle, 2003; Sarfati, Hardy-Bayle, Besche, & Widlocher, 1997), identifying the mental state of another individual (Kelemen et al., 2005; Kington, Jones, Watt, Hopkin, & Williams, 2000), and understanding faux pas (Martino, Bucay, Butman, & Allegri, 2007). More recent meta-analyses also provide clear evidence for impairments in individuals with schizophrenia relative to healthy individuals, with large effect sizes ranging from .99 to 1.25 across the mentalizing domain (Bora, Yucel, & Pantelis, 2009; Chung, Barch, & Strube, 2014; Sprong, Schothorst, Vos, Hox, & van Engeland, 2007) and for individuals with bipolar disorder relative to healthy individuals, with an effect size of .5 in euthymic patients and 1.23 during acute episodes (Bora, Bartholomeusz, & Pantelis, 2016).

Areas of focus within the mentalizing literature include how performance in this domain relates to symptoms and how it relates to non-social cognitive ability. In regard to symptoms, the meta-analyses cited above demonstrate that impairments do not seem to be related to symptom severity (Chung et al., 2014) but rather that they are likely to represent a more stable, trait-like deficit, which is evident even in remitted patients (Bora et al., 2009; Sprong et al., 2007). Emerging evidence is also beginning to suggest that the types of mentalizing errors one makes may be related to the predominance of certain symptoms. For example, under-mentalizing errors (i.e., failing to attribute intentions to another individual) appear to be more common in individuals with negative symptoms, whereas over-mentalizing errors (i.e., generating too many possible intentions and then choosing the wrong one) are more pronounced in individuals with predominately positive symptoms (Fretland et al., 2015; Montag et al., 2011).

Mentalizing has also been linked to non-social cognitive ability, or neurocognition, such that greater mentalizing impairments are seen in those individuals who also show greater neurocognitive deficits (Bora, Yucel, & Pantelis, 2009). Additionally, while all domains of neurocognition (e.g., attention, memory, etc.) appear to contribute somewhat equally to mentalizing deficits in schizophrenia (Thibaudeau, Achim, Parent, Turcotte, & Cellard, 2020), poor executive function may be most predictive of impaired mentalizing (Bechi et al., 2018; Catalan et al., 2018).

Attributional style/bias

Attributional style has received relatively less research attention compared to the other social cognitive domains. This is largely due to the same reasons that social perception has not been as widely studied, namely that attributional style is difficult to measure and the lack of psychometrically sound assessment tools (Pinkham et al., 2016b). Nevertheless, early work honedin on two patterns of thinking that seemed to be more prominent in psychosis – the externalizing bias and the personalizing bias. The externalizing bias refers to the tendency to make external attributions for negative outcomes (Janssen et al., 2006; Langdon, Ward, & Coltheart, 2010), and the personalizing bias primarily clarifies this tendency to externalize by noting that external causes of events can either be another individual (i.e., an external personal attribution) or a situational factor (i.e., an external situational attribution). Several studies suggest that the personalizing form of the externalizing bias is more common in individuals with psychosis and particularly those with more severe persecutory ideation (Aakre, Seghers, St-Hilaire, & Docherty, 2009; Langdon et al., 2010; Mehl et al., 2014). The robustness of these findings, however, is currently unclear as a recent meta-analysis failed to support the presence of either bias in schizophrenia, even when limiting the analyses to individuals with persecutory delusions (Savla et al., 2013).

A relatively newer emphasis within the attributional style area has focused on the hostile attribution bias, which is defined as the tendency to interpret others' actions as antagonistic and intentional (Combs, Penn, Wicher, & Waldheter, 2007a). Buck et al. (2020) recently reviewed the growing literature regarding the hostility bias in psychosis and offered two primary conclusions: (1) individuals with schizophrenia make more hostile attributions than healthy individuals, and (2) the hostility bias is strongly related to levels of paranoia, which has been demonstrated both across the schizophrenia spectrum (Buck, Pinkham, Harvey, & Penn, 2016; Darrell-Berry et al., 2017) and in healthy individuals (Combs, Penn, Wicher, & Waldheter, 2007b). Indeed, in direct group comparisons, patients with high levels of paranoia show a greater hostility bias than non-paranoid patients (Combs et al., 2009; Pinkham, Harvey, & Penn, 2016a). The hostility bias, therefore, seems to have high clinical significance and may offer important clues as to which symptoms manifest during psychotic episodes. Also noted by Buck and colleagues, however, a number of questions remain regarding the nature of this bias. These include whether this tendency is more trait- or state-like and whether the hostility bias contributes causally to paranoia. Thus, it is expected that the hostility bias will continue to gain attention within the domain of attributional style.

The importance of social cognition

When social cognition first emerged as an area of study within psychosis, a prevailing question was whether or not it represented an independent construct or just a downstream consequence of the neurocognitive impairments that are so prevalent in psychosis. The current consensus on this question is that while social cognition has clear areas of overlap with neurocognition, it does seem to be relatively independent. Correlational studies suggest only modest relations between social and neurocognition (Ventura, Wood, & Hellemann, 2011), and factor analyses consistently note that the two load on different factors (Sergi et al., 2007; Van Hooren et al., 2008). Further, results from studies using differential deficit designs support the specificity of social cognitive impairments in schizophrenia by demonstrating impaired performance on social cognitive tasks but intact performance on comparable, non-social tasks (Kosmidis et al., 2007; Pinkham, Sasson et al., 2014).

Another key question within the literature has been whether or not social cognitive impairments matter in terms of the real-world functioning of individuals with psychosis. Two separate meta-analyses, the first utilizing 52 studies comprising 2,692 participants (Fett, Viechtbauer, Penn, van Os, & Krabbendam, 2011) and the second using 166 studies comprising 12,868 participants (Halverson, Orleans-Pobee et al., 2019), both demonstrate that social cognition explains more unique variance in functional outcomes than neurocognition. It also appears that social cognition mediates the relation between neurocognition and functioning (Halverson, Orleans-Pobee et al., 2019). Thus, social cognition appears to be critically important for community and social functioning, which highlights social cognition as an important target for treatment and remediation (see Box 6.1: Case Study for a real-world example).

Box 6.1   Case 1: RL: Young women with schizophrenia

History:

RL is a 22-year-old woman who was diagnosed with schizophrenia at the age of 19. She had been attending university when her symptoms began but discontinued her schooling due to repeated hospitalizations and difficulties maintaining her grades. She currently lives at home with her parents and younger siblings.

Relationship with family and friends:

RL reports that her relationship with her parents is contentious and that she often feels like she cannot understand what her parents want to her to do. This tends to lead to arguments when RL has failed to meet her parents' expectations. Most recently, both RL and her parents acknowledge arguing about RL's failure to look for a job. RL's parents indicate that they hinted multiple times that RL should not spend all of her time at home and that she needed to engage in productive activities. However, RL did not connect these comments to finding employment and instead just started spending more time away from home. Similarly, RL indicates that relationships with friends have been difficult and that she has recently felt like her one remaining friend was intentionally ignoring her when she did not immediately return a call or text message.

As part of her treatment program, RL was encouraged to think of potential reasons why her friend may not respond right away and then to "check-in" with her friend to inquire about the reasons for the delay. In doing so, RL was surprised to learn that her friend had recently started a new job that prevented her from immediately calling back. This information made RL feel much better about the relationship.

Opinion:

As exemplified here, social cognitive difficulties with inferring the thoughts of others and the reasons for their behaviour can contribute to considerable difficulties in social functioning.

Finally, investigators have asked about the generalizability of social cognitive impairments across the clinical spectrum. As noted above, social cognitive impairments are now viewed as transdiagnostic and are seen in multiple disorders including bipolar disorder (de Siqueira Rotenberg, Beraldi, Okawa

Belizario, & Lafer, 2020), major depression (Bora & Berk, 2016), anxiety disorders (Lavoie, Battaglia, & Achim, 2014), and substance use disorders (Bora & Zorlu, 2017). Evidence is also building in support of social cognition as an endophenotype, particularly within the psychosis spectrum (Green, Horan, & Lee, 2015; Gur & Gur, 2016). For example, emotion processing impairments are evident in individuals experiencing their first psychotic episode (Barkl, Lah, Harris, & Williams, 2014), individuals identified as being at clinical high risk for developing psychosis (Kohler et al., 2014), and first-degree relatives of individuals with psychosis (Allott et al., 2015). Mentalizing and social perception show similar patterns (Barbato et al., 2015; Bora & Pantelis, 2013). Additionally, both cross-sectional (Comparelli et al., 2013) and longitudinal studies (Horan et al., 2012; Piskulic et al., 2016) demonstrate that social cognitive impairment is stable across phases of illness and time. These studies therefore demonstrate that social cognitive impairments are longstanding and widespread, and when viewed within the context of their negative impact on functioning, the importance of social cognition is clear.

Neurobiological correlates of social cognitive impairments

Given the strong foundation of work demonstrating that social cognition is significantly impaired in psychosis and that it relates to functioning, the field has also attempted to identify a potential neural mechanism for these impairments. Neuroscience research investigating social information processing in healthy individuals has long supported the hypothesis of a "social brain", or the idea that some brain regions and networks are specialized for social information (Brothers, 1990). Early work emphasized the roles of the *orbitofrontal cortex, superior temporal sulcus,* and *amygdala*; however, the field now focuses on much broader networks that involve multiple neural regions with reciprocal connections between them (Stanley & Adolphs, 2013). These networks generally map onto the core social cognitive domains that have been discussed here (Kennedy & Adolphs, 2012), including a "social perception" network important for emotion processing, centered on the *amygdala* and including the *orbitofrontal cortex, striatum, nucleus accumbens,* and *visual cortices* (Adolphs, 2010) and a "mentalizing" network comprised of *medial prefrontal cortex (MPFC), superior temporal sulcus* and surrounding *superior temporal gyrus,* and *temporoparietal junction* (Amodio & Frith, 2006; Saxe, 2006) (see also Chapter 1 for further discussion).

Over the last 20 years, these networks have been studied extensively in psychosis, and there is now ample evidence demonstrating that individuals with psychosis show abnormal activation and connectivity of these networks as compared to healthy individuals. For example, meta-analyses of neural activation during tasks of facial emotion recognition demonstrate reduced activation in the *amygdala, fusiform gyrus, anterior cingulate cortex,* and *thalamus* in individuals with schizophrenia and individuals with bipolar disorders (Delvecchio, Sugra-nyes, & Frangou, 2013; Taylor et al., 2012). Similar findings of hypoactivation have been reported during mentalizing tasks for *medial prefrontal cortex, orbito-frontal cortex,* and a portion of the *temporoparietal junction* (TPJ) (Kronbichler, Tschernegg, Martin, Schurz, & Kronbichler, 2017; Vucurovic, Caillies, & Kaladjian, 2020). Reduced functional connectivity within these networks has also been reported, specifically, reduced *amygdala-medial prefrontal cortex* con-nectivity while processing negative emotional images (Bjorkquist, Olsen, Nel-son, & Herbener, 2016) and reduced *TPJ-hippocampus* connectivity during a complex mentalizing task (Bitsch, Berger, Nagels, Falkenberg, & Straube, 2019). Taken together, this body of work indicates that aberrant functioning of these neural networks may indeed be a viable mechanism for social cognitive impairment, and this conclusion is further bolstered by growing evidence that social cognitive training leads to increased activation within social cognitive neural circuits as well as performance improvements (Campos et al., 2016).

As a final note on neurobiological correlates, a growing number of neu-roimaging studies have demonstrated that greater levels of activation within social cognitive neural networks are associated with better social behavior and functioning (e.g., Pinkham, Loughead et al., 2011) (Dodell-Feder, Tully, Lin-coln, & Hooker, 2014). Likewise, reduced functional connectivity has also been found to be related to poorer social functioning (Bjorkquist et al., 2016). These data provide a compelling argument for causal links between neural processing, social cognitive abilities, and overall functioning that will likely continue to be a focus of social cognitive research. These data also suggest that one avenue for improving social functioning in psychosis and related disorders is to improve social cognition and normalize neural functioning.

Social cognitive treatment approaches

The strong research interest in, and functional significance of, social cognition provided a springboard for the rapid development and testing of numerous treatment approaches. As it was demonstrated relatively early that antipsychotic medications do little to improve social cognitive abilities (Penn et al., 2009), the majority of interventions have adopted psychosocial techniques. Additional approaches utilizing novel pharmacological agents and neurostimulation have also been investigated, but these are less developed and the evidence for efficacy is more tenuous.

Psychosocial interventions

Existing psychosocial interventions can be generally categorized as "bottom-up" or "top-down." Bottom-up approaches focus on clearly definable social cognitive abilities, like facial emotion recognition, and attempt to improve them via traditional learning techniques such as drill and practice. These approaches are sometimes also referred to as "targeted" interventions and are thought to improve performance by strengthening the neural networks assumed to underlie these skills. Indeed, such approaches have resulted in improved performance on measures of face emotion perception (Silver, Goodman, Knoll, & Isakov, 2004), social perception (Corrigan, Hirschbeck, & Wolfe, 1995), and mentalizing (Sarfati, Passerieux, & Hardy-Baylé, 2000).

Top-down approaches, on the other hand, tend to be less intensive and more integrative, in that they focus on the application of social information processing strategies to complex stimuli and real-life social situations. Social cognitive skills training (SCST; Horan et al., 2011) and social cognition and interaction training (SCIT; Roberts, Penn, & Combs, 2015) are excellent examples of top-down approaches, and both typically use a group format in which participants evaluate social images, videos, and scenarios, as well as social interactions and relationships in their own day-to-day lives. Both SCST and SCIT also target multiple domains of social cognition and are therefore often referred to as "comprehensive" interventions. Such top-down approaches are generally considered to be insufficient for retraining very specific neural circuits, and instead, they focus on the development of compensatory cognitive strategies that may be more easily generalized to an individual's day-to-day life. A relatively recent meta-analysis examining the efficacy of comprehensive interventions found large weighted effect sizes for improvements in facial affect perception (d = 0.84, across 12 studies) and medium-to-large effect sizes for mentalizing (d = 0.70, across 13 studies). Fewer studies were available to assess efficacy for improving social perception (n = 4) and attributional bias (n = 7); however, these yielded large (d = 1.29) and small-to-medium (d = 0.30–0.52) effect sizes, respectively (Kurtz, Gagen, Rocha, Machado, & Penn, 2016).

Despite the promise of these interventions, the research in this area is still relatively new and plagued by methodological limitations that prevent strong conclusions and leave several unanswered questions. As recently reviewed by Horan and Green (2019), the majority of sample sizes are small, only a minority of studies have used randomized controlled trial designs, and the outcome measures that have been employed vary widely and largely lack psychometric validation. In addition, the majority of psychosocial treatment studies have also failed to use blinded assessment, monitor treatment fidelity, or examine the durability of treatment gains. It is hoped that more rigorous and well-powered clinical trials will continue to provide support for these intervention strategies; however, this currently remains unseen.

Pharmacological agents

Almost in parallel to the development of the psychosocial approaches discussed above, another branch of research has focused on oxytocin (OT), a neuropeptide that is linked to pro-social behavior (MacDonald & MacDonald, 2010) and that appears to increase the perceived salience of social cues (Rosenfeld,

Lieberman, & Jarskog, 2010). The majority of studies investigating the effects of oxytocin in schizophrenia have utilized intranasal administration that is either implemented as a single dose or repeatedly over several days or weeks. Initial studies reported modest improvements in social cognitive performance after acute OT administration (Davis et al., 2013) and improvements in both social cognition and symptoms after two- or three-week trials of daily OT administration (Feifel et al., 2010; Pedersen et al., 2011). Likewise, early efforts to augment psychosocial treatment approaches with OT seemed promising in that OT appeared to enhance the effectiveness of social cognitive training (Davis et al., 2014).

More recent evidence, however, has been considerably mixed, with larger, well-controlled trials failing to show an effect for oxytocin alone (Halverson, Jarskog, Pedersen, & Penn, 2019) or in conjunction with a psychosocial treatment (Strauss et al., 2019). A meta-analysis of 12 studies has suggested that OTs effects may be limited to improving higher-level social cognitive skills such as mentalizing, but the magnitude of the effect is quite small (SMD = 0.20), which calls into question its clinical relevance (Bürkner, Williams, Simmons, & Woolley, 2017). Additionally, some have also suggested that the effects of OT may vary pending important individual differences in the type of social cognitive impairment shown and that OT may actually be harmful for certain subgroups of patients. Zik and Roberts (2015) note that OT's effect of increasing the salience of social cues may be detrimental to individuals with prominent paranoia or persecutory delusions who already tend to interpret benign cues as self-relevant and threatening. Thus, while OT may be beneficial for individuals who show deficits in social cognitive ability, it may be counterproductive for those who show social cognitive bias. This important caveat regarding the use of OT, and the overall mixed findings, indicate that caution is warranted when considering OT as a treatment for social cognitive impairment, but it remains possible that OT may yet be found to be a useful and viable treatment option for some individuals.

Neurostimulation techniques

Building on the research linking social cognitive impairments to hypoactivation within social brain networks, researchers have very recently begun to investigate whether neural activity can be normalized via direct electrical stimulation and whether this results in behavioral improvements. These studies have used transcranial direct current stimulation (tDCS), which allows for noninvasive, transient excitation of neural responses via the administration of low-level electrical signals. Single and repeated tDCS to the *dorsolateral prefrontal cortex* in schizophrenia has shown positive, but modest, effects on attention and working memory (Mervis, Capizzi, Boroda, & MacDonald, 2017), and it is therefore unsurprising that this work has been expanded to social cognition. While still in its infancy, there is some room for optimism with this approach. An early pilot study reported better emotion recognition ability in participants with schizophrenia who received active stimulation of the dorsolateral prefrontal cortex relative to patients receiving sham stimulation, and in another study, stimulation of the left frontal lobe improved social cue perception in individuals with schizophrenia spectrum disorders (Schülke & Straube, 2019). Many methodological questions remain unanswered (e.g., should stimulation be repeated or is a single session sufficient for change, what is the duration of stimulation effects, which brain regions should be targeted, etc.); however, this will likely be an area of continued interest for psychosis and psychiatric disorders more broadly. Chapter 11 provides a more detailed discussion of trans-diagnostic remediation techniques.

Current challenges and areas of growth in social cognitive research

Unresolved issues and challenges within the field of social cognitive research have been emphasized throughout this chapter and include questions regarding the factor structure of social cognition in psychiatric disorders, the need for a better understanding of how neural activity and connectivity contribute to social cognitive difficulties, and the need for well-validated treatment programs. A significant issue that has not yet been discussed in detail is how social cognition is measured, although Chapters 9 and 10 provide an extensive discussion. Many of the most widely used tasks either have very limited psychometric information or show poor psychometric properties, which compromises the validity of many studies and limits treatment development and evaluation by rendering it difficult to accurately evaluate treatment response (Pinkham, Penn et al., 2014; Pinkham et al., 2016b). Unfortunately, efforts to identify psychometrically sound tasks have yielded relatively few candidate measures. The Social Cognition Psychometric Evaluation Study (SCOPE) recommended only three tasks for use in clinical trials that addressed the domains of emotion processing and mentalizing (Pinkham, Harvey, & Penn, 2018), and the Social Cognition and Functioning in Schizophrenia (SCAF) study endorsed only a single measure of empathic accuracy (Kern et al., 2013). Thus, the field is still lacking adequate measures of social perception and attributional style/bias, and as attributional style often loads on a different factor from social cognitive ability, it is critically important that a comprehensive social cognitive battery include an assessment of attributional bias.

Another related challenge is the cross-cultural validity of the existing social cognitive assessments. The vast majority of social cognitive tasks were developed in English speaking, Western cultures. It seems unlikely that these tasks would retain their same psychometric properties when administered across cultures and language, and indeed, current evidence does demonstrate that culture impacts social cognitive performance among individuals with psychosis (Pinkham, Kelsven, Kouros, Harvey, & Penn, 2017; Pinkham et al., 2008;

Wu & Keysar, 2007). However, despite a call for culturally specific assessments (Mehta, Thirthalli, Gangadhar, & Keshavan, 2011), almost no studies have investigated the potential role of cultural differences on performance or how the culture reflected within a specific social cognitive assessment may affect performance (Hajdúk, Achim, Brunet-Gouet, Mehta, & Pinkham, 2020). See Chapter 2 for a further discussion of these issues. A clear area of growth within the field is therefore to consider an international/transcultural perspective in measure development and validation and to continue to develop novel measures that will allow for the assessment of the full spectrum of social cognitive domains.

Finally, the boundaries of social cognition (i.e., the skills/abilities/biases that are prioritized within this construct) continue to represent both a challenge and a promising area for growth. As alluded to previously, empathy has yet to be fully integrated into the larger social cognitive construct; however, impairments in empathy have clear neural substrates (Vucurovic et al., 2020) that are linked to functional outcomes in psychosis (Smith et al., 2015). Thus, clarifying how empathy overlaps with, and is distinct from the other, more well-established social cognitive domains could substantially advance our understanding of social cognition (see Chapter 1). An additional area that offers significant promise for better understanding functional outcomes in psychosis is social cognitive introspective accuracy (IA), or the ability to accurately evaluate one's own social cognitive skills and abilities (Harvey & Pinkham, 2015). A growing literature demonstrates that: (1) social cognitive IA is impaired in schizophrenia (Harvey, Twamley, Pinkham, Depp, & Patterson, 2017; Pinkham, Shasteen, & Ackerman, 2019), (2) individuals with schizophrenia show reduced IA-specific neural activity in the *right rostrolateral prefrontal cortex*, a region that is critical for successful IA (Pinkham, Klein, Hardaway, Kemp, & Harvey, 2018), and (3) most importantly, social cognitive IA predicts real-world functioning above and beyond social cognitive task performance (Silberstein, Pinkham, Penn, & Harvey, 2018). Social cognitive IA therefore likely represents an important and novel target for intervention that may improve the functional significance of the social cognitive construct. The construct of IA also overlaps considerably with the notion of self-awareness and/or meta-cognition that is often described in relation to brain lesions (see Chapter 1), and so cross fertilization between fields may be particularly informative. Thus, while it is tempting to think of social cognition as clearly defined and firmly established, the field may be best served by viewing social cognition as an evolving area that is open to expansion and the integration of new concepts.

Conclusions

The study of social cognition is a vibrant and rapidly evolving area that has contributed greatly to our understanding of the social impairments that are commonly seen in psychiatric disorders. While the field still faces a number of challenges, it now seems clear that social cognitive impairments are evident in numerous disorders and that these impairments are critically related to social and vocational functioning, particularly in psychosis. Abnormal functioning and connectivity of the "social brain" is a highly viable mechanism for social cognitive impairments, and there is considerable evidence that social cognition can be improved via psychosocial interventions. Social cognition is therefore a critical area of investigation within psychiatric disorders.

References

Aakre, J. M., Seghers, J. P., St-Hilaire, A., & Docherty, N. (2009). Attributional style in delusional patients: A comparison of remitted paranoid, remitted nonparanoid, and current paranoid patients with nonpsychiatric controls. *Schizophrenia Bulletin, 35*(5), 994–1002. www.ncbi.nlm.nih.gov/entrez/query.fcgi?cmd=Retrieve&db=PubMed&dopt=Citation&list_uids=18495648

Addington, J., Saeedi, H., & Addington, D. (2006). Influence of social perception and social knowledge on cognitive and social functioning in early psychosis. *British Journal of Psychiatry, 189*, 373–378. www.ncbi.nlm.nih.gov/entrez/query.fcgi?cmd=Retrieve&db=PubMed&dopt=Citation&list_uids=17012662

Adolphs, R. (2010). What does the amygdala contribute to social cognition? *Annals of the New York Academy of Sciences, 1191*, 42–61. www.ncbi.nlm.nih.gov/entrez/query.fcgi?cmd=Retrieve&db=PubMed&dopt=Citation&list_uids=20392275

Allott, K. A., Rice, S., Bartholomeusz, C. F., Klier, C., Schlögelhofer, M., Schäfer, M. R., & Amminger, G. P. (2015). Emotion recognition in unaffected first-degree relatives of individuals with first-episode schizophrenia. *Schizophrenia Research, 161*(2), 322–328.

American Psychiatric Association (2013). *Diagnostic and Statistical Manual of Mental Disorders (DSM-5®)*. Washington, DC: American Psychiatric Pub.

Amodio, D. M., & Frith, C. D. (2006). Meeting of minds: The medial frontal cortex and social cognition. *Nature Reviews Neuroscience, 7*(4), 268–277. www.ncbi.nlm.nih.gov/entrez/query.fcgi?cmd=Retrieve&db=PubMed&dopt=Citation&list_uids=16552413

Barbato, M., Liu, L., Cadenhead, K. S., Cannon, T. D., Cornblatt, B. A., McGlashan, T. H., . . . Walker, E. F. (2015). Theory of mind, emotion recognition and social perception in individuals at clinical high risk for psychosis: Findings from the NAPLS-2 cohort. *Schizophrenia Research: Cognition, 2*(3), 133–139.

Barkl, S. J., Lah, S., Harris, A. W., & Williams, L. M. (2014). Facial emotion identification in early-onset and first-episode psychosis: A systematic review with meta-analysis. *Schizophrenia Research, 159*(1), 62–69.

Bechi, M., Bosia, M., Agostoni, G., Spangaro, M., Buonocore, M., Bianchi, L., . . . Cavallaro, R. (2018). Can patients with schizophrenia have good mentalizing skills? Disentangling heterogeneity of theory of mind. *Neuropsychology, 32*(6), 746.

Bell, M. D., Fiszdon, J. M., Greig, T. C., & Wexler, B. E. (2010). Social attribution test – multiple choice (SAT-MC) in schizophrenia: Comparison with community sample and relationship to neurocognitive, social cognitive and symptom measures. *Schizophrenia Research, 122*(1–3), 164–171.

Bigelow, N. O., Paradiso, S., Adolphs, R., Moser, D. J., Arndt, S., Heberlein, A., . . . Andreasen, N. C. (2006). Perception of socially relevant stimuli in schizophrenia.

Schizophrenia Research, *83*(2–3), 257–267. www.ncbi.nlm.nih.gov/entrez/query.fcgi?cm d=Retrieve&db=PubMed&dopt=Citation&list_uids=16497483

Bitsch, F., Berger, P., Nagels, A., Falkenberg, I., & Straube, B. (2019). Impaired right temporoparietal junction – hippocampus connectivity in schizophrenia and its relevance for generating representations of other minds. *Schizophrenia Bulletin*, *45*(4), 934–945.

Bjorkquist, O. A., Olsen, E. K., Nelson, B. D., & Herbener, E. S. (2016). Altered amygdala-prefrontal connectivity during emotion perception in schizophrenia. *Schizophrenia Research*, *175*(1–3), 35–41.

Bonfils, K. A., Lysaker, P. H., Minor, K. S., & Salyers, M. P. (2016). Affective empathy in schizophrenia: a meta-analysis. *Schizophrenia Research*, *175*(1–3), 109–117.

Bora, E., Bartholomeusz, C., & Pantelis, C. (2016). Meta-analysis of theory of mind (ToM) impairment in bipolar disorder. *Psychological Medicine*, *46*(2), 253–264.

Bora, E., & Berk, M. (2016). Theory of mind in major depressive disorder: A meta-analysis. *Journal of Affective Disorders*, *191*, 49–55.

Bora, E., & Pantelis, C. (2013). Theory of mind impairments in first-episode psychosis, individuals at ultra-high risk for psychosis and in first-degree relatives of schizophrenia: Systematic review and meta-analysis. *Schizophrenia Research*, *144*(1), 31–36.

Bora, E., & Pantelis, C. (2016). Social cognition in schizophrenia in comparison to bipolar disorder: A meta-analysis. *Schizophrenia Research*, *175*(1–3), 72–78.

Bora, E., Yucel, M., & Pantelis, C. (2009). Theory of mind impairment in schizophrenia: Meta-analysis. *Schizophrenia Research*, *109*(1–3), 1–9. www.ncbi.nlm.nih.gov/entrez/query.fcgi?cmd=Retrieve&db=PubMed&dopt=Citation&list_uids=19195844

Bora, E., & Zorlu, N. (2017). Social cognition in alcohol use disorder: A meta-analysis. *Addiction*, *112*(1), 40–48.

Bortolon, C., Capdevielle, D., & Raffard, S. (2015). Face recognition in schizophrenia disorder: A comprehensive review of behavioral, neuroimaging and neurophysiological studies. *Neuroscience & Biobehavioral Reviews*, *53*, 79–107.

Brothers, L. (1990). The social brain: A project for integrating primate behavior and neurophysiology in a new domain. *Concepts in Neuroscience*, *1*, 27–51.

Browne, J., Penn, D. L., Raykov, T., Pinkham, A. E., Kelsven, S., Buck, B., & Harvey, P. D. (2016). Social cognition in schizophrenia: Factor structure of emotion processing and theory of mind. *Psychiatry Research*, *242*, 150–156.

Brune, M., Abdel-Hamid, M., Lehmkamper, C., & Sonntag, C. (2007). Mental state attribution, neurocognitive functioning, and psychopathology: What predicts poor social competence in schizophrenia best? *Schizophrenia Research*, *92*(1–3), 151–159. www.ncbi.nlm.nih.gov/entrez/query.fcgi?cmd=Retrieve&db=PubMed&dopt=Citation&list_uids=17346931

Brunet, E., Sarfati, Y., & Hardy-Bayle, M. C. (2003). Reasoning about physical causality and other's intentions in schizophrenia. *Cognitive Neuropsychiatry*, *8*(2), 129–139. www.ncbi.nlm.nih.gov/entrez/query.fcgi?cmd=Retrieve&db=PubMed&dopt=Citation&list_uids=16571555

Buck, B. E., Browne, J., Gagen, E. C., & Penn, D. L. (2020). Hostile attribution bias in schizophrenia-spectrum disorders: Narrative review of the literature and persisting questions. *Journal of Mental Health*, 1–18.

Buck, B. E., Healey, K. M., Gagen, E. C., Roberts, D. L., & Penn, D. L. (2016). Social cognition in schizophrenia: Factor structure, clinical and functional correlates. *Journal of Mental Health*, *25*(4), 330–337.

Buck, B. E., Pinkham, A. E., Harvey, P. D., & Penn, D. L. (2016). Revisiting the validity of measures of social cognitive bias in schizophrenia: Additional results from the social cognition psychometric evaluation (SCOPE) study. *British Journal of Clinical Psychology, 55*(4), 441–454.

Bürkner, P.-C., Williams, D. R., Simmons, T. C., & Woolley, J. D. (2017). Intranasal oxytocin may improve high-level social cognition in schizophrenia, but not social cognition or neurocognition in general: A multilevel bayesian meta-analysis. *Schizophrenia Bulletin, 43*(6), 1291–1303.

Campos, C., Santos, S., Gagen, E., Machado, S., Rocha, S., Kurtz, M. M., & Rocha, N. B. (2016). Neuroplastic changes following social cognition training in schizophrenia: A systematic review. *Neuropsychology Review, 26*(3), 310–328.

Catalan, A., Angosto, V., Díaz, A., Martínez, N., Guede, D., Pereda, M., . . . Osa, L. (2018). The relationship between theory of mind deficits and neurocognition in first episode-psychosis. *Psychiatry Research, 268*, 361–367.

Chung, Y. S., Barch, D., & Strube, M. (2014). A meta-analysis of mentalizing impairments in adults with schizophrenia and autism spectrum disorder. *Schizophrenia Bulletin, 40*(3), 602–616.

Combs, D. R., Penn, D. L., Michael, C. O., Basso, M. R., Wiedeman, R., Siebenmorgan, M., . . . Chapman, D. (2009). Perceptions of hostility by persons with and without persecutory delusions. *Cognitive Neuropsychiatry, 14*(1), 30–52.

Combs, D. R., Penn, D. L., Wicher, M., & Waldheter, E. (2007a). The ambiguous intentions hostility questionnaire (AIHQ): A new measure for evaluating hostile social-cognitive biases in paranoia. *Cognitive Neuropsychiatry, 12*(2), 128–143.

Combs, D. R., Penn, D. L., Wicher, M., & Waldheter, E. (2007b). The ambiguous intentions hostility questionnaire (AIHQ): A new measure for evaluating hostile social-cognitive biases in paranoia. *Cognitive Neuropsychiatry, 12*(2), 128–143.

Comparelli, A., Corigliano, V., De Carolis, A., Mancinelli, I., Trovini, G., Ottavi, G., . . . Girardi, P. (2013). Emotion recognition impairment is present early and is stable throughout the course of schizophrenia. *Schizophrenia Research, 143*(1), 65–69.

Constantino, J. N., Przybeck, T., Friesen, D., & Todd, R. D. (2000). Reciprocal social behavior in children with and without pervasive developmental disorders. *Journal of Developmental and Behavioral Pediatrics, 21*(1), 2–11.

Corcoran, R., & Frith, C. D. (2003). Autobiographical memory and theory of mind: Evidence of a relationship in schizophrenia. *Psychological Medicine, 33*(5), 897–905. www.ncbi.nlm.nih.gov/entrez/query.fcgi?cmd=Retrieve&db=PubMed&dopt=Citation&list_uids=12877404

Corrigan, P. W., Garman, A., & Nelson, D. (1996). Situational feature recognition in schizophrenic outpatients. *Psychiatry Research, 62*(3), 251–257.

Corrigan, P. W., & Green, M. F. (1993a). Schizophrenic patients' sensitivity to social cues: The role of abstraction. *The American Journal of Psychiatry, 150*(4), 589–594. www.ncbi.nlm.nih.gov/pubmed/8465875

Corrigan, P. W., & Green, M. F. (1993b). The situational feature recognition test: A measure of schema comprehension for schizophrenia. *International Journal of Methods in Psychiatric Research, 31*(3), 29–35.

Corrigan, P. W., Hirschbeck, J. N., & Wolfe, M. (1995). Memory and vigilance training to improve social perception in schizophrenia. *Schizophrenia Research, 17*(3), 257–265.

Corrigan, P. W., & Nelson, D. R. (1998). Factors that affect social cue recognition in schizophrenia. *Psychiatry Research, 78*(3), 189–196.

Darrell-Berry, H., Bucci, S., Palmier-Claus, J., Emsley, R., Drake, R., & Berry, K. (2017). Predictors and mediators of trait anger across the psychosis continuum: The role of attachment style, paranoia and social cognition. *Psychiatry Research, 249*, 132–138.

Davis, M. C., Green, M. F., Lee, J., Horan, W. P., Senturk, D., Clarke, A. D., & Marder, S. R. (2014). Oxytocin-augmented social cognitive skills training in schizophrenia. *Neuropsychopharmacology, 39*(9), 2070.

Davis, M. C., Lee, J., Horan, W. P., Clarke, A. D., McGee, M. R., Green, M. F., & Marder, S. R. (2013). Effects of single dose intranasal oxytocin on social cognition in schizophrenia. *Schizophrenia Research, 147*(2), 393–397.

Delvecchio, G., Sugranyes, G., & Frangou, S. (2013). Evidence of diagnostic specificity in the neural correlates of facial affect processing in bipolar disorder and schizophrenia: A meta-analysis of functional imaging studies. *Psychological Medicine, 43*(03), 553–569.

de Siqueira Rotenberg, L., Beraldi, G. H., Okawa Belizario, G., & Lafer, B. (2020). Impaired social cognition in bipolar disorder: A meta-analysis of theory of mind in euthymic patients. *Australian & New Zealand Journal of Psychiatry*, 0004867420924109.

Dodell-Feder, D., Tully, L. M., Lincoln, S. H., & Hooker, C. I. (2014). The neural basis of theory of mind and its relationship to social functioning and social anhedonia in individuals with schizophrenia. *NeuroImage: Clinical, 4*, 154–163.

Etchepare, A., & Prouteau, A. (2018). Toward a two-dimensional model of social cognition in clinical neuropsychology: A systematic review of factor structure studies. *Journal of the International Neuropsychological Society: JINS, 24*(4), 391.

Feifel, D., Macdonald, K., Nguyen, A., Cobb, P., Warlan, H., Galangue, B., . . . Perry, W. (2010). Adjunctive intranasal oxytocin reduces symptoms in schizophrenia patients. *Biological Psychiatry, 68*(7), 678–680.

Fett, A.-K. J., Viechtbauer, W., Penn, D. L., van Os, J., & Krabbendam, L. (2011). The relationship between neurocognition and social cognition with functional outcomes in schizophrenia: A meta-analysis. *Neuroscience & Biobehavioral Reviews, 35*(3), 573–588.

Fretland, R. A., Andersson, S., Sundet, K., Andreassen, O. A., Melle, I., & Vaskinn, A. (2015). Theory of mind in schizophrenia: Error types and associations with symptoms. *Schizophrenia Research, 162*(1), 42–46.

Frith, C. D. (1992). *The Cognitive Neuropsychology of Schizophrenia*. London: Psychology Press.

Green, M. F., Horan, W. P., & Lee, J. (2015). Social cognition in schizophrenia. *Nature Reviews Neuroscience, 16*(10), 620–631.

Green, M. F., Penn, D. L., Bentall, R., Carpenter, W. T., Gaebel, W., Gur, R. C., . . . Heinssen, R. (2008). Social cognition in schizophrenia: An NIMH workshop on definitions, assessment, and research opportunities. *Schizophrenia Bulletin, 34*(6), 1211–1220. doi:10.1093/schbul/sbm145

Gur, R. C., & Gur, R. E. (2016). Social cognition as an RDoC domain. *American Journal of Medical Genetics Part B: Neuropsychiatric Genetics, 171*(1), 132–141.

Gur, R. E., Kohler, C. G., Ragland, J. D., Siegel, S. J., Lesko, K., Bilker, W. B., & Gur, R. C. (2006). Flat affect in schizophrenia: Relation to emotion processing and neurocognitive measures. *Schizophrenia Bulletin, 32*(2), 279–287. www.ncbi.nlm.nih.gov/entrez/query.fcgi?cmd=Retrieve&db=PubMed&dopt=Citation&list_uids=16452608

Hajdúk, M., Achim, A. M., Brunet-Gouet, E., Mehta, U. M., & Pinkham, A. E. (2020). How to move forward in social cognition research? Put it into an international perspective. *Schizophrenia Research, 215*, 463.

Hajdúk, M., Klein, H. S., Bass, E. L., Springfield, C. R., & Pinkham, A. E. (2020). Implicit and explicit processing of bodily emotions in schizophrenia. *Cognitive Neuropsychiatry*, *25*(2), 139–153.

Halverson, T. F., Jarskog, L. F., Pedersen, C., & Penn, D. (2019). Effects of oxytocin on empathy, introspective accuracy, and social symptoms in schizophrenia: A 12-week twice-daily randomized controlled trial. *Schizophrenia Research*, *204*, 178–182.

Halverson, T. F., Orleans-Pobee, M., Merritt, C., Sheeran, P., Fett, A.-K., & Penn, D. L. (2019). Pathways to functional outcomes in schizophrenia spectrum disorders: Meta-analysis of social cognitive and neurocognitive predictors. *Neuroscience & Biobehavioral Reviews*, *105*, 212–219.

Harvey, P. D., & Pinkham, A. (2015). Impaired self-assessment in schizophrenia: Why patients misjudge their cognition and functioning: Observations from caregivers and clinicians seem to have the most validity. *Current Psychiatry*, *14*(4), 53.

Harvey, P. D., Twamley, E. W., Pinkham, A. E., Depp, C. A., & Patterson, T. L. (2017). Depression in schizophrenia: Associations with cognition, functional capacity, everyday functioning, and self-assessment. *Schizophrenia Bulletin*, *43*(3), 575–582.

Horan, W. P., & Green, M. F. (2019). Treatment of social cognition in schizophrenia: Current status and future directions. *Schizophrenia Research*, *203*, 3–11.

Horan, W. P., Green, M. F., DeGroot, M., Fiske, A., Hellemann, G., Kee, K., . . . Subotnik, K. L. (2012). Social cognition in schizophrenia, part 2: 12-month stability and prediction of functional outcome in first-episode patients. *Schizophrenia Bulletin*, *38*(4), 865–872.

Horan, W. P., Kern, R. S., Tripp, C., Hellemann, G., Wynn, J. K., Bell, M., . . . Green, M. F. (2011). Efficacy and specificity of social cognitive skills training for outpatients with psychotic disorders. *Journal of Psychiatric Research*, *45*(8), 1113–1122.

Janssen, I., Versmissen, D., Campo, J. A., Myin-Germeys, I., Van Os, J., & Krabbendam, L. (2006). Attribution style and psychosis: Evidence for an externalizing bias in patients but not individuals at high risk. *Psychological Medicine*, *36*, 771–778.

Kelemen, O., Erdelyi, R., Pataki, I., Benedek, G., Janka, Z., & Keri, S. (2005). Theory of mind and motion perception in schizophrenia. *Neuropsychology*, *19*(4), 494–500. www.ncbi.nlm.nih.gov/entrez/query.fcgi?cmd=Retrieve&db=PubMed&dopt=Citation&list_uids=16060824

Kennedy, D. P., & Adolphs, R. (2012). The social brain in psychiatric and neurological disorders. *Trends in Cognitive Sciences*, *16*(11), 559–572.

Kern, R. S., Penn, D. L., Lee, J., Horan, W. P., Reise, S. P., Ochsner, K. N., . . . Green, M. F. (2013). Adapting social neuroscience measures for schizophrenia clinical trials, part 2: Trolling the depths of psychometric properties. *Schizophrenia Bulletin*, *39*(6), 1201–1210. doi:10.1093/schbul/sbt127

Kimhy, D., Vakhrusheva, J., Jobson-Ahmed, L., Tarrier, N., Malaspina, D., & Gross, J. J. (2012). Emotion awareness and regulation in individuals with schizophrenia: Implications for social functioning. *Psychiatry Research*, *200*(2), 193–201.

Kington, J. M., Jones, L. A., Watt, A. A., Hopkin, E. J., & Williams, J. (2000). Impaired eye expression recognition in schizophrenia. *Journal of Psychiatric Research*, *34*(4–5), 341–347. www.ncbi.nlm.nih.gov/entrez/query.fcgi?cmd=Retrieve&db=PubMed&dopt=Citation&list_uids=11104848

Kohler, C. G., Richard, J. A., Brensinger, C. M., Borgmann-Winter, K. E., Conroy, C. G., Moberg, P. J., . . . Calkins, M. E. (2014). Facial emotion perception differs in young persons at genetic and clinical high-risk for psychosis. *Psychiatry Research*, *216*(2), 206–212.

Kohler, C. G., Turner, T. H., Bilker, W. B., Brensinger, C. M., Siegel, S. J., Kanes, S. J., . . . Gur, R. C. (2003). Facial emotion recognition in schizophrenia: Intensity effects and error pattern. *The American Journal of Psychiatry*, *160*(10), 1768–1774. www.ncbi.nlm.nih.gov/entrez/query.fcgi?cmd=Retrieve&db=PubMed&dopt=Citation&list_uids=14514489

Kohler, C. G., Walker, J. B., Martin, E. A., Healey, K. M., & Moberg, P. J. (2010). Facial emotion perception in schizophrenia: A meta-analytic review. *Schizophrenia Bulletin*, *36*(5), 1009–1019. www.ncbi.nlm.nih.gov/entrez/query.fcgi?cmd=Retrieve&db=PubMed&dopt=Citation&list_uids=19329561

Kosmidis, M. H., Bozikas, V. P., Giannakou, M., Anezoulaki, D., Fantie, B. D., & Karavatos, A. (2007). Impaired emotion perception in schizophrenia: A differential deficit. *Psychiatry Research*, *149*(1–3), 279–284.

Kring, A. M., Siegel, E. H., & Barrett, L. F. (2014). Unseen affective faces influence person perception judgments in schizophrenia. *Clinical Psychological Science*, *2*(4), 443–454. doi:10.1177/2167702614536161

Kronbichler, L., Tschernegg, M., Martin, A. I., Schurz, M., & Kronbichler, M. (2017). Abnormal brain activation during theory of mind tasks in schizophrenia: A meta-analysis. *Schizophrenia Bulletin*, *43*(6), 1240–1250.

Kurtz, M. M., Gagen, E., Rocha, N. B., Machado, S., & Penn, D. L. (2016). Comprehensive treatments for social cognitive deficits in schizophrenia: A critical review and effect-size analysis of controlled studies. *Clinical Psychology Review*, *43*, 80–89.

Langdon, R., Ward, P. B., & Coltheart, M. (2010). Reasoning anomalies associated with delusions in schizophrenia. *Schizophrenia Bulletin*, *36*(2), 321–330. www.ncbi.nlm.nih.gov/entrez/query.fcgi?cmd=Retrieve&db=PubMed&dopt=Citation&list_uids=18622010

Lavoie, M.-A., Battaglia, M., & Achim, A. M. (2014). A meta-analysis and scoping review of social cognition performance in social phobia, posttraumatic stress disorder and other anxiety disorders. *Journal of Anxiety Disorders*, *28*(2), 169–177.

Lee, P., & Van Meter, A. (2020). Emotional body language: Social cognition deficits in bipolar disorder. *Journal of Affective Disorders*, *272*, 231–238.

Lin, Y. C., Ding, H., & Zhang, Y. (2018). Emotional prosody processing in schizophrenic patients: A selective review and meta-analysis. *Journal of Clinical Medicine*, *7*(10), 363.

Lin, Y. C., Wynn, J. K., Hellemann, G., & Green, M. F. (2012). Factor structure of emotional intelligence in schizophrenia. *Schizophrenia Research*, *139*(1–3), 78–81. doi:10.1016/j.schres.2012.04.013

Lysaker, P. H., Dimaggio, G., Carcione, A., Procacci, M., Buck, K. D., Davis, L. W., & Nicolò, G. (2010). Metacognition and schizophrenia: The capacity for self-reflectivity as a predictor for prospective assessments of work performance over six months. *Schizophrenia Research*, *122*(1–3), 124–130.

MacDonald, K., & MacDonald, T. M. (2010). The peptide that binds: A systematic review of oxytocin and its prosocial effects in humans. *Harvard Review of Psychiatry*, *18*(1), 1–21.

Mancuso, F., Horan, W. P., Kern, R. S., & Green, M. F. (2011). Social cognition in psychosis: Multidimensional structure, clinical correlates, and relationship with functional outcome. *Schizophrenia Research*, *125*(2–3), 143–151. doi:10.1016/j.schres.2010.11.007

Marjoram, D., Gardner, C., Burns, J., Miller, P., Lawrie, S. M., & Johnstone, E. C. (2005). Symptomatology and social inference: A theory of mind study of schizophrenia and psychotic affective disorder. *Cognitive Neuropsychiatry*, *10*(5), 347–359. www.ncbi.nlm.nih.gov/entrez/query.fcgi?cmd=Retrieve&db=PubMed&dopt=Citation&list_uids=16571466

Martino, D. J., Bucay, D., Butman, J. T., & Allegri, R. F. (2007). Neuropsychological frontal impairments and negative symptoms in schizophrenia. *Psychiatry Research, 152*(2–3), 121–128. www.ncbi.nlm.nih.gov/entrez/query.fcgi?cmd=Retrieve&db=PubMed&dopt=Citation&list_uids=17507100

Mehl, S., Landsberg, M. W., Schmidt, A.-C., Cabanis, M., Bechdolf, A., Herrlich, J., . . . Klingberg, S. (2014). Why do bad things happen to me? Attributional style, depressed mood, and persecutory delusions in patients with schizophrenia. *Schizophrenia Bulletin, 40*(6), 1338–1346.

Mehta, U. M., Thirthalli, J., Gangadhar, B. N., & Keshavan, M. S. (2011). Need for culture specific tools to assess social cognition in schizophrenia. *Schizophrenia Research, 133*(1–3), 255.

Mervis, J. E., Capizzi, R. J., Boroda, E., & MacDonald III, A. W. (2017). Transcranial direct current stimulation over the dorsolateral prefrontal cortex in schizophrenia: A quantitative review of cognitive outcomes. *Frontiers in Human Neuroscience, 11*, 44.

Montag, C., Dziobek, I., Richter, I. S., Neuhaus, K., Lehmann, A., Sylla, R., . . . Gallinat, J. (2011). Different aspects of theory of mind in paranoid schizophrenia: Evidence from a video-based assessment. *Psychiatry Research, 186*(2), 203–209.

Moritz, S., & Lysaker, P. H. (2018). Metacognition – what did James H. Flavell really say and the implications for the conceptualization and design of metacognitive interventions. *Schizophrenia Research, 201*, 20–26.

Okruszek, Ł., & Pilecka, I. (2017). Biological motion processing in schizophrenia – systematic review and meta-analysis. *Schizophrenia Research, 190*, 3–10.

Pedersen, C. A., Gibson, C. M., Rau, S. W., Salimi, K., Smedley, K. L., Casey, R. L., . . . Penn, D. L. (2011). Intranasal oxytocin reduces psychotic symptoms and improves theory of mind and social perception in schizophrenia. *Schizophrenia Research, 132*(1), 50–53.

Penn, D. L., Addington, J., & Pinkham, A. (2006). Social cognitive impairments. In J. A. Lieberman, T. S. Stroup, & D. O. Perkins (Eds.), *A Textbook of Schizophrenia*. Washington: American Psychiatry Press.

Penn, D. L., Keefe, R. S., Davis, S. M., Meyer, P. S., Perkins, D. O., Losardo, D., & Lieberman, J. A. (2009). The effects of antipsychotic medications on emotion perception in patients with chronic schizophrenia in the CATIE trial. *Schizophrenia Research, 115*(1), 17–23.

Penn, D. L., Ritchie, M., Francis, J., Combs, D., & Martin, J. (2002). Social perception in schizophrenia: The role of context. *Psychiatry Research, 109*(2), 149–159. www.ncbi.nlm.nih.gov/pubmed/11927140

Perry, Y., Henry, J. D., & Grisham, J. R. (2011). The habitual use of emotion regulation strategies in schizophrenia. *British Journal of Clinical Psychology, 50*(2), 217–222.

Pickup, G. J., & Frith, C. D. (2001). Theory of mind impairments in schizophrenia: Symptomatology, severity and specificity. *Psychological Medicine, 31*(2), 207–220. www.ncbi.nlm.nih.gov/entrez/query.fcgi?cmd=Retrieve&db=PubMed&dopt=Citation&list_uids=11232909

Pinkham, A. E., Brensinger, C., Kohler, C., Gur, R. E., & Gur, R. C. (2011). Actively paranoid patients with schizophrenia over attribute anger to neutral faces. *Schizophrenia Research, 125*(2–3), 174–178. www.ncbi.nlm.nih.gov/entrez/query.fcgi?cmd=Retrieve&db=PubMed&dopt=Citation&list_uids=21112186

Pinkham, A. E., Gur, R. E., & Gur, R. C. (2007). Affect recognition deficits in schizophrenia: Neural substrates and psychopharmacological implications. *Expert Review of*

Neurotherapeutics, 7(7), 807–816. www.ncbi.nlm.nih.gov/entrez/query.fcgi?cmd=Retrie ve&db=PubMed&dopt=Citation&list_uids=17610388

Pinkham, A. E., Harvey, P. D., & Penn, D. L. (2016a). Paranoid individuals with schizophrenia show greater social cognitive bias and worse social functioning than non-paranoid individuals with schizophrenia. *Schizophrenia Research: Cognition, 3*, 33–38.

Pinkham, A. E., Harvey, P. D., & Penn, D. L. (2018). Social cognition psychometric evaluation: Results of the final validation study. *Schizophrenia Bulletin, 44*(4), 737–748.

Pinkham, A. E., Kelsven, S., Kouros, C., Harvey, P. D., & Penn, D. L. (2017). The effect of age, race, and sex on social cognitive performance in individuals with schizophrenia. *The Journal of Nervous and Mental Disease, 205*(5), 346.

Pinkham, A. E., Klein, H. S., Hardaway, G. B., Kemp, K. C., & Harvey, P. D. (2018). Neural correlates of social cognitive introspective accuracy in schizophrenia. *Schizophrenia Research, 202*, 166–172.

Pinkham, A. E., Loughead, J., Ruparel, K., Overton, E., Gur, R. E., & Gur, R. C. (2011). Abnormal modulation of amygdala activity in schizophrenia in response to direct-and averted-gaze threat-related facial expressions. *American Journal of Psychiatry, 168*(3), 293–301.

Pinkham, A. E., & Penn, D. L. (2006). Neurocognitive and social cognitive predictors of interpersonal skill in schizophrenia. *Psychiatry Research, 143*(2–3), 167–178. www.ncbi.nlm.nih.gov/entrez/query.fcgi?cmd=Retrieve&db=PubMed&dopt=Citation&list_uids=16859754

Pinkham, A. E., Penn, D. L., Green, M. F., Buck, B., Healey, K., & Harvey, P. D. (2014). The social cognition psychometric evaluation study: Results of the expert survey and RAND panel. *Schizophrenia Bulletin, 40*(4), 813–823. doi:10.1093/schbul/sbt081

Pinkham, A. E., Penn, D. L., Green, M. F., & Harvey, P. D. (2016b). Social cognition psychometric evaluation: Results of the initial psychometric study. *Schizophrenia Bulletin, 42*(2), 494–504. doi:10.1093/schbul/sbv056

Pinkham, A. E., Sasson, N. J., Calkins, M. E., Richard, J., Hughett, P., Gur, R. E., & Gur, R. C. (2008). The other-race effect in face processing among African American and Caucasian individuals with schizophrenia. *American Journal of Psychiatry, 165*(5), 639–645.

Pinkham, A. E., Sasson, N. J., Kelsven, S., Simpson, C. E., Healey, K., & Kohler, C. (2014). An intact threat superiority effect for nonsocial but not social stimuli in schizophrenia. *Journal of Abnormal Psychology, 123*(1), 168.

Pinkham, A. E., Shasteen, J. R., & Ackerman, R. A. (2019). Metaperception of personality in schizophrenia. *Journal of Experimental Psychopathology, 10*(2), 2043808719840915.

Piskulic, D., Liu, L., Cadenhead, K. S., Cannon, T. D., Cornblatt, B. A., McGlashan, T. H., . . . Walker, E. F. (2016). Social cognition over time in individuals at clinical high risk for psychosis: Findings from the NAPLS-2 cohort. *Schizophrenia Research, 171*(1), 176–181.

Roberts, D. L., Penn, D. L., & Combs, D. R. (2015). *Social Cognition and Interaction Training (SCIT): Group Psychotherapy for Schizophrenia and other Psychotic Disorders, Clinician Guide.* Oxford: Oxford University Press.

Rosenfeld, A. J., Lieberman, J. A., & Jarskog, L. F. (2010). Oxytocin, dopamine, and the amygdala: A neurofunctional model of social cognitive deficits in schizophrenia. *Schizophrenia Bulletin, 37*(5), 1077–1087.

Rosenthal, R., DePaulo, B. M., & Jall, J. A. (1979). *The PONS Test Manual: Profile of Nonverbal Sensitivity.* Irvington Pub.

Ruocco, A. C., Reilly, J. L., Rubin, L. H., Daros, A. R., Gershon, E. S., Tamminga, C. A., . . . Sweeney, J. A. (2014). Emotion recognition deficits in schizophrenia-spectrum disorders and psychotic bipolar disorder: Findings from the bipolar-schizophrenia network on intermediate phenotypes (B-SNIP) study. *Schizophrenia Research*, *158*(1–3), 105–112. doi:10.1016/j.schres.2014.07.001

Sachs, G., Steger-Wuchse, D., Kryspin-Exner, I., Gur, R. C., & Katschnig, H. (2004). Facial recognition deficits and cognition in schizophrenia. *Schizophrenia Research*, *68*(1), 27–35. www.ncbi.nlm.nih.gov/entrez/query.fcgi?cmd=Retrieve&db=PubMed&dopt=Citation &list_uids=15037337

Sarfati, Y., Hardy-Bayle, M. C., Besche, C., & Widlocher, D. (1997). Attribution of intentions to others in people with schizophrenia: A non-verbal exploration with comic strips. *Schizophrenia Research*, *25*(3), 199–209. www.ncbi.nlm.nih.gov/entrez/query.fcgi?cmd= Retrieve&db=PubMed&dopt=Citation&list_uids=9264175

Sarfati, Y., Passerieux, C., & Hardy-Baylé, M.-C. (2000). Can verbalization remedy the theory of mind deficit in schizophrenia? *Psychopathology*, *33*(5), 246–251.

Sasson, N. J., Pinkham, A. E., Carpenter, K. L., & Belger, A. (2011). The benefit of directly comparing autism and schizophrenia for revealing mechanisms of social cognitive impairment. *Journal of Neurodevelopmental Disorders*, *3*(2), 87–100.

Sasson, N. J., Pinkham, A. E., Weittenhiller, L. P., Faso, D. J., & Simpson, C. (2016). Context effects on facial affect recognition in schizophrenia and autism: Behavioral and eye-tracking evidence. *Schizophrenia Bulletin*, *42*(3), 675–683. doi:10.1093/schbul/sbv176

Sasson, N. J., Tsuchiya, N., Hurley, R., Couture, S. M., Penn, D. L., Adolphs, R., & Piven, J. (2007). Orienting to social stimuli differentiates social cognitive impairment in autism and schizophrenia. *Neuropsychologia*, *45*(11), 2580–2588. www.ncbi.nlm.nih.gov/entrez/ query.fcgi?cmd=Retrieve&db=PubMed&dopt=Citation&list_uids=17459428

Savla, G. N., Vella, L., Armstrong, C. C., Penn, D. L., & Twamley, E. W. (2013). Deficits in domains of social cognition in schizophrenia: A meta-analysis of the empirical evidence. *Schizophrenia Bulletin*, *39*(5), 979–992. doi:10.1093/schbul/sbs080

Saxe, R. (2006). Uniquely human social cognition. *Current Opinion in Neurobiology*, *16*(2), 235–239. www.ncbi.nlm.nih.gov/entrez/query.fcgi?cmd=Retrieve&db=PubMed&dopt =Citation&list_uids=16546372

Schülke, R., & Straube, B. (2019). Transcranial direct current stimulation improves semantic speech – gesture matching in patients with schizophrenia spectrum disorder. *Schizophrenia Bulletin*, *45*(3), 522–530.

Sellers, R., Varese, F., Wells, A., & Morrison, A. P. (2017). A meta-analysis of metacognitive beliefs as implicated in the self-regulatory executive function model in clinical psychosis. *Schizophrenia Research*, *179*, 75–84.

Sergi, M. J., Fiske, A. P., Horan, W. P., Kern, R. S., Kee, K. S., Subotnik, K. L., . . . Green, M. F. (2009). Development of a measure of relationship perception in schizophrenia. *Psychiatry Research*, *166*(1), 54–62.

Sergi, M. J., & Green, M. F. (2003). Social perception and early visual processing in schizophrenia. *Schizophrenia Research*, *59*(2–3), 233–241. www.ncbi.nlm.nih.gov/ pubmed/12414080

Sergi, M. J., Rassovsky, Y., Widmark, C., Reist, C., Erhart, S., Braff, D. L., . . . Green, M. F. (2007). Social cognition in schizophrenia: Relationships with neurocognition and negative symptoms. *Schizophrenia Research*, *90*(1–3), 316–324. www.ncbi.nlm.nih.gov/entrez/ query.fcgi?cmd=Retrieve&db=PubMed&dopt=Citation&list_uids=17141477

Shamay-Tsoory, S. G. (2011). The neural bases for empathy. *Neuroscientist, 17*(1), 18–24. doi:10.1177/1073858410379268

Shasteen, J. R., Pinkham, A. E., Kelsven, S., Ludwig, K., Payne, B. K., & Penn, D. L. (2016). Intact implicit processing of facial threat cues in schizophrenia. *Schizophrenia Research, 170*(1), 150–155. doi:10.1016/j.schres.2015.11.029

Silberstein, J. M., Pinkham, A. E., Penn, D. L., & Harvey, P. D. (2018). Self-assessment of social cognitive ability in schizophrenia: Association with social cognitive test performance, informant assessments of social cognitive ability, and everyday outcomes. *Schizophrenia research, 199*, 75–82.

Silver, H., Goodman, C., Knoll, G., & Isakov, V. (2004). Brief emotion training improves recognition of facial emotions in chronic schizophrenia. A pilot study. *Psychiatry research, 128*(2), 147–154.

Simpson, C., Pinkham, A. E., Kelsven, S., & Sasson, N. J. (2013). Emotion recognition abilities across stimulus modalities in schizophrenia and the role of visual attention. *Schizophrenia Research, 151*(1–3), 102–106. doi:10.1016/j.schres.2013.09.026

Smith, M. J., Schroeder, M. P., Abram, S. V., Goldman, M. B., Parrish, T. B., Wang, X., . . . Reilly, J. L. (2015). Alterations in brain activation during cognitive empathy are related to social functioning in schizophrenia. *Schizophrenia Bulletin, 41*(1), 211–222.

Sprong, M., Schothorst, P., Vos, E., Hox, J., & van Engeland, H. (2007). Theory of mind in schizophrenia: Meta-analysis. *British Journal of Psychiatry, 191*, 5–13. www.ncbi.nlm.nih.gov/entrez/query.fcgi?cmd=Retrieve&db=PubMed&dopt=Citation&list_uids=17602119

Stanley, D. A., & Adolphs, R. (2013). Toward a neural basis for social behavior. *Neuron, 80*(3), 816–826.

Strauss, G. P., Granholm, E., Holden, J. L., Ruiz, I., Gold, J. M., Kelly, D. L., & Buchanan, R. W. (2019). The effects of combined oxytocin and cognitive behavioral social skills training on social cognition in schizophrenia. *Psychological Medicine, 49*(10), 1731–1739.

Taylor, S. F., Kang, J., Brege, I. S., Tso, I. F., Hosanagar, A., & Johnson, T. D. (2012). Meta-analysis of functional neuroimaging studies of emotion perception and experience in schizophrenia. *Biological Psychiatry, 71*(2), 136–145.

Thibaudeau, É., Achim, A. M., Parent, C., Turcotte, M., & Cellard, C. (2020). A meta-analysis of the associations between theory of mind and neurocognition in schizophrenia. *Schizophrenia Research, 216*, 118–128.

Toomey, R., Schuldberg, D., Corrigan, P., & Green, M. F. (2002). Nonverbal social perception and symptomatology in schizophrenia. *Schizophrenia Research, 53*(1–2), 83–91. www.ncbi.nlm.nih.gov/pubmed/11728841

Van Hooren, S., Versmissen, D., Janssen, I., Myin-Germeys, I., à Campo, J., Mengelers, R., . . . Krabbendam, L. (2008). Social cognition and neurocognition as independent domains in psychosis. *Schizophrenia Research, 103*(1–3), 257–265.

Ventura, J., Wood, R. C., & Hellemann, G. S. (2011). Symptom domains and neurocognitive functioning can help differentiate social cognitive processes in schizophrenia: A meta-analysis. *Schizophrenia Bulletin.* www.ncbi.nlm.nih.gov/entrez/query.fcgi?cmd=Retrieve&db=PubMed&dopt=Citation&list_uids=21765165

Ventura, J., Wood, R. C., Jimenez, A. M., & Hellemann, G. S. (2013). Neurocognition and symptoms identify links between facial recognition and emotion processing in schizophrenia: Meta-analytic findings. *Schizophrenia Research, 151*(1–3), 78–84. doi:10.1016/j.schres.2013.10.015

Vucurovic, K., Caillies, S., & Kaladjian, A. (2020). Neural correlates of theory of mind and empathy in schizophrenia: An activation likelihood estimation meta-analysis. *Journal of Psychiatric Research, 120,* 163–174.

Walss-Bass, C., Fernandes, J. M., Roberts, D. L., Service, H., & Velligan, D. (2013). Differential correlations between plasma oxytocin and social cognitive capacity and bias in schizophrenia. *Schizophrenia Research, 147*(2–3), 387–392.

World Health Organization. (2018). *International Classification of Diseases for Mortality and Morbidity Statistics* (11th Rev.). https://icd.who.int/browse11/l-m/en

Wu, S., & Keysar, B. (2007). The effect of culture on perspective taking. *Psychological Science, 18*(7), 600–606.

Zik, J. B., & Roberts, D. L. (2015). The many faces of oxytocin: Implications for psychiatry. *Psychiatry Research, 226*(1), 31–37.

Chapter 7

Social cognition in dementia syndromes

Stephanie Wong and Fiona Kumfor

Dementia is an umbrella term used to describe various conditions which are characterised by progressive cognitive decline. While decline in memory is often emphasised, several dementia subtypes are characterised by changes in social cognition, either early in the disease process or with disease progression. The extent that social cognition is affected in dementia is variable and depends on the pattern of atrophy and disease stage. This chapter considers some of the most common dementia syndromes, with a particular focus on those characterised by social cognition impairment. First, we focus on subtypes of frontotemporal dementia; a group of dementia syndromes where social cognition is affected early in the disease course and is increasingly recognised as central to the clinical profile. Then we turn to Alzheimer's disease, which is the most common dementia syndrome. Finally, we consider atypical, frontal presentations of Alzheimer's disease where social cognition tends to be affected early in the disease stage. For each syndrome, we outline the typical clinical features and describe current knowledge about the social cognition profile of each dementia subtype.

Frontotemporal dementia

Frontotemporal dementia refers to a group of dementia syndromes associated with atrophy of the frontal and/or temporal lobes. Onset of symptoms of frontotemporal dementia typically occurs at a younger age than for Alzheimer's disease (i.e., < 65 years of age), with frontotemporal dementia accounting for around the same number of cases as Alzheimer's disease in people under age 65 years (Coyle-Gilchrist et al., 2016; Harvey, 2003; Mercy, Hodges, Dawson, Barker, & Brayne, 2008; Ratnavalli, Brayne, Dawson, & Hodges, 2002). Three main clinical variants of frontotemporal dementia are recognised: the behavioural variant, and two language variants, termed semantic dementia and progressive nonfluent aphasia. Each clinical variant is characterised by distinct profiles of cognitive and behavioural symptoms and patterns of brain atrophy (Gorno-Tempini et al., 2011; Rascovsky et al., 2011).

DOI: 10.4324/9781003027034-7

Behavioural variant frontotemporal dementia

Patients with behavioural variant frontotemporal dementia (bvFTD) present with predominant changes in social behaviour and personal conduct (see Box 7.1). Hallmark clinical features of this dementia syndrome include disinhibition, apathy, motor and verbal stereotypies, altered eating habits, loss of empathy and emotional blunting. Insight into the presence and severity of these symptoms is also often impaired (Mendez & Shapira, 2011; Muñoz-Neira, Tedde, Coulthard, Thai, & Pennington, 2019). In terms of cognition, current diagnostic criteria for bvFTD mandate a primarily dysexecutive profile, with relative sparing of episodic memory and visuospatial functions (Rascovsky et al., 2011). The diagnostic utility of this criterion has been questioned, however, in light of evidence that executive dysfunction is not specific to bvFTD (Harciarek & Cosentino, 2013) and that episodic memory is indeed impaired in these patients (Hornberger, Piguet, Graham, Nestor, & Hodges, 2010). As such, increasing emphasis is placed on the characterisation of other cognitive deficits in the neuropsychological profile of bvFTD, particularly impairments in social cognition. This is because tests of social cognition are sensitive to early deficits in bvFTD, especially in comparison to traditional measures of executive dysfunction that are commonly used in the clinic (Funkiewiez, Bertoux, de Souza, Levy, & Dubois, 2012; Torralva, Roca, Gleichgerrcht, Bekinschtein, & Manes, 2009). See Box 7.1 for a case study of an individual with bvFTD.

From the earliest disease stage, patients with bvFTD show atrophy in a network of *frontal* (*orbitofrontal, dorsolateral* and *ventromedial prefrontal* and *frontopolar cortices*) and *paralimbic* (*anterior cingulate* and *insular cortices*) regions, together with the *hippocampus, striatum* and *thalamus* (Schroeter, Stein, Maslowski, & Neumann, 2009; Seeley et al., 2008). Atrophy in these frontal-paralimbic regions continues to spread over time, encroaching into the *basal ganglia, subcortical limbic regions* and the *parietal cortex* (Landin-Romero et al., 2017; Seeley et al., 2008). Degeneration of white matter tracts has also been documented, with those tracts connecting the frontal and temporal regions particularly affected (Frings et al., 2014; Lam, Halliday, Irish, Hodges, & Piguet, 2013; Whitwell et al., 2010).

Box 7.1 Case 1: Mr K: Adult with behavioural variant frontotemporal dementia

History:

Mr K is a 56-year-old man, who completed 15 years of formal education and worked as an accountant for 33 years before taking early retirement two years ago.

Presentation:

On interview, Mr K presented as a friendly and garrulous man. His spontaneous speech was fluent and there were no obvious phonological or syntactical errors, though he tended to be tangential and repeated certain 'catch-phrases'. He self-reported problems with short-term memory and word-finding difficulties. He denied any changes in his behaviour or social interactions.

In contrast, his wife described a five-year history of changes in personality and behaviour. In the 18 months leading up to his retirement, his colleagues had raised concerns regarding his poor organisation and increasingly inappropriate behaviour at work. He frequently mislaid paperwork, missed deadlines, talked over others during conversations and bragged about his sexual exploits. He had previously been a tidy, efficient, polite and reserved man. According to his wife, Mr K showed increasing tactlessness and reduced empathy and awareness for others. He used crude language in front of his grandchildren. He was very gullible and signed up for an online dating website. Over a period of 12 months, he paid increasing sums of money to access online chat services. He bragged that he had formed a relationship with a woman and that he was leaving his wife to live with his new girlfriend. On several occasions, he packed his bags and drove more than five hours to meet his new girlfriend, but nobody showed up. He did not tell anyone where he was going and did not appear to be concerned about the distress he had caused his family. Mr K's wife and son discovered that the website was a scam and attempted to reason with him, but he refused to believe them. Mr K's son has enduring power of attorney and placed daily limits on his credit card. However, Mr K continued to spend money on the dating website to chat to women. In the past six months, his wife noticed declines in personal hygiene and table manners, as well as an increased preference for sweet foods. He also became increasingly rigid and insisted on following his preferred daily routine.

Testing:

On cognitive testing, he scored 73/100 on the Addenbrooke's Cognitive Examination, 3rd Edition (ACE-III), losing most points on verbal fluency, but also across the areas of attention, memory and language. On formal neuropsychological assessment, he showed mild reductions in working memory and impaired executive functioning. On memory tests, he showed poor recall of verbal and non-verbal information, and endorsed a high number of false positives on recognition tests. Confrontation naming, word repetition and comprehension were within normal limits. He scored poorly on a static facial emotion recognition test (28/42) and on Part 1 of TASIT (16/28). An informant-report version of the Cambridge Behavioural Inventory indicated difficulties in self-care, abnormal behaviour (including socially inappropriate and impulsive behaviour), bizarre beliefs, changes in eating habits, apathy and stereotypic behaviours.

On neurological examination, Mr K did not show any evidence of apraxia, Parkinsonism, gait disorder, postural instability, disordered eye movement or other motor or frontal release signs. His MRI scan revealed bilateral frontal atrophy with relative preservation of medial temporal and parietal regions.

Summary and comment:

Mr K's presentation is consistent with bvFTD. His symptoms have been present for at least five years, and his MRI revealed bilateral frontal atrophy. The earliest reported symptoms involve striking changes in personality, behaviour and social comportment. In addition, he presents with reduced empathy, verbal stereotypies, altered eating habits and executive dysfunction. As patients with bvFTD often show limited insight, collateral information gained from clinical observations, interviews with family members and informant-rated measures of behaviour are crucial in correctly diagnosing bvFTD.

Emotion perception

Impairments in emotion recognition are well documented in bvFTD. Difficulties in perceiving and recognising these social-emotional cues are thought to at least partially account for the overt emotional changes and socially-inappropriate behaviour seen in this patient group (Kumfor et al., 2012; Lavenu et al., 2005; Lavenu et al., 1999). The majority of studies to date have focused on emotion recognition from facial stimuli, with bvFTD patients showing deficits in facial recognition accuracy for negative emotions (e.g., anger, fear, sadness and disgust) relative to positive emotions (e.g., happiness, surprise) (Fernandez-Duque et al., 2005; Kipps et al., 2009; Kumfor et al., 2013). On the other hand, some studies suggest that recognition deficits extend beyond negative emotions to include positive emotions as well (Hutchings et al., 2018; Rosen et al., 2004). A meta-analysis of facial emotion recognition performance in bvFTD confirmed widespread impairments, though the most severe deficits were for negative emotions, particularly anger and disgust, while milder deficits in recognition of positive emotions (e.g., happiness) were also evident (Bora et al., 2016). Given that emotion recognition tests typically overrepresent negative compared to positive emotions, however, it is possible that this negative–positive distinction reflects a methodological artefact (see also Chapter 1), rather than a specific deficit in recognising negative emotions per se.

Deficits in emotion recognition appear to be especially pronounced for more subtle facial emotional expressions. In particular, studies using morphed facial expressions that manipulate emotion intensity show greater impairment for emotions at lower intensity levels (Jiskoot et al., 2020; Kumfor et al., 2011). Given that some bvFTD patients show slight improvements in recognition accuracy for emotional expressions presented at higher intensities, it is possible that increasing the salience of certain facial features (i.e., by exaggerating the eyebrows or mouth) may help improve facial emotion recognition (Kumfor et al., 2011). This also suggests that emotion recognition deficits in bvFTD may be partly due to inattention or perceptual difficulties.

Breakdown in the brain's face processing network likely also contributes to the social and emotional impairments in bvFTD (Hutchings et al., 2017). Abnormal visual scanning of facial stimuli and reduced fixation to the eyes has been documented across a range of other clinical disorders that are characterised by social dysfunction (e.g., autism, schizophrenia and other focal anterior brain lesions) and appears to contribute to emotion recognition deficits in these syndromes (Sasson et al., 2007; Spezio et al., 2006; Wolf et al., 2014). In bvFTD, one study employed eye-tracking to record visual scanning patterns. Surprisingly, bvFTD patients showed increased, rather than decreased, fixations to the eye region of static facial stimuli (Hutchings et al., 2018). Importantly, bvFTD patients' gaze patterns were modulated by emotional content (i.e., more fixations to the eyes of fearful compared to happy faces), but these abnormal fixation patterns were not associated with greater emotion recognition performance (as was the case in controls). The authors reasoned that the automatic visual mechanisms to 'look in the right place' appeared to be intact, but patients were unable to efficiently utilise this information in order to interpret and respond to emotional cues (Hutchings et al., 2018).

A small number of studies have investigated auditory emotion recognition in bvFTD. In a study contrasting emotion recognition accuracy for positive (e.g., cheering for happiness) and negative (e.g., retching for disgust) non-verbal vocalisations, patients showed impaired performance irrespective of valence (Hsieh et al., 2013a). In another study that examined subjective affective ratings (i.e., 'How pleasant was the sound?') and pupillary responses to 'negative' (e.g., a person spitting, a mosquito), 'neutral' (e.g., telephone, throat clearing), and 'positive' (e.g., baby laughing, stream burbling) sounds, bvFTD patients showed subjective ratings of pleasantness that varied appropriately according to emotional valence, and were in-line with controls (Fletcher et al., 2015). Unlike controls, however, pupillary responses in bvFTD were not modulated in accordance with emotional valence, suggesting reduced physiological reactivity to emotionally salient auditory stimuli.

Nonetheless, accurate social and emotional perception and recognition in everyday life requires the integration of information across multiple modalities. While the majority of research in bvFTD has employed tests that assess a single modality (e.g., pictures of faces, audio recordings), performance on these tasks may not necessarily reflect behaviour in real life (Ibáñez et al., 2012). As such, research approaches that incorporate contextual information and multiple modalities are increasingly favoured. Contextual information, such as emotional body language, has been shown to improve facial emotional recognition in bvFTD, but only when the face and body language stimuli are congruent (e.g., an angry face paired with a body with raised fists) (Kumfor, Ibanez et al., 2018). On the other hand, bvFTD patients showed poor emotion recognition when presented with facial or body expressions alone, or when facial and body language stimuli are incongruent (e.g., a sad face paired with a body with raised fists), with responses indicating an over-reliance on external contextual information. Findings from studies that employ dynamic video stimuli in the assessment of emotion recognition (e.g., The Awareness of Social Inference Test; TASIT; (McDonald et al., 2003)) also confirm the widespread emotion recognition impairments in bvFTD (Goodkind et al., 2015; Kipps et al., 2009; Kumfor et al., 2017). Importantly, while performance on such video-based measures appears to be highly correlated with performance on emotion recognition tasks that use static facial stimuli (Goodkind et al., 2015), the former has greater ecological validity. Future studies that compare the sensitivity of these dynamic vs. static stimuli for detecting emotion recognition deficits in bvFTD will provide valuable insights to optimising test selection in clinical settings.

Empathy

Considering their widespread deficits in emotion perception and recognition, it is unsurprising that impairments in emotional empathy are widely recognised in bvFTD (Carr et al., 2018; Dermody et al., 2016). The patients themselves typically show a lack of insight regarding their reduced emotional responsiveness and inability to connect emotionally with others, which can place significant strains on partner and familial relationships and lead to relationship breakdowns (Hsieh et al., 2013b; Takeda et al., 2019).

In bvFTD, emotional empathy may be disrupted due to altered responsivity to emotional stimuli. For example, in a study where participants were shown a disgust-eliciting video clip, videotaped observations of emotional facial responses (e.g., wrinkled nose, raised upper lip, tongue moving forward in the mouth) and self-reported emotional experience revealed reduced disgust reactions (Eckart et al., 2012). Psychophysiological responses also appear to be compromised. In bvFTD patients, skin conductance (Eckart et al., 2012; Kumfor et al., 2019), cardiac reactivity (Eckart et al., 2012; Marshall et al., 2018a) and pupil dilation (Fletcher et al., 2015) are attenuated in response to emotionally salient stimuli. Dampening of these autonomic processes is thought to play a key role in bvFTD patients' difficulties interpreting their own emotions, leading to emotional blunting as well as reduced reactivity to other people's emotions (Van den Stock & Kumfor, 2019).

Studies of facial mimicry in bvFTD have shown an overall reduction in facial electromyographical responses to emotional videos (Kumfor et al., 2019). Importantly, bvFTD patients showed limited variation in their facial electromyographical responses according to emotional valence, unlike healthy older controls (Kumfor et al., 2019; Marshall et al., 2018b). Another study found abnormal increases in facial motor mimicry in bvFTD, with greater smiling responses to positive, negative and neutral faces than healthy controls (Hua et al., 2018). Notably, however, these increases in facial emotional reactivity were found to be predictive of poorer recognition of negative emotions and lower empathy in everyday life. Taken together, these findings suggest that bvFTD patients have difficulty appropriately attuning their emotional reactions to that of their current social context, which may impact on their ability to respond to others' emotions.

Theory of mind

The ability to adopt and understand another's' perspective (also referred to as cognitive empathy, mentalising or theory of mind; ToM) is also impacted in bvFTD (Dermody et al., 2016; Oliver et al., 2015). These impairments have been well documented across several clinical and experimental tasks. Patients show clear deficits on first-order false belief tasks (Eslinger et al., 2011; Gregory et al., 2002; Lough et al., 2001; Lough et al., 2002; Poletti et al., 2012) and struggle to correctly identify faux pas from scenarios (Bertoux et al., 2015a; Funkiewiez et al., 2012; Gleichgerrcht et al., 2010; Torralva et al., 2015; Torralva et al., 2009). More recently, however, Le Bouc et al. (2012) further distinguished between difficulty inferring someone else's (false) belief versus difficulty inhibiting one's own belief, showing that bvFTD patients' poor performance on false belief tasks is mainly attributable to the latter. These deficits were also associated with more a more general impairment in verbal inhibitory control (i.e., on a Stroop task). ToM appears to worsen with disease severity from mild to moderate bvFTD and is associated with poorer performance on tests of executive function (Baez et al., 2014; Torralva et al., 2015). Importantly, tasks such as the Story-based Empathy Task (Dodich et al., 2015) and Animated Shapes task (White et al., 2011), which rely on nonverbal cartoons and moving shapes to assess attribution of intention, have also been employed and have confirmed robust cognitive ToM deficits in this patient group (Cerami et al., 2014; Dodich et al., 2016; Synn et al., 2018). Interpretation of indirect language, such as sarcasm and lies, is also affected in bvFTD, whereas the ability to interpret sincere exchanges is largely intact (Kipps et al., 2009; Kumfor et al., 2017; Rankin et al., 2009; Shany-Ur et al., 2012). Thus, a large body of evidence has demonstrated impaired theory of mind in bvFTD across a range of methodologies.

Disorders of social behaviour

Social disinhibition

Behavioural disinhibition with socially inappropriate behaviour and declines in social comportment are key diagnostic criteria for bvFTD (Mendez et al., 2014; Rascovsky et al., 2011). Carers and family members often report that individuals with bvFTD seem to lack a 'filter' and appear unconcerned about how their actions might impact on others. Overall, their social interactions and behaviours seem to reflect a disregard for social norms. Indeed, bvFTD patients demonstrate poorer knowledge of social norms and score lower than controls on measures such as the Social Norms Questionnaire (Panchal et al., 2015; Strikwerda-Brown et al., 2020). Self-conscious emotions, such as embarrassment, are also reduced in bvFTD. On a task designed to elicit feelings of embarrassment, where participants viewed video recordings of themselves singing karaoke, bvFTD patients showed decreased physiological reactivity and self-conscious emotional behaviours relative to controls (Sturm et al., 2013a). Furthermore, sensitivity to social feedback appears to be diminished in bvFTD (Grossman et al., 2010; Perry et al., 2015), though this may also reflect broader deficits in reward processing and incentive motivation (Perry et al., 2013; Wong et al., 2018). Altogether, changes in social norm knowledge, self-conscious emotions and sensitivity to social rewards likely contribute to increased social disinhibition in bvFTD.

Emotional apathy

Apathy is a key symptom in the clinical diagnosis of bvFTD (Rascovsky et al., 2011). While previously considered to be a unidimensional construct, more recent conceptualisations of apathy subdivide symptoms into three dimensions: cognitive, emotional and behavioural apathy (Levy et al., 2006). Each apathy subtype is associated with disruption to distinct neurocognitive processes (Radakovic et al., 2018). Of relevance here, emotional apathy, which manifests as emotional blunting and diminished interest or concern for others, is elevated early in the disease course, particularly in relation to other dementia subtypes such as Alzheimer's disease (Kumfor, Zhen et al., 2018; Wei et al., 2019). As mentioned above, sensitivity to the rewarding (or punishing) nature of social and emotional stimuli may be attenuated in bvFTD, which may, in turn, contribute to reduced social engagement and concern for others (Kumfor, Zhen et al., 2018; Wong et al., 2018).

Reduced prosocial behaviour

Changes in prosocial functioning are evident early in the disease course. Reports of antisocial behaviour range from reduced social tact and crude language to shoplifting, trespass, traffic violations, unsolicited sexual approaches, indecent exposure and physical assault (Liljegren et al., 2015; Mendez, 2010; Mendez et al., 2005b). When interviewed, patients express remorse and demonstrate awareness that their behaviour is wrong but do not seem to be able to refrain from acting impulsively or show concern for the consequences (Mendez et al., 2005b). While they show intact knowledge of moral rules and norms, bvFTD patients are more likely to have a 'utilitarian' approach to moral reasoning tasks such as the 'trolley car' and 'footbridge' dilemmas (Mendez et al., 2005a). Notably, individuals who choose the utilitarian option show significantly poorer emotion recognition (Gleichgerrcht et al., 2011), less autonomic arousal and self-report less conflict and subjective discomfort regarding their decision (Fong et al., 2016). On more detailed moral reasoning tasks, bvFTD patients make similar decisions as controls but, importantly, their emotional responses to these decisions are strikingly abnormal (Strikwerda-Brown et al., 2020). This is consistent with reports of diminished self-conscious moral emotions such as guilt, regret and embarrassment in this patient group (Darby et al., 2016; Sturm et al., 2006).

BvFTD patients also score highly on measures of 'antisocial' moral emotions, such as schadenfreude (i.e., pleasure for others' misfortunes) and envy (Santamaría-García et al., 2017). Furthermore, reductions in prosocial behaviour have been demonstrated on novel neuroeconomic tasks in which participants are required to share resources when personal gain is not at stake, or give money to less-fortunate others (O'Callaghan et al., 2016; Sturm et al., 2017). When required to integrate social contextual information to guide these decisions, bvFTD patients are particularly impaired (O'Callaghan et al., 2016). In a similar vein, bvFTD patients appear to have difficulty applying socially relevant information to modulate monetary decisions in everyday life (Wong et al., 2017). Together with deficits in inferring the intentions, thoughts and feelings of others (i.e., ToM), difficulties in using social contextual information to guide decision-making may contribute to higher gullibility and susceptibility to interpersonal solicitation, which are commonly noticed in patients with bvFTD (Chiong et al., 2014).

Summary

BvFTD represents a prototypical disorder of social cognition, with deficits in the above-mentioned areas pervading the majority of not only patients' everyday lives, but also that of their family and friends. From a clinical perspective, increasing efforts have focused on methods of earlier diagnosis, as the earliest symptoms of bvFTD are often misdiagnosed as psychiatric disorders (Woolley et al., 2011). Within the clinic setting, abnormal interpersonal behaviours typically associated with bvFTD can sometimes be undetected, as the patient is placed in a highly structured environment. Similarly, tests of social cognition often involve the patient responding to stimuli that bear limited resemblance to typical social interactions in everyday life. As such, studies that employ naturalistic observations or 'second-person' approaches to examining changes in real-world social behaviour have shed new light on the nature of social cognitive deficits in bvFTD (Mendez et al., 2014; Visser et al., 2020). Finally, although considerable efforts have been devoted to examining and delineating social cognitive impairments in bvFTD, the clinicopathological specificity of such symptoms remains to be elucidated (Dodich, Crespi, Santi, Cappa, & Cerami, 2021) and empirical evidence for the efficacy of intervention and management strategies remains a critical area of future enquiry.

Semantic dementia

As mentioned above, frontotemporal dementia is an umbrella term, with three clinical subtypes typically recognised. The two language variants fall under the broader term of primary progressive aphasia. The first language variant, semantic dementia (SD) (also known as semantic-variant primary progressive aphasia), is characterised by word-finding difficulty, empty speech and poor single word comprehension, although language remains fluent with respect to production, including prosody and grammar (Gorno-Tempini et al., 2011; Hodges et al., 2007; Hodges et al., 1992). These clinical features reflect the gradual loss of semantic knowledge associated with progressive *anterior temporal lobe* atrophy, which tends to be asymmetrical with the left hemisphere more affected than the right hemisphere (Kumfor et al., 2016; Mion et al., 2010). When it was initially described, the clinical presentation of SD emphasised its language features; however, a large body of evidence has now demonstrated that these patients also show impairment in aspects of social cognition (Fittipaldi et al., 2019).

Emotion perception

A large body of work has demonstrated that SD patients show profoundly impaired emotion perception. Importantly, this extends to both positive and negative emotions, basic as well as more complex emotions (e.g., embarrassment, pride) and on both static and dynamic stimuli (Bertoux et al., 2020; Kumfor et al., 2011; Rosen et al., 2002; Rosen et al., 2004). Converging evidence has shown that these impairments cannot be accounted for by other cognitive impairments, such as attention or perceptual deficits, or verbal ability alone (Bertoux et al., 2020; Irish et al., 2013; Kumfor et al., 2011). Rather, these patients seem to experience an insidious and increasingly widespread loss of the conceptual knowledge of emotions (Bertoux et al., 2020; Kumfor,

Ibanez et al., 2018; Kumfor et al., 2016). Indeed, even psychophysiological responses to non-verbal emotional stimuli are abnormal in this syndrome (Kumfor et al., 2019). Impaired emotion perception from other types of stimuli have also been reported, including emotion from music (Hsieh et al., 2012; Omar et al., 2011), prosody (Perry et al., 2001a) and non-verbal sounds (Omar et al., 2011).

Empathy and theory of mind

Unsurprisingly, pervasive loss of empathy has also been reported, using a variety of different (largely questionnaire) measures (Binney et al., 2016; Hutchings et al., 2015; Marshall et al., 2017; Sollberger et al., 2014). Notably, SD patients have poor insight into their reduced empathy (Hutchings et al., 2015; Sollberger et al., 2014). With respect to theory of mind, widespread impairments are also observed, irrespective of the task employed, although evidence in this domain is considerably less than evidence on emotion perception. SD patients have reduced ability to correctly attribute intentions (Duval et al., 2012), accurately interpret false-belief tasks (Duval et al., 2012), understand others' mental states to correctly interpret humorous cartoons (Irish et al., 2014) and are impaired on the Reading the Mind in the Eyes Test (Duval et al., 2012). Understanding of sarcasm is also compromised (Rankin et al., 2009).

Disorders of social behaviour

Thus, social cognition impairment in SD is profound and widespread and often observed to a similar extent as seen in bvFTD. Severe social behaviour changes are also common and may include apathy, disinhibition, loss of empathy and antisocial behaviours (Diehl-Schmid et al., 2013; Kamminga et al., 2015; Kumfor et al., 2016; Van Langenhove et al., 2016). However, clinically, and even in terms of research, the emphasis is still largely on the language impairment. Hence, family members and carers are often blindsided by social cognition impairment and the associated behavioural changes, leading to significant levels of carer burden (Hsieh et al., 2013b) and inadequate support. It is therefore essential that clinicians consider social cognition in the assessment and management of SD.

Right temporal variant frontotemporal dementia

While the syndrome of SD is relatively well characterised, it is also recognised that a proportion of patients present with asymmetrical right-, rather than left-lateralised, temporal lobe atrophy. This syndrome has been variably referred to as right SD, right temporal variant frontotemporal dementia and right-sided frontotemporal lobar degeneration. Here, we use the term 'right temporal variant frontotemporal dementia (rtvFTD)' as recently proposed (Ulugut Erkoyun et al., 2020). Approximately 30% of patients who present with a neurodegenerative syndrome with anterior temporal lobe atrophy will show right greater than left hemisphere involvement (Chan et al., 2009; Kumfor et al., 2016). Clinically, these patients present with prosopagnosia, memory deficits, difficulties with navigation and behavioural changes (Chan et al., 2009; Kamminga et al., 2015; Thompson et al., 2003). These behavioural symptoms can be profound and include disinhibition, increased obsessive personality features, apathy, compulsiveness, decreased empathy and dietary changes (Kamminga et al., 2015). Furthermore, some individuals develop hyperreligiosity (Chan et al., 2009). In many cases, differentiation of rtvFTD from bvFTD is challenging (Kamminga et al., 2015), and how social cognition is affected in rtvFTD is increasingly a topic of interest. See Box 7.2 for a case with rtvFTD.

Box 7.2   Case 2: Mrs P: Adult with right temporal variant frontotemporal dementia

History:

Mrs P is a 74-year-old right-handed lady who completed nine years of education before training to become a hairdresser. She worked as a hairdresser/beautician up until the assessment, although her number of clients had substantially reduced.

Presentation:

On interview, she was unable to provide a clear history. Her speech was repetitive and empty with a reduction in vocabulary and reduced comprehension. She had a two-year history of incorrect word use (e.g., "Are we going to the 'pool' today?" when she was referring to the club) and also remarkable prosopagnosia. For example, at a recent wedding, she was unable to recognise her cousin who she had known all her life. She had been prosecuted for shoplifting, which was out of character. She had also begun approaching strangers and asking them where they came from. During an at home occupational therapy assessment, she was noted to be drinking shampoo in the shower (in spite of her previous occupation as a hairdresser). She had also developed rigid eating behaviours, insisting on eating the same food for virtually all her meals. Notably, her basic self-care remained good, and she was remarkably well groomed when she presented for the assessment. Her husband reported he had noticed some change in functioning approximately three to four years prior, although there had been a more rapid decline in the preceding 12 months. He noted that her moods had changed and that on occasion she could be quite nasty, which was unlike her former self.

Testing:

On the Addenbrooke's Cognitive Examination of general cognition, she scored 50/100. On formal neuropsychological assessment, she showed impaired attention, verbal memory, naming and executive functioning. Visual memory was comparatively spared. Social cognition was profoundly impaired. On the Ekman 60 test, she scored 18/60 ($z = -6.44$) and on TASIT Part 1, she scored 11/28 ($z = -4.99$).

Summary and comment:

Mrs P's presentation is consistent with rtvFTD. Her symptoms have been present for at least four years, and it is likely that atrophy has now progressed from the right to the left hemisphere, accounting for the emerging language deficits. Patients with rtvFTD are often diagnosed quite late in the disease course. This is in part because the earliest symptoms of prosopagnosia and behavioural changes may go unnoticed, a lack of awareness of clinicians about this relatively rare syndrome, as well as difficulty detecting impairments on standard neuropsychological assessments. Supplementing assessment of traditional cognitive domains with assessment of social cognition and face recognition is helpful in the early and accurate diagnosis of rtvFTD.

The earliest studies of social cognition focused on emotion perception and emotional expression. Perry et al. (2001a) described four patients who presented with anterior temporal lobe atrophy. The patients with right lateralised atrophy generally showed impaired emotion perception from both faces and voices, loss of empathy and abnormal interpersonal skills. Interestingly, their expression of emotion was also affected. They were reported as having a 'frozen' facial expression with only slight movement of the zygomaticus facial muscle resulting in a fixed smile. They were also reported as showing a Duchenne (unfelt or non-genuine) smile with no involvement of the orbicularis oculi muscle (see Figure 7.1) (Perry et al., 2001a).

Subsequent studies have demonstrated that rtvFTD patients show greater impairments in social cognition than patients with SD. Unsurprisingly, given that prosopagnosia is a hallmark feature of rtvFTD, memory for faces is impaired, and this impairment seems to be greater than what is seen in SD (Kumfor et al., 2015). Other aspects of face perception and processing of identity are compromised (Kumfor et al., 2016), as well as recognition and naming of famous

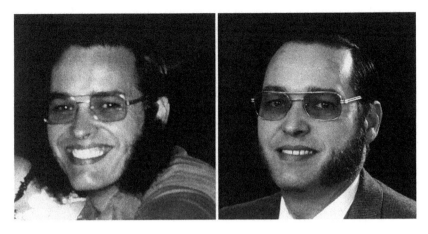

Figure 7.1 Facial expression of a man diagnosed with rtvFTD in 1980 (left) and 1993 (right)

Source: As depicted in Perry et al. (2001b)

faces (Luzzi et al., 2017). When compared to patients with SD, patients with rtvFTD show disproportionate impairments in emotion perception from faces, especially for the emotions anger and happiness (Irish et al., 2013). Notably, deficits in recognition of anger remain significant, even when face processing and semantic processing ability are accounted for (Irish et al., 2013). RtvFTD patients also show reduced empathy on the Interpersonal Reactivity Index (IRI), particularly on the empathic concern subscale (Irish et al., 2013). To our knowledge, theory of mind has not been specifically explored in this syndrome, although this may reflect the fact that currently no diagnostic criteria exist for rtvFTD, and even agreement in nosology has only just been reached. Hence, many research studies include rtvFTD either as part of the left-lateralised SD group, or as part of the bvFTD group given their overlapping symptom profile. Nevertheless, it would be expected that theory of mind is also compromised in this group in light of evidence that the right *anterior temporal lobe* is implicated in theory of mind in related disorders (Irish et al., 2014). At the behavioural level, rtvFTD patients show increased apathy as well as displaying more abnormal behaviours when compared with other dementia syndromes such as Alzheimer's disease (Kumfor et al., 2016). These abnormal behaviours include laughing at things others do not find funny, showing socially embarrassing behaviours, making tactless or suggestive remarks, being uncooperative, having temper outbursts and acting impulsively. With disease progression, emotion perception and social behaviour continues to decline (Kumfor et al., 2016).

It should be noted that as with other syndromes, the presentation of SD and rtvFTD is dependent on lateralisation of language function. One of the cases reported by Perry et al. (2001a) had predominant *right temporal lobe* atrophy and was left-handed and showed predominantly social cognition impairment, but the other left-handed case with right-hemisphere atrophy showed a predominantly language based clinical profile. It is agreed that ~15–30% of left-handed people show lateralisation of language function to the right hemisphere. Hence, classification of SD and rtvFTD cannot be made on neuroimaging evidence alone. Handedness and lateralisation of language function must be considered together with the clinical profile when classifying these dementia syndromes. While both SD and rtvFTD have social cognition impairments, the behavioural disturbances tend to be more severe in rtvFTD than SD, even with disease progression. From a neurobiological perspective, the extent of right temporal lobe involvement appears to be key in determining the degree of social cognition impairment (Kumfor et al., 2016).

Progressive non-fluent aphasia

The non-fluent/agrammatic variant of primary progressive aphasia (Gorno-Tempini et al., 2011), referred to here as progressive non-fluent aphasia (PNFA), can be seen as the opposite side of the coin to SD. Patients with PNFA present with laboured and effortful speech; however, semantic knowledge is generally well-preserved, with single word comprehension remaining intact, at least early in the disease course. Like the other primary progressive aphasia syndromes, historically, research focused on characterising the language impairment. However, more recent studies have suggested that social cognition is also affected to a degree in this dementia syndrome.

Emotion perception

We were the first to describe emotion perception impairments in PNFA almost a decade ago. Patients with PNFA showed impaired ability to recognise sadness, anger and fear, while recognition of positive emotions was within normal limits (Kumfor et al., 2011). Subsequent studies have confirmed that facial emotion perception is impaired in this syndrome (Couto et al., 2013; Hazelton et al., 2017; Johnen et al., 2018; Kumfor et al., 2013; Piguet et al., 2015) and emotional enhancement of memory is also compromised (Kumfor, Hodges et al., 2014). Interestingly, some evidence suggests that other cognitive abilities, such as face processing, inattention or language, may in part contribute to reduced performance on emotion perception tasks (Couto et al., 2013; Hutchings et al., 2017; Kumfor et al., 2011).

Empathy

In PNFA, evidence for the extent that empathy is affected is somewhat mixed and based largely on informant-rated questionnaires. When compared to healthy older controls, emotional empathy appears to be intact (Hazelton et al., 2017; Rankin et al., 2006; Sollberger et al., 2009). However, when patients' current level of empathy is compared with levels of empathy prior to disease onset (as retrospectively reported), a decline is observed (Hazelton et al., 2017). Longitudinal studies are rare, but one study reported a decline in empathy with disease progression (Van Langenhove et al., 2016). Together, these studies suggest that changes in empathy early in the disease are relatively subtle, although empathy may become compromised with disease progression. Findings that facial emotion recognition correlates with emotional empathy support this position (Hazelton et al., 2017). To date, studies which examine emotional contagion in these patients (e.g., via psychophysiological measures) or other objective measures of emotional empathy are lacking. Future studies that redress this gap in the literature will help clarify the extent that emotional empathy is affected in PNFA.

Theory of mind

Turning to ToM, again, studies are relatively scarce. One study which used the Reading the Mind in the Eyes Test found that patients with PNFA were impaired compared to controls and performed at a similar level to patients with bvFTD (Couto et al., 2013). A second study using TASIT found no significant reduction in understanding sincere or sarcastic exchanges (Rankin et al., 2009). The limited evidence available suggests that some aspects of ToM may be compromised in these patients, although this area of research clearly needs further exploration.

Disorders of social behaviour

Aside from formal assessment of social cognition, while overt social behavioural abnormalities are not common, social interaction in PNFA is undoubtedly compromised as a result of their expressive speech impairment. Fluent conversation is an essential component of social interactions. From a clinical perspective, patients with PNFA often withdraw from participating in social interactions, due to embarrassment or the overwhelming effort required to engage. This appears to lead to social isolation and reduced quality of life (despite many other aspects of cognition remaining remarkably well preserved). Interventions which assist social interactions, such as script training (El-Wahsh et al., 2020; Henry et al., 2018), are therefore likely to be of considerable benefit for this patient group.

Alzheimer's disease

Alzheimer's disease (AD) is the most common form of dementia. Clinically, patients show pervasive impairments in episodic memory, with particular deficits in learning and recall of new information (see Box 7.3). This memory impairment typically manifests as difficulties remembering events or appoint-ments, misplacing personal belongings, getting lost on familiar routes and repetitive questions or conversations. In addition, deficits are present in at least one other cognitive domain, such as reasoning/judgement (e.g., diffi-culty understanding safety risks, financial management and decision-making problems, inability to plan complex or multi-step activities), visuospatial abili-ties (e.g., difficulties finding objects in direct view despite good visual acuity, operating simple implements and orienting clothing to the body) or language abilities (e.g., word difficulties, hesitations, errors in speech, spelling and writ-ing), (McKhann et al., 2011). As the disease progresses, impairment invariably spreads across multiple cognitive domains, with changes in aspects of personal-ity, behaviour or comportment (e.g., agitation, apathy, social withdrawal, and to a lesser extent, loss of empathy, compulsive or obsessive behaviours, and other socially inappropriate behaviours) also being reported.

The earliest stage of AD is associated with atrophy in the medial temporal lobe (particularly the *hippocampus* and *transentorhinal cortex*), as well as hypome-tabolism in the *inferior parietal lobule* and *precuneus* (Schroeter et al., 2009). With disease progression, atrophy spreads from the *medial temporal lobe* to *lateral tem-poral, parietal* and *frontal regions*, and this spread is closely related to progressive cognitive decline (Eskildsen et al., 2013; Thompson et al., 2007).

Social cognition remains relatively intact in AD, particularly during the ear-lier stages of the disease. As seen in the Case Study in Box 7.3, changes in social and emotional functions are not typically reported as the predominant presenting symptom, and if reported, these changes appear secondary to gen-eral cognitive decline. In contrast to other dementia subtypes (e.g., bvFTD), various aspects of socio-emotional functioning, including empathy, emotion recognition, social conformity, antisocial behaviour and sociability, are rated by carers and family members to be within normal limits (Hutchings et al., 2015). Nonetheless, impaired performance on tests of social cognition have been documented in AD. We discuss these findings in more detail below.

Box 7.3   Case 3: Mr R: Adult with Alzheimer's disease

History:

Mr R is a 59-year-old man who had completed 15 years of formal education and worked as a teacher for 22 years. He retired from teach-ing approximately three years ago, after concerns were raised regarding his ability to keep up with paperwork and remember the names of his students.

Presentation:

On interview, Mr R presented as a pleasant and polite man. No obvious speech production errors were noted, though he tended to pause when thinking of the right word. He reported experiencing lapses in attention, difficulty processing multiple or complex pieces of information and handling money.

Mr R's wife reported a four-year history of cognitive changes, with progressive decline in memory, attention and planning capacity. She also described a slowness in learning new skills. Mr R had always enjoyed cooking and previously prepared all of their family meals. In the past two years, he began to experience difficulty keeping track of complex recipes and misplaced kitchen items. He gradually reverted to cooking simpler and more familiar recipes and, due to safety concerns, his wife had taken over the majority of cooking responsibilities. Over the past year, his wife noticed that he had become increasingly socially withdrawn. He engaged less with his teenage grandchildren, who visit most weekends. He tended to lose track of conversations and to stare off into space. No other changes in personality or behaviour were noted.

Testing:

On the ACE-III, Mr R scored 74/100, losing the majority of points on attention and memory as well as some points across the language and visuospatial subscales. On formal neuropsychological assessment, he showed impairments in working memory, language, processing of visual information and mental flexibility. He had great difficulty in learning and retaining new information across both verbal and visual modalities. In contrast, he scored within normal limits on a static facial emotion recognition test (41/42) and on Part 1 of TASIT (25/28).

Mr R's motor neurological examination was unremarkable. He did not show any signs of tremor, postural instability, disordered eye movements or abnormal motor reflexes. His MRI scan showed mild to moderate atrophy in the hippocampus and medial temporal lobes, extending posteriorly to the precuneus and parietal lobes. A PiB-PET scan revealed positive binding to amyloid.

Summary and comment:

Mr R's presentation is consistent with Alzheimers disease (AD). His symptoms have been present for at least four years, with progressive decline noted by his family and colleagues. His MRI scan revealed predominantly medial temporal and parietal lobe atrophy, and his PiB-PET scan results support a diagnosis of AD. While Mr R has shown some signs of reduced social engagement, this is likely due to the high working memory and language demands of conversations and social interactions, which would be taxing given Mr R's current level of cognitive functioning.

Emotion perception

In AD, the majority of studies have reported lower emotion recognition performance in patients than controls, though the nature and extent of this impairment remains controversial (De Melo Fádel et al., 2018). While some studies suggest that emotion recognition worsens with disease progression (Lavenu et al., 2005) and severity (Bertoux et al., 2015b), as well as a decline in other cognitive domains (Spoletini et al., 2008), others suggest that these deficits remain relatively stable. In particular, one meta-analysis of emotion recognition performance in AD found significant impairment relative to controls, regardless of disease severity, as well as task type or modality, emotional valence, or cognitive status (Klein-Koerkamp et al., 2012). Emotion recognition impairments have also been reported in the prodromal stages of AD (i.e., amnestic mild cognitive impairment) (McCade et al., 2011), and these deficits appear to be as severe as those in clinical AD (Kessels et al., 2020). Moreover, on a longitudinal study of emotion recognition performance, AD patients showed lower performance relative to controls at baseline, but no significant declines were evident over the subsequent two years (Kumfor, Irish et al., 2014).

Notably, impaired recognition of fearful expressions in AD improves when patients are instructed to direct their attention to the eye region (Hot et al., 2013). This suggests that the emotion recognition deficits in AD may partly be explained by visuo-perceptual deficits. Of relevance, recognition of emotions from auditory stimuli appears to be intact in AD (Hsieh et al., 2013a) and the provision of additional auditory and social contextual cues ameliorates emotion recognition deficits (Duclos et al., 2018; Goodkind et al., 2015). Taken together, evidence from a large body of literature indicates that performance on emotion recognition tests is reduced in AD relative to controls. Nonetheless, these deficits may be attenuated with the provision of additional contextual and multi-modal information. From a clinical diagnostic perspective, it is widely accepted that emotion recognition deficits in AD are not as severe as those seen in bvFTD (Bertoux et al., 2015a; Bora et al., 2016).

Empathy

The ability to emotionally empathise with others remains largely intact in AD (Bartochowski et al., 2018). On questionnaire measures, empathy is typically rated by carers or family members to be similar to controls (Dermody et al., 2016; Hutchings et al., 2015). In an observational study of patients' facial expressions, the majority of patients demonstrated intact and appropriate emotional responsivity during interactions with family members (Magai et al., 1996). In the same vein, AD patients show heightened emotional states in response to viewing sad or happy films, which persist despite poor conscious recollection of the films on memory testing (Guzmán-Vélez et al., 2014). Interestingly, emotional contagion appears to be elevated in AD, which may function as a low-level mechanism for affect sharing when higher-order cognitive empathic abilities decline with disease progression (Sturm et al., 2013b).

Theory of mind

In contrast, impaired performance on theory of mind (ToM) tasks are more widely documented and closely linked to cognitive decline in AD. Patients show clear deficits on ToM tasks, such as the Story-based Empathy and Animated Shapes tasks (Dodich et al., 2016; Synn et al., 2018), as well as on informant-rated measures of perspective taking (Dermody et al., 2016). On false-belief tasks, AD patients perform within normal limits on first-order false belief items, but perform worse on the more cognitively-demanding second-order false belief items (Fernandez-Duque et al., 2009; Gregory et al., 2002). Furthermore, AD patients show intact identification of faux pas from scenarios, but also fail the control questions which assess comprehension (Gregory et al., 2002). Thus, AD patients' performance on ToM tasks appears to be modulated by cognitive load, and deficits have been shown to be ameliorated when controlling for other variables such as general cognitive dysfunction, disease severity and progression (Dermody et al., 2016; Dodich et al., 2016; Synn et al., 2018). Similarly, while the ability to interpret indirect language (e.g., sarcasm) may be intact in the earlier stages of AD, significant declines become evident with disease progression (Kumfor, Irish et al., 2014). These findings are further supported by evidence of intact ToM performance in patients with prodromal AD (Dodich et al., 2016; Yi et al., 2020).

Disorders of social behaviour

Despite severe cognitive impairments, day-to-day social functioning and social graces remain relatively preserved in AD. Their knowledge of social norms remains intact (Panchal et al., 2015; Strikwerda-Brown et al., 2020) and sensitivity to social feedback is similar to controls (Perry et al., 2015). Symptoms of emotional apathy (e.g., social withdrawal, emotional blunting) are uncommon in AD (Kumfor, Zhen et al., 2018) but may manifest in later disease stages (Wei et al., 2019). In terms of prosocial behaviour, AD patients behave similarly to controls on measures of moral reasoning (Fong et al., 2016; Strikwerda-Brown et al., 2020), schadenfreude, envy (Santamaría-García et al., 2017) and prosocial giving (Sturm et al., 2017).

Summary

In summary, although patients with AD can show impaired performance on some measures of social cognition, such as emotion recognition and theory of mind, these deficits are at least partially due to generalised cognitive decline and disease progression, rather than a primary impairment in social cognition. We turn now to the atypical frontal presentation of AD, where unlike in typical AD, impairments in social cognition may be present, even early in the disease course.

Frontal AD

As discussed previously, most patients with AD present with predominant memory impairment. However, a small but not trivial subset of patients present with non-amnestic symptoms. In these patients, the initial and most prominent cognitive deficits are in language, visuospatial or executive functions, depending on the pattern of atrophy in the initial stages of the disease (McKhann et al., 2011). Of relevance to this chapter is the dysexecutive or frontal presentation of AD, where patients present with disproportionate impairments in executive function, including deficits in reasoning, judgement and problem-solving (McKhann et al., 2011). Patients with frontal AD show patterns of pathology and therefore atrophy, which deviate from the typical sequence of neurodegeneration described above, with greater involvement of the frontal lobes (Blennerhassett, Lillo, Halliday, Hodges, & Kril, 2014; Johnson, Head, Kim, Starr, & Cotman, 1999).

In comparison to typical AD, frontal AD patients present with disproportionate executive dysfunction and behavioural changes (see Box 7.4) (Lam, Masellis, Freedman, Stuss, & Black, 2013; Ossenkoppele et al., 2015). While most studies have emphasised the dysexecutive cognitive profile of frontal AD, including deficits in working memory, cognitive flexibility, planning and problem-solving (Binetti et al., 1996; Johnson et al., 1999; Woodward et al., 2010), increasing evidence indicates additional changes in personality and behaviour, including apathy, disinhibition and social cognition impairment (Blennerhassett et al., 2014; Duclos et al., 2016; Larner, 2006; Taylor, Probst, Miserez, Monsch, & Tolnay, 2008). However, studies of social cognition in frontal AD remain scarce, and the majority are based on single case studies or case series. We highlight below the main findings. See Box 7.4 for a Case Study example.

Box 7.4   Case 4: Mr P: Adult with frontal Alzheimer's Disease

History:

Mr P is a 57-year-old man who had completed 15 years of formal education. He worked as a groundsman for the majority of his career and had recently retired.

Presentation:

Mr P presented as a talkative and good-humoured man. His speech was fluent and no overt language errors were evident at a conversational level. He did not self-report any particular cognitive or behavioural concerns and only provided vague details regarding his personal history.

His wife reported that in the past two years, he had become increasingly forgetful, having lost his wallet and keys on multiple occasions, and experienced difficulty following plots of television shows. She described progressive withdrawal from social events and a reduced level of affection for family members. He occasionally responded impulsively or in ways which were not applicable to the situation and became agitated when confronted. In addition, she stated that he had always tended to be eccentric, but that this had noticeably worsened. He developed strange habits (e.g., tapping things repeatedly and rearranging old photographs) and had become very routine in his everyday life. More recently, he had begun to hoard stationary items, and his wife had noticed him take items from public spaces (e.g., pens and pencils from the public library and post office). Furthermore, his eating had become more impulsive, such that he often started eating before others and would quickly cram his mouth full of food.

Testing:

On cognitive testing, he scored 81/100 on the ACE-III, losing points on attention, memory and verbal fluency. On formal neuropsychological assessment, he showed impaired working memory, verbal inhibitory control and mental flexibility. On memory tests, he showed poor recall and recognition of verbal and non-verbal information. Confrontation naming, word repetition and comprehension were within normal limits. He scored poorly on a static facial emotion recognition test (23/42) and on Part 1 of TASIT (13/28).

Neurological examination was unremarkable. He did not show any evidence of apraxia, Parkinsonism, gait disorder, postural instability, disordered eye movement or other motor or frontal release signs. His MRI brain scan showed evidence of marked frontal lobe atrophy. A PiB-PET scan revealed a positive uptake of the ligand for amyloid indicating underlying AD pathology. He commenced Donepezil shortly thereafter (a cholinesterase inhibitor treatment specific for AD), and has derived noticeable benefit.

Summary and comment:

Given the two-year history of cognitive and behavioural decline, Mr P's presentation is consistent with dementia. His clinical symptoms and MRI scan closely resemble the presentation and neuroimaging findings associated with behavioural-variant frontotemporal dementia. However, results from his PiB-PET scan and reported improvements after taking a cholinesterase inhibitor support a diagnosis of dementia with Alzheimer-type pathology. As the clinical and neuropsychological profile of frontal AD and bvFTD patients can overlap considerably, there is a high risk of misdiagnosis. In these cases, additional neuroimaging and biomarker investigations are highly informative, but are often not widely available especially in clinical settings.

Emotion perception

Evidence from a case series (de Souza et al., 2013) and two single case studies (Duclos et al., 2016; Wong et al., 2019) of frontal AD indicates significant impairment on tests of emotion recognition, although another case study reported marked deficits on recognition of fear only (de Souza et al., 2019). Notably, one case showed intact emotion recognition performance at baseline, but scored within the impaired range one year later (Duclos et al., 2016).

Empathy and theory of mind

To our knowledge, empathy has not been studied in this rare patient group. On the other hand, impairment on false belief and faux pas tasks has been reported (de Souza et al., 2013; Duclos et al., 2016), suggesting that theory of mind is impaired in frontal AD.

Disorders of social behaviour

The majority of cases of frontal AD have a history of decline in social behaviour, interpersonal conduct and apathy (de Souza et al., 2013; Duclos et al., 2016; Wong et al., 2019). One case study examined knowledge of social norms using a novel visual task, demonstrating marked impairments at both baseline and follow-up (Duclos et al., 2016).

Summary

Although only a limited number of studies have examined social cognition in frontal AD, overall findings support the notion that profiles of social cognitive impairment in these patients are considerable. Although preliminary, these results highlight the challenges in accurate diagnosis of frontal AD, particularly when biomarker investigations are limited. Accurate clinical diagnosis of frontal AD is crucial, given the availability of pharmacotherapies that target underlying Alzheimer-type pathology. In order to improve diagnosis and management,

Table 7.1 Summary of profiles of social cognition impairment in dementia

	Clinical presentation	Pattern of atrophy	Social cognition profile
Behavioural-variant frontotemporal dementia	Early and insidious change in behaviour and personality. Symptoms include apathy, loss of empathy, disinhibition, perseveration, changes in eating behaviour and executive dysfunction	Ventromedial, orbitofrontal and insula	❖ Widespread impairment in emotion perception, empathy and theory of mind. ❖ Prominent disorders of social behaviour.
Semantic dementia	Loss of semantic knowledge which manifests as anomia and impaired single word comprehension in the context of fluent speech production	Asymmetric left anterior temporal lobe	❖ Widespread impairment in emotion perception, empathy and theory of mind. ❖ Profile similar to that seen in bvFTD.
Right temporal lobe variant frontotemporal dementia	Prosopagnosia, difficulties with navigation, behavioural changes, variable episodic memory impairment	Asymmetric right anterior temporal lobe	❖ Impaired emotional perception and expression; ❖ memory for faces < object memory; ❖ reduced empathy; ❖ emergence of abnormal social behaviours
Progressive non-fluent aphasia	Effortful and laboured speech production, which may be agrammatic, in the context of preserved language comprehension	Left inferior frontal and peri-sylvian region	❖ Reduced emotion perception, most evident from facial stimuli; ❖ subtle decline in empathy which increases with disease progression
Alzheimer's disease	Early impairment of episodic memory. Deficits are also present in at least one other cognitive domain (reasoning/judgement, visuospatial abilities, language or personality/behaviour/comportment)	Medial temporal and parietal lobes	❖ Impaired emotion perception and theory of mind. ❖ Preserved social graces, particularly during early disease stages.
Frontal Alzheimer's disease	Disproportionate executive dysfunction and behavioural changes relative to memory impairment	Medial and lateral frontal lobes	❖ Preliminary evidence indicates impaired emotion perception, theory of mind and prominent disorders of social behaviour.

further characterisation of the social cognitive impairments in frontal AD represents an important area of future investigation.

Conclusions

Dementia is associated with progressive decline in cognitive functioning, which may also extend to social cognition. Importantly, as summarised in Table 7.1, profiles of social cognition impairment vary across dementia subtypes, and are closely linked to underlying patterns of neurodegeneration. Importantly, these profiles reflect the *location*, rather than *type*, of brain pathology. While social cognition impairments are central to the clinical profile of some dementia subtypes (i.e., frontotemporal dementia), these deficits may also arise in other dementia subtypes (e.g., Alzheimer's disease) either secondary to cognitive impairment, or as atrophy extends to brain regions which underpin social cognition. Hence, assessment of social cognition is an essential component of dementia diagnosis. From a clinical viewpoint, a deeper understanding of the nature of social cognition impairments in dementia will help guide personally tailored intervention and management strategies.

Acknowledgements/Funding

SW is supported by an NHMRC Investigator Grant (GNT1196904). FK is supported by an NHMRC Career Development Fellowship (GNT1158762).

References

Baez, S., Manes, F., Huepe, D., Torralva, T., Fiorentino, N., Richter, F., . . . Ibanez, A. (2014). Primary empathy deficits in frontotemporal dementia. *Frontiers in Aging Neuroscience*, *6*, 262.

Bartochowski, Z., Gatla, S., Khoury, R., Al-Dahhak, R., & Grossberg, G. (2018). Empathy changes in neurocognitive disorders: A review. *Annals of Clinical Psychiatry*, *30*(3), 220–232.

Bertoux, M., de Souza, L. C., O'Callaghan, C., Greve, A., Sarazin, M., Dubois, B., & Hornberger, M. (2015a). Social cognition deficits: The key to discriminate behavioral variant frontotemporal dementia from Alzheimer's disease regardless of amnesia? *Journal of Alzheimer's Disease*, *49*(4), 1065–1074.

Bertoux, M., de Souza, L. C., Sarazin, M., Funkiewiez, A., Dubois, B., & Hornberger, M. (2015b). How preserved is emotion recognition in Alzheimer disease compared with behavioral variant frontotemporal dementia? *Alzheimer Disease and Associated Disorders*, *29*(2), 154–157.

Bertoux, M., Duclos, H., Caillaud, M., Segobin, S., Merck, C., de La Sayette, V., . . . Laisney, M. (2020). When affect overlaps with concept: Emotion recognition in semantic variant of primary progressive aphasia. *Brain*, *143*(12), 3850–3864.

Binetti, G., Magni, E., Padovani, A., Cappa, S., Bianchetti, A., & Trabucchi, M. (1996). Executive dysfunction in early Alzheimer's disease. *Journal of Neurology, Neurosurgery & Psychiatry*, *60*(1), 91–93.

Binney, R., Henry, M., Babiak, M., Pressman, P., Santos-Santos, M., Narvid, J., ... Gorno-Tempini, M. (2016). Reading words and other people: A comparison of exception word, familiar face and affect processing in the left and right temporal variants of primary progressive aphasia. *Cortex*, *82*, 147–163.

Blennerhassett, R., Lillo, P., Halliday, G., Hodges, J., & Kril, J. (2014). Distribution of pathology in frontal variant Alzheimer's disease. *Journal of Alzheimer's Disease: JAD*, *39*(1), 63–70.

Bora, E., Velakoulis, D., & Walterfang, M. (2016). Meta-analysis of facial emotion recognition in behavioral variant frontotemporal dementia. *Journal of Geriatric Psychiatry and Neurology*, *29*(4), 205–211.

Carr, A., & Mendez, M. (2018). Affective empathy in behavioral variant frontotemporal dementia: A meta-analysis. *Frontiers in Neurology*, *9*, 2456–2458.

Cerami, C., Dodich, A., Canessa, N., Crespi, C., Marcone, A., Cortese, F., ... Cappa, S. (2014). Neural correlates of empathic impairment in the behavioral variant of frontotemporal dementia. *Alzheimer's & Dementia*, 1–8.

Chan, D., Anderson, V., Pijnenburg, Y., Whitwell, J., Barnes, J., Scahill, R., ... Fox, N. (2009). The clinical profile of right temporal lobe atrophy. *Brain*, *132*(5), 1287–1298.

Chiong, W., Hsu, M., Wudka, D., Miller, B. L., & Rosen, H. (2014). Financial errors in dementia: Testing a neuroeconomic conceptual framework. *Neurocase*, *20*(4), 389–396.

Couto, B., Manes, F., Montañés, P., Matallana, D., Reyes, P., Velasquez, M., ... Ibáñez, A. (2013). Structural neuroimaging of social cognition in progressive non-fluent aphasia and behavioral variant of frontotemporal dementia. *Frontiers in Human Neuroscience*, *7*, 467.

Coyle-Gilchrist, I. T., Dick, K. M., Patterson, K., Rodríguez, P. V., Wehmann, E., Wilcox, A., ... Mead, S. (2016). Prevalence, characteristics, and survival of frontotemporal lobar degeneration syndromes. *Neurology*, *86*(18), 1736–1743.

Darby, R., Edersheim, J., & Price, B. (2016). What patients with behavioral-variant frontotemporal dementia can teach us about moral responsibility. *AJOB Neuroscience*, *7*(4), 193–201.

De Melo Fádel, B., De Carvalho, R., Dos Santos, T., & Dourado, M. (2018). Facial expression recognition in Alzheimer's disease: A systematic review. *Journal of Clinical and Experimental Neuropsychology (Neuropsychology, Development and Cognition: Section A)*, *41*(2), 192–203.

Dermody, N., Wong, S., Ahmed, R., Piguet, O., Hodges, J., & Irish, M. (2016). Uncovering the neural bases of cognitive and affective empathy deficits in Alzheimer's disease and the behavioral-variant of frontotemporal dementia. *Journal of Alzheimer's Disease*, *53*(3), 801–816.

de Souza, L., Bertoux, M., Funkiewiez, A., Samri, D., Azuar, C., Habert, M., ... Dubois, B. (2013). Frontal presentation of Alzheimer's disease: A series of patients with biological evidence by CSF biomarkers. *Dementia & Neuropsychologia*, *7*(1), 66–74.

de Souza, L., Mariano, L., de Moraes, R., & Caramelli, P. (2019). Behavioral variant of frontotemporal dementia or frontal variant of Alzheimer's disease? A case study. *Dementia & Neuropsychologia*, *13*(3), 356–360.

Diehl-Schmid, J., Perneczky, R., Koch, J., Nedopil, N., & Kurz, A. (2013). Guilty by Suspicion? Criminal behavior in frontotemporal lobar degeneration. *Cognitive and Behavioral Neurology*, *26*(2), 73–77.

Dodich, A., Cerami, C., Crespi, C., Canessa, N., Lettieri, G., Iannaccone, S., ... Cacioppo, J. (2015). A novel task assessing intention and emotion attribution: Italian standardization and normative data of the story-based empathy task. *Neurological Sciences*, *36*(10), 1907–1912.

Dodich, A., Cerami, C., Crespi, C., Canessa, N., Lettieri, G., Iannaccone, S., . . . Cacioppo, J. (2016). Differential impairment of cognitive and affective mentalizing abilities in neurodegenerative dementias: Evidence from behavioral variant of frontotemporal dementia, Alzheimer's disease, and mild cognitive impairment. *Journal of Alzheimer's disease: JAD*, *50*(4), 1011–1022.

Dodich, A., Crespi, C., Santi, G. C., Cappa, S. F., & Cerami, C. (2021). Evaluation of discriminative detection abilities of social cognition measures for the diagnosis of the behavioral variant of frontotemporal dementia: A systematic review. *Neuropsychology Review*, *31*(2), 251–266.

Dodich, A., Cerami, C., Crespi, C., Canessa, N., Lettieri, G., Iannaccone, S., . . . Cacioppo, J. (2018). Role of context in affective theory of mind in Alzheimer's disease. *Neuropsychologia*, *119*, 363–372.

Duclos, H., de la Sayette, V., Bonnet, A.-L., Viard, A., Eustache, F., Desgranges, B., & Laisney, M. (2016). Social cognition in the frontal variant of Alzheimer's disease: A case study. *Journal of Alzheimer's Disease*, *55*(2), 459–463.

Duval, C., Bejanin, A., Piolino, P., Laisney, M., de la Sayette, V., Belliard, S., . . . Desgranges, B. (2012). Theory of mind impairments in patients with semantic dementia. *Brain*, *135*(1), 228–241.

Eckart, J. A., Sturm, V. E., Miller, B. L., & Levenson, R. (2012). Diminished disgust reactivity in behavioral variant frontotemporal dementia. *Neuropsychologia*, *50*(5), 786–790.

El-Wahsh, S., Monroe, P., Kumfor, F., & Ballard, K. (2020). Communication interventions for people with dementia and their communication partners. In L. F. Low & K. Laver (Eds.), *Dementia Rehabilitation: Evidence-Based Interventions and Clinical Recommendations*. United Kingdom: Academic Press.

Eskildsen, S., Coupé, P., García-Lorenzo, D., Fonov, V., Pruessner, J., Collins, D., & Alzheimer's Disease Neuroimaging Initiative. (2013). Prediction of Alzheimer's disease in subjects with mild cognitive impairment from the ADNI cohort using patterns of cortical thinning. *NeuroImage*, *65*, 511–521.

Eslinger, P. J., Moore, P., Anderson, C., & Grossman, M. (2011). Social cognition, executive functioning, and neuroimaging correlates of empathic deficits in frontotemporal dementia. *The Journal of Neuropsychiatry and Clinical Neurosciences*, *23*(1), 74–82.

Fernandez-Duque, D., Baird, J. A., & Black, S. (2009). False-belief understanding in frontotemporal dementia and Alzheimer's disease. *Journal of Clinical and Experimental Neuropsychology (Neuropsychology, Development and Cognition: Section A)*, *31*(4), 489–497.

Fernandez-Duque, D., & Black, S. (2005). Impaired recognition of negative facial emotions in patients with frontotemporal dementia. *Neuropsychologia*, *43*(11), 1673–1687.

Fittipaldi, S., Ibáñez, A., Baez, S., Manes, F., Sedeño, L., & García, A. (2019). More than words: Social cognition across variants of primary progressive aphasia. *Neuroscience and Biobehavioral Reviews*, *100*, 263–284.

Fletcher, P., Nicholas, J., Shakespeare, T., Downey, L., Golden, H., Agustus, J., . . . Warren, J. (2015). Physiological phenotyping of dementias using emotional sounds. *Alzheimer's & Dementia: Diagnosis, Assessment & Disease Monitoring*, *1*(2), 170–178.

Fong, S., Navarrete, C., Perfecto, S., Carr, A., Jimenez, E., & Mendez, M. (2016). Behavioral and autonomic reactivity to moral dilemmas in frontotemporal dementia versus Alzheimer's disease. *Social Neuroscience*, *5*(11), 1–10.

Frings, L., Yew, B., Flanagan, E., Lam, B., Hüll, M., Huppertz, H., . . . Hornberger, M. (2014). Longitudinal grey and white matter changes in frontotemporal dementia and Alzheimer's disease. *PLoS One*, *9*(3), e90814–e90818.

Funkiewiez, A., Bertoux, M., de Souza, L., Levy, R., & Dubois, B. (2012). The SEA (social cognition and emotional assessment): A clinical neuropsychological tool for early diagnosis of frontal variant of frontotemporal lobar degeneration. *Neuropsychology, 26*(1), 81–90.

Gleichgerrcht, E., Torralva, T., Roca, M., & Manes, F. (2010). Utility of an abbreviated version of the executive and social cognition battery in the detection of executive deficits in early behavioral variant frontotemporal dementia patients. *Journal of the International Neuropsychological Society: JINS, 16*(04), 687–694.

Gleichgerrcht, E., Torralva, T., Roca, M., Pose, M., & Manes, F. (2011). The role of social cognition in moral judgment in frontotemporal dementia. *Social Neuroscience, 6*(2), 113–122.

Goodkind, M., Sturm, V., Ascher, E., Shdo, S., Miller, B., Rankin, K., & Levenson, R. (2015). Emotion recognition in frontotemporal dementia and Alzheimer's disease: A new film-based assessment. *Emotion, 15*(4), 416–427.

Gorno-Tempini, M., Hillis, A., Weintraub, S., Kertesz, A., Mendez, M., Cappa, S., . . . Grossman, M. (2011). Classification of primary progressive aphasia and its variants. *Neurology, 76*(11), 1006–1014.

Gregory, C., Lough, S., Stone, V., Erzinclioglu, S., Martin, L., Baron-Cohen, S., & Hodges, J. (2002). Theory of mind in patients with frontal variant frontotemporal dementia and Alzheimer's disease: Theoretical and practical implications. *Brain, 125*(Pt 4), 752–764.

Grossman, M., Eslinger, P., Troiani, V., Anderson, C., Avants, B., Gee, J., . . . Antani, S. (2010). The role of ventral medial prefrontal cortex in social decisions: Converging evidence from fMRI and frontotemporal lobar degeneration. *Neuropsychologia, 48*(12), 3505–3512.

Guzmán-Vélez, E., Feinstein, J., & Tranel, D. (2014). Feelings without memory in Alzheimer disease, *27*(3), 117–129.

Harciarek, M., & Cosentino, S. (2013). Language, executive function and social cognition in the diagnosis of frontotemporal dementia syndromes. *International Review of Psychiatry, 25*(2), 178–196.

Harvey, R. (2003). The prevalence and causes of dementia in people under the age of 65 years. *Journal of Neurology, Neurosurgery & Psychiatry, 74*(9), 1206–1209.

Hazelton, J., Irish, M., Hodges, J., Piguet, O., & Kumfor, F. (2017). Cognitive and affective empathy disruption in non-fluent primary progressive aphasia syndromes. *Brain Impairment, 18*(1), 117–129.

Henry, M., Hubbard, H., Grasso, S., Mandelli, M., Wilson, S., Sathishkumar, M., . . . Gorno-Tempini, M. (2018). Retraining speech production and fluency in non-fluent/agrammatic primary progressive aphasia. *Brain, 141*(6), 1799–1814.

Hodges, J., & Patterson, K. (2007). Semantic dementia: A unique clinicopathological syndrome. *The Lancet Neurology, 6*(11), 1004–1014.

Hodges, J., Patterson, K., Oxbury, S., & Funnell, E. (1992). Semantic dementia: Progressive fluent aphasia with temporal-lobe atrophy. *Brain, 115*(6), 1783–1806.

Hornberger, M., Piguet, O., Graham, A., Nestor, P., & Hodges, J. (2010). How preserved is episodic memory in behavioral variant frontotemporal dementia? *Neurology, 74*(6), 472–479.

Hot, P., Klein-Koerkamp, Y., Borg, C., Richard-Mornas, A., Zsoldos, I., Adeline, A. P., . . . Baciu, M. (2013). Fear recognition impairment in early-stage Alzheimer's disease: When focusing on the eyes region improves performance. *Brain and Cognition, 82*(1), 25–34.

Hsieh, S., Hodges, J., & Piguet, O. (2013a). Recognition of positive vocalizations is impaired in behavioral-variant frontotemporal dementia. *Journal of the International Neuropsychological Society, 19*(4), 483–487.

Hsieh, S., Hornberger, M., Piguet, O., & Hodges, J. (2012). Brain correlates of musical and facial emotion recognition: Evidence from the dementias. *Neuropsychologia, 50*(8), 1814–1822.

Hsieh, S., Irish, M., Daveson, N., Hodges, J., & Piguet, O. (2013b). When one loses empathy: Its effect on carers of patients with dementia. *Journal of Geriatric Psychiatry and Neurology, 26*(3), 174–184.

Hua, A., Sible, I., Perry, D., Rankin, K., Kramer, J., Miller, B., . . . Sturm, V. (2018). Enhanced positive emotional reactivity undermines empathy in behavioral variant frontotemporal dementia. *Frontiers in Neurology, 9*, 402.

Hutchings, R., Hodges, J., Piguet, O., Kumfor, F., & Boutoleau-Bretonniere, C. (2015). Why should I care? Dimensions of socio-emotional cognition in younger-onset dementia. *Journal of Alzheimer's Disease, 48*(1), 135–147.

Hutchings, R., Palermo, R., Bruggemann, J., Hodges, J., Piguet, O., & Kumfor, F. (2018). Looking but not seeing: Increased eye fixations in behavioural-variant frontotemporal dementia. *Cortex, 103*, 71–81.

Hutchings, R., Palermo, R., Piguet, O., & Kumfor, F. (2017). Disrupted face processing in frontotemporal dementia: A review of the clinical and neuroanatomical evidence. *Neuropsychology Review, 27*(1), 18–30.

Ibañez, A., & Manes, F. (2012). Contextual social cognition and the behavioral variant of frontotemporal dementia. *Neurology, 78*(17), 1354–1362.

Irish, M., Hodges, J., & Piguet, O. (2014). Right anterior temporal lobe dysfunction underlies theory of mind impairments in semantic dementia. *Brain, 137*(4), 1241–1253.

Irish, M., Kumfor, F., Hodges, J., & Piguet, O. (2013). A tale of two hemispheres: Contrasting socioemotional dysfunction in right- versus left-lateralised semantic dementia. *Dementia & Neuropsychologia, 7*(1), 88–95.

Jiskoot, L., Poos, J., Vollebergh, M., Franzen, S., van Hemmen, J., Papma, J., . . . van den Berg, E. (2020). Emotion recognition of morphed facial expressions in presymptomatic and symptomatic frontotemporal dementia, and Alzheimer's dementia. *Journal of Neurology*, 1–12.

Johnen, A., Reul, S., Wiendl, H., Meuth, S., & Duning, T. (2018). Apraxia profiles-A single cognitive marker to discriminate all variants of frontotemporal lobar degeneration and Alzheimer's disease. *Alzheimer's & Dementia (Amsterdam, Netherlands), 10*, 363–371.

Johnson, J., Head, E., Kim, R., Starr, A., & Cotman, C. (1999). Clinical and pathological evidence for a frontal variant of Alzheimer disease. *Archives of Neurology, 56*(10), 1233–1239.

Kamminga, J., Kumfor, F., Burrell, J., Piguet, O., Hodges, J., & Irish, M. (2015). Differentiating between right-lateralised semantic dementia and behavioural-variant frontotemporal dementia: An examination of clinical characteristics and emotion processing. *Journal of Neurology, Neurosurgery, and Psychiatry, 86*(10), 1082–1088.

Kessels, R., Waanders Oude Elferink, M., & Tilborg, I. (2020). Social cognition and social functioning in patients with amnestic mild cognitive impairment or Alzheimer's dementia. *Journal of Neuropsychology, 29*(1), 154–118.

Kipps, C., Nestor, P., Acosta-Cabronero, J., Arnold, R., & Hodges, J. (2009). Understanding social dysfunction in the behavioural variant of frontotemporal dementia: The role of emotion and sarcasm processing. *Brain, 132*(3), 592–603.

Klein-Koerkamp, Y., Beaudoin, M., Baciu, M., & Hot, P. (2012). Emotional decoding abilities in Alzheimer's disease: A meta-analysis. *Journal of Alzheimer's Disease, 32*(1), 109–125.

Kumfor, F., & Piguet, O. (2012). Disturbance of emotion processing in frontotemporal dementia: A synthesis of cognitive and neuroimaging findings. *Neuropsychology Review, 22*(3), 280–297.

Kumfor, F., Hazelton, J., Rushby, J., Hodges, J., & Piguet, O. (2019). Facial expressiveness and physiological arousal in frontotemporal dementia: Phenotypic clinical profiles and neural correlates. *Cognitive, Affective, & Behavioral Neuroscience, 19*(1), 197–210.

Kumfor, F., Hodges, J., & Piguet, O. (2014). Ecological assessment of emotional enhancement of memory in progressive nonfluent aphasia and Alzheimer's disease. *Journal of Alzheimer's Disease, 42*(1), 201–210.

Kumfor, F., Honan, C., McDonald, S., Hazelton, J., Hodges, J., & Piguet, O. (2017). Assessing the "social brain" in dementia: Applying TASIT-S. *Cortex, 93*, 166–177.

Kumfor, F., Hutchings, R., Irish, M., Hodges, J., Rhodes, G., Palermo, R., & Piguet, O. (2015). Do I know you? Examining face and object memory in frontotemporal dementia. *Neuropsychologia, 71*(C), 101–111.

Kumfor, F., Ibanez, A., Hutchings, R., Hazelton, J., Hodges, J., & Piguet, O. (2018). Beyond the face: How context modulates emotion processing in frontotemporal dementia subtypes. *Brain, 141*(4), 1172–1185.

Kumfor, F., Irish, M., Hodges, J., & Piguet, O. (2013). Discrete neural correlates for the recognition of negative emotions: Insights from frontotemporal dementia. *PLoS One, 8*(6), e67457.

Kumfor, F., Irish, M., Leyton, C., Miller, L., Lah, S., Devenney, E., . . . Piguet, O. (2014). Tracking the progression of social cognition in neurodegenerative disorders. *Journal of Neurology, Neurosurgery, and Psychiatry, 85*(10), 1076–1083.

Kumfor, F., Landin-Romero, R., Devenney, E., Hutchings, R., Grasso, R., Hodges, J., & Piguet, O. (2016). On the right side? A longitudinal study of left- versus right-lateralized semantic dementia. *Brain, 139*(Pt 3), 986–998.

Kumfor, F., Miller, L., Lah, S., Hsieh, S., Savage, S., Hodges, J., & Piguet, O. (2011). Are you really angry? The effect of intensity on facial emotion recognition in frontotemporal dementia. *Social Neuroscience, 6*(5–6), 502–514.

Kumfor, F., Zhen, A., Hodges, J., Piguet, O., & Irish, M. (2018). Apathy in Alzheimer's disease and frontotemporal dementia: Distinct clinical profiles and neural correlates. *Cortex, 103*, 350–359.

Lam, B., Halliday, G., Irish, M., Hodges, J., & Piguet, O. (2013). Longitudinal white matter changes in frontotemporal dementia subtypes. *Human Brain Mapping, 35*(7), 3547–3557.

Lam, B., Masellis, M., Freedman, M., Stuss, D., & Black, S. (2013). Clinical, imaging, and pathological heterogeneity of the Alzheimer's disease syndrome. *Alzheimer's Research & Therapy, 5*(1), 1.

Landin-Romero, R., Kumfor, F., Leyton, C., Irish, M., Hodges, J., & Piguet, O. (2017). Disease-specific patterns of cortical and subcortical degeneration in a longitudinal study of Alzheimer's disease and behavioural-variant frontotemporal dementia. *NeuroImage, 151*, 72–80.

Larner, A. (2006). "Frontal variant Alzheimer's disease": A reappraisal. *Clinical Neurology and Neurosurgery, 108*(7), 705–708.

Lavenu, I., & Pasquier, F. (2005). Perception of emotion on faces in frontotemporal dementia and Alzheimer's disease: A longitudinal study. *Dementia and Geriatric Cognitive Disorders, 19*(1), 37–41.

Lavenu, I., Pasquier, F., Lebert, F., Petit, H., & der Linden, M. (1999). Perception of emotion in frontotemporal dementia and Alzheimer disease. *Alzheimer Disease and Associated Disorders, 13*(2), 96–101.

Le Bouc, R., Lenfant, P., Delbeuck, X., Ravasi, L., Lebert, F., Semah, F., & Pasquier, F. (2012). My belief or yours? Differential theory of mind deficits in frontotemporal dementia and Alzheimer's disease. *Brain, 135*(10), 3026–3038.

Levy, R., & Dubois, B. (2006). Apathy and the functional anatomy of the prefrontal cortex-basal ganglia circuits. *Cerebral Cortex, 16*(7), 916–928.

Liljegren, M., Naasan, G., Temlett, J., Perry, D., Rankin, K., Merrilees, J., . . . Miller, B. (2015). Criminal behavior in frontotemporal dementia and Alzheimer disease. *JAMA Neurology, 72*(3), 295–300.

Lough, S., Gregory, C., & Hodges, J. (2001). Dissociation of social cognition and executive function in frontal variant frontotemporal dementia. *Neurocase, 7*(2), 123–130.

Lough, S., & Hodges, J. (2002). Measuring and modifying abnormal social cognition in frontal variant frontotemporal dementia. *Journal of Psychosomatic Research, 53*(2), 639–646.

Luzzi, S., Baldinelli, S., Ranaldi, V., Fabi, K., Cafazzo, V., Fringuelli, F., . . . Gainotti, G. (2017). Famous faces and voices: Differential profiles in early right and left semantic dementia and in Alzheimer's disease. *Neuropsychologia, 94*, 118–128.

Magai, C., Cohen, C., Gomberg, D., Malatesta, C., & Culver, C. (1996). Emotional expression during mid- to late-stage dementia. *International Psychogeriatrics, 8*(3), 383–395.

Marshall, C., Hardy, C., Allen, M., Russell, L., Clark, C., Bond, R., . . . Warren, J. (2018a). Cardiac responses to viewing facial emotion differentiate frontotemporal dementias. *Annals of Clinical and Translational Neurology, 347*(Pt 5), f4827–f4810.

Marshall, C., Hardy, C., Russell, L., Clark, C., Bond, R., Dick, K., . . . Warren, J. (2018b). Motor signatures of emotional reactivity in frontotemporal dementia. *Scientific Reports*, 1–13.

Marshall, C., Hardy, C., Russell, L., Clark, C., Dick, K., Brotherhood, E., . . . Rohrer, J. (2017). Impaired interoceptive accuracy in semantic variant primary progressive aphasia. *Frontiers in Neurology, 8*, 610.

McCade, D., Savage, G., & Naismith, S. (2011). Review of emotion recognition in mild cognitive impairment. *Dementia and Geriatric Cognitive Disorders, 32*(4), 257–266.

McDonald, S., Flanagan, S., Rollins, J., & Kinch, J. (2003). TASIT: A new clinical tool for assessing social perception after traumatic brain injury. *The Journal of Head Trauma Rehabilitation, 18*(3), 219–238.

McKhann, G., Knopman, D., Chertkow, H., Hyman, B., Jack, C., Kawas, C., . . . Phelps, C. (2011). The diagnosis of dementia due to Alzheimer's disease: Recommendations from the National Institute on Aging-Alzheimer's Association workgroups on diagnostic guidelines for Alzheimer's disease. *Alzheimer's & Dementia, 7*(3), 263–269.

Mendez, M. (2010). The unique predisposition to criminal violations in frontotemporal dementia. *Journal of the American Academy of Psychiatry and the Law, 38*(3), 318–323.

Mendez, M., Anderson, E., & Shapira, J. (2005a). An investigation of moral judgement in frontotemporal dementia. *Cognitive and Behavioral Neurology, 18*(4), 193–197.

Mendez, M., Chen, A., Shapira, J., & Miller, B. (2005b). Acquired sociopathy and frontotemporal dementia. *Dementia and Geriatric Cognitive Disorders, 20*(2–3), 99–104.

Mendez, M., Fong, S., Shapira, J., Jimenez, E., Kaiser, N., Kremen, S., & Tsai, P. (2014). Observation of social behavior in frontotemporal dementia. *American Journal of Alzheimer's Disease & Other Dementias, 29*(3), 215–221.

Mendez, M., & Shapira, J. (2011). Loss of emotional insight in behavioral variant frontotemporal dementia or "frontal anosodiaphoria". *Consciousness and Cognition, 20*(4), 1690–1696.

Mercy, L., Hodges, J., Dawson, K., Barker, R., & Brayne, C. (2008). Incidence of early-onset dementias in Cambridgeshire, United Kingdom. *Neurology, 71*(19), 1496–1499.

Mion, M., Patterson, K., Acosta-Cabronero, J., Pengas, G., Izquierdo-Garcia, D., Hong, Y., . . . Nestor, P. (2010). What the left and right anterior fusiform gyri tell us about semantic memory. *Brain, 133*(11), 3256–3268.

Muñoz-Neira, C., Tedde, A., Coulthard, E., Thai, N., & Pennington, C. (2019). Neural correlates of altered insight in frontotemporal dementia_ a systematic review. *YNICL, 24*, 102066.

O'Callaghan, C., Bertoux, M., Irish, M., Shine, J., Wong, S., Spiliopoulos, L., . . . Hornberger, M. (2016). Fair play: Social norm compliance failures in behavioural variant frontotemporal dementia. *Brain, 139*(Pt 1), 204–216.

Oliver, L., Mitchell, D., Dziobek, I., MacKinley, J., Coleman, K., Rankin, K., & Finger, E. (2015). Parsing cognitive and emotional empathy deficits for negative and positive stimuli in frontotemporal dementia. *Neuropsychologia, 67*, 14–26.

Omar, R., Henley, S., Bartlett, J., Hailstone, J., Gordon, E., Sauter, D., . . . Warren, J. (2011). The structural neuroanatomy of music emotion recognition: Evidence from frontotemporal lobar degeneration. *Neuroimage, 56*(3), 1814–1821.

Ossenkoppele, R., Pijnenburg, Y., Perry, D., Cohn-Sheehy, B., Scheltens, N., Vogel, J., . . . Rabinovici, G. (2015). The behavioural/dysexecutive variant of Alzheimer's disease: Clinical, neuroimaging and pathological features. *Brain, 138*(Pt 9), 2732–2749.

Panchal, H., Paholpak, P., Lee, G., Carr, A., Barsuglia, J., Mather, M., . . . Mendez, M. (2015). Neuropsychological and neuroanatomical correlates of the social norms questionnaire in frontotemporal dementia versus Alzheimer's disease. *American Journal of Alzheimer's Disease and Other Dementias, 31*(4), 326–332.

Perry, D., & Kramer, J. (2013). Reward processing in neurodegenerative disease. *Neurocase, 21*(1), 120–133.

Perry, R., Rosen, H., Kramer, J., Beer, J., Levenson, R., & Miller, B. (2001a). Hemispheric dominance for emotions, empathy and social behaviour: Evidence from right and left handers with frontotemporal dementia. *Neurocase, 7*(2), 145–160.

Perry, R., Rosen, H., Kramer, J., Beer, J., Levenson, R., & Miller, B. (2001b). Hemispheric dominance for emotions, empathy and social behaviour: Evidence from right and left handers with frontotemporal dementia. *Neurocase, 7*(2), 145–160.

Perry, D., Sturm, V., Wood, K., Miller, B., & Kramer, J. (2015). Divergent processing of monetary and social reward in behavioral variant frontotemporal dementia and Alzheimer disease. *Alzheimer Disease and Associated Disorders, 29*(2), 161–164.

Piguet, O., Leyton, C., Gleeson, L., Hoon, C., & Hodges, J. (2015). Memory and emotion processing performance contributes to the diagnosis of non-semantic primary progressive aphasia syndromes. *Journal of Alzheimer's Disease, 44*(2), 541–547.

Poletti, M., Enrici, I., & Adenzato, M. (2012). Cognitive and affective theory of mind in neurodegenerative diseases: Neuropsychological, neuroanatomical and neurochemical levels. *Neuroscience and Biobehavioral Reviews, 36*(9), 2147–2164.

Radakovic, R., & Abrahams, S. (2018). Multidimensional apathy: Evidence from neurodegenerative disease. *Current Opinion in Behavioral Sciences 22*, 42–49.

Rankin, K., Gorno-Tempini, M., Allison, S., Stanley, C., Glenn, S., Weiner, M., & Miller, B. (2006). Structural anatomy of empathy in neurodegenerative disease. *Brain, 129*(Pt 11), 2945–2956.

Rankin, K., Salazar, A., Gorno-Tempini, M., Sollberger, M., Wilson, S., Pavlic, D., . . . Miller, B. (2009). Detecting sarcasm from paralinguistic cues: Anatomic and cognitive correlates in neurodegenerative disease. *NeuroImage, 47*(4), 2005–2015.

Rascovsky, K., Hodges, J., Knopman, D., Mendez, M., Kramer, J., Neuhaus, J., . . . Miller, B. (2011). Sensitivity of revised diagnostic criteria for the behavioural variant of fronto-temporal dementia. *Brain, 134*(Pt 9), 2456–2477.

Ratnavalli, E., Brayne, C., Dawson, K., & Hodges, J. (2002). The prevalence of frontotem-poral dementia. *Neurology, 58*(11), 1615–1621.

Rosen, H., Gorno-Tempini, M., Goldman, W., Perry, R., Schuff, N., Weiner, M., . . . Miller, B. (2002). Patterns of brain atrophy in frontotemporal dementia and semantic dementia. *Neurology, 58*(2), 198–208.

Rosen, H., Pace-Savitsky, K., Perry, R., Kramer, J., Miller, B., & Levenson, R. (2004). Recognition of emotion in the frontal and temporal variants of frontotemporal dementia. *Dementia and Geriatric Cognitive Disorders, 17*(4), 277–281.

Santamaría-García, H., Baez, S., Reyes, P., Santamaría-García, J., Santacruz-Escudero, J., Matallana, D., . . . Ibáñez, A. (2017). A lesion model of envy and Schadenfreude: Legal, deservingness and moral dimensions as revealed by neurodegeneration. *Brain, 140*(12), 3357–3377.

Sasson, N., Tsuchiya, N., Hurley, R., Couture, S. M., Penn, D., Adolphs, R., & Piven, J. (2007). Orienting to social stimuli differentiates social cognitive impairment in autism and schizophrenia. *Neuropsychologia, 45*(11), 2580–2588.

Schroeter, M., Stein, T., Maslowski, N., & Neumann, J. (2009). Neural correlates of Alzhei-mer's disease and mild cognitive impairment: A systematic and quantitative meta-analysis involving 1351 patients. *NeuroImage, 47*(4), 1196–1206.

Seeley, W., Crawford, R., Rascovsky, K., Kramer, J., Weiner, M., Miller, B., & Gorno-Tempini, M. (2008). Frontal paralimbic network atrophy in very mild behavioral variant frontotemporal dementia. *Archives of Neurology, 65*(2), 249–255.

Shany-Ur, T., Poorzand, P., Grossman, S., Growdon, M., Jang, J., Ketelle, R., . . . Rankin, K. (2012). Comprehension of insincere communication in neurodegenerative disease: Lies, sarcasm, and theory of mind. *Cortex, 48*(10), 1329–1341.

Sollberger, M., Rosen, H. J., Shany-Ur, T., Ullah, J., Stanley, C., Laluz, V., . . . Rankin, K. (2014). Neural substrates of socioemotional self-awareness in neurodegenerative disease. *Brain and Behavior, 4*(2), 201–214.

Sollberger, M., Stanley, C., Wilson, S., Gyurak, A., Beckman, V., Growdon, M., . . . Rankin, K. (2009). Neural basis of interpersonal traits in neurodegenerative diseases. *Neuropsychologia, 47*(13), 2812–2827.

Spezio, M., Adolphs, R., Hurley, R., & Piven, J. (2006). Abnormal use of facial information in high-functioning autism. *Journal of autism and developmental disorders, 37*(5), 929–939.

Spoletini, I., Marra, C., Di Iulio, F., Gianni, W., Giubilei, F., Trequattrini, A., . . . Spalletta, G. (2008). Facial emotion recognition deficit in amnestic mild cognitive impairment and Alzheimer disease. *American Journal of Geriatric Psychiatry, 16*, 389–398.

Strikwerda-Brown, C., Ramanan, S., Goldberg, Z.-L., Mothakunnel, A., Hodges, J., Ahmed, R., . . . Irish, M. (2020). The interplay of emotional and social conceptual processes during moral reasoning in frontotemporal dementia – a role for the uncinate fasiculus. *Brain*, 1–32.

Sturm, V., Perry, D., Wood, K., Hua, A., Alcantar, O., Datta, S., . . . Kramer, J. (2017). Prosocial deficits in behavioral variant frontotemporal dementia relate to reward network atrophy. *Brain and Behavior, 7*(10), e00807.

Sturm, V., Rosen, H., Allison, S., Miller, B., & Levenson, R. (2006). Self-conscious emo-tion deficits in frontotemporal lobar degeneration. *Brain, 129*(Pt 9), 2508–2516.

Sturm, V., Sollberger, M., Seeley, W., Rankin, K., Ascher, E., Rosen, H., . . . Levenson, R. (2013a). Role of right pregenual anterior cingulate cortex in self-conscious emotional reactivity. *Social Cognitive and Affective Neuroscience, 8*(4), 468–474.

Sturm, V., Yokoyama, J., Seeley, W., Kramer, J., Miller, B., & Rankin, K. (2013b). Heightened emotional contagion in mild cognitive impairment and Alzheimer's disease is associated with temporal lobe degeneration. *Proceedings of the National Academy of Science, 110*(24), 9944–9949.

Synn, A., Mothakunnel, A., Kumfor, F., Chen, Y., Piguet, O., Hodges, J., & Irish, M. (2018). Mental states in moving shapes: Distinct cortical and subcortical contributions to theory of mind impairments in dementia. *Journal of Alzheimer's Disease, 61*(2), 521–535.

Takeda, A., Sturm, V., Rankin, K., Ketelle, R., Miller, B., & Perry, D. (2019). Relationship turmoil and emotional empathy in frontotemporal dementia. *Alzheimer Disease and Associated Disorders, 33*(3), 260–265.

Taylor, K., Probst, A., Miserez, A., Monsch, A., & Tolnay, M. (2008). Clinical course of neuropathologically confirmed frontal-variant Alzheimer's disease. *Nature Clinical Practice Neurology*, 1–7.

Thompson, P., Hayashi, K., Dutton, R., Chiang, M.-C., Leow, A., Sowell, E., . . . Toga, A. (2007). Tracking Alzheimers' disease. *Annals of the New York Academy of Sciences, 1097*, 183–214.

Thompson, S., Patterson, K., & Hodges, J. (2003). Left/right asymmetry of atrophy in semantic dementia: Behavioral – cognitive implications. *Neurology,* (61), 1196–1203.

Torralva, T., Gleichgerrcht, E., Torres Ardila, M., Roca, M., & Manes, F. (2015). Differential cognitive and affective theory of mind abilities at mild and moderate stages of behavioral variant frontotemporal dementia. *Cognitive and Behavioral Neurology, 28*(2), 63–70.

Torralva, T., Roca, M., Gleichgerrcht, E., Bekinschtein, T., & Manes, F. (2009). A neuropsychological battery to detect specific executive and social cognitive impairments in early frontotemporal dementia. *Brain, 132*(Pt 5), 1299–1309.

Ulugut Erkoyun, H., Groot, C., Heilbron, R., Nelissen, A., van Rossum, J., Jutten, R., . . . Pijnenburg, Y. (2020). A clinical-radiological framework of the right temporal variant of frontotemporal dementia. *Brain, 143*(9), 2831–2843.

Van den Stock, J., & Kumfor, F. (2019). Behavioural variant frontotemporal dementia: At the interface of interoception, emotion and social cognition? *Cortex, 115*, 335–340.

Van Langenhove, T., Leyton, C., Piguet, O., & Hodges, J. (2016). Comparing longitudinal behavior changes in the primary progressive aphasias. *Journal of Alzheimer's Disease, 53*(3), 1033–1042.

Visser, M., Wong, S., Simonetti, S., Hazelton, J., Devenney, E., Ahmed, R., . . . Kumfor, F. (2020). Using a second-person approach to identify disease-specific profiles of social behavior in frontotemporal dementia and Alzheimer's disease. *Cortex, 133*, 236–246.

Wei, G., Irish, M., Hodges, J., Piguet, O., & Kumfor, F. (2019). Disease-specific profiles of apathy in Alzheimer's disease and behavioural-variant frontotemporal dementia differ across the disease course. *Journal of Neurology*, 1–11.

White, S., Coniston, D., Rogers, R., & Frith, U. (2011). Developing the Frith-Happé animations: A quick and objective test of theory of mind for adults with autism. *Autism Research: Official Journal of the International Society for Autism Research, 4*(2), 149–154.

Whitwell, J., Avula, R., Senjem, M., Kantarci, K., Weigand, S., Samikoglu, A., . . . Jack, C. (2010). Gray and white matter water diffusion in the syndromic variants of frontotemporal dementia. *Neurology, 74*(16), 1279–1287.

Wolf, R., Philippi, C., Motzkin, J., Baskaya, M., & Koenigs, M. (2014). Ventromedial pre-frontal cortex mediates visual attention during facial emotion recognition. *Brain, 137*(6), 1772–1780.

Wong, S., Balleine, B., & Kumfor, F. (2018). A new framework for conceptualizing symptoms in frontotemporal dementia: From animal models to the clinic. *Brain, 141*(8), 2245–2254.

Wong, S., Irish, M., O'Callaghan, C., Kumfor, F., Savage, G., Hodges, J., . . . Hornberger, M. (2017). Should I trust you? Learning and memory of social interactions in dementia. *Neuropsychologia, 104*, 157–167.

Wong, S., Strudwick, J., Devenney, E., Hodges, J., Piguet, O., & Kumfor, F. (2019). Frontal variant of Alzheimer's disease masquerading as behavioural-variant frontotemporal dementia: A case study comparison. *Neurocase, 25*(1–2), 48–58.

Woodward, M., Brodaty, H., Boundy, K., Ames, D., Blanch, G., & Balshaw, R. (2010). Does executive impairment define a frontal variant of Alzheimer's disease? *International Psychogeriatrics, 22*(08), 1280–1290.

Woolley, J., Khan, B., Murthy, N., Miller, B., & Rankin, K. (2011). The diagnostic challenge of psychiatric symptoms in neurodegenerative disease: Rates of and risk factors for prior psychiatric diagnosis in patients with early neurodegenerative disease. *The Journal of Clinical Psychiatry, 72*(2), 126–133.

Yi, Z., Zhao, P., Zhang, H., Shi, Y., Shi, H., Zhong, J., & Pan, P. (2020). Theory of mind in Alzheimer's disease and amnestic mild cognitive impairment: A meta-analysis. *Neurological Science, 41*(5), 1027–1039.

Chapter 8

Social cognition in neurodegenerative diseases

Huntington's disease, Parkinson's disease and multiple sclerosis

Katherine Osborne-Crowley, Cynthia Honan and Helen M Genova

There is increasing interest in social cognitive dysfunction in neurodegenerative diseases that compromise the subcortical regions of the brain and/or the neural connections involving the brain's frontal-striatal networks. These diseases, which include Huntington's disease (HD), Parkinson's disease (PD) and multiple sclerosis (MS), affect the brain structures and networks involved in social communication as a consequence of their neuropathology. In the current chapter, we will review the types of social cognitive dysfunction that have been most studied in these three disorders, including difficulties in emotion recognition and theory of mind (ToM) abilities. We will also review contributing factors to this dysfunction, how this may impact on everyday functioning, and provide future directions for social cognition research in patients with HD, PD and MS.

What are HD, PD and MS?

HD is an inherited neurodegenerative movement disorder that is caused by an expanded CAG trinucleotide repetition on chromosome 4. Characterised by progressive motor dysfunction, cognitive decline and affective disturbance (Walker, 2007), its worldwide prevalence is 2.71 per 100,000 (Pringsheim et al., 2012). With no available effective treatment, patients typically die within 15 years of disease onset (Folstein, 1989). The presence of unequivocal motor signs determines disease onset, yet subtle cognitive and affective symptoms may occur 10 to 20 years before the appearance of these motor signs, in what is known as the prodromal disease stage (Paulsen et al., 2008). The average age of onset is 40 years, although there is large variation with onset known to also occur in childhood or in late adulthood (Myers, 2004). In HD studies, groups of participants are often divided into *manifest HD*, those who have a diagnosis of HD based on the presence of unequivocal motor signs, and *pre-manifest HD*, those individuals who have a positive genetic test for HD but are not yet exhibiting unequivocal motor signs. Neurodegeneration in HD begins in the *striatum* decades before symptoms appear, affecting functioning

DOI: 10.4324/9781003027034-8

of corticostriatal circuits from early in the disease course (Aylward et al., 2000; Lawrence, Sahakian, & Robbins, 1998). While striatal atrophy continues to be a prominent feature as the disease progresses, there is also increasing dysfunction and neuronal death in subcortical regions, the cerebral cortex and white matter (Vonsattel, Keller, & Ramirez, 2011). Although the clinical diagnosis of HD relies on the manifestation of motor symptoms, the cognitive and behavioural changes are not only debilitating but also are highly associated with functional decline and increased family burden (Hamilton et al., 2003; Williams et al., 2010).

PD is a diverse neurodegenerative movement disorder characterised by rigidity, tremor, bradykinesia and impaired postural reflexes. While traditionally thought to predominantly affect motor functioning, non-motor symptoms, including cognitive impairments, sleep problems and neuropsychiatric symptoms, are not only present early in the disease course but also are known to significantly affect everyday functioning (Poewe, 2008). The onset of PD typically occurs age 65 to 70 years, although onset can occur before the age of 40 years in 5% of cases (Tysnes & Storstein, 2017). Its prevalence ranges from 100 to 200 per 100,000 people, and it occurs slightly more frequently in men than women. Both genetic and/or environmental factors may contribute to disease onset. PD arises from the depletion of dopaminergic neurons in the *substantia nigra*, resulting in abnormal functioning of the nigrostriatal and mesocortical dopaminergic systems (McNamara & Durso, 2018). Whereas the nigrostriatal system terminates in the *striatum*, the mesocortical system terminates in the *ventral striatum, limbic system* and cortical areas of the brain, particularly the *motor* and *prefrontal* areas. While PD in its milder form may involve impaired executive function and memory due to reduced activity of the brain's dopamine-mediated fronto-striatal circuit (Chiaravalloti et al., 2014; Kudlicka, Clare, & Hindle, 2011), in PD with dementia (PDD), more extensive cognitive impairments are usually present, the first sign of which is attributable to the extended involvement of posterior cortical regions (O'Callaghan & Lewis, 2017).

Multiple sclerosis (MS) is a chronic autoimmune disease of the central nervous system, involving demyelination and inflammation (Weinshenker, 1996). The disease course is highly variable, with most individuals first diagnosed with a relapsing-remitting disease subtype in which periods of neuropathology and neurologic deficits occur, followed by episodes of little to no disease activity. However, many patients transition to a progressive disease course in which neurological deterioration occurs without suspension. Still others are diagnosed with a progressive disease course at onset in which there is only neurologic deterioration (Mahad, Trapp, & Lassmann, 2015). The typical age of onset is late-20s to mid-30s, although pediatric MS is possible. Over 2.2 million people have MS worldwide (NMSS: Wallin et al., 2019). While the cause of MS is largely unknown, both genetic and non-genetic (environmental; viral infection) factors are likely contributors. Individuals with MS experience a host of physical, cognitive and emotional symptoms. For many, the first noticeable and presenting symptoms are physical (spasticity, numbness or weakness). In addition to physical symptoms, 40–70% will experience cognitive impairments (Chiaravalloti & DeLuca, 2008). Most will also report debilitating mental and physical fatigue, which may further affect their daily functioning. Finally, many also report worsening mood symptomatology, including depression and anxiety, over the course of their disease.

In addition to motor, cognitive and affective symptoms, impairments in social cognition are common in HD, PD and MS. These impairments include difficulty in recognising emotions from the face, voice or body (Bora, Velakoulis, & Walterfang, 2016; Coundouris, Adams, Grainger, & Henry, 2019; Cotter et al., 2016; de Gelder, Van den Stock, de Diego Balaguer, & Bachoud-Lévi, 2008; Zarotti, Fletcher, & Simpson, 2019), impaired ToM (Coundouris, Adams, & Henry et al., 2020; Eddy & Rickards, 2015), alterations in the way emotions are experienced (Ille, Holl et al., 2011; Péron et al., 2012), emotional blunting (Craufurd et al., 2001; Leroi et al., 2014), impaired emotion regulation and emotional awareness (Ille et al., 2016; Zarotti, Simpson, Fletcher, Squitieri, & Migliore, 2018; Zarotti et al., 2019) and a tendency to draw incorrect inferences from social situations (Pell et al., 2014; Snowden et al., 2003). In HD, impairments in emotion recognition are widely considered to be one of the earliest signs of the disease, typically occurring years before motor signs appear (Paulsen, 2011). These impairments are subtle and selective at first but worsen as the disease progresses. In PD and MS, there is also evidence that social cognitive difficulties can occur early in the disease course (Kraemer, Herold, Uekermann, Kis, Wiltfang et al., 2013; Palmeri et al., 2017) and tend to worsen with disease severity (Coundouris et al., 2019; Dulau et al., 2017; Isernia et al., 2019).

Emotion recognition

The most widely studied aspect of social cognition in HD, PD and MS is the ability to recognise emotions from facial expressions. Recent meta-analyses provide a useful overview of the extent to which emotion recognition ability may be impaired in these disorders. In HD, Bora, Velakoulis et al. (2016) summarised the results of 18 studies incorporating 413 participants with *manifest* HD and found reduced performance across all basic emotions, with the largest effect sizes found for anger, disgust and fear. On the other hand, in participants with *premanifest* HD (1,502 participants across 17 studies), reduced performance was found only for anger, disgust, fear and sadness, and with much smaller effect sizes than those seen in *manifest* HD. In PD, Coundouris et al. (2019) presented the findings of 79 studies incorporating 4,148 participants and found reduced performance across all basic emotion types, with the largest effect sizes found for anger, fear, sadness and disgust. Cotter et al. (2016) summarised results from 13 studies incorporating 473 participants with MS and found reduced ability to recognise anger, fear and sadness. In another study with MS patients, however, Bora, Özakbaş, Velakoulis, and Walterfang (2016) found reduced performance across all basic emotion types based on the results from 17 studies incorporating 596 participants, with the largest effects found for anger, fear, sadness and surprise. Overall, these meta-analyses not only highlight that emotion recognition difficulties are an important feature of all three disorders, but also that the recognition of *negative* facial emotions appears to be particularly impaired.

Many authors have argued that there is a *specific impairment* in the processing of negatively valenced facial emotion expressions in these disorders, implying that the brain regions subserving the recognition of negative emotions are more affected than those subserving positive emotions (Chalah & Ayache, 2017; Coundouris et al., 2019; Kordsachia, Labuschagne, & Stout, 2017). However, it also has been argued that negative expressions in typical emotion recognition tasks are more difficult to recognise, which may account for the greater impairment (Montagne, Kessels, De Haan, & Perrett, 2007). This difficulty is attributable to the shared similar features in negative emotions that make these emotions more difficult to distinguish; and conversely, the high salience of happiness attributable to its distinctiveness as the only positive emotion. To account for the differential levels of difficulty, some studies have varied the intensity of emotional expressions with mixed results. While in one study of PD, difficulty in recognising happiness did emerge when the expression was displayed at lower intensity (Buxton, MacDonald, & Tippett, 2013), no such impairment was found in a HD study, even after accounting for difficulty (Montagne et al., 2006). The question of whether emotion recognition difficulties in HD, PD and MS are genuinely unique to negative emotions needs to be more systematically examined, either by controlling for recognition difficulty across emotions or by including more positive emotions in emotion recognition tests.

There is also evidence for impaired emotion recognition ability in other modalities, including vocal prosody and body language. In their meta-analysis, Bora, Velakoulis et al. (2016) found that, similarly to facial emotion recognition, *manifest* HD participants were less able to accurately detect basic emotion types through voice prosody, with the greatest effect sizes found for anger, disgust and fear, smaller effect sizes for surprised and sad voices, and the smallest effect size for happy voices. In PD, two meta-analyses have moderate-to-large effect sizes for the reduced ability to recognise negative emotions through voice prosody, with smaller effect sizes reported for positive emotions (Coundouris et al., 2019; Gray & Tickle-Degnen, 2010). Preliminary evidence also suggests that there is reduced ability to detect emotions through voice prosody in MS (Beatty, Orbelo, Sorocco, & Ross, 2003; Kraemer, Herold, Uekermann, Kis, Daum et al., 2013), with one study indicating these impairments may be specific only to anger and fear (Kraemer, Herold, Uekermann, Kis, Daum et al., 2013). While there is negligible research examining emotion recognition via body language in MS, there is preliminary evidence of such difficulties from two small studies in HD (de Gelder et al., 2008; Zarotti et al., 2019). In PD, there is some evidence of such difficulties based on the findings of one study where individuals with PD were found not to have a reduced ability to describe communicative gestures (Jaywant, Wasserman, Kemppainen, Neargarder, & Cronin-Golomb, 2016).

As indicated above, there is much support for the existence of emotion recognition impairments across all three diseases. However, it should be noted that such findings have not been consistently demonstrated. In HD, while reduced emotion recognition ability has been found consistently in *manifest* individuals (Kordsachia et al., 2017), results have been mixed for *premanifest* individuals, with some studies finding no such difficulties (e.g. van Asselen et al., 2012). This is likely because deficits are more subtle at this early disease stage and occur at lower prevalence. In PD, several studies have suggested intact emotion recognition abilities (e.g., Wabnegger et al., 2015). Further, whereas some studies have found difficulty recognising emotion from *both* prosody and facial expressions (e.g., Yip, Lee, Ho, Tsang, & Li, 2003), others have detected only select difficulties in prosody (Kan, Kawamura, Hasegawa, Mochizuki, & Nakamura, 2002), and yet others have reported select difficulties in facial emotion recognition (Clark, Neargarder, & Cronin-Golomb, 2008). In MS, at least five studies to date have found intact emotion recognition abilities (Di Bitonto et al., 2011; Jehna et al., 2010, 2011; Passamonti et al., 2009; Pinto et al., 2012). These findings may be owing to participants being in the relapsing-remitting disease course (or having a "clinically isolated syndrome") or being early in disease progression. This mixed evidence may, in part, be an indicator that not all individuals with these disorders exhibit impairments in the ability to recognise emotions. Additionally, the mixed results may be owing to a complex combination of differences in sample characteristics (e.g., comorbid depression, the use of medications and disease severity/progression) and research methodology, particularly with regard to the type of emotion perception task used. More systematic evidence about the prevalence of emotion perception impairments in these diseases is needed.

What mechanisms underpin emotion processing problems in subcortical disorders?

While emotion recognition difficulties are well documented among HD, PD and MS patients, the underlying mechanisms remain unclear. Next we explore potential mechanisms of these difficulties.

Relationship to disease progression, general cognitive difficulties and general face processing abilities

In HD, emotion recognition difficulties are typically associated with disease progression (e.g. Tabrizi et al., 2013). Bora, Velakoulis et al. (2016) in their recent meta-analysis also found that emotion recognition difficulties are associated with greater illness duration, disease burden, motor symptoms, age and

CAG repeat length. Further, in *premanifest* HD, the emergence of emotion recognition difficulties is associated with a higher likelihood of motor onset of HD within the next five years. In MS, there is evidence to suggest that although emotion recognition deficits *can* occur early in the disease course, disease progression is a likely contributor, with those later in the disease course being more likely to exhibit deficits. This is suggested by studies that show a relationship between increasing neuropathology and emotion recognition ability in MS (e.g. Pitteri et al., 2019). Further, those with a progressive disease course appear to show more difficulties compared to those with relapsing-remitting MS (Dulau et al., 2017). There is also research that indicates emotion recognition difficulties are associated with increasing physical disability in MS (Prochnow et al., 2011).

Severity of PD is also likely to be associated with emotion recognition ability. Using a sensitive indicator of disease progression, Marneweck and Hammond (2014) found large reductions in emotion recognition ability on both discrimination and labelling tasks in high-severity PD, but negligible reduction in low-severity PD. Coundouris et al. (2019) in their meta-analysis found that neither disease duration nor severity accounted variance in emotion recognition ability. However, given prior studies have predominantly included individuals with mild-to-moderate levels of motor symptomology and/or used a severity rating scale thought to be insensitive to broader elements of disease progression, the association with disease severity in this meta-analysis is likely masked (Argaud, Vérin, Sauleau, & Grandjean, 2018).

Whether emotion recognition impairments in HD, PD and MS are, at least partially, due to broad cognitive impairments has been the subject of debate (Bäckman, Robins-Wahlin, Lundin, Ginovart, & Farde, 1997; Paulsen, 2011). Individuals with HD and MS typically experience changes in a wide range of cognitive functions including attention, working memory, executive functions and inhibitory control (e.g., Chiaravalloti & DeLuca, 2008; Paulsen, 2011), which may contribute to emotion recognition abilities. Indeed, a meta-analysis showed that emotion recognition performance in HD was significantly related to verbal fluency, a domain of functioning that is thought to be sensitive to early cognitive decline in HD (Bora, Velakoulis et al., 2016). An alternative meta-analysis in MS has also showed general cognitive abilities to be related to emotion recognition ability (Bora, Özakbaş et al., 2016). Evidence of an association between emotion recognition and general cognitive functioning, particularly for learning and memory, verbal fluency and executive functioning has also been found in PD (e.g., Hipp, Diederich, Pieria, & Vaillant, 2014). There is a need for future research to elucidate how much general cognitive decline contributes to poor emotion recognition across these three diseases.

General face processing deficits linked to perceptual abnormalities might also contribute to facial emotion recognition difficulties. General face processing ability is typically measured with a test of facial identity recognition such as the Benton Facial Recognition Task (BFRT). In both HD and MS, while the majority of emotion recognition studies that have included a test of general face processing have found no impairments on these tests (e.g. Di Bitonto et al., 2011; Henley et al., 2012; Pinto et al., 2012), emotion recognition abilities have been found to be related to performance on the BFRT (Beatty et al., 1989; Bora, Velakoulis et al., 2016; Di Bitonto et al., 2011). In PD, configural face processing has been found to be both impaired and related to the ability to recognise negative emotions (Narme, Bonnet, Dubois, & Chaby, 2011). A recent study has also shown poorer face discrimination ability is related to slower reaction times on dynamic emotion recognition tasks in PD (Ho et al., 2020). These findings indicate that facial processing difficulties may partly undermine the ability to recognise facial emotions in HD, PD and MS.

Further, given that oculomotor impairments are a common feature of HD, PD and MS, some studies have used eye tracking to investigate whether abnormal visual scanning patterns contribute to emotion recognition difficulty. In HD, van Asselen et al. (2012) found no differences between HD patients and controls on fixations or fixation duration for the eyes, nose and mouth regions of emotional faces. However, Kordsachia, Labuschagne, and Stout (2018) found that participants with HD spent less time looking at the eyes and nose/mouth regions and made fewer fixations on these regions. Further, visual scanning of the eye area predicted the participants' performance on an emotion recognition task. In PD, while facial emotion recognition impairments have been linked to visuospatial abilities (e.g., Hipp et al., 2014), only one study has used eye tracking to measure visual processing. This study found a reduced number of fixations and time spent fixated on upper facial regions was associated with reduced ability to recognise sad faces (Clark, Neargarder, & Cronin-Golomb, 2010). To date, eye tracking has not been used to examine facial affect recognition in MS, but given the visual impairment frequently reported in this population, such an investigation would be worthwhile.

In summary, there is evidence that non-social cognitive dysfunction and perceptual abnormalities (i.e., face processing) may contribute to, but not fully explain, social cognitive difficulties in HD, PD and MS.

The role of motor impairment

Simulation theories (or embodiment theories) of emotion recognition posit that there is a reciprocal relationship between how emotions are expressed in the face and body and how the emotions of others are interpreted. For instance, when perceiving emotional expressions of others, people tend to subtly mimic the expression, and this sensorimotor simulation is believed to facilitate recognition of the other persons' emotion (Hess & Fischer, 2013; Wood, Rychlowska, Korb, & Niedenthal, 2016) (see Chapter 1 for further discussion). Motor impairments are a key feature of HD, PD and MS and, thus, may contribute to poor emotion recognition by compromising this mimicry mechanism (Kordsachia et al., 2017; Prenger & MacDonald, 2018). Indeed, hypomimia (the reduced expression of emotion in the face) is one of the most frequent and distinctive motor symptoms of PD (Bologna et al., 2013). Impairments in the production of emotional facial expressions have also been shown in HD (Hayes, Stevenson, & Coltheart, 2009). Further, in HD, a number of studies have found a relationship between patients' abilities to produce emotional facial expressions (for instance voluntary imitation of a facial expression) and their accuracy in identifying emotional expressions (Ricciardi et al., 2017; Trinkler, de Langavant, & Bachoud-Lévi, 2013; Trinkler et al., 2017), providing evidence that emotion recognition may be linked to a motoric mechanism. In PD, however, Bologna et al. (2016) found impairments in both expressivity and recognition in patients but found no correlation between the two.

Spontaneous facial mimicry and its relationship to emotion recognition has also been examined in a few studies in HD and PD. Spontaneous facial mimicry is the automatic activation of facial muscles congruent with the observed facial expression, measured using electromyography (EMG), which has been shown in healthy controls to facilitate recognition of the observed expression (Oberman, Winkielman, & Ramachandran, 2007; Ponari, Conson, D'Amico, Grossi, & Trojano, 2012). Two EMG studies in PD patients found decreased mimicry overall but there were particularly profound difficulties in the mimicry in the zygomaticus (smile) muscle of happy faces (Argaud et al., 2016; Livingstone, Vezer, McGarry, Lang, & Russo, 2016). While Livingstone et al. (2016) found an association between mimicry of happy faces and response times for emotional ratings, Argaud et al. (2016) found a relationship between the mimicry and recognition of happy faces. In HD, two studies have found reduced facial mimicry to emotional faces (Kordsachia, Labuschagne, Andrews, & Stout, 2018; Trinkler et al., 2017), but only one of these found a correlation with emotion recognition ability (Trinkler et al., 2017). The ability to produce facial emotional expressions or spontaneous mimicry of the expressions of others has not been examined in MS. The simulation theory of emotion recognition also posits that physiological responsivity is an important part of the simulation process, which helps people identify the emotions of others. Although physiological responsivity (measured through skin conductance, heart rate, pupil dilation and startle blink reflexes) and their relationship to emotion recognition have been extensively studied in other clinical groups, it has not been widely investigated in patients with HD, PD or MS.

This evidence suggests that motor impairments affecting the ability to produce facial emotional expressions may be a contributing factor in emotion recognition impairments in PD and HD, although this body of research is still in its infancy. One problem with the simulation theory in relation to HD, specifically, is that it does not account for the early detectable emotion recognition deficits that might occur prior to any motor symptoms (Yitzhak et al., 2020). On the other hand, dysfunction in motor mental representations may precede pronounced motor symptoms, and therefore may underlie early emotion perception impairments (Kordsachia et al., 2017). This hypothesis warrants further investigation.

Relationship to neuropsychiatric symptoms

Emotion recognition difficulties may also be associated with neuropsychiatric syndromes that affect general emotional functioning, such as apathy and depression. Emotion recognition may be mechanistically linked with emotional apathy because an inability to affectively engage with social rewards may reduce motivation for social behaviour as well as preclude the proper processing of social stimuli such as facial expressions (Osborne-Crowley et al., 2019). Indeed, an association between apathy and emotion recognition has been demonstrated in PD (Martínez-Corral et al., 2010) and in HD (Kempnich et al., 2018; Osborne-Crowley et al., 2019) but remains unexamined in MS. Depression, which is known to be associated with emotion recognition difficulty in the general population (Dalili, Penton-Voak, Harmer, & Munafò, 2015), may also contribute to the emotion recognition difficulties in neurological patient groups. In PD, Gray and Tickle-Degnen (2010) compared emotion recognition performance reported in studies of PD patients with comorbid depressive symptoms with those reported in studies of patients with normal depression scores and concluded that emotion recognition deficits occur regardless of the level of depressive symptoms present. Although some studies have reported a correlation between depression and social cognitive abilities in MS (Ciampi et al., 2018; Genova, Lancaster et al., 2020), a meta-analysis by Bora, Özakbaş et al. (2016) concluded that emotion recognition difficulties occur regardless of depression status. This link has not been systematically examined in HD (Kordsachia et al., 2017). Thus, while there is evidence for an association between emotion recognition and apathy, there is little evidence for a similar relationship with depressive symptoms. In summary, a number of mechanisms that might underlie emotion perception impairments have been explored in HD, PD and MS. It is likely that a range of non-specific factors (e.g., cognitive dysfunction, visual processing, neuropsychiatric symptomology) combine with specific brain pathology factors (discussed later) to produce emotion recognition impairments in these disorders. It is also likely that these factors intensify and interact as the diseases progress, contributing to worsening emotion recognition performance.

Ecological validity in emotion recognition assessment

The vast majority of studies that have examined emotion recognition in patients with HD, PD and MS have used static images of stereotypical facial emotions expressed at full intensity (e.g., the Ekman faces; Ekman & Friesen, 1976). However, real emotions are expressed dynamically and often fleetingly and occur within a social context where multiple cues are available to help a person interpret an emotion (Osborne-Crowley, 2020). Further, emotion recognition tasks have typically required participants to assess emotions in one modality or another (i.e., face, voice or body language), whereas in everyday settings people have access to information in multiple modalities simultaneously. Ecologically valid tests of emotion recognition attempt to more closely replicate the ways emotions are expressed in real social settings. In such tasks, because patients have multiple sources of information to guide their perceptions, they may actually be less impaired compared with more typical emotion recognition tasks. For instance, Baez et al. (2015) has found that while emotion recognition performance is reduced in tasks using decontextualised faces, it is not reduced on a video-based test, The Awareness of Social Inference Test (TASIT; McDonald, Flanagan, & Rollins, 2017) among HD patients. Similarly, Kan et al. (2002) found that PD patients were better at recognising emotions from dynamic compared with statically displayed faces. If patients can successfully use dynamic, multi-modal and contextual information to compensate for emotion recognition impairments, it may mean that the impairments measured on typical emotion recognition tasks have little impact in real-life social settings (Pell et al., 2014). However, the extent to which compensation may occur through the use of external cues warrants further research.

Further, while it is reasonable to assume that deficits identified on more ecologically valid emotion recognition tasks will be more predictive of real-world deficits, this has not been empirically tested in HD, PD or MS. In HD, some studies have demonstrated impairments in emotion recognition on TASIT among *manifest* patients (Larsen et al., 2015; Philpott, Andrews, Staios, Churchyard, & Fisher, 2016), while others have not (Baez et al., 2015). No impairments on emotion recognition on TASIT have been demonstrated in *premanifest* HD (Larsen et al., 2015). While impairments in progressive MS have been demonstrated on this task (Genova & McDonald, 2020), none have been found in PD (Pell et al., 2014). Based on findings from TASIT, there is some evidence that emotion recognition impairments may extend to real-world impairments in PD and MS, but further studies should seek to explicitly test this link.

Theory of mind

Theory of mind (ToM) refers to the ability to understand the content of another persons' mind as distinct from the content of one's own mind. It is another important aspect of social cognitive functioning that may be impaired in HD, PD and MS. ToM is often divided in two component processes, *cognitive ToM*, used to infer other's beliefs, intentions and desires, and *affective ToM*, used to understand others' emotional states and feelings.

Cognitive ToM

Individuals with HD, PD and MS have well-documented difficulties on tests of cognitive ToM (Bora, Velakoulis et al., 2016; Coundouris et al., 2020; Cotter et al., 2016). Cognitive ToM is often assessed using tasks containing simple picture or written vignettes, which require a person to ascribe 'false beliefs' to story characters by recognising that the characters may possess incomplete or erroneous knowledge about the situation. One particularly common false belief task is the Faux Pas test. In this test, participants receive all the information needed to understand a given social situation. However, one character in the story who does not have the same full information commits a social faux pas (i.e., they say/do something unintentionally awkward or hurtful) and participants are required to make judgements about the intentionality of the character. Reduced performance on the Faux Pas test has been found in individuals with *manifest* HD in a meta-analysis (Bora, Velakoulis et al., 2016) and in one study in individuals with *premanifest* HD (Eddy & Rickards, 2015). The Faux Pas test has also been used in multiple studies in PD, with one meta-analysis study showing moderate effects for reduced performance (Bora, Walterfang, & Velakoulis, 2015). Interestingly, several studies indicate that while individuals with PD remained capable of detecting inappropriate remarks, they were unable to interpret them correctly (Kawamura & Koyama, 2007; Narme et al., 2013). In MS, based on the results of a meta-analysis examining seven studies that reported a small effect for reduced performance ($g = 0.26$), the sensitivity of the Faux Pas test has been questioned in this population (Cotter et al., 2016). However, more recent studies have reported reduced performance in MS (e.g. Isernia et al., 2019). Interestingly, Isernia et al. (2019) found that those with progressive, but not relapsing-remitting, MS were impaired on the task. A similar relationship was recently reported by Ignatova et al. (2020) who found poorer task performance in those with higher disability scores. This same association between disease course and reduced performance on the Faux Pas task has been noted in PD (Péron et al., 2009). Hence, this task may be more sensitive to more advanced disease states.

Accurately understanding such social inferences requires ToM and is highly important for successful social interaction. Other tasks similar to the false belief tasks have also been used to assess the participant's ability to understand a social inference, such as a joke, lie, sarcastic remark or figure of speech. The Strange Stories task (Happé, 1994) consists of a series of vignettes whereby the participant must understand a particular type of social inference. Individuals with MS are reported to have reduced ability recognising a range of social inference types (Isernia et al., 2019; Ouellet, 2010). One small study in HD has found reduced performance on the Strange Stories task in *manifest* HD patients (Bayliss et al., 2019). In PD, while one study has detected reduced performance on this task (Díez-Cirarda, 2015), recent studies have failed to detect such difficulties (e.g., Del Prete et al., 2020).

In summary, all three disorders exhibit reduced ability to utilise cognitive ToM, as assessed across multiple tasks such as false belief tasks and those which require understanding of social inference. While studies utilizing these tests have provided mixed evidence of impairments across all three populations, they have suggested that certain elements of cognitive ToM are affected, and that these abilities may become worse as the neurological disease progress over time.

Affective ToM

While related to emotion recognition ability, affective ToM is a broader concept that extends to the ability to understand the feelings of others. The Reading in the Mind Eyes Test (RMET; Baron-Cohen, Wheelwright, Hill, Raste, & Plumb, 2001) is a commonly used test requiring participants to infer complex mental states (e.g., serious, ashamed, alarmed, irritated) from viewing photos of the eye region of a face. A meta-analysis summarising the results of eight studies in a total of 159 *manifest* HD participants found evidence for a significantly reduced performance on the RMET (Bora, Velakoulis et al., 2016). Mason et al. (2015) further found that performance on the RMET deteriorated significantly with disease phase (early, moderate and late-stage HD). Since this meta-analysis, additional studies have found reduced performance on the RMET in participants with *manifest* HD (Lagravinese et al., 2017) and *premanifest* HD (e.g. Eddy & Rickards, 2015). Although Mason et al. (2015) and Larsen et al. (2015) did not find reduced performance in *premanifest* participants, they did find that performance on the RMET correlated with disease burden and estimated time to onset of motor symptoms. In PD, a meta-analysis summarising the results of 10 studies found evidence of reduced performance on the RMET, but no relationship with disease severity (Bora et al., 2015). Finally, in MS, RMET is impaired relative to controls according to a meta-analysis summarizing five studies (Cotter et al., 2016). Thus, the RMET is sensitive to changes in affective ToM across HD, PD and MS. In HD, but not in PD, it appears to be related to disease progression.

Empathy

Empathy, a construct related to ToM, is typically measured using self-report questionnaires. Empathy is often divided into emotional and cognitive components. Whereas *cognitive empathy* refers to one's ability to *understand* how another person is feeling, *emotional empathy* refers to the ability to *resonate with* or feel how another person is feeling. In HD, there is mixed evidence for changes in empathy. Clinically, patients are often described as being self-centered and as lacking sympathy or empathy (Snowden et al., 2003). In *manifest* HD, two studies have found reduced self-reported cognitive but not emotional empathy (Eddy, Mahalingappa, & Rickards, 2014; Maurage et al., 2016), yet other studies have found no reductions at all (e.g. Trinkler et al., 2013). In participants with *premanifest* HD, although some reduced self-reported emotional empathy has been found, it is cognitive empathy where the largest reductions are reported (Eddy & Rickards, 2015). Interestingly, self-reported cognitive empathy in this study was related to RMET performance. Other studies, however, have found no reduced empathy in premanifest HD (Maurage et al., 2016).

In PD, no overall reduction in self-reported empathy was found in a recent meta-analysis (Coundouris et al., 2020). However, in one specific study in advanced PD participants, self-reported reductions in cognitive, but not affective, empathy were found (Schmidt, Paschen, Deuschl, & Witt, 2017). In MS, changes in empathy are not well understood and studies examining empathy have been highly inconsistent. Specifically, whereas some studies have found low levels of self-reported empathy (Kraemer, Herold, Uekermann, Kis, Wiltfang et al., 2013), others have found high levels of self-reported empathy (Banati et al., 2010.

Thus, it appears that across HD, PD and MS, findings of reduced empathy are not consistently reported. An important consideration in the use of self-report scales is that patients may have impaired insight, a reported feature of all three conditions (e.g., Benedict, Priore, Miller, Munschauer, & Jacobs, 2001; Ho et al., 2006; Sitek, Sławek, & Wieczorek, 2008). Additionally, the presence of alexithymia (an inability to understand one's own emotions), mood disturbances and cognitive impairments all might contribute to inaccurate self-reflection on questionnaire measures. Given the discrepancy between self- and other- reported empathy (e.g., Benedict et al., 2001), scientists should begin to explore objective methods to assess empathy.

ToM and executive functioning

In HD, cognitive ToM has been consistently linked to executive function (e.g., Eddy et al., 2014). Indeed, a 2016 meta-analysis found a significant relationship across a number of studies with verbal fluency in HD (Bora, Velakoulis et al., 2016). In one study, difficulties in the attribution of intention were ameliorated when deficits in cognitive flexibility were controlled for (Brüne et al., 2011). However, a published case study has indicated that impairments in second-order cognitive ToM can be present in the early stages of HD when performance on cognitive tests are within the normal range (Caillaud et al., 2020). Similarly, Eddy and Rickards (2015) found reduced performance among *premanifest* participants in three ToM tasks despite intact executive skills. This evidence suggests that while a proportion of ToM impairment in *manifest* HD may be attributable to executive impairments, ToM impairments can emerge independently earlier in disease course, potentially representing a specific social cognitive deficit. As in HD, a meta-analysis in patients with PD found that reductions in ToM were related to poorer verbal fluency (Bora et al., 2015). Other studies have found relationships between ToM and working memory, inhibition and cognitive flexibility (Del Prete et al., 2020; Monetta et al., 2009; Santangelo et al., 2012). In MS, a relationship has also been found between inhibition ability and ToM (Dulau et al., 2017; Genova & McDonald, 2020).

The interaction between executive functioning and ToM is likely highly complex and may depend on the type of ToM task being used. In traumatic brain injury for example, differential relationships between ToM and executive functioning have been detected depending on whether the task involves mere comprehension of information and making judgements about this information or production of speech as required for social interaction (Honan et al., 2015; McDonald et al., 2014). This delineation is yet to be explored in HD, PD and MS. Case 1 (Box 8.1) illustrates the possible unique interaction between the ability to inhibit self-referential thoughts and the ability to understand the perspective of another that may affect communication.

Box 8.1   Case 1: LN: Adult with MS

History:

LN is a 60-year-old woman with primary progressive MS. She had phoned a researcher to make enquiries about participating in an MS research study.

Presentation:

The researcher found LN to be particularly chatty. She spoke at length about her differential diagnosis difficulties, her past breast cancer and her son who was studying abroad in Canada. Obtaining responses to essential screening questions proved challenging. Four weeks later, the researcher ran into LN at an MS support group, to which LN announced, "You're the person who uses us as lab rats". While LN was previously seen by the researcher as very "chatty" and someone who was easy to develop a good rapport with, it now appeared that LN was rather "disinhibited". Her "blunt" comments continued throughout the MS support group session. LN displayed a pattern of behaviour that included reduced ability to take on new information that challenged her negative beliefs (e.g., that rehabilitation strategies would be of any help). There were also clear difficulties in her ability to judge how her comments would be interpreted by others and in adjusting her responses so that they were "socially acceptable".

Opinion:

While LN's behaviours showed evidence of ToM difficulties, her behaviours also demonstrated the potential for these difficulties to interact with executive processes (e.g., inhibition and cognitive flexibility) and undermine her ability to form meaningful relationships.

3.4 Ecological validity of ToM assessment

The ecological validity of ToM tasks such as the Strange Stories task can be criticised because they do not reflect communication in real-life contexts. TASIT, a dynamic video-based task that assesses the ability to understand the use of sarcasm, is an example of a more ecologically valid task of social inference. Reduced TASIT performance on sarcasm items has been found in *manifest*, but not *premanifest* HD (Larsen et al., 2015; Philpott et al., 2016). Reduced TASIT performance has also been demonstrated in PD; however, this was found only for items embedded in contextually enriched environments (Pell et al., 2014). Individuals with relapsing-remitting and progressive MS have also demonstrated reduced performance on TASIT (Genova et al., 2016; Genova, Lancaster et al., 2020), on both a sub-test in which they are given contextual information which should make interpretation easier, as well as a sub-test in which that information is not provided. Reduced performance on alternative, ecologically valid tasks assessing ToM including the Movie for the Assessment of Social Cognition (Pöttgen et al., 2013) and the Virtual Assessment of Mentalizing Ability has also been found (Lancaster et al., 2019). Taken together these findings suggest that individuals with HD, PD and MS may show reduced performance in ecological ToM tasks. This indicates that, in contrast to emotion perception where difficulties in everyday contexts appear unlikely (due to the ability to use contextual cues), difficulties in ToM appear more apparent in everyday contexts. ToM impairments will, therefore, likely impact the social functioning in those with HD, PD and MS by leading to misunderstandings and challenges in navigating the social world.

4. Neurobiological basis of social cognition in HD, PD and MS

HD, PD and MS are different in terms of both their neuropathological mechanisms and symptomatology. What is common is the disruption to regions commonly referred to as "the social brain network". These disruptions can be structural (assessed via measures of atrophy, lesion load and damage to white matter) or functional (assessed via measures of brain activity or functional connectivity) in nature.

One of the most widely examined brain regions underlying emotion recognition is the *amygdala*, and both structural and functional disruption to the amygdala have been studied across the three disorders. Regarding functional disruptions, aberrant amygdala activity and connectivity appears to be associated with emotion recognition across all three populations of HD, PD and MS (Dogan et al., 2014; Passamonti et al., 2009; Tessitore et al., 2002). In terms of structural damage, reduced grey matter of the *amygdala* is associated with impairments in the recognition of expressions in both patients with HD (Kipps et al., 2007) and PD (Ibarretxe-Bilbao et al., 2009). In MS, cortical lesion volume in the *amygdala* is reported to be predictive of emotion perception deficits (Pitteri et al., 2019). Hence, both structural and functional damage to the amygdala appears to play a role in emotion recognition difficulties across all three populations.

Damage in other subcortical regions may also contribute to emotion recognition difficulties. Reduced activation of the *striatum* is related to emotion perception deficits in both *manifest* (Dogan et al., 2014) and *premanifest* HD (Hennenlotter et al., 2004; Novak et al., 2012) as well as PD (Heller et al., 2018). Grey matter volume of the striatum is also related to emotion perception deficits in HD (Harrington et al., 2014; Henley et al., 2008, Scahill et al., 2013). Finally, the striatum is also thought to play a role in emotion recognition in both HD and PD through its functional connectivity with other structures involved in emotion recognition (e.g., Argaud et al., 2018; Dogan et al., 2014).

Frontal damage, both structural and functional, is also reported to be related to emotion recognition impairments across all three disorders. Decreased activation of the *ventrolateral prefrontal cortex* has been found in MS patients who are impaired in facial affect recognition compared to unimpaired patients (Krause et al., 2009). Interestingly, *enhanced* activation of frontal regions has been reported in participants with *premanifest* HD during implicit emotion perception, which was interpreted by the authors as a compensatory mechanism (Novak et al., 2012). Structurally, atrophy of frontal regions (such as *orbitofrontal* and *dorsolateral prefrontal cortex*) is related to poor emotion recognition in HD (Baggio et al., 2012; Henley et al., 2008; Ille, Schäfer et al., 2011), PD (Ibarretxe-Bilbao et al., 2009) and MS (Ciampi et al., 2018). Reduced ability to recognise fear has also been associated with fractional anisotropy levels in the frontal portion of the *right inferior fronto-occipital fasciculus* in PD (Baggio et al., 2012), indicating structural damage to white matter connectivity stemming from or leading to frontal regions.

As visual processing is essential to emotion perception tasks requiring examination of facial features, the occipital lobes are often considered an essential part of the social brain. Thus, in each of the disorders, occipital lobe damage appears to play a role in facial emotion recognition abilities. For example, Golde et al. (2020) reported a positive relationship between connectivity of the *fusiform gyrus* and emotion perception in MS, indicating reduced connectivity was associated with worse emotion perception. FMRI studies have shown reduced activity in occipital regions in participants with *manifest* (Dogan et al., 2014) and *premanifest* HD when processing emotional facial expressions (Hennenlotter et al., 2004; Novak et al., 2012). Across all three disorders, emotion recognition difficulties have been related to atrophy in different regions of the occipital lobe (Baggio et al., 2012; Harrington et al., 2014; Scahill et al., 2013).

The *somatosensory cortex* has previously been found to be important for the recognition of facial emotional expressions in previous research and is consistent with the idea that recognition of another's emotional state occurs by internally generating somatosensory representations that simulate how others would feel (Adolphs, Damasio, Tranel, Cooper, & Damasio, 2000). In PD, both reduced performance accuracy and perceived emotion intensity is related to reduced activation in the secondary somatosensory cortex for the emotions of disgust, anger and fear. Similarly, in HD, Dogan et al. (2014) found evidence of reduced activation in sensorimotor and somatosensory cortices during emotion recognition in patients. In the *insula* (a somatosensory region involved in subjective emotional perception), decreased activity has been found in persons with MS with impairments in facial affect recognition compared to those without such impairments (Krause et al., 2009). Similarly, lower activation of the insula has also been reported in *manifest* HD (Dogan et al., 2014) and in *premanifest* HD during an implicit emotion perception task (Hennenlotter et al., 2004; Novak et al., 2012). Regarding structural damage, reduced grey matter volume of the insula is correlated with emotion perception deficits in HD (Henley et al., 2008; Ille, Schäfer et al., 2011; Kipps et al., 2007) and MS (Ciampi et al., 2018). The insula has been hypothesised to be involved in emotion recognition deficits in PD as well (Christopher et al., 2014; Ricciardi et al., 2017), although at least two studies have not identified a relationship either through structural or functional imaging (Baggio et al., 2012; Wabnegger et al., 2015).

In summary, it appears that damage to 'social brain' regions plays a significant role in social cognition impairments. Across all three diseases, it appears that before obvious structural damage occurs to these brain regions (such as atrophy), disruption to neural networks can be observed functionally from early in the disease course. One potential hypothesis is that in the early stages of HD, MS and PD, functional disruptions begin to occur. However, as pathology increases, the brain can no longer compensate for social cognitive difficulties using broader connective networks. It is at this time that structural damage to core regions of the social brain is associated with social cognition impairments.

Psychosocial outcomes of social cognitive deficits

Few studies have examined the impact of social cognitive impairments on everyday social functioning in HD, PD and MS. It is often speculated in the literature that deficits in emotion recognition contribute to reduced social quality of life (e.g. Yitzhak et al., 2020). For instance, changes in the subjective experience of emotions could affect well-being, impairments in expression recognition could affect communication and changes in social motivation could affect social opportunities (Kordsachia et al., 2017). In HD, studies show that patients commonly experience reduced social quality of life, including social isolation, social withdrawal, disrupted relationships and disturbances in social interactions (Hayden et al., 1980; Helder et al., 2001; Kempnich et al., 2018). They also discuss compromised social health as occurring more frequently than mental or physical health difficulties (Carlozzi & Tulsky, 2013). As shown in MT's case outlined in Case Study 2 (see Box 8.2), behavioural changes which disrupt social relationships can be a key complaint of those close to people with HD. However, it is not known what relationship these social outcomes have with social cognitive impairments. In PD, impaired emotion recognition has been linked to frustration in social relationships, social disconnection, interpersonal distress and social behaviour disorders (Clark et al., 2008; Narme et al., 2013). In MS, social cognitive abilities have been related to poorer psychological and social aspects of quality of life (Phillips et al., 2011) and psychosocial fatigue (Genova, Lancaster et al., 2020). Thus, the limited evidence available suggests that social cognitive impairments may have a negative impact on psychosocial functioning in HD, PD and MS. Critically, more research is needed to determine these impacts.

Box 8.2   Case 2: MT: Adult with Huntington's disease

History:

MT is a 49-year-old woman. She is a successful lawyer, has a wide social network and enjoys many physical hobbies. Because MT does not know her father, she is unaware that she is genetically at risk of Huntington's disease.

Presentation:

MT was brought to see a GP by her husband who had noticed that despite her successful career, her mental health was deteriorating and was exhibiting subtle behavioural changes. She had depressive symptoms including low mood, agitation, problems sleeping and poor concentration. In conversation, she had become voluble and often tangential. Increased irritability with infrequent angry outburst was her most impactful change, which was very distressing for her husband and children.

Assessment:

MT was referred to a neurologist who noted some minor motor abnormalities and that MT had difficulty in sitting still. A neuropsychologist reported a mild deficit in processing speed and in the recognition of negative emotions but performance in the normal range on tests of executive function. An MRI scan was normal. After learning about her estranged father, the neurologist recommended a genetic test for Huntington's disease. The test confirmed the diagnosis. The presence of subtle motor changes in combination with mild cognitive decline and an unremarkable MRI indicated that MT was likely in the late stages of prodromal HD.

Summary and comment:

This case study highlights how social cognitive functioning may be impaired, even in the early stages of HD. While this was identifiable through formal neuropsychological testing, it was the input of MT's close family and friends that highlighted how social-cognitive difficulties manifested in her daily life. MT's diagnosis may not have been made if it weren't for the recognition of social behavioural changes by her husband.

Summary and future directions

While social cognition dysfunction is apparent across HD, PD and MS and appears to be related to reduced social quality of life, there is a significant paucity of research on how this dysfunction can be treated. When considering treatment, a number of factors must be considered. First, what is the deficit that is being treated? While the obvious answer is "social cognition", one thing identified in this chapter is the role of other factors that contribute to social cognition. For example, general cognitive difficulties may undermine social cognitive abilities. In all three diseases, processing speed is one of the most well-documented cognitive impairments. If slowed processing is an issue, then the recognition of fleeting emotions on the faces of others, for instance, would pose a significant difficulty. Second, what is the best method of treatment? For instance, research should elucidate whether rehabilitation of the processing speed deficit or emotion recognition specific training is most effective. Alternatively, perhaps a combination of these two rehabilitative approaches is most effective. Comorbidity of mood disorders which may exacerbate social cognitive deficits represent another potential avenue for treatment. That is, it may be that by improving mood symptoms, social cognition abilities also improve. In summary, treatment studies for social cognition deficits in individuals with MS, PD, and HD are much needed and should consider multiple potential contributing factors.

Other future directions include the use of innovative techniques to study social cognitive difficulties in these disorders. As mentioned previously, the use of more laboratory-based social cognition measures (e.g., with static facial expressions) calls into question whether the difficulties detected in many studies are truly representative of any difficulties that occur in everyday functioning. New techniques, such as virtual reality, represent an exciting avenue for the future assessment of social cognitive abilities, as the participant can more fully engaged in the stimuli in simulated real-world environments. The application of virtual reality to the assessment of social cognition is in its infancy; however, such tasks are now being used in the field of autism and schizophrenia, and the application of these tasks to HD, PD and MS is worth exploring.

While the development of new ecologically valid measures of social cognition are important, the field should work towards creating a common bank of measures that can be shared across studies, facilitating comparisons. Currently, several different measures are being used to assess social cognition across multiple studies, with few studies offering any psychometric data on their validity, reliability or sensitivity in these populations. A concerted effort is needed to identify valid measures of social cognition, sensitive to deficits in each population, so that they can be added to batteries of cognitive ability given to patients (similar to the MACFIMS in the case of MS). Chapter 9 provides a full discussion of the current measures of social cognition.

References

Adolphs, R., Damasio, H., Tranel, D., Cooper, G., & Damasio, A. (2000). A role for somatosensory cortices in the visual recognition of emotion as revealed by three-dimensional lesion mapping. *Journal of Neuroscience, 20*, 2683–2690.

Argaud, S., Delplanque, S., Houvenaghel, J., Auffret, M., Duprez, J., Vérin, M., . . . Sauleau, P., (2016). Does facial amimia impact the recognition of facial emotions? An EMG study in Parkinson's disease. *PLoS One, 11*, e0160329.

Argaud, S., Vérin, M., Sauleau, P., & Grandjean, D. (2018). Facial emotion recognition in Parkinson's disease: A review and new hypotheses. *Movement Disorders, 33*(4), 554–567.

Aylward, E. H., Codori, A. M., Rosenblatt, A., Sherr, M., Brandt, J., Stine, O. C., . . . Ross, C. A. (2000). Rate of caudate atrophy in presymptomatic and symptomatic stages of Huntington's disease. *Movement Disorders, 15*(3), 552–560.

Bäckman, L., Robins-Wahlin, T. B., Lundin, A., Ginovart, N., & Farde, L. (1997). Cognitive deficits in Huntington's disease are predicted by dopaminergic PET markers and brain volumes. *Brain, 120*(12), 2207–2217.

Baez, S., Herrera, E., Gershanik, O., Garcia, A. M., Bocanegra, Y., Kargieman, L., . . . Ibanez, A. (2015). Impairments in negative emotion recognition and empathy for pain in Huntington's disease families. *Neuropsychologia, 68*, 158–167.

Baggio, H. C., Segura, B., Ibarretxe-Bilbao, N., Valldeoriola, F., Marti, M. J., Compta, Y., . . . Junque, C. (2012). Structural correlates of facial emotion recognition deficits in Parkinson's disease patients. *Neuropsychologia, 50*(8), 2121–2128.

Banati, M., Sandor, J., Mike, A., Illes, E., Bors, L., Feldmann, A., . . . Illes, Z. (2010). Social cognition and theory of mind in patients with relapsing-remitting multiple sclerosis. *European Journal of Neurology : The Official Journal of the European Federation of Neurological Societies, 17*(3), 426–433.

Baron-Cohen, S., Wheelwright, S., Hill, J., Raste, Y., & Plumb, I. (2001). The "reading the mind in the eyes" test revised version: A study with normal adults, and adults with Asperger syndrome or high-functioning autism. *The Journal of Child Psychology and Psychiatry and Allied Disciplines, 42*(2), 241–251.

Bayliss, L., Galvez, V., Ochoa-Morales, A., Chávez-Oliveros, M., Rodríguez-Agudelo, Y., Delgado-García, G., & Boll, M. C. (2019). Theory of mind impairment in Huntington's disease patients and their relatives. *Arquivos de Neuro-Psiquiatria, 77*(8), 574–578.

Beatty, W., Goodkin, D., Weir, W., Statin, R., Monson, N., & Beatty, P. (1989). Affective judgments by patients with Parkinson's disease or chronic progressive multiple sclerosis. *Bulletin of the Psychonomic Society, 27*, 361–364.

Beatty, W., Orbelo, D., Sorocco, K., & Ross, E. D. (2003). Comprehension of affective prosody in multiple sclerosis. *Multiple Sclerosis, 9*, 148–153.

Benedict, R. H., Priore, R. L., Miller, C., Munschauer, F., & Jacobs, L. (2001). Personality disorder in multiple sclerosis correlates with cognitive impairment. *The Journal of Neuropsychiatry and Clinical Neurosciences, 13*(1), 70–76.

Bologna, M., Berardelli, I., Paparella, G., Marsili, L., Ricciardi, L., Fabbrini, G., & Berardelli, A. (2016). Altered kinematics of facial emotion expression and emotion recognition deficits are unrelated in Parkinson's disease. *Frontiers in Neurology, 7*, 230.

Bologna, M., Fabbrini, G., Marsili, L., Defazio, G., Thompson, P. D., & Berardelli, A. (2013). Facial bradykinesia. *Journal of Neurology, Neurosurgery & Psychiatry, 84*(6), 681–685.

Bora, E., Özakbaş, S., Velakoulis, D., & Walterfang, M. (2016). Social cognition in multiple sclerosis: A meta-analysis. *Neuropsychology Review, 26*(2), 160–172.

Bora, E., Velakoulis, D., & Walterfang, M. (2016). Social cognition in Huntington's disease: A meta-analysis. *Behavioural Brain Research, 297*, 131–140.

Bora, E., Walterfang, M., & Velakoulis, D. (2015). Theory of mind in Parkinson's disease: A meta-analysis. *Behavioural Brain Research, 292*, 515–520.

Brüne, M., Blank, K., Witthaus, H., & Saft, C. (2011). "Theory of mind" is impaired in Huntington's disease. *Movement Disorders, 26*(4), 671–678.

Buxton, S. L., MacDonald, L., & Tippett, L. J. (2013). Impaired recognition of prosody and subtle emotional facial expressions in Parkinson's disease. *Behavioral Neuroscience, 127*(2), 193.

Caillaud, M., Laisney, M., Bejanin, A., Scherer-Gagou, C., Bonneau, D., Duclos, H., . . . Allain, P. (2020). Specific cognitive theory of mind and behavioral dysfunctions in early manifest Huntington disease: A case report. *Neurocase, 26*(1), 36–41.

Carlozzi, N. E., & Tulsky, D. S. (2013). Identification of health-related quality of life (HRQOL) issues relevant to individuals with Huntington disease. *Journal of Health Psychology, 18*(2), 212–225.

Chalah, M. A., & Ayache, S. S. (2017). Deficits in social cognition: An unveiled signature of multiple sclerosis. *JINS, 23*(3), 266–286.

Chiaravalloti, N. D., & DeLuca, J. (2008). Cognitive impairment in multiple sclerosis. *The Lancet Neurology, 7*(12), 1139–1151.

Chiaravalloti, N. D., Ibarretxe-Bilbao, N., DeLuca, J., Rusu, O., Pena, J., García-Gorostiaga, I., & Ojeda, N. (2014). The source of the memory impairment in Parkinson's disease: Acquisition versus retrieval. *Movement Disorders, 29*(6), 765–771.

Christopher, L., Koshimori, Y., Lang, A. E., Criaud, M., & Strafella, A. P. (2014). Uncovering the role of the insula in non-motor symptoms of Parkinson's disease. *Brain, 137*(8), 2143–2154.

Ciampi, E., Uribe-San-Martin, R., Vásquez, M., Ruiz-Tagle, A., Labbe, T., Cruz, J. P., . . . Cárcamo-Rodríguez, C. (2018). Relationship between social cognition and traditional cognitive impairment in progressive multiple sclerosis and possible implicated neuroanatomical regions. *Multiple Sclerosis and Related Disorders, 20*, 122–128.

Clark, U. S., Neargarder, S., & Cronin-Golomb, A. (2008). Specific impairments in the recognition of emotional facial expressions in Parkinson's disease. *Neuropsychologia, 46*(9), 2300–2309.

Clark, U. S., Neargarder, S., & Cronin-Golomb, A. (2010). Visual exploration of emotional facial expressions in Parkinson's disease. *Neuropsychologia, 48*(7), 1901–1913.

Cotter, J., Firth, J., Enzinger, C., Kontopantelis, E., Yung, A. R., Elliott, R., & Drake, R. J. (2016). Social cognition in multiple sclerosis: A systematic review and meta-analysis. *Neurology, 87*(16), 1727–1736.

Coundouris, S. P., Adams, A. G., Grainger, S. A., & Henry, J. D. (2019). Social perceptual function in parkinson's disease: A meta-analysis. *Neuroscience & Biobehavioral Reviews, 104,* 255–267.

Coundouris, S. P., Adams, A. G., & Henry, J. D. (2020). Empathy and theory of mind in Parkinson's disease: A meta-analysis. *Neuroscience & Biobehavioral Reviews, 109,* 92–102.

Craufurd, D., Thompson, J. C., & Snowden, J. S. (2001). Behavioral changes in Huntington disease. *Cognitive and Behavioral Neurology, 14*(4), 219–226.

Dalili, M. N., Penton-Voak, I. S., Harmer, C. J., & Munafò, M. R. (2015). Meta-analysis of emotion recognition deficits in major depressive disorder. *Psychological Medicine, 45*(6), 1135–1144.

de Gelder, B., Van den Stock, J., de Diego Balaguer, R., & Bachoud-Lévi, A. C. (2008). Huntington's disease impairs recognition of angry and instrumental body language. *Neuropsychologia, 46*(1), 369–373.

Del Prete, E., Turcano, P., Unti, E., Palermo, G., Pagni, C., Frosini, D., . . . Ceravolo, R. (2020). Theory of mind in Parkinson's disease: Evidences in drug-naïve patients and longitudinal effects of dopaminergic therapy. *Neurological Sciences,* 1–6.

Di Bitonto, L., Longato, N., Jung, B., Fleury, M., Marcel, C., Collongues, N., . . . Blanc, F. (2011). Reduced emotional reactivity to negative stimuli in multiple sclerosis, preliminary results. *Revue Neurologique, 167*(11), 820–826.

Díez-Cirarda, M., Ojeda, N., Peña, J., Cabrera-Zubizarreta, A., Gómez-Beldarrain, M. Á., Gómez-Esteban, J. C., & Ibarretxe-Bilbao, N. (2015). Neuroanatomical correlates of theory of mind deficit in Parkinson's disease: A multimodal imaging study. *PLoS One, 10*(11), e0142234.

Dogan, I., Saß, C., Mirzazade, S., Kleiman, A., Werner, C. J., Pohl, A., . . . Reetz, K. (2014). Neural correlates of impaired emotion processing in manifest Huntington's disease. *Social Cognitive and Affective Neuroscience, 9*(5), 671–680.

Dulau, C., Deloire, M., Diaz, H., Saubusse, A., Charre-Morin, J., Prouteau, A., & Brochet, B. (2017). Social cognition according to cognitive impairment in different clinical phenotypes of multiple sclerosis. *Journal of Neurology, 264*(4), 740–748.

Eddy, C. M., Mahalingappa, S. S., & Rickards, H. E. (2014). Putting things into perspective: The nature and impact of theory of mind impairment in Huntington's disease. *European Archives of Psychiatry and Clinical Neuroscience, 264*(8), 697–705.

Eddy, C. M., & Rickards, H. E. (2015). Theory of mind can be impaired prior to motor onset in Huntington's disease. *Neuropsychology, 29*(5), 792.

Ekman, P., & Friesen, W. V. (1976). *Pictures of Facial Affect.* Palo Alto, CA: Consulting Psychologists Press.

Folstein, S. E. (1989). *Huntington's Disease: A Disorder of Families.* Baltimore, MA: Johns Hopkins University Press.

Genova, H. M., Cagna, C. J., Chiaravalloti, N. D., DeLuca, J., & Lengenfelder, J. (2016). Dynamic assessment of social cognition in individuals with multiple sclerosis: A pilot study. *JINS, 22*(1), 83–88.

Genova, H. M., & McDonald, S. (2020). Social cognition in individuals with progressive multiple sclerosis: A pilot study using TASIT-S. *Journal of the International Neuropsychological Society, 26*(5), 539–544.

Genova, H. M., Lancaster, K., Lengenfelder, J., Bober, C. P., DeLuca, J., & Chiaravalloti, N. D. (2020). Relationship between social cognition and fatigue, depressive symptoms, and anxiety in multiple sclerosis. *Journal of Neuropsychology, 14*(2), 213–225.

Golde, S., Heine, J., Pöttgen, J., Mantwill, M., Lau, S., Wingenfeld, K., . . . Stellmann, J. P. (2020). Distinct functional connectivity signatures of impaired social cognition in multiple sclerosis. *Frontiers in Neurology*, *11*, 507.

Gray, H. M., & Tickle-Degnen, L. (2010). A meta-analysis of performance on emotion recognition tasks in Parkinson's disease. *Neuropsychology*, *24*(2), 176.

Hamilton, J. M., Salmon, D. P., Corey-Bloom, J., Gamst, A., Paulsen, J. S., Jerkins, S., . . . Peavy, G. (2003). Behavioural abnormalities contribute to functional decline in Huntington's disease. *Journal of Neurology, Neurosurgery & Psychiatry*, *74*(1), 120–122.

Happé, F. G. (1994). An advanced test of theory of mind: Understanding of story characters' thoughts and feelings by able autistic, mentally handicapped, and normal children and adults. *Journal of Autism and Developmental Disorders*, *24*(2), 129–154.

Harrington, D. L., Liu, D., Smith, M. M., Mills, J. A., Long, J. D., Aylward, E. H., . . . PREDICT-HD Investigators Coordinators of the Huntington Study Group. (2014). Neuroanatomical correlates of cognitive functioning in prodromal Huntington disease. *Brain and Behavior*, *4*(1), 29–40.

Hayden, M. R., Ehrlich, R., Parker, H., & Ferera, S. J. (1980). Social perspectives in Huntington's chorea. *SA Medical Journal*, *58*(5), 201–203.

Hayes, C. J., Stevenson, R. J., & Coltheart, M. (2009). Production of spontaneous and posed facial expressions in patients with Huntington's disease: Impaired communication of disgust. *Cognition and Emotion*, *23*(1), 118–134.

Helder, D. I., Kaptein, A. A., Van Kempen, G. M. J., Van Houwelingen, J. C., & Roos, R. A. C. (2001). Impact of Huntington's disease on quality of life. *Movement Disorders*, *16*(2), 325–330.

Heller, J., Mirzazade, S., Romanzetti, S., Habel, U., Derntl, B., Freitag, N. M., . . . Reetz, K. (2018). Impact of gender and genetics on emotion processing in Parkinson's disease-a multimodal study. *NeuroImage: Clinical*, *18*, 305–314.

Henley, S. M., Novak, M. J., Frost, C., King, J., Tabrizi, S. J., & Warren, J. D. (2012). Emotion recognition in Huntington's disease: A systematic review. *Neuroscience & Biobehavioral Reviews*, *36*(1), 237–253.

Henley, S. M., Wild, E. J., Hobbs, N. Z., Warren, J. D., Frost, C., Scahill, R. I., . . . Tabrizi, S. J. (2008). Defective emotion recognition in early HD is neuropsychologically and anatomically generic. *Neuropsychologia*, *46*(8), 2152–2160.

Hennenlotter, A., Schroeder, U., Erhard, P., Haslinger, B., Stahl, R., Weindl, A., . . . Ceballos-Baumann, A. O. (2004). Neural correlates associated with impaired disgust processing in pre-symptomatic Huntington's disease. *Brain*, *127*(6), 1446–1453.

Hess, U., & Fischer, A. (2013). Emotional mimicry as social regulation. *Personality and Social Psychology Review*, *17*(2), 142–157.

Hipp, G., Diederich, N. J., Pieria, V., & Vaillant, M. (2014). Primary vision and facial emotion recognition in early Parkinson's disease. *Journal of the Neurological Sciences*, *338*(1–2), 178–182.

Ho, A. K., Robbins, A. O., & Barker, R. A. (2006). Huntington's disease patients have selective problems with insight. *Movement Disorders*, *21*(3), 385–389.

Ho, M. W. R., Chien, S. H. L., Lu, M. K., Chen, J. C., Aoh, Y., Chen, C. M., . . . Tsai, C. H. (2020). Impairments in face discrimination and emotion recognition are related to aging and cognitive dysfunctions in Parkinson's disease with dementia. *Scientific Reports*, *10*(1), 1–8.

Honan, C. A., McDonald, S., Gowland, A., Fisher, A., & Randall, R. K. (2015). Deficits in comprehension of speech acts after TBI: The role of theory of mind and executive function. *Brain and Language*, *150*, 69–79.

Ibarretxe-Bilbao, N., Junque, C., Tolosa, E., Marti, M. J., Valldeoriola, F., Bargallo, N., & Zarei, M. (2009). Neuroanatomical correlates of impaired decision-making and facial emotion recognition in early Parkinson's disease. *European Journal of Neuroscience, 30*(6), 1162–1171.

Ignatova, V. G., Surchev, J. K., Stoyanova, T. G., Vassilev, P. M., Haralanov, L. H., & Todorova, L. P. (2020). Social cognition impairments in patients with multiple sclerosis: Comparison with grade of disability. *Neurology India, 68*(1), 94.

Ille, R., Holl, A. K., Kapfhammer, H. P., Reisinger, K., Schäfer, A., & Schienle, A. (2011). Emotion recognition and experience in Huntington's disease: Is there a differential impairment? *Psychiatry Research, 188*(3), 377–382.

Ille, R., Schäfer, A., Scharmüller, W., Enzinger, C., Schöggl, H., Kapfhammer, H. P., & Schienle, A. (2011). Emotion recognition and experience in Huntington disease: A voxel-based morphometry study. *Journal of Psychiatry & Neuroscience, 36*(6), 383.

Ille, R., Wabnegger, A., Schwingenschuh, P., Katschnig-Winter, P., Kögl-Wallner, M., Wenzel, K., & Schienle, A. (2016). Intact emotion recognition and experience but dysfunctional emotion regulation in idiopathic Parkinson's disease. *Journal of the Neurological Sciences, 361*, 72–78.

Isernia, S., Baglio, F., d'Arma, A., Groppo, E., Marchetti, A., & Massaro, D. (2019). Social mind and long-lasting disease: Focus on affective and cognitive theory of mind in multiple sclerosis. *Frontiers in Psychology, 10*, 218.

Jaywant, A., Wasserman, V., Kemppainen, M., Neargarder, S., & Cronin-Golomb, A. (2016). Perception of communicative and non-communicative motion-defined gestures in Parkinson's disease. *JINS, 22*(5), 540.

Jehna, M., Langkammer, C., Wallner-Blazek, M., Neuper, C., Loitfelder, M., Ropele, S., . . . Enzinger, C. (2011). Cognitively preserved MS patients demonstrate functional differences in processing neutral and emotional faces. *Brain Imaging and Behavior, 5*(4), 241–251.

Jehna, M., Neuper, C., Petrovic, K., Wallner-Blazek, M., Schmidt, R., Fuchs, S., . . . Enzinger, C. (2010). An exploratory study on emotion recognition in patients with a clinically isolated syndrome and multiple sclerosis. *Clinical Neurology and Neurosurgery, 112*(6), 482–484.

Kan, Y., Kawamura, M., Hasegawa, Y., Mochizuki, S., & Nakamura, K. (2002). Recognition of emotion from facial, prosodic and written verbal stimuli in Parkinson's disease. *Cortex, 38*(4), 623–630.

Kawamura, M., & Koyama, S. (2007). Social cognitive impairment in Parkinson's disease. *Journal of Neurology, 254*(4), IV49–IV53.

Kempnich, C. L., Andrews, S. C., Fisher, F., Wong, D., Georgiou-Karistianis, N., & Stout, J. C. (2018). Emotion recognition correlates with social-neuropsychiatric dysfunction in Huntington's disease. *JINS, 24*(5), 417.

Kipps, C. M., Duggins, A. J., McCusker, E. A., & Calder, A. J. (2007). Disgust and happiness recognition correlate with anteroventral insula and amygdala volume respectively in preclinical Huntington's disease. *Journal of Cognitive Neuroscience, 19*(7), 1206–1217.

Kordsachia, C. C., Labuschagne, I., Andrews, S. C., & Stout, J. C. (2018). Diminished facial EMG responses to disgusting scenes and happy and fearful faces in Huntington's disease. *Cortex, 106*, 185–199.

Kordsachia, C. C., Labuschagne, I., & Stout, J. C. (2017). Beyond emotion recognition deficits: A theory guided analysis of emotion processing in Huntington's disease. *Neuroscience & Biobehavioral Reviews, 73*, 276–292.

Kordsachia, C. C., Labuschagne, I., & Stout, J. C. (2018). Visual scanning of the eye region of human faces predicts emotion recognition performance in Huntington's disease. *Neuropsychology, 32*(3), 356.

Kraemer, M., Herold, M., Uekermann, J., Kis, B., Daum, I., Wiltfang, J., . . . Abdel-Hamid, M. (2013). Perception of affective prosody in patients at an early stage of relapsing-remitting multiple sclerosis. *Journal of Neuropsychology, 7*(1), 91–106.

Kraemer, M., Herold, M., Uekermann, J., Kis, B., Wiltfang, J., Daum, I., . . . Abdel-Hamid, M. (2013). Theory of mind and empathy in patients at an early stage of relapsing remitting multiple sclerosis. *Clinical Neurology and Neurosurgery, 115*(7), 1016–1022.

Krause, M., Wendt, J., Dressel, A., Berneiser, J., Kessler, C., Hamm, A. O., & Lotze, M. (2009). Prefrontal function associated with impaired emotion recognition in patients with multiple sclerosis. *Behavioural Brain Research, 205*(1), 280–285.

Kudlicka, A., Clare, L., & Hindle, J. V. (2011). Executive functions in Parkinson's disease: Systematic review and meta-analysis. *Movement Disorders, 26*(13), 2305–2315.

Lagravinese, G., Avanzino, L., Raffo De Ferrari, A., Marchese, R., Serrati, C., Mandich, P., . . . Pelosin, E. (2017). Theory of mind is impaired in mild to moderate Huntington's disease independently from global cognitive functioning. *Frontiers in Psychology, 8*, 80.

Lancaster, K., Stone, E. M., & Genova, H. M. (2019). Cognitive but not affective theory of mind deficits in progressive MS. *JINS*, 1–5.

Larsen, I. U., Vinther-Jensen, T., Gade, A., Nielsen, J. E., & Vogel, A. (2015). Do I misconstrue? Sarcasm detection, emotion recognition, and theory of mind in Huntington disease. *Neuropsychology, 30*(2), 181.

Lawrence, A. D., Sahakian, B. J., & Robbins, T. W. (1998). Cognitive functions and corticostriatal circuits: Insights from Huntington's disease. *Trends in Cognitive Sciences, 2*(10), 379–388.

Leroi, I., Perera, N., Harbishettar, V., & Robert, P. (2014). Apathy and emotional blunting in Parkinson's disease. *Brain Disorders & Therapy, 3*(5), 2.

Livingstone, S. R., Vezer, E., McGarry, L. M., Lang, A. E., & Russo, F. A. (2016). Deficits in the mimicry of facial expressions in Parkinson's disease. *Frontiers in Psychology, 7*, 780.

Mahad, D. H., Trapp, B. D., & Lassmann, H. (2015). Pathological mechanisms in progressive multiple sclerosis. *The Lancet Neurology, 14*, 183–193.

Marneweck, M., & Hammond, G. (2014). Discriminating facial expressions of emotion and its link with perceiving visual form in Parkinson's disease. *Journal of the Neurological Sciences, 346*(1–2), 149–155.

Martínez-Corral, M., Pagonabarraga, J., Llebaria, G., Pascual-Sedano, B., García-Sánchez, C., Gironell, A., & Kulisevsky, J. (2010). Facial emotion recognition impairment in patients with Parkinson's disease and isolated apathy. *Parkinson's Disease, 2010*.

Mason, S. L., Zhang, J., Begeti, F., Guzman, N. V., Lazar, A. S., Rowe, J. B., . . . Hampshire, A. (2015). The role of the amygdala during emotional processing in Huntington's disease: From premanifest to late stage disease. *Neuropsychologia, 70*, 80–89.

Maurage, P., Lahaye, M., Grynberg, D., Jeanjean, A., Guettat, L., Verellen-Dumoulin, C., . . . Constant, E. (2016). Dissociating emotional and cognitive empathy in pre-clinical and clinical Huntington's disease. *Psychiatry Research, 237*, 103–108.

McDonald, S., Flanagan, S., & Rollins, J. (2017). *The Awareness of Social Inference Test (TASIT) Manual* (3rd ed.). Sydney: ASSBI Resources.

McDonald, S., Gowland, A., Randall, R., Fisher, A., Osborne-Crowley, K., & Honan, C. (2014). Cognitive factors underpinning poor expressive communication skills after traumatic brain injury: Theory of mind or executive function? *Neuropsychology, 28*(5), 801.

McNamara, P., & Durso, R. (2018). The dopamine system, Parkinson's disease and language function. *Current Opinion in Behavioral Sciences, 21*, 1–5.

Monetta, L., Grindrod, C. M., & Pell, M. D. (2009). Irony comprehension and theory of mind deficits in patients with Parkinson's disease. *Cortex, 45*(8), 972–981.

Montagne, B., Kessels, R. P., De Haan, E. H., & Perrett, D. I. (2007). The emotion recognition task: A paradigm to measure the perception of facial emotional expressions at different intensities. *Perceptual and Motor Skills, 104*(2), 589–598.

Montagne, B., Kessels, R. P., Kammers, M. P., Kingma, E., de Haan, E. H., Roos, R. A., & Middelkoop, H. A. (2006). Perception of emotional facial expressions at different intensities in early-symptomatic Huntington's disease. *European Neurology, 55*(3), 151–154.

Myers, R. H. (2004). Huntington's disease genetics. *NeuroRx, 1*(2), 255–262.

Narme, P., Bonnet, A. M., Dubois, B., & Chaby, L. (2011). Understanding facial emotion perception in Parkinson's disease: The role of configural processing. *Neuropsychologia, 49*(12), 3295–3302.

Narme, P., Mouras, H., Roussel, M., Duru, C., Krystkowiak, P., & Godefroy, O. (2013). Emotional and cognitive social processes are impaired in Parkinson's disease and are related to behavioral disorders. *Neuropsychology, 27*(2), 182.

Novak, M. J., Warren, J. D., Henley, S. M., Draganski, B., Frackowiak, R. S., & Tabrizi, S. J. (2012). Altered brain mechanisms of emotion processing in premanifest Huntington's disease. *Brain, 135*(4), 1165–1179.

Oberman, L. M., Winkielman, P., & Ramachandran, V. S. (2007). Face to face: Blocking facial mimicry can selectively impair recognition of emotional expressions. *Social Neuroscience, 2*(3–4), 167–178.

O'Callaghan, C., & Lewis, S. J. (2017). Cognition in Parkinson's disease. *International Review of Neurobiology, 133*, 557–583.

Osborne-Crowley, K. (2020). Social cognition in the real world: Reconnecting the study of social cognition with social reality. *Review of General Psychology, 24*(2), 144–158.

Osborne-Crowley, K., Andrews, S. C., Labuschagne, I., Nair, A., Scahill, R., Craufurd, D., . . . Stout, J. C. (2019). Apathy associated with impaired recognition of happy facial expressions in Huntington's disease. *JINS, 25*(5), 453.

Ouellet, J., Scherzer, P. B., Rouleau, I., Metras, P., Bertrand-Gauvin, C., Djerroud, N., . . . Duquette, P. (2010). Assessment of social cognition in patients with multiple sclerosis. *JINS, 16* (2), 287–296.

Palmeri, R., Lo Buono, V., Corallo, F., Foti, M., Di Lorenzo, G., Bramanti, P., & Marino, S. (2017). Nonmotor symptoms in Parkinson disease: A descriptive review on social cognition ability. *Journal of Geriatric Psychiatry and Neurology, 30*(2), 109–121.

Passamonti, L., Cerasa, A., Liguori, M., Gioia, M. C., Valentino, P., Nistico, R., . . . Fera, F. (2009). Neurobiological mechanisms underlying emotional processing in relapsing-remitting multiple sclerosis. *Brain, 132*(12), 3380–3391.

Paulsen, J. S. (2011). Cognitive impairment in Huntington disease: Diagnosis and treatment. *Current Neurology and Neuroscience Reports, 11*(5), 474.

Paulsen, J. S., Langbehn, D. R., Stout, J. C., Aylward, E., Ross, C. A., Nance, M., . . . Duff, K. (2008). Detection of Huntington's disease decades before diagnosis: The Predict-HD study. *Journal of Neurology, Neurosurgery & Psychiatry, 79*(8), 874–880.

Pell, M. D., Monetta, L., Rothermich, K., Kotz, S. A., Cheang, H. S., & McDonald, S. (2014). Social perception in adults with Parkinson's disease. *Neuropsychology, 28*(6), 905.

Péron, J., Dondaine, T., Le Jeune, F., Grandjean, D., & Vérin, M. (2012). Emotional processing in Parkinson's disease: A systematic review. *Movement Disorders, 27*(2), 186–199.

Péron, J., Vicente, S., Leray, E., Drapier, S., Drapier, D., Cohen, R., . . . Vérin, M. (2009). Are dopaminergic pathways involved in theory of mind? A study in Parkinson's disease. *Neuropsychologia*, 47(2), 406–414.

Phillips, L. H., Henry, J. D., Scott, C., Summers, F., Whyte, M., & Cook, M. (2011). Specific impairments of emotion perception in multiple sclerosis. *Neuropsychology*, 25(1), 131.

Philpott, A. L., Andrews, S. C., Staios, M., Churchyard, A., & Fisher, F. (2016). Emotion evaluation and social inference impairments in Huntington's disease. *Journal of Huntington's Disease*, 5(2), 175–183.

Pinto, C., Gomes, F., Moreira, I., Rosa, B., Santos, E., & Silva, A. M. (2012). Emotion recognition in multiple sclerosis. *JETVCE*, 2, 76–81.

Pitteri, M., Genova, H., Lengenfelder, J., DeLuca, J., Ziccardi, S., Rossi, V., & Calabrese, M. (2019). Social cognition deficits and the role of amygdala in relapsing remitting multiple sclerosis patients without cognitive impairment. *Multiple Sclerosis and Related Disorders*, 29, 118–123.

Poewe, W. (2008). Non-motor symptoms in Parkinson's disease. *European Journal of Neurology*, 15, 14–20.

Ponari, M., Conson, M., D'Amico, N. P., Grossi, D., & Trojano, L. (2012). Mapping correspondence between facial mimicry and emotion recognition in healthy subjects. *Emotion*, 12(6), 1398.

Pöttgen, J., Dziobek, I., Reh, S., Heesen, C., & Gold, S. M. (2013). Impaired social cognition in multiple sclerosis. *Journal of Neurology, Neurosurgery, and Psychiatry*, 84(5), 523–528.

Prenger, M., & MacDonald, P. A. (2018). Problems with facial mimicry might contribute to emotion recognition impairment in Parkinson's Disease. *Parkinson's Disease*, 2018.

Pringsheim, T., Wiltshire, K., Day, L., Dykeman, J., Steeves, T., & Jette, N. (2012). The incidence and prevalence of Huntington's disease: A systematic review and meta-analysis. *Movement Disorders*, 27(9), 1083–1091.

Prochnow, D., Donell, J., Schäfer, R., Jörgens, S., Hartung, H. P., Franz, M., & Seitz, R. J. (2011). Alexithymia and impaired facial affect recognition in multiple sclerosis. *Journal of Neurology*, 258(9), 1683–1688.

Ricciardi, L., Visco-Comandini, F., Erro, R., Morgante, F., Bologna, M., Fasano, A., . . . Kilner, J. (2017). Facial emotion recognition and expression in Parkinson's disease: An emotional mirror mechanism? *PLoS One*, 12(1), e0169110.

Santangelo, G., Vitale, C., Trojano, L., Errico, D., Amboni, M., Barbarulo, A. M., . . . Barone, P. (2012). Neuropsychological correlates of theory of mind in patients with early Parkinson's disease. *Movement Disorders*, 27(1), 98–105.

Scahill, R. I., Hobbs, N. Z., Say, M. J., Bechtel, N., Henley, S. M., Hyare, H., . . . Durr, A. (2013). Clinical impairment in premanifest and early Huntington's disease is associated with regionally specific atrophy. *Human Brain Mapping*, 34(3), 519–529.

Schmidt, N., Paschen, L., Deuschl, G., & Witt, K. (2017). Reduced empathy scores in patients with Parkinson's disease: A non-motor symptom associated with advanced disease stages. *Journal of Parkinson's Disease*, 7(4), 713–718.

Sitek, E. J., Sławek, J., & Wieczorek, D. (2008). Self-awareness of deficits in Huntington's and Parkinson's disease. *Psychiatria Polska*, 42(3), 393–403.

Snowden, J. S., Gibbons, Z. C., Blackshaw, A., Doubleday, E., Thompson, J., Craufurd, D., . . . Neary, D. (2003). Social cognition in frontotemporal dementia and Huntington's disease. *Neuropsychologia*, 41(6), 688–701.

Tabrizi, S. J., Scahill, R. I., Owen, G., Durr, A., Leavitt, B. R., Roos, R. A., . . . Craufurd, D. (2013). Predictors of phenotypic progression and disease onset in premanifest and early-stage Huntington's disease in the TRACK-HD study: Analysis of 36-month observational data. *The Lancet Neurology, 12*(7), 637–649.

Tessitore, A., Hariri, A. R., Fera, F., Smith, W. G., Chase, T. N., Hyde, T. M., . . . Mattay, V. S. (2002). Dopamine modulates the response of the human amygdala: A study in Parkinson's disease. *Journal of Neuroscience, 22*(20), 9099–9103.

Trinkler, I., de Langavant, L. C., & Bachoud-Lévi, A. C. (2013). Joint recognition – expression impairment of facial emotions in Huntington's disease despite intact understanding of feelings. *Cortex, 49*(2), 549–558.

Trinkler, I., Devignevielle, S., Achaibou, A., Ligneul, R. V., Brugières, P., de Langavant, L. C., . . . Bachoud-Lévi, A. C. (2017). Embodied emotion impairment in Huntington's disease. *Cortex, 92*, 44–56.

Tysnes, O.-B., & Storstein, A. (2017). Epidemiology of Parkinson's disease. *Journal of Neural Transmission, 124*(8), 901–905.

van Asselen, M., Júlio, F., Januário, C., Bobrowicz Campos, E., Almeida, I., Cavaco, S., & Castelo-Branco, M. (2012). Scanning patterns of faces do not explain impaired emotion recognition in Huntington disease: Evidence for a high-level mechanism. *Frontiers in Psychology, 3*, 31.

Vonsattel, J. P. G., Keller, C., & Ramirez, E. P. C. (2011). Huntington's disease – neuropathology. In *Handbook of Clinical Neurology* (Vol. 100, pp. 83–100). Amsterdam: Elsevier.

Wabnegger, A., Ille, R., Schwingenschuh, P., Katschnig-Winter, P., Kögl-Wallner, M., Wenzel, K., & Schienle, A. (2015). Facial emotion recognition in Parkinson's disease: An fMRI investigation. *PLoS One, 10*(8), e0136110.

Walker, F. O. (2007). Huntington's disease. *The Lancet, 369*(9557), 218e228.

Wallin, M. T., Culpepper, W. J., Nichols, E., Bhutta, Z. A., Gebrehiwot, T. T., Hay, S. I., . . . Murray, C. J. L. (2019). Global, regional, and national burden of multiple sclerosis 1990–2016: A systematic analysis for the Global Burden of Disease Study 2016. *The Lancet Neurology, 18*(3), 269–285.

Weinshenker, B. G. (1996). Epidemiology of multiple sclerosis. *Neurologic Clinics, 14*(2), 291–308.

Williams, J. K., Barnette, J. J., Reed, D., Sousa, V. D., Schutte, D. L., McGonigal-Kenney, M., . . . Paulsen, J. S. (2010). Development of the Huntington disease family concerns and strategies survey from focus group data. *Journal of Nursing Measurement, 18*(2), 83–99.

Wood, A., Rychlowska, M., Korb, S., & Niedenthal, P. (2016). Fashioning the face: Sensorimotor simulation contributes to facial expression recognition. *Trends in Cognitive Sciences, 20*(3), 227–240.

Yip, J. T., Lee, T. M., Ho, S. L., Tsang, K. L., & Li, L. S. (2003). Emotion recognition in patients with idiopathic Parkinson's disease. *Movement Disorders, 18*(10), 1115–1122.

Yitzhak, N., Gurevich, T., Inbar, N., Lecker, M., Atias, D., Avramovich, H., & Aviezer, H. (2020). Recognition of emotion from subtle and non-stereotypical dynamic facial expressions in Huntington's disease. *Cortex, 126*, 343–354.

Zarotti, N., Fletcher, I., & Simpson, J. (2019). New perspectives on emotional processing in people with symptomatic Huntington's disease: Impaired emotion regulation and recognition of emotional body language. *Archives of Clinical Neuropsychology, 34*(5), 610–624.

Zarotti, N., Simpson, J., Fletcher, I., Squitieri, F., & Migliore, S. (2018). Exploring emotion regulation and emotion recognition in people with presymptomatic Huntington's disease: The role of emotional awareness. *Neuropsychologia, 112*, 1–9.

Chapter 9

Assessing social cognition in adults

Michelle Kelly, Skye McDonald and Amy Pinkham

Historically, impairments in social cognition were inferred from performance on neuropsychological tests, such as those assessing executive function, with attention, inhibition and memory (Godfrey & Shum, 2000). However, there is convincing evidence, across multiple populations, that social cognitive impairments occur independently of general cognitive deficits (Shimokawa et al., 2000; Spikman et al., 2012). In light of this, tools are being developed across all the traditional categories of measurement including self- and informant-report questionnaires, behavioural observation and performance-based tests, with some being augmented with physiological measurement and neuroimaging techniques. Different aspects of social cognition lend themselves to different kinds of assessment (see Chapter 1 for a full discussion of the different facets of social cognition). For example, empathy is often assessed via self-report, or physiological measurement of changes in arousal, while emotion perception, face identity, attributional bias (e.g., attributing ambiguous events to hostile intentions) and theory of mind (ToM) are normally assessed with performative tasks. Despite the proliferation of measurement tool development, there is still reticence among clinicians to assess social cognitive deficits, suggesting awareness of their value is yet to be recognized, and/or there are other barriers to their use (Kelly et al., 2017a; Kelly et al., 2017b). Here we discuss measurement tools and techniques, domains for assessment in different clinical conditions and psychometric properties of various measures, as well as their utility in research and clinical practice.

Self- and informant-report measures of social cognition

Self- and informant-report measures of social cognition are typically quick, easily adapted to online formats and inexpensive to use in both research and clinical settings, making them an attractive option. They are used to measure both internal states (feelings about a situation) and behaviour in a person with a clinical disorder, as rated by an informant, often a family member. While there are many benefits of using self- and informant-report questionnaires,

DOI: 10.4324/9781003027034-9

there are also shortcomings. The first is lack of insight. For example, people with frontotemporal dementia (FTD) have severe loss of empathy as rated by their caregiver; however, their own ratings differ markedly (Hsieh et al., 2013), highlighting the impact of poor self-awareness (e.g., Clare et al., 2012).

Self-report measures are also susceptible to social desirability biases (Schieman & Van Gundy, 2000; Watson & Morris, 1991) as well as cohort differences (Konrath et al., 2010; O'Brien et al., 2013). Meta-cognition, i.e., self-reflection, changes with age, meaning older adults will self-report differently than younger individuals (Mecacci & Righi, 2006). There can also be biases in caregiver response. Caregivers (often family and friends) can experience stress and burden associated with their role, resulting in negativity biases and elevated reports of impairment in the person they care for (Clare et al., 2011; Martyr & Clare, 2018; Martyr et al., 2019) or alternatively, may play down deficits in function. These issues make it necessary to consider the timing of informant-reports on social function in relation to what is happening for the patient and their family at that time.

Despite drawbacks, self- and informant-report measures of social cognition and behaviour represent three of the top five instruments used most commonly by clinicians in the field of brain injury (Kelly et al., 2017a) and are the most common means to assess empathy and social communication in brain injury research (Wallis et al., in press). Because self-report measures often fail to correlate with behavioural measures in both clinical populations and healthy adults (Francis et al., 2017; Healey et al., 2015; Kelly et al., under review; Murphy & Lilienfeld, 2019), performance-based measures are critical to increase objectivity of measurement.

Performance-based measures of social cognition

Similar to other neuropsychological tests, performance-based measures of social cognition compare an individual's task performance to normative standards. Emotion recognition (or perception) has overwhelmingly relied on Ekman and Friesen's set of black and white photos of actors posing six basic emotion expressions as well as neutral (Ekman & Friesen, 1976). However, many contemporary emotion recognition stimuli are now available. Tests assessing vocal affect (prosody) and body language have also been developed to assess different modalities of emotion perception, such as the Florida Affect Battery (Bowers et al., 1991) or the Comprehensive Affect Test System (CATS) (Froming et al., 2006). There are also tests using videoed emotions such as The Awareness of Social Inference test (TASIT) (McDonald et al., 2003). Scoring of these tests is simple and objective, usually obtained by summing the number of stimuli correctly labelled, or in some cases, matched to another image or voice. Similarly, face identity recognition is often measured by selecting the same identity as a target face from different angles or recognising familiar (famous) faces (Benton et al., 1983; Duchaine & Nakayama, 2006).

Tests of ToM were originally developed for use in children with autism spectrum disorder (ASD) using cartoons or puppets to assess understanding of the beliefs and motives of story characters (Wimmer & Perner, 1983). Cartoon stories are also used for assessment of adults but, more typically, text-based scenarios with questions about the thoughts, beliefs and motives of various characters are used (Stone et al., 1998). Other behavioural measures assess language nuance such as detection of sarcasm, lies and jokes (Happe, 1994; McDonald, Flanagan et al., 2011). More recently, with the goal of making tests more ecologically valid, both audiovisual tests and tests based in a virtual environment have been developed (Canty et al., 2017; Dziobek et al., 2006; McDonald, Flanagan et al., 2011; Samson et al., 2005).

Although there are a few performance-based tests of empathy, such as the Multifaceted Empathy Test (MET), mostly this is assessed using self-report questionnaires. Attributional bias, a construct examined predominately in individuals with schizophrenia spectrum disorder (SSD), is typically assessed by providing written examples of situations where bias is inherent and asking the participant to interpret this using either a fixed or open response (Combs et al., 2007a; Rosset, 2008). Similarly, social perception and moral judgement tasks mostly involve written passages and vignettes, followed by questions (Chiasson et al., 2017; Costanzo & Archer, 1989; Sergi et al., 2009).

Augmenting measures of social cognition with physiological and imaging technology

As Discussed in Chapter 2, the use of technologies including physiological measures and brain imaging has provided new opportunities to examine social cognition and provided supporting evidence for the construct validity of both self-report and behavioural tests (Neumann & Westbury, 2011). Physiological measurement is useful for detecting correlates of emotional experience (Cacioppo et al., 2007) such as changes in *autonomic nervous system* activation, indexed by heart rate, respiration, pupil constriction and dilation, eye gaze direction, skin conductance and skin temperature. Most of the social cognitive constructs we describe, including emotion recognition, theory of mind and empathy, have an inherent emotional component. By measuring the physiological response of the participant, we can validate their self-reported emotional changes when these occur or reveal changes in emotional arousal that the participant is unaware of or unable to describe.

Skin conductance (electrodermal activity) has been used to augment self-report and behavioural measures of emotion perception, empathy, trustworthiness judgements and in response to moral transgressions (for example see Cecchetto et al., 2018; de Sousa et al., 2012; Mathersul et al., 2013b; Neumann & Westbury, 2011) across multiple clinical populations. For example, in people with brain injuries, atypical skin conductance responses are linked to lowered empathic response to emotions (de Sousa et al., 2011) possibly as a result of more general blunting of physiological responses (de Sousa et al., 2010). Eye gaze direction and pupil dilation is frequently used in research into ASD to determine whether this is a factor in emotion perception difficulties, both in relation to time spent paying attention to particular regions of the face and how rewarding or aversive this experience is (e.g., Black et al., 2017; Sepeta et al., 2012).

Likewise, electromyography (EMG: measurement of muscles in the face that reflect mimicry and emotional expression), has also been used to help explain social impairments. Individuals with ASD and those with acquired brain injury show differential facial mimicry to emotional stimuli when compared to age-matched controls (de Sousa et al., 2011; Mathersul et al., 2013a; McDonald, Li et al., 2011). These various physiological indices of social processes have, together, informed understanding of the processes underlying impairments in social cognition in clinical populations. This information is useful for guid-ing where interventions should be targeted and what type of intervention is possible. While physiological measurement has been an invaluable research tool, it is important to stress that such measurement is less useful for individual assessments such as may be required for clinical work. Physiological measures are inherently variable, making them unreliable for routine, within-subject assessments.

Brain imaging techniques such as structural and functional magnetic reso-nance imaging (MRI), positron emission tomography (PET) and single photon emission computed tomography (SPECT) have also advanced the assessment and understanding of social cognition (see Chapter 2 for further discussion). Via MRI, the field of social neuroscience has been able to develop several tasks and paradigms that have clearly identified neural substrates to task performance which can inform both diagnosis and treatment approaches. Recently, research-ers have evaluated the clinical utility of several of these tasks (Green et al., 2013), and while the results were not as positive as initially hoped, these efforts did identify a promising measure of empathy. The empathic accuracy paradigm was sensitive to clinical impairment in schizophrenia and showed adequate reliability (Kern et al., 2013) while also showing significant associations with functional outcomes (Olbert et al., 2013). As noted above, there are few well-validated behavioral assessments of empathy, and thus, this direct translation of a social neuroscience measure to the clinical arena may provide a roadmap for similar strategies to improve and expand social cognitive assessment.

Beyond these contributions to assessment, neuroimaging of social cognition in healthy and clinical populations has supported the relative independence of social cognition. While it is acknowledged that several of the same brain struc-tures critical for cognitive processes such as perception, memory and attention are involved in social cognition, the preponderance of evidence also demon-strates neural specialization for social cognition (Adolphs, 2009). Identifica-tion of such specialized neural systems provides fertile ground for hypotheses suggesting that impaired functioning of these systems may underlie behavioral impairments in social cognition and social interaction (e.g., Pinkham et al., 2003). By and large, imaging investigations of clinical populations have found reduced/impaired activity and functional connectivity of social cognitive networks in clinically impaired groups (Bjorkquist et al., 2016; Cusi et al., 2012; Taylor et al., 2012). Thus, MRI has helped to identify a potential mechanism for social cognitive impairment that may be able to be targeted via pharmacology or neurostimulation. As an alternate method of measuring brain activity, electroencephalography (EEG) also holds promise. For example, in individuals with a diagnosis of schizophrenia, EEG has been beneficial for elucidating electrophysiological differences in brain function during joint-tasks (De La Asuncion et al., 2015).

Psychometric standards required in tests of social cognition

While psychophysiological and brain imaging techniques provide an important adjunct to more traditional approaches to assessing cognition and emotion, it is likely that self-report and performance-based tasks will remain pivotal to both research and clinical assessment. In order to have confidence in such instruments, they need to be reliable (test consistently across varying conditions), valid (test what we think they test) and have utility for people with clinical disorders in terms of both length and content, with minimal demands on verbal and executive functioning skills and with normative data (see Table 9.1 for key psychometric attributes). To date, few tests have adequately demonstrated evidence for all of these attributes (Kelly et al., 2017b).

Reliability refers to the consistency of the test to measure the targeted construct and is typically examined using various correlational analyses with the statistic falling between -1 and 1. Scores closer to 0 in either direction indicate smaller associations. Most of the tests itemized in Table 9.2 demonstrates reasonable internal reliability, i.e., the items within the test consistently measure the social cognition construct. *The Reading the Mind in the Eyes Test*, however, has consistently been criticized for having poor internal reliability (Prevost et al., 2014; Voracek & Dressler, 2006). Most tests in Table 9.2 also have adequate test-retest reliability when this is reported. Only *TASIT* and the *Social Attribution Task (SAT)* have parallel versions to allow for testing on multiple occasions, and of these two, reliability of alternative forms have only been demonstrated for *TASIT* (McDonald et al., 2006). Even if a test is shown to be reliable, it also needs to demonstrate that it is sensitive to change if it is to be used for clinical assessment to document deterioration (for people with deteriorating conditions) or improvement, due to recovery or remediation. Very few tests of social cognition (with the exception of TASIT (Bornhofen & McDonald, 2008b)) have demonstrated sensitivity to change.

Reliability can be negatively affected if scoring is complex or ambiguous. Many social cognitive tests require categorical responses (e.g., yes/no, happy/

Table 9.1 Psychometric standards for tests of social cognition

For a test to be reliable, it needs to demonstrate that it has

❖ Simple unambiguous scoring methods
❖ Consistency across raters when items require subjective scoring (inter-rater reliability, e.g., intraclass correlations: ICC)
❖ All items measuring the same construct (internal reliability, e.g., coefficient alpha or split half reliability) is 0.7 or greater (Nunnally & Bernstein, 1994).
❖ Consistency across time (test-retest reliability, pearson r or ICC is 0.7 or greater (Nunnally & Bernstein, 1994).
❖ Strong correlations between parallel versions if these are used.

For a test to be valid, it has to demonstrate that it

❖ Has minimal floor and ceiling effects for target group, ensuring adequate range
❖ Correlates with other measures of a similar construct (convergent validity)
❖ Does not correlate with other measures of dissimilar constructs (divergent validity)
❖ Discriminates people with known social cognitive impairment from those who do not have impairment (discriminant validity)
❖ Is predictive of real-world function (ecological validity)

For a test to have clinical utility, it has to have

❖ Appropriate length and content for the target clinical group
❖ Minimal verbal and executive demands
❖ A control task to parse out non-social cognitive demands
❖ Normative data that are demographically similar to the person being assessed

For a test to be fit for purpose, it may require

❖ Sensitivity to small changes that represent improvement/decline in individuals
❖ The ability to separate out separate components of social cognitive processes

sad), making scoring simple and objective. However, some tests of ToM and empathy rely on subjectivity in scoring criterion. In this case, estimates of inter-rater reliability are needed and raters may need to be trained beforehand to achieve this. For example, the SAT (Klin & Jones, 2006) asks the examinee to describe what they observe to be happening in a scene, the responses are then transcribed and scored against a complex set of criteria, increasing the likelihood of unreliable data. The SAT developers have also designed multiple choice type questions to reduce this risk (Bell et al., 2010). The Strange Stories Test, Faux Pas Recognition Tests, Movie for the Assessment of Social Cognition and the SAT all demonstrate adequate consistency of scores between raters (Dziobek et al., 2006; Gregory et al., 2002; Klin & Jones, 2006; McKown et al., 2013).

The validity of social cognitive tests reflects the extent to which they measure the construct they were designed to measure. One way of measuring this is by determining whether the test differentiates between the clinical group and a demographically matched control group (*discriminant validity*) and most tests in Table 9.2 meet this criterion. However, the majority of tools used to assess social cognition are also influenced by intellectual ability, memory, language or executive function (Eddy, 2019), which suggests poor *divergent validity*. This is a problem for most of the populations known to experience social cognitive deficits, such as schizophrenia, brain injury and dementia (Rabinowitz & Levin, 2014; Tate et al., 1989), all of whom have cognitive impairment and may, therefore, have poorer performances on social cognitive tests due to the ancillary demands of the tests. One solution to this is for the tasks to include a 'control' condition. This provides a way of parsing out the role of general cognitive skills such as memory from social cognitive ability. For example, the Strange Stories task, a test that requires the individual to explain a speaker's intention where the literal meaning is not true (i.e., irony, white lies) has demonstrated that children and adults with autism spectrum disorders (ASD) perform poorly on the mentalising stories but within the normal range on control stories (Happe, 1994; Spek et al., 2010). Likewise, on TASIT, people with brain injury understand the meanings and intentions of actors in video vignettes where they are making sincere utterances, but fail to understand sarcasm and lies (McDonald & Flanagan, 2004).

Validity of an instrument can also be diminished by test length, which taxes clinical populations who suffer from cognitive fatigue (Johnson et al., 1997; Schultz et al., 2018) and which may, therefore, influence test scores. Tests such as TASIT (McDonald, Flanagan et al., 2011) and the MASC (Dziobek et al., 2006) take 45–75 minutes to administer, which can be impractical, especially in conjunction with standard neuropsychological assessment battery. Another 'ideal' for social cognitive tests is an absence of ceiling and floor effects, although this may differ between the clinical and the normative groups. Criterion referenced tests, for example, assess whether a client falls below a specific cut-off (criteria) indicative of impairment. Tests such as TASIT (McDonald, Flanagan et al., 2011) and the BASS-D (Kelly & McDonald, 2020) are designed in this way so that normally functioning adults perform close to, or at ceiling. While tests such as these have shown clinical sensitivity across a range of populations including brain injury, schizophrenia and dementia (Bliksted et al., 2017; Kipps et al., 2009; McDonald & Flanagan, 2004), convergent validity can be difficult to demonstrate, at least in the normal population, because of the restricted range of scores.

Tests designed to assess individual differences pose a different challenge to validity because in this case, the items need to be sensitive to a range of levels of ability within the normal population. One way to vary difficulty is to reduce the time allowed to respond by increasing the perceptual demands of the task, e.g., showing faces on an angle, removing extraneous features such as hair and accessories and switching between labelling and matching (Matsumoto et al., 2000; Palermo et al., 2013). ToM tasks have proven more challenging to design

Table 9.2 Details of tests of social cognition in each of the seven domains[1]

Test	Verbal demands	Control	Time mins	Simple to score	Internal reliability	Test-Retest	Convergent validity	Ecological validity	Clinical Sensitivity	Norms
TESTS OF FACE IDENTITY RECOGNITION										
BFRT (long & short)	Point to face	No	9m	✓	long✗ short✗	long✓ short✗	✓	N/A	✗	A ✓ 20–90 yrs C N/A
CFRT	Point to/sort faces	No	10–15m	✓	✓	✓	✓	✓	✓	A ✓ 20–88 yrs C N/A
TESTS OF EMOTION PERCEPTION										
FEEST	Choose b/w labels	No	10m	✓	✗	N/A	✓	N/A	✓	A ✓ 20–70 yrs C N/A
CATS	Listen to sentences/ Choose b/w labels	Identity matching	??	✓	✓	✓	✓	N/A	✓	A ✓ 20–79 yrs C N/A
ERT (long & short)	Choose b/w labels	No	20m & 10m	✓	✓[1]	N/A	✓[1]	✓	✓	A ✓ <75 yrs C ✓ >7 yrs
TASIT & TASIT-S: Part 1	Watch dialogue Choose b/w labels	No	20m & 10m	✓	✓	✓	✓	✓		A ✓ 16–75 yrs C ✓ 13–19 yrs

ER-40	Choose b/w labels	No	3.5m	✓	✓	✓	✓	✓	A ✓ M:39 yrs C N/A
BLERT	Choose b/w labels	No	7m	✓	✓	✓	✓	✓	A ✓ M:39 yrs C N/A
TESTS OF THEORY OF MIND									
RMET	Choose b/w labels	No	6.6m	✓	✗	✗	N/A	✓	A ✓ M:39 yrs C✓ 9–15 yrs
SST	Read text, answer questions	Control stories	15–20m	✓	✓	✓	✓	✓	A ✗ C ✓ 4–14 yrs
FPT	Read text. Answer questions	Memory questions	15–20m	✗	✓	✓	✓	✓	A ✓ 18–35 yrs C ✓ 7,9,11yrs
HT	Read text. Answer questions	No	6m	✓	✓	✓	✓	✓	A ✓ M:39 yrs C N/A
TASIT & TASIT-S: Pt 2 & Pt 3.	Watch dialogue Answer Y/N questions	Part 2: Sincere items	50m & 20m	✓	✓	✓	✓	✓	A ✓ 16–75 yrs C ✓ 13–19 yrs

(Continued)

Table 9.2 (Continued)

Test	Verbal demands	Control	Time mins	Simple to score	Internal reliability	Test-Retest	Convergent validity	Ecological validity	Clinical Sensitivity	Norms
MASC	Watch dialogue Answer Y/N questions	No	45 m	✓	✓	✗	✓	N/A	✓	A ✓ M:29–39 yrs C N/A
SAT	Verbally explain/ read MC items	No	10m	✗	✓	N/A	✓	✓	✓	A ✓ M:42 yrs C N/A
Yoni Task	Listen to questions and point	physical judgement	??	✓	N/A	N/A	✓	N/A	✓	A ✓ M:23 yrs C N/A
TESTS OF EMPATHY										
IRI	Read 28 statements	No	3–5m	✓	✓	✓	✓	✓	✓	A ✓ M:17 yrs C ✓ 11th grade
QCAE	Read 31 statements	No	3–5m	✓	✓	✓	✓	✓	✓	A ✓ 17–65 yrs C N/A
BEES	Read 30 statements	No	3–5 m	✓	✓	✓	✓	✓	✓	A ✓ 25–45 yrs C N/A

EQ	No	Read 40 statements	3–5 m	✓	✓	✓	✓	✓	A ✓ 18–75 yrs C ✓ 7–16 yrs
MET (original and short)	No	Choose b/w labels, use Likert scales	35m & 3–5m	✓	✓	N/A	✓	N/A	A ✓ 20–79 yrs C N/A

TESTS OF ATTRIBUTIONAL BIAS

AIHQ	No	Read vignettes and write responses	5–7 m	✗	✓	✓	N/A	✓	A ✓ M:19.6 yrs M: 39.2 yrs C: N/A

TESTS OF SOCIAL COMMUNICATION[2]

LCQ	No	Read 30 statements	15m	✓	✓	✓	✓	✓	A ✓ 16–39 yrs C: N/A

TESTS OF SOCIAL PERCEPTION

RAD	No	Read 14 vignettes, answer Y/N	16m	✓	✓	✓	✓	✗	A ✓ M:39 yrs C: N/A

1 Adapted, with permission, from Haaland, K., Brown, G., Crossen, B., & King, T. (Eds) APA Handbook of Neuropsychology: Volume 2: Assessment: Emerging methods. APA

BFRT =The Benton Facial Recognition Test (Benton et al., 1983). Available from Psychological Assessment resources: PAR.
CFRT = Cambridge Face Recognition Tasks: (Duchaine & Nakayama, 2006) including the Face Memory test and the Face Perception test (Duchaine et al., 2007). For availability, contact the authors.

(Continued)

Table 9.2 (Continued)

FEEST = Facial Expression of Emotion: Stimuli and Tests (Young et al., 2002). For availability, contact the authors.

CATS = The Comprehensive Affect Test System (Froming et al., 2006). No longer available.

ERT = Emotion Recognition Test (Kessels, Montagne, Hendriks, Perrett, & de Haan, 2014). For availability, contact the first author.

TASIT = The Awareness of Social Inference Test (McDonald, Flanagan et al., 2017b) & TASIT-S = TASIT Short version (McDonald, Honan et al., 2017). Available from ASSBI Resources www.assbi.com.au/ASSBI-Online-store.

ER-40 = The Penn Emotion Recognition Test (Kohler et al., 2003) Available from developers. See https://penncnp.med.upenn.edu/request.pl.

BLERT = The Bell-Lysaker Emotion Recognition Test (Bryson et al., 1997b). Available from first author.

RMET = Reading the Mind in the Eyes – Revised (Baron-Cohen, Wheelright et al., 2001). Available from the Autism Research Centre: www.autism-researchcentre.com/arc_tests.

SST = Strange Stories Test (Happe, 1994). For availability, contact the authors.

FPT = Faux Pas Recognition Test (Stone et al., 1998). Available from the Autism Research Centre: www.autismresearchcentre.com/arc_tests.

HT = The Hinting Task (Corcoran et al., 1995b). Available from first author upon request. Revised scoring criteria from Dr. A. Pinkham (amy.pinkham@utdallas.edu).

MASC = Movie for the Assessment of Social Cognition (Dziobek et al., 2006). Available from the authors.

SAT = The Social Attribution Task (Klin & Jones, 2006). For availability, contact the authors.

The Yoni task (Shamay-Tsoory & Aharon-Peretz, 2007). For availability, contact the authors.

IRI = Interpersonal Reactivity Index (Davis, 1980). For availability, contact the authors.

QCAE = Questionnaire of Cognitive and Affective Empathy (Reniers et al., 2011). Available from the authors.

BEES = The Balanced Emotional Empathy Scale (Mehrabian, 2000). Available from the author.

EQ = Empathy Quotient (Baron-Cohen & Wheelright, 2004). Available from the Autism Research Centre: www.autismresearchcentre.com/arc_tests.

MET = The Multifaceted Empathy Test (Dziobek et al., 2008; Foell et al., 2018). Available from the authors.

AIHQ = Attributional Bias and Hostility Questionnaire (Combs et al., 2007a). Available from the authors.

LCQ = LaTrobe Communication Questionnaire (Douglas, Bracy, & Snow, 2007). Available from the authors.

RAD = Relationship Across Domains (Sergi et al., 2009). Available from the authors.

B/W = between; Y/N = Yes/No; MC= Multiple Choice; [1] values based on unpublished data analysis; ✗ = values from majority of sources unacceptable; ✓ values reported from majority of source are acceptable; N/A No information available; Note that acceptable reliability (internal consistency, test retest, inter-rater) >.70, acceptable normative data either in manual or published independently > N =50. A = adults; C = children/adolescents. Acceptable convergent validity: majority of research finds that the test is significantly associated with others purported to measure the same construct. Acceptable sensitivity: test demonstrated to discriminate between clinical disorders with social cognition impairment and healthy control participants. Acceptable ecological validity: Evidence that test predicts functional outcomes. [2] TASIT is also a test of social communication and the SST is also used for this purpose.

for individual differences. Most already load highly on working memory (Schneider et al., 2012), and increasing task difficulty by increasing the complexity or ambiguity of the scenarios presented, or the questions that assess understanding, risks both the validity and reliability of the task, a problem also seen in other domains of social cognition.

Social cognitive tests should also be associated with real-life outcomes, i.e., *ecological validity*. For example, TASIT performance is related to social skills demonstrated during an in vivo encounter with a confederate (McDonald et al., 2004). However, evidence for ecological validity of many other tests outlined in Table 9.2 is lacking. Given one goal for tests of social cognition is to guide remediation, a higher standard for demonstrating ecological validity is required. There is also a need for assessments that can identify specific processes in isolation, such as the sound of an angry voice. Isolating key processes can be important for both research and when targeting a process for intervention (Bornhofen & McDonald, 2008a). However, the use of deconstructed social situations can remove non-trivial task demands and reduce ecological validity. Real life does not occur in still, black and white images (e.g., Ekman and Friesen's photos) but, rather, is dynamic, fast and noisy. Compared to static images, moving facial expressions require additional neural systems to process (Adolphs et al., 2003), and the distracting environment in which these social situations take place provides additional challenges. Actual emotional responses are also usually influenced by the social expectations of the environment. For example, despite feeling angry in a workplace meeting, a person may hide that emotion, producing a softened or mixed expression that is ambiguous. The use of audiovisual or dynamic stimuli such as those in the TASIT and the Bell Lysaker Emotion Recognition Test (Bryson et al., 1997b) overcomes some of these limitations by replicating real-world social scenarios while providing the option to break down component processes of social processing sound versus vision.

Normative data

To have value in clinical contexts, tests of social cognition need to have suitable normative data available, i.e., the examinee can be compared to the performance of a normative population that is comparable in terms of age, race, education and in some cases, gender. Culture is an important consideration in social cognitive performance and is considered in detail in Chapter 2. Many tests of social cognition do not provide normative data and, where it is available, it is often based on university students (typically aged 18–22 and highly educated), thus, not suitable for older adults or those from more varied socioeconomic backgrounds. The Balanced Emotional Empathy Scale (Mehrabian, 2000) is a good example of this, with the majority of normative data having been collected in the 18–40 year old age range (Dehning et al., 2013; Toussaint & Webb, 2005).

When normative data is available, the sample is also often small, from 25 or less through to a few hundred, reflecting the challenges of labour-intensive face-to-face testing. As tests are increasingly developed and reimagined to be delivered online, some tools provide normative data for samples in the thousands (3000+ Cambridge Face Memory Test: Wilmer et al., 2010). Many of these larger samples are collected using platforms such as Prolific and Mechanical Turk in which participants from around the world are accessed and paid for their responses. Participants remain completely anonymous and unknown to the researcher (Goodman & Paolacci, 2017). This breeds its own problems as the data may be skewed by responders who are not truthful or diligent in their responses.

Social cognition assessment tools in adults

A number of reviews in different clinical fields have identified a broad range of social cognitive measures. In the neuropsychiatric field, a review of 48 studies (Eddy, 2019) identified 78 measures, 12 of which were used in more than 10% of studies, mostly assessing emotion perception and ToM. In brain injury, a review of 367 studies identified over 200 measures, mainly focused on emotion perception, ToM, social communication, identity recognition and empathy (Wallis et al., in press). In SSD (Pinkham et al., 2014; Pinkham et al., 2016) and early psychosis (Ludwig et al., 2017), 108 measures were identified assessing emotion processing, social perception, ToM and attributional style with seven measures of social cognition (schizophrenia) and one (early psychosis) being recommended. In ASD, eight measures of social cognition have been identified as having adequate psychometric properties focused on emotion perception and ToM (Morrison et al., 2019). Finally, in dementia, and predominately FTD, emotion perception, ToM and empathy are the domains most frequently examined in the literature (e.g., Bora et al., 2016; Bora et al., 2015; Carr & Mendez, 2018). In sum, measures have been reported for seven domains of social cognition: face identity, emotion perception, ToM, empathy, attributional bias, social communication and social perception. Across these various reviews, data has been reported on test popularity, validity and reliability. Here, we will provide an overview of the research and clinical suitability of measures that we have selected for each of the seven identified domains. Selection was based on the published reviews, expert recommendations and our own research. A summary of these can be found in Table 9.2, while full details and additional tools are referenced in the Appendix.

Face identification

Facial identification tasks require examinees to match faces from different angles, or name/ describe familiar or famous individuals based on photographs. A long-standing and widely used instrument for assessing face perception *per se* is the *Benton Face Recognition Test* (Benton et al., 1983). The original relied on a flip chart with the target black and white face on one page and foils on another. Recently, a computerised form has been developed (Rossion & Michel, 2018). The *BFRT* has been criticised for failing to detect congenital prosopagnosia but performance is improved if response times are scored (Busigny & Rossion, 2010). The newer *Cambridge Facial Recognition Test (CFMT)* (Duchaine & Nakayama, 2006) has a perceptual and a memory component. In the *CFMT*, examinees match morphed facial images for similarity, and they must pick out a previously seen identity from distractors. The *CFMT* has good reliability and it is more sensitive to prosopagnosia than the *BFRT* (Albonico et al., 2017) and has quite extensive norms (e.g., Wilmer et al., 2010). Memory for faces is also tested as part of neuropsychological batteries such as the *Wechsler Memory Scale III* (WMS-III; Wechsler, 1997) and the *Rivermead Behavioural Memory Test* (Wilson et al., 2008). Newer, briefer tasks have also been included in social cognitive batteries (Kelly & McDonald, 2020). Face identity recognition was examined in 14% (53 independent studies) with of papers reporting on brain injury, with the BFRT being most frequently used (62%), followed by the WMS-III. Face recognition is also commonly tested in dementia in research and clinical settings (Greene & Hodges, 1996; Kelly & McDonald, 2020; Snowden et al., 2004). Further, in a meta-analysis of 112 included studies, Griffin and colleagues (Griffin et al., 2020) demonstrated that those with ASD (across lifespan) performed close to one standard deviation below the normative comparison group on both face identity recognition (Hedge's g = 0.86) and discrimination (Hedge's g = 0.82).

Emotion perception

Tests of facial emotion perception typically rely on still images; however, there are a range of dynamic and audiovisual stimuli now available. Most tools assess the six emotions (sadness, happiness, fear, anger, surprise and disgust) that are believed to be universal across cultures (Ekman & Friesen, 1971). Typically, examinees choose a label from a list of alternatives or spontaneously verbalise the emotion. In some cases, examinees are required to match the emotion to another or discriminate between expressions. The most commonly used tool is the Ekman and Friesen *Pictures of Face Affect* (Ekman & Friesen, 1976), which was later developed into a standardised test of emotion labelling, the *Facial Expression of Emotion: Stimuli and Tests* (FEEST: Young et al., 2002). The *FEEST* includes 10 still, black and white images of faces posing each of the six basic emotions. The *FEEST* has established validity and reliability and has normative data for adults aged 20–70 years (Table 9.2). The *Pictures of Face Affect* were also later developed into the *Comprehensive Affect Test System* (Froming et al., 2006), which assesses facial and vocal affect recognition, non-emotional prosody and the ability to decode semantic cues in 13 subtests. The tool examines each of these skills separately and integrated. A short version is available

(Schaffer et al., 2009), and information on test reliability as well as normative data for the long-form is available in the manual. The *Ekman* faces have frequently been used in dementia and brain injury research (see Bora et al., 2016; Wallis et al., under review), and some subtests demonstrate clinical sensitivity in SSD (Martins et al., 2011).

In SSD and ASD, expert consensus points to alternative emotion perception tests. The *Penn Emotion Recognition Test* (ER-40: Kohler et al., 2003) uses 40 posed still images representing four emotions (happiness, sadness, anger and fear) across two levels of intensity as well as neutral expressions. The ER-40 uses modern, colour images of faces representative of a range of ages and ethnicities. This tool is suitable for schizophrenia research, though less so as an outcome measure for clinical trials (Pinkham et al., 2014; Pinkham et al., 2016). It is also recommended for ASD (Morrison et al., 2019). Normative data is available (Pinkham et al., 2018; Pinkham et al., 2016). Tools with greater potential ecological validity use audiovisual stimuli to assess emotion perception. The *Bell Lysaker Emotion Recognition Test* (BLERT: Bryson et al., 1997a) presents 21 video clips of male actors (~10 seconds each) representing seven emotional states. This test is valid, reliable, tolerable and sensitive to emotion perception difficulties in SSD (also suitable for clinical trials) and ASD (Morrison et al., 2019; Pinkham et al., 2014; Pinkham et al., 2016).

The *Emotion Recognition Test* (ERT: Kessels et al., 2014) presents 96 video clips of faces morphing from neutral into one of six emotions. Items finish morphing at different intensities of emotion (40%, 60%, 80% and 100%), ensuring varying levels of difficulty. Preliminary evidence attests to the validity and reliability of this task, and it has normative data in 373 individuals aged 8–75 years (Kessels et al., 2014). Clinical sensitivity has also been demonstrated for FTD (Kessels et al., 2007), SSD (Scholten et al., 2005), brain injury (Rosenberg et al., 2015), ASD (Evers et al., 2015), Huntington's disease (Montagne et al., 2006) and stroke (Montagne et al., 2007).

TASIT (McDonald, Flanagan et al., 2011, 2017a) and it's abbreviated version *TASIT-S* (Honan et al., 2016) were designed as ecologically valid tools for assessing *emotion perception* and *ToM* (or social inference) in people with brain injury. *TASIT has apparent ecological validity* in its likeness to real-world social interactions where the social cues are available from the face, body language and tone of voice, as well as subtleties in spoken language. It thus has a significant advantage over tests using still images. Part 1 (with alternate forms) require examinees to watch short audiovisual vignettes of actors in scenes, followed by multiple-choice questions regarding the emotion expressed. *TASIT* has been extensively used (Eddy, 2019; Wallis et al., in press) and is sensitive to many clinical conditions in adults including ASD (Mathersul et al., 2013c; Morrison et al., 2019), stroke (Cooper et al., 2014), dementia (Kipps et al., 2009; Kumfor et al., 2017), acquired brain injury (McDonald & Flanagan, 2004), SSD (Green et al., 2011), multiple sclerosis (Genova et al., 2016) and Parkinson's Disease (Pell et al., 2014). Reviews in brain injury (Honan,

McDonald et al., 2017; Wallis et al., in press) recommend it for use in early recovery, outcome and intervention studies. It is also recommended for assessment in SSD (Pinkham et al., 2014) and ASD (Morrison et al., 2019), though the alternative forms are less reliable as outcome measurement (Pinkham et al., 2016). Normative data is available for 13–75+ year olds for both short and long forms of the test (McDonald, Flanagan et al., 2017a; McDonald, Honan et al., 2017), and there is strong evidence for validity and reliability of the measures (Table 9.2).

Theory of mind (ToM)

Tests of ToM (also known as social inference or mentalising) vary from written text to cartoons and audiovisual content, typically followed by probes ranging from simple questions about a character's beliefs (first order theory of mind) to complex questions regarding the beliefs of one character about another character's thoughts or feelings.

The *Hinting Task* (Corcoran et al., 1995a) assesses an individual's ability to infer intentions. Ten short stories where one character makes a hint to another are presented verbally, and examinees are asked what the character *truly* meant. If the first response is inaccurate, an additional *hint* is provided to the examinee (total score 0–20). The *Hinting Task* has been used in at least 10% of studies identified in Eddy's review (Eddy, 2019). It is specifically recommended for people with SSD (Pinkham et al., 2014), is useful as a clinical outcome measure (Pinkham et al., 2016), has ecological validity, i.e., associated with functional outcomes (Pinkham et al., 2017), and is also recommended for use in psychosis (Ludwig et al., 2017) and ASD (Morrison et al., 2019). Modest normative data is available (Corcoran et al., 1995a; Pinkham et al., 2017; Pinkham et al., 2016).

Across the broader social cognition literature (Eddy, 2019) and in brain injury (Wallis et al., in press), the *Faux Pas Recognition Test* (FPT: Stone et al., 1998) is a commonly used tool to examine ToM. Examinees are required to read 20 short passages, half of which contain an unintentional faux pas and half of which do not (control stories). Follow-up questions tap whether the examinee recognises the faux pas, knows why it was a faux pas and how the target of the faux pas may feel. A final question taps understanding of general content. The *FPT* is sensitive to impairment in ASD (Zalla et al., 2009), dementia (Gregory et al., 2002), acquired brain injury (Martin-Rodriguez & Leon-Carrion, 2010) and SSD (Pijnenborg et al., 2013). While it has been used in more than 20% of published studies (Eddy, 2019) and also frequently in brain injury research (Wallis et al., in press), experts did not specifically recommend it for SSD (Pinkham et al., 2014) or brain injury (Honan, McDonald et al., 2017). It has been used with those with behavioural variant FTD demonstrating large effect sizes ($d = 2.28$) compared to healthy controls. Meta-analysis revealed no impairment for those with Alzheimer's disease (Bora et al., 2015).

While the short, written passages remain available to examinees while they answer questions, the test does tap memory and attentional processes (Gregory et al., 2002) and relies on knowledge of social norms (Bora et al., 2015). The tool has been translated into many languages, though normative data is not available.

The *Reading the Mind in the Eyes Test* (RMET: Baron-Cohen, Wheelwright et al., 2001) is cited in over 20% of reviewed studies (Eddy, 2019). The examinee views 36 photographs of the eye region that were sourced from magazines. They select the apparent mental state from options, e.g., 'playful' or 'pensive'. The *RMET* demonstrates clinical sensivity in ASD (Baron-Cohen et al., 2015), brain injury (Muller et al., 2010), SSD (Pinkham et al., 2016) and behavioural variant FTD (Bora et al., 2015; Gregory et al., 2002). While it has been used in more than 20% of published studies (Eddy, 2019), it is not recommended as an outcome measure in brain injury (Honan, McDonald et al., 2017), early psychosis or schizophrenia (Ludwig et al., 2017; Pinkham et al., 2016), but was deemed acceptable for use in ASD (Morrison et al., 2019). The test is freely available from the authors and some normative data is available in various studies. Like the *FPT*, the *RMET* demonstrates reliance on other non-social cognitive skills, specifically vocabulary (Olderbak et al., 2015; Pinkham et al., 2017), and it does not correlate with other measures of ToM (Ahmed & Miller, 2011; Duval et al., 2011).

TASIT (McDonald, Flanagan et al., 2011, 2017a) and its abbreviated version TASIT-S (Honan et al., 2016) also provide an assessment of ToM. In Parts 2–3 (with alternate forms), examinees watch short audiovisual vignettes of actors in conversations that are sincere, contain lies or are sarcastic, followed by a number of multiple-choice questions regarding the emotion, thoughts and intentions of those speakers. As above, *TASIT* has been extensively used (Eddy, 2019; Wallis et al., in press), is sensitive to many clinical conditions and has extensive norms.

There are also emerging theory of mind tasks (Eddy, 2019) that, as yet, have limited psychometric information. The *Movie for the Assessment of Social Cognition* (MASC: Dziobek et al., 2006) requires individuals to watch audiovisual clips of movies of people interacting. Videos are paused periodically, and examinees answer questions about the characters' beliefs and intentions. The MASC was originally developed for use in ASD, though it has also been used in SSD (e.g., Martinez et al., 2017). The MASC is available in several languages including English, German, French and Italian. The *Yoni Task* (Shamay-Tsoory & Aharon-Peretz, 2007) displays a number of schematic faces in the centre of a computer screen. Examinees answer questions about mental processes as well as relationships to objects based on eye gaze, mouth shape and distance between images. The first study examined people with brain lesions (Shamay-Tsoory & Aharon-Peretz, 2007) followed by people with SSD (Shamay-Tsoory et al., 2007). It also discriminates people with mild cognitive impairment, Parkinson's disease (Shamay-Tsoory et al., 2007) and Huntington's disease (Adjeroud et al., 2015) from healthy controls. Due to limited requirements on language, translations have been developed (e.g., French and Italian). Finally, the *Social Attribution Task* (Klin, 2000) and the *Animation Task* (Abell et al., 2000) require examinees to view animated films of geometric shapes and interpret the actions of those shapes. The shapes either move randomly, demonstrate simple 'pushing' behaviour or complex interactions where one shape appears to 'coax' the other (*Animation Task*) or 'in synchrony', 'against' or in 'response' to the other (*SAT*). Scoring is somewhat complex with publishers suggesting the need for multiple blinded raters. These tasks were, again, developed in ASD research but have extended use across a number of other clinical populations including Huntington's disease (Eddy & Rickards, 2015) and SSD (Horan et al., 2009).

Empathy

Empathy is most commonly assessed using self-report measures in order to garner an examinee's subjective emotional response. Given empathy typically refers to both cognitive and affective judgements, many of the tests examined in the above section are also argued to measure cognitive empathy, i.e., ToM and/or perspective taking. However, most research into empathy relies on self-reported empathy measures.

The *Interpersonal Reactivity Index* (IRI: Davis, 1980, 1983) measures four facets of empathy: perspective taking, empathic concern, personal distress and fantasy. Examinees read 28 items and rate each on a five-point Likert scale. The *IRI* is sensitive to brain injury (Zupan et al., 2018), ASD (Mathersul et al., 2013c) and behavioural variant FTD (based on relative report) (Sollberger et al., 2014). It has been used in more than 20% of reviewed published studies in neuropsychiatry (Eddy, 2019) and frequently in brain injury (Wallis et al., in press) and is specifically recommended in brain injury outcome studies (Honan, McDonald et al., 2017). In a meta-analysis in SSD, the *IRI* was the most frequently examined tool, with the Empathic Concern scale, specifically, differentiating those with SSD from matched controls (Bonfils et al., 2016). Due to problems with validity (Davis, 1983), it is recommended that the Personal Distress and Fantasy subscales be excluded (Cliffordson, 2001; De Corte et al., 2007), with many researchers opting to just include the Empathic Concern and Perspective Taking scales. Data for normative comparisons can be extracted from the many published studies in healthy people.

There are many other self-report questionnaires of cognitive and/or affective empathy. The *Balanced Emotional Empathy Scale* (BEES: Mehrabian, 2000) focuses on the emotional component of empathy and was the second most frequently used tool in brain injury studies (Wallis et al., in press). It has 30 items and normative data (predominately based on younger samples) available in the manual. The *Empathy Quotient* (EQ: Baron-Cohen & Wheelwright,

2004) has 60 items (40 empathy, 20 filler) with factor analysis identifying three components: cognitive empathy, affective empathy and social skills (Lawrence et al., 2004). There are suitable versions for adults and children (Auyeung et al., 2009), and it has been translated into French, Italian and Korean among others. Normative data is available for males and females separately and on large samples (e.g., 5490 aged 18–75 years; Cassidy et al., 2016). It has predominately been used in ASD research. The *Questionnaire of Cognitive and Emotional Empathy* (QCAE: Reniers et al., 2011) assesses both cognitive and affective empathy in 31 items derived from factor analyses of items from other well-established scales including the IRI. The *QCAE* (cognitive empathy) is sensitive to impairment in SSD and also predicts better community functioning (Horan et al., 2015). Normative data from the original validation study and later, online studies yield relative large samples although these are skewed to include mostly university students (Powell, 2018).

There are also some emerging performance-based tests of empathy. The *Multifaceted Empathy Test* (Dziobek et al., 2008) requires individuals to view a number of images of people in social scenes and make judgements about the emotional state of the character, as well as the concern they feel for the character (empathic concern) and how it affects the examinee (also see below).

Attributional bias

Attributional bias is the lens through which individuals view their social world, and how they attribute causes to events. For example, a hostility bias is characteristic of paranoid thinking (Combs et al., 2007a). Attributional bias has predominately been investigated in individuals with a diagnosis of schizophrenia (see Pinkham et al., 2014) with some evaluation in brain injury also (Neumann et al., 2020). The *Ambiguous Intentions and Hostility Questionnaire*, abbreviated version (Combs et al., 2007b), has been frequently used and requires examinees to read five ambiguous situations which have negative outcomes. Examinees rate, on a Likert scale, the degree to which the perpetrator's action was deliberate, how angry they would feel, the extent of blame and how they would respond. Pinkham and colleagues (Buck et al., 2016, Pinkham et al., 2014) reported the tool to be suitable to assess attribution bias in SSD but insufficiently sensitive for use as an outcome measure in clinical trials (Pinkham et al., 2016). Attributional bias has also been measured behaviourally via trustworthy ratings of ambiguous faces such as the *Trustworthiness/Approachability Task* (Adolphs et al., 1998), which comprises 84 unfamiliar grayscale photographs. Such trustworthiness ratings are associated with structures within the 'social brain' (see Chapter 1) in people with *amygdala* lesions (Adolphs et al., 1998) and SSD (Pinkham et al., 2008). However, this task, and other similar ones, do not reliably differentiate people with clinical disorders including dementia, SSD and ASD (Blessing et al., 2010; Mathersul et al., 2013b; Morrison et al., 2019; Pinkham et al., 2008; Pinkham et al., 2016).

Social communication

Social communication, also referred to as cognitive communication or pragmatic language, refer to the ability to use language in context, for example, understand sarcasm, humour and irony, and has overlapping features with ToM assessment. In brain injury research, the *La Trobe Communication Questionnaire* (Douglas et al., 2007) and *TASIT* are the most frequently used tools (Wallis et al., in press), and both are recommended for use in early recovery, outcome and intervention studies (see Honan, McDonald et al., 2017). *TASIT* has also been used for this purpose in people with dementia (Kumfor et al., 2017). *TASIT*, along with other tools, has shown discernible impairments in people with behavioural variant FTD and AD (Luzzi et al., 2020). In dementia research, proverb and metaphor comprehension tasks are also frequently used (see Rapp & Wild, 2011 for review). In ASD, the *Strange Stories Task* (Happe, 1994) is frequently used (Loukusa & Moilanen, 2009).

Social perception

In the schizophrenia literature, social perception refers to social knowledge and assumptions one would need to successfully interact. The *Interpersonal Perception Task* (Mah et al., 2004) assesses knowledge of social status, intimacy, kinship, competition and deception. *The Relationships Across Domains* (RAD) examines implicit knowledge of four relational models (i.e., communal sharing, authority ranking, equality matching and market pricing – contribution to social interaction and return) (Sergi et al., 2009). The *RAD* is recommended for assessment (but not outcome measurement) in schizophrenia (Pinkham et al., 2014; Pinkham et al., 2016) and in autism research (Morrison et al., 2019). Moral reasoning is also relevant to this domain, and deficits in moral reasoning have been documented in people with brain lesions. However, adult assessment tasks have been limited to the 'trolley' task (Mendez et al., 2005). In the developmental literature, the *So-Moral* task has been developed specifically for individual assessment (see Chapter 10).

Omnibus tests

There are a few measures that target a number of domains of social cognition within one test. This reduces the need to acquire multiple tests and also gives the option of focusing on the domain of interest, thus reducing time required for administration. The following examples are considered emerging tests with limited evidence for reliability and validity.

The *Social Cognition and Emotional Assessment* (SEA: Funkiewiez et al., 2012) was designed for the differential diagnosis of behavioural variant FTD (Bertoux, Delavest et al., 2012; Bertoux, Volle et al., 2012). The *SEA* is a combination of five existing tools of social cognition, varied slightly or shortened for this purpose. Domains include facial emotion perception (Ekman and Fre-isen images), ToM (*Faux Pas Recognition Test*), behavioural control and reversal learning (computer administered tasks) and a carer-rated apathy scale (Starkstein et al., 1992). The *SEA* takes approximately 60 minutes to administer, while a short version (Emotion Perception and Faux Pas only) takes 30 minutes.

The *Brief Assessment of Social Skills* (BASS: Kelly & McDonald, 2020) is a short screening tool also developed for assessing people with dementia. The BASS measures face emotion perception, face identification, empathy/ToM, social disinhibition, social reasoning and memory for new faces. The stimuli are a combination of photos and drawings of social scenes. The BASS differenti-ates people with dementia and controls, and five of the six domains of social cognition show good convergent validity. As a relatively new tool designed for clinical use, normative data are not yet available. Studies are underway to provide normative data across the adult lifespan, and to determine sensitivity to other clinical populations such as those with brain injury and schizophre-nia. Research is also underway to determine whether the BASS is suitable for remote administration.

Additional domains relevant to social cognition

Self-awareness

Self-awareness is not typically included among measures of social cognition but is pivotal to good social awareness, and indeed self-awareness *of* social cognitive ability has been shown to be a better predictor of functioning than social cog-nitive ability alone (Silberstein et al., 2018). In disorders such as alexithymia, i.e., impaired awareness of emotion and internal states (Larsen et al., 2003), poor self-awareness will directly affect emotional empathy. Impaired meta-cognition, causing difficulty reflecting on one's own mental processes (Boake et al., 1995; Godfrey et al., 1993), is also implicated in perspective taking and empathy.

Alexithymia is commonly assessed using the 20 item *Toronto Alexithymia Scale* (Taylor et al., 2003). In regards to self-awareness, four measures have been generally recommended (Tate, 2010). One is the *Patient Competency Rating Scale* (PCRS) (30 items) (Prigatano & Altman, 1990), with three versions (self, relative, clinician) that assesses current competency on a Likert scale (1 = Can't do, to 5 = Can do with ease) in cognition, interpersonal function, emotional behaviour and living skills. Discrepancies between self and informant are used to index lack of self-awareness. Similar discrepancies between self and inform-ant are derived on the *Awareness Questionnaire* (AQ) (17 items) (Sherer et al., 1998) and the *Mayo Portland Adaptability Index* (MPAI-4) (12 items) (Malec & Thompson, 1994), which assess changes in motor/sensory, cognition, commu-nication and emotional/behavioural domains. Alternatively, the *Self-Awareness of Deficits Interview* (SADI) (Fleming et al., 1996) is a semi-structured interview that assesses the individual's awareness of changes in functioning, associated implications and the capacity to set realistic goals. Collateral ratings from the clinician yield scores ranging from 0 (no impairment) to 9 (severe impairment). There is generally good concordance between these measures (Ownsworth et al., 2019).

Social behaviour

Disorders of social cognition will impact behaviour as the person with impaired social cognition will become less sensitive and able to deal with social cues. There are also disorders of social behaviour that may arise directly from brain pathology (see Chapter 1). Abnormal social behaviour can manifest when someone fails to demonstrate manners (e.g., cannot wait their turn to speak) and/or behave in line with social conventions such as placing feet on the table or demonstrate poor interpersonal boundaries or present in an apathetic and disinterested way. Assessment of such behaviour usually takes the form of informant report and a number of these questionnaires have been developed for specific populations but with clear relevance to others. Some of the most widely used include the *Frontal Systems Behavior Scale* (Grace et al., 2001), the *Frontal Behavioural Inventory* (Kertesz et al., 2000), the *Overt Behaviour Scale* (Kelly et al., 2006), the *Dysexecutive Questionnaire* (Burgess et al., 1996), and the *Behaviour Rating Inventory of Executive Function – Adult* (Roth, Isquith, & Gioia, 2005). There are also newer questionnaires that have been designed specifically to tap into social aspects of behaviour, including those that reflect social cognition. Two such scales, the *Social Functioning in Dementia Scale* (Sommerlad et al., 2017) and the *Social Skills Questionnaire-TBI* (Francis et al., 2017) have been designed for assessing people with dementia and traumatic brain injury respectively.

Due to some of the inherent limitations of self and informant questionnaires discussed above, there has been a push to develop performance-based measures that can capture aspects of poor social behaviour, specifically, poor decision-making and poor behavioural inhibition. Decision-making has typically been measured using experimental tasks such as the *Iowa Gambling task (IGT)* (Bechara et al., 2005; Damasio et al., 1991). While popular, the *IGT* has many drawbacks conceptually and has been criticised as a test which is not actually social in nature (Torralva et al., 2013; Torralva et al., 2007). An alternate *Social Decision Making Task* was developed in brain injury, though has gained little traction to date (Kelly et al., 2014). Several tasks have been developed to assess social disinhibition, including an observational measure using an interview format while scoring the degree of inappropriate self-disclosure observed (Osborne-Crowley et al., 2016), a task that comprises images of social scenarios and questions (Honan, Allen et al., 2017) and a simple Stroop-like task encompassing socially relevant material designed for dementia (BASS: Kelly & McDonald, 2020).

Benefits of assessment of social cognition in adult clinical populations

The social cognitive assessments that have been detailed in this chapter herald a new way of assessing and understanding neuropsychological impairment. Social cognition is pivotal to interpersonal function, and therefore assessment of impairment has direct relevance to functional outcomes and targets for remediation. Difficulties reading emotions from the face, tone of voice and posture will have downstream effects on the ability of the individual to understand the complexities behind what their communication partner may be both feeling and thinking, leaving them unable to respond appropriately and in many cases unable to respond empathically. Further, and much more obvious when it occurs, disinhibited behaviour extends from saying something socially inappropriate or rude to engaging in sexually explicit or other behaviours inappropriate to the setting. All such social impairments have significant impacts on the person afflicted but also on those around them.

The assessment of social cognition speaks directly to the rights and benefits of patients, and in the right circumstances, their family or formal/informal carers to have knowledge of the condition they are managing as well as its symptoms and prognosis (Kiser et al., 2012; Shinan-Altman, & Werner, 2017). Understanding the diagnosis reduces societal stigma (Herrmann et al., 2018) and enables formal and informal carers to provide compassionate care for longer (Quinn et al., 2019). As outlined in Case Studies 1 and 2 (see Boxes 9.1 and 9.2), simple acknowledgement of the symptoms, labelling of those symptoms and normalizing of the impact and experience of that symptom on family carers is sometimes all that is needed for beneficial outcomes for the patient and their family carer, and this communication need extend beyond the medical features to psychological and social features of disease.

Box 9.1   Case 1: Mr L: Adult with Parkinson's dementia

History:

Mr L had advancing Parkinson's dementia. He lived at home with his second wife and also has a daughter with a young family.

Presentation:

His daughter reported that her stepmother found it distressing that her father seemed to 'no longer care' about how she was feeling.

Intervention:

The clinician discussed with the daughter the likely social cognitive impairments that Mr L might be experiencing, including the loss of ability to recognise emotions in others, also the impact of these changes on the ability to understand how others are feeling, and show empathy.

The clinician also discussed how providing the language to describe these impairments and attributing them to the disease, not the person alone, can help with family coping. The next time the clinician spoke with the daughter, she reported that she had provided her stepmother with the language to describe the social changes, simply "he was now struggling to show empathy", and that these changes were not uncommon with dementia.

The daughter explained that she saw visible relief come over her stepmother's face, just to know there are words to describe the changes, that others experience this and that it is part of the disease.

Comment:

While we cannot, at this stage, do a lot to ameliorate social cognition impairments in people with dementia, arming families with the knowledge that these changes are indeed part of the symptomology is sometimes enough to reduce some of the stress associated with the caring role.

Box 9.2   Case 2: Mr J: Adult with probable dementia

History:

Mr J is a 73-year-old man who was diagnosed with probable dementia when he was 67. There was no familial history. He had 10 years of education and previously worked as a butcher, retiring when he was 65 years of age.

Presentation:

Mr J lived at home with his wife who was concerned that he was becoming increasingly agitated at home and that he no longer cared about her feelings or the feelings of others, and that the family relationships have been affected by his indifference. His wife reported that their friends no longer invite them out. She was feeling demoralized and alone, and no longer knew how to connect with her husband.

Assessment:

Five years after his initial diagnosis of probably dementia, Mr J was given the BASS (Kelly & McDonald, 2020), a screening tool of social cognition designed for people with dementia. Mr J. demonstrated impairments in face emotion perception (2.5 SD below norms), social reasoning (3.5 SD below norms) and empathy/ToM (2 SD below norms).

Comment:

These impairments in social cognition would explain a lot of the problems that his wife and family were experiencing day-to-day. Had these assessments (1) been available, (2) been administered at the time of diagnosis or during ongoing care periods after diagnosis and (3) this feedback and education provided early on in the disease process, the family may have been better prepared to manage the changes in social cognition and been able to attribute these changes to the disease.

While we have detailed a large number of tests in this chapter, the field of social cognitive assessment is in its infancy. Most tests were designed for research rather than clinical applications. In the clinical space, we lack a range of social cognition measures that have good clinical utility, reliability and normative data. In particular, as discussed in Chapter 2, we need a much better understanding of the cultural influences on social cognition measures. In the research space, we need to move towards instruments that have greater ecological validity and truly measure social cognition as it occurs, in real time and in complex environments. See Chapter 2 for a further discussion of this.

References

Abell, F., Happe, F., & Frith, U. (2000). Do triangles play tricks? Attribution of mental states to animated shapes in normal and abnormal development. *Cognitive Development, 15*(1), 1–16.

Adjeroud, N., Besnard, J., Massioui, N. E., Verny, C., Prudean, A., Scherer, C., Gohier, B., Bonneau, D., & Allain, P. (2015). Theory of mind and empathy in preclinical and clinical Huntington's disease. *Social Cognitive and Affective Neuroscience, 11*(1), 89–99. doi:10.1093/scan/nsv093

Adolphs, R. (2009). The social brain: Neural basis of social knowledge. *Annual Review of Psychology, 60,* 693–716.

Adolphs, R., Tranel, D., & Damasio, A. R. (1998). The human amygdala in social judgment. *Nature, 393*(6684), 470–474.

Adolphs, R., Tranel, D., & Damasio, A. R. (2003). Dissociable neural systems for recognizing emotions. *Brain & Cognition, 52*(1), 61–69.

Ahmed, F. S., & Miller, L. S. (2011). Executive function mechanisms of theory of mind. *Journal of Autism and Developmental Disorders, 41*(5), 667–678.

Albonico, A., Malaspina, M., & Daini, R. (2017). Italian normative data and validation of two neuropsychological tests of face recognition: Benton facial recognition test and Cambridge face memory test. *Neurological Sciences, 38*(9), 1637–1643. doi:10.1007/s10072-017-3030-6

Auyeung, B., Wheelwright, S., Allison, C., Atkinson, M., Samarawickrema, N., & Baron-Cohen, S. (2009). The children's empathy quotient and systemizing quotient: Sex differences in typical development and in autism spectrum conditions. *Journal of Autism and Developmental Disorders, 39*(11), 1509.

Baron-Cohen, S., Bowen, D. C., Holt, R. J., Allison, C., Auyeung, B., Lombardo, M. V., Smith, P., & Lai, M.-C. (2015). The "reading the mind in the eyes" test: Complete absence of typical sex difference in~400 men and women with autism. *PLoS One, 10*(8), e0136521.

Baron-Cohen, S., & Wheelwright, S. (2004). The empathy quotient: An investigation of adults with Asperger syndrome or high functioning autism, and normal sex differences. *Journal of Autism and Developmental Disorders, 34*(2), 163–175.

Baron-Cohen, S., Wheelright, S., Hill, J., Raste, Y., & Plumb, I. (2001). The "reading the mind in the eyes" test revised version: A study with normal adults and adults with Aspergers syndrome or high functioning autism. *Journal of Child Psychology and Psychiatry, 42,* 241–251. doi:10.1111/1469-7610.00715

Bechara, A., Damasio, H., Tranel, D., & Damasio, A. (2005). The Iowa Gambling task and the somatic marker hypothesis: Some questions and answers. *Trends in Cognitive Sciences, 9*(4), 159–162. www.sciencedirect.com/science/article/B6VH9-4FH0DK1-1/2/d7a8eff60fff25f8553caf1cfa8f7b97

Bell, M. D., Fiszdon, J. M., Greig, T. C., & Wexler, B. E. (2010). Social attribution test – multiple choice (SAT-MC) in schizophrenia: Comparison with community sample and relationship to neurocognitive, social cognitive and symptom measures. *Schizophrenia Research, 122*(1–3), 164–171. doi:10.1016/j.schres.2010.03.024

Benton, A. L., Sivan, A. B., Hamsher, K. D. S., Varney, N. R., & Spreen, O. (1983). Facial recognition: Stimulus and multiple choice pictures. In A. L. Benton, A. B. Sivan, K. D. S. Hamsher, N. R. Varney, & O. Spreen (Eds.), *Contribution to Neuropsychological Assessment* (pp. 30–40). Oxford: Oxford University Press.

Bertoux, M., Delavest, M., de Souza, L. C., Funkiewiez, A., Lepine, J. P., Fossati, P., Dubois, B., & Sarazin, M. (2012). Social cognition and emotional assessment differentiates frontotemporal dementia from depression. *Journal of Neurology, Neurosurgery, and Psychiatry, 83*(4), 411–416. doi:10.1136/jnnp-2011-301849

Bertoux, M., Volle, E., Funkiewiez, A., de Souza, L. C., Leclercq, D., & Dubois, B. (2012). Social cognition and emotional assessment (SEA) is a marker of medial and orbital frontal functions: A voxel-based morphometry study in behavioral variant of frontotemporal degeneration. *Journal of the International Neuropsychological Society: JINS, 18*(6), 972–985. doi:10.1017/S1355617712001300

Bjorkquist, O. A., Olsen, E. K., Nelson, B. D., & Herbener, E. S. (2016). Altered amygdala-prefrontal connectivity during emotion perception in schizophrenia. *Schizophrenia Research, 175*(1–3), 35–41.

Black, M. H., Chen, N. T., Iyer, K. K., Lipp, O. V., Bölte, S., Falkmer, M., Tan, T., & Girdler, S. (2017). Mechanisms of facial emotion recognition in autism spectrum disorders: Insights from eye tracking and electroencephalography. *Neuroscience & Biobehavioral Reviews, 80*, 488–515.

Blessing, A., Zöllig, J., Dammann, G., & Martin, M. (2010). Accurate judgment by dementia patients of neutral faces with respect to trustworthiness and valence. *GeroPsych: The Journal of Gerontopsychology and Geriatric Psychiatry, 23*(1), 33.

Bliksted, V., Videbech, P., Fagerlund, B., & Frith, C. (2017). The effect of positive symptoms on social cognition in first-episode schizophrenia is modified by the presence of negative symptoms. *Neuropsychology, 31*(2), 209–219.

Boake, C., Freelands, J. C., Ringholz, G. M., Nance, M. L., & Edwards, K. E. (1995). Awareness of memory loss after severe close head injury. *Brain Injury, 9*(3), 273–283.

Bonfils, K. A., Lysaker, P. H., Minor, K. S., & Salyers, M. P. (2016). Affective empathy in schizophrenia: A meta-analysis. *Schizophrenia Research, 175*(1), 109–117. doi:10.1016/j.schres.2016.03.037

Bora, E., Velakoulis, D., & Walterfang, M. (2016). Meta-analysis of facial emotion recognition in behavioral variant frontotemporal dementia: Comparison with Alzheimer disease and healthy controls. *Journal of Geriatric Psychiatry and Neurology, 29*(4), 205–211. doi:10.1177/0891988716640375

Bora, E., Walterfang, M., & Velakoulis, D. (2015). Theory of mind in behavioural-variant frontotemporal dementia and Alzheimer's disease: A meta-analysis. *Journal of Neurology, Neurosurgery, and Psychiatry, 86*(7), 714–719. doi:10.1136/jnnp-2014-309445

Bornhofen, C., & McDonald, S. (2008a). Emotion perception deficits following traumatic brain injury: A review of the evidence and rationale for intervention. *Journal of the International Neuropsychological Society, 14*(04), 511–525. doi:10.1017/S1355617708080703

Bornhofen, C., & McDonald, S. (2008b). Treating deficits in emotion perception following traumatic brain injury *Neuropsychological Rehabilitation, 18*(1), 22–44.

Bowers, D., Blonder, L. X., & Heilman, K. M. (1991). *Florida Affect Battery*. Gainsville, FL: Centre for Neuropsychological Studies, University of Florida.

Bryson, G., Bell, M., & Lysaker, P. (1997a). Affect recognition in schizophrenia: A function of global impairment or a specific cognitive deficit. *Psychiatry Research, 71*(2), 105–113.

Bryson, G., Bell, M., & Lysaker, P. (1997b). Affect recognition in schizophrenia: A function of global impairment or a specific cognitive deficit. *Psychiatry Research, 71*(2), 105–113. doi:10.1016/s0165-1781(97)00050-4

Buck, B. E., Pinkham, A. E., Harvey, P. D., & Penn, D. L. (2016). Revisiting the validity of measures of social cognitive bias in schizophrenia: Additional results from the social cognition psychometric evaluation (SCOPE) study. *British Journal of Clinical Psychology, 55*(4), 441–454. doi:10.1111/bjc.12113

Burgess, P., Alderman, N., Wilson, B., Evans, J., & Emslie, H. (1996). The dysexecutive questionnaire. In *Behavioural Assessment of the Dysexecutive Syndrome*. Bury St. Edmunds, UK: Thames Valley Test Company.

Busigny, T., & Rossion, B. (2010). Acquired prosopagnosia abolishes the face inversion effect. *Cortex, 46*(8), 965–981. doi:10.1016/j.cortex.2009.07.004

Cacioppo, J. T., Tassinary, L. G., & Berntson, G. (2007). *Handbook of Psychophysiology*. Cambridge: Cambridge University Press.

Canty, A. L., Neumann, D. L., Fleming, J., & Shum, D. H. K. (2017). Evaluation of a newly developed measure of theory of mind: The virtual assessment of mentalising ability. *Neuropsychological Rehabilitation, 27*(5), 834–870. doi:10.1080/09602011.2015.1052820

Carr, A. R., & Mendez, M. F. (2018). Affective empathy in behavioral variant frontotemporal dementia: A meta-analysis [systematic review]. *Frontiers in Neurology, 9*(417). doi:10.3389/fneur.2018.00417

Cassidy, S., Hannant, P., Tavassoli, T., Allison, C., Smith, P., & Baron-Cohen, S. (2016). Dyspraxia and autistic traits in adults with and without autism spectrum conditions. *Molecular Autism, 7*(1), 48.

Cecchetto, C., Korb, S., Rumiati, R. I., & Aiello, M. (2018). Emotional reactions in moral decision-making are influenced by empathy and alexithymia. *Social Neuroscience, 13*(2), 226–240.

Chiasson, V., Vera-Estay, E., Lalonde, G., Dooley, J. J., & Beauchamp, M. H. (2017). Assessing social cognition: Age-related changes in moral reasoning in childhood and adolescence. *The Clinical Neuropsychologist, 31*(3), 515–530. doi:10.1080/13854046.2016.1268650

Clare, L., Nelis, S. M., Martyr, A., Whitaker, C. J., Marková, I. S., Roth, I., Woods, R. T., & Morris, R. G. (2012). Longitudinal trajectories of awareness in early-stage dementia. *Alzheimer Disease and Associated Disorders, 26*(2), 140–147. doi:10.1097/WAD.0b013e31822c55c4

Clare, L., Whitaker, C. J., Nelis, S. M., Martyr, A., Markova, I. S., Roth, I., Woods, R. T., & Morris, R. G. (2011). Multidimensional assessment of awareness in early-stage dementia: A cluster analytic approach. *Dementia and Geriatric Cognitive Disorders, 31*(5), 317–327. doi:10.1159/000327356

Cliffordson, C. (2001). Parents' judgments and students' self-judgments of empathy: The structure of empathy and agreement of judgments based on the interpersonal reactivity index (IRI). *European Journal of Psychological Assessment, 17*(1), 36.

Combs, D. R., Penn, D. L., Wicher, M., & Waldheter, E. (2007a). The ambiguous intentions hostility questionnaire (AIHQ): A new measure for evaluating hostile social-cognitive biases in paranoia. *Cognitive Neuropsychiatry, 12*(2), 128–143. doi:10.1080/13546800600787854

Combs, D. R., Penn, D. L., Wicher, M., & Waldheter, E. (2007b). The ambiguous intentions hostility questionnaire (AIHQ): A new measure for evaluating hostile social-cognitive biases in paranoia. *Cognitive Neuropsychiatry, 12*(2), 128–143.

Cooper, C. L., Phillips, L. H., Johnston, M., Radlak, B., Hamilton, S., & McLeod, M. J. (2014). Links between emotion perception and social participation restriction following stroke. *Brain Injury, 28*(1), 122–126.

Corcoran, R., Mercer, G., & Frith, C. D. (1995a). Schizophrenia, symptomatology and social inference: Investigating theory of mind in people with schizophrenia. *Schizophrenia Research, 17*, 5–13.

Corcoran, R., Mercer, G., & Frith, C. D. (1995b). Schizophrenia, symptomology and social inference: Investigating "theory of mind" in people with schizophrenia. *Schizophrenia Research, 17*, 5–13.

Costanzo, M., & Archer, D. (1989). Interpreting the expressive behavior of others: The interpersonal perception task. *Journal of Nonverbal Behavior, 13*, 225–245.

Cusi, A. M., Nazarov, A., Holshausen, K., MacQueen, G. M., & McKinnon, M. C. (2012). Systematic review of the neural basis of social cognition in patients with mood disorders. *Journal of Psychiatry & Neuroscience, 37*(3), 154–169.

Damasio, A., Tranel, D., & Damasio, H. (1991). Somatic markers and the guidance of behavior: Theory and preliminary testing. In H. S. Levin, H. M. Eisenberg, & A. L.

Benton (Eds.), *Frontal Lobe Function and Dysfunction* (pp. 217–229). Oxford: Oxford University Press, Inc.

Davis, M. H. (1980). A multidimensional approach to individual differences in empathy. *JSAS Catalog of Selected Documents in Psychology, 10*, 85.

Davis, M. H. (1983). Measuring individual differences in empathy: Evidence for a multidimensional approach. *Journal of Personality and Social Psychology, 44*(1), 113–126.

De Corte, K., Buysse, A., Verhofstadt, L. L., Roeyers, H., Ponnet, K., & Davis, M. H. (2007). Measuring empathic tendencies: Reliability and validity of the Dutch version of the interpersonal reactivity index. *Psychologica Belgica, 47*(4), 235–260.

De La Asuncion, J., Bervoets, C., Morrens, M., Sabbe, B., & De Bruijn, E. (2015). EEG correlates of impaired self-other integration during joint-task performance in schizophrenia. *Social Cognitive and Affective Neuroscience, 10*(10), 1365–1372.

de Sousa, A., McDonald, S., & Rushby, J. (2012). Changes in emotional empathy, affective responsivity, and behavior following severe traumatic brain injury. *Journal of Clinical and Experimental Neuropsychology, 34*(6), 606–623. doi:10.1080/13803395.2012.667067

de Sousa, A., McDonald, S., Rushby, J., Li, S., Dimoska, A., & James, C. (2010). Why don't you feel how I feel? Insight into the absence of empathy after severe traumatic brain injury. *Neuropsychologia, 48*(12), 3585–3595. doi:10.1016/j.neuropsychologia.2010.08.008

de Sousa, A., McDonald, S., Rushby, J., Li, S., Dimoska, A., & James, C. (2011). Understanding deficits in empathy after traumatic brain injury: The role of affective responsivity. *Cortex, 47*(5), 526–535. doi:10.1016/j.cortex.2010.02.004

Dehning, S., Gasperi, S., Krause, D., Meyer, S., Reiß, E., Burger, M., Jacobs, F., Buchheim, A., Müller, N., & Siebeck, M. (2013). Emotional and cognitive empathy in first-year medical students. *International Scholarly Research Notices, 2013*.

Douglas, J. M., Bracy, C. A., & Snow, P. C. (2007). Measuring perceived communicative ability after traumatic brain injury: Reliability and validity of the La Trobe communication questionnaire. *Journal of Head Trauma Rehabilitation, 22*(1), 31–38.

Duchaine, B., & Nakayama, K. (2006). The Cambridge face memory test: Results for neurologically intact individuals and an investigation of its validity using inverted face stimuli and prosopagnosic participants. *Neuropsychologia, 44*(4), 576–585. doi:10.1016/j.neuropsychologia.2005.07.001

Duchaine, B., Germine, L., & Nakayama, K. (2007). Family resemblance: Ten family members with prosopagnosia and within-class object agnosia. *Cognitive Neuropsychology, 24*(4), 419–430. doi:10.1080/02643290701380491

Duval, C., Piolino, P., Bejanin, A., Eustache, F., & Desgranges, B. (2011). Age effects on different components of theory of mind. *Consciousness and Cognition, 20*(3), 627–642.

Dziobek, I., Fleck, S., Kalbe, E., Rogers, K., Hassenstab, J., Brand, M., Kessler, J., Woike, J. K., Wolf, O. T., & Convit, A. (2006). Introducing MASC: A movie for the assessment of social cognition. *Journal of Autism and Developmental Disorders, 36*(5), 623–636. doi:10.1007/s10803-006-0107-0

Dziobek, I., Rogers, K., Fleck, S., Bahnemann, M., Heekeren, H. R., Wolf, O. T., & Convit, A. (2008). Dissociation of cognitive and emotional empathy in adults with Asperger syndrome using the multifaceted empathy test (MET). *Journal of Autism and Developmental Disorders, 38*(3), 464–473. doi:10.1007/s10803-007-0486-x

Eddy, C. M. (2019). What do you have in mind? Measures to assess mental state reasoning in neuropsychiatric populations. *Frontiers in Psychiatry, 10*.

Eddy, C. M., & Rickards, H. E. (2015). Interaction without intent: The shape of the social world in Huntington's disease. *Social Cognitive and Affective Neuroscience, 10*(9), 1228–1235.

Ekman, P., & Friesen, W. V. (1971). Constants across cultures in the face and emotion. *Journal of Personality and Social Psychology, 17*(2), 124–129. www.ncbi.nlm.nih.gov/pubmed/5542557

Ekman, P., & Friesen, W. V. (1976). *Pictures of Facial Affect*. Palo Alto, CA: Consulting Psychologists Press.

Evers, K., Steyaert, J., Noens, I., & Wagemans, J. (2015). Reduced recognition of dynamic facial emotional expressions and emotion-specific response bias in children with an Autism spectrum disorder [article]. *Journal of Autism and Developmental Disorders, 45*(6), 1774–1784. doi:10.1007/s10803-014-2337-x

Fleming, J. M., Strong, J., & Ashton, R. (1996). Self-awareness of deficits in adults with traumatic brain injury: How best to measure? *Brain Injury, 10*, 1–15.

Foell, J., Brislin, S. J., Drislane, L. E., Dziobek, I., & Patrick, C. J. (2018). Creation and validation of an english-language version of the multifaceted empathy test (MET). *Journal of Psychopathology and Behavioral Assessment, 40*(3), 431–439. doi:10.1007/s10862-018-9664-8

Francis, H. M., Osborne-Crowley, K., & McDonald, S. (2017). Validity and reliability of a questionnaire to assess social skills in traumatic brain injury: A preliminary study. *Brain Injury, 31*(3), 336–343. doi:10.1080/02699052.2016.1250954

Froming, K., Levy, M., Schaffer, S., & Ekman, P. (2006). *The Comprehensive Affect Testing System*. Gainsville, FL: Psychology Software, Inc.

Funkiewiez, A., Bertoux, M., de Souza, L. C., Levy, R., & Dubois, B. (2012). The SEA (social cognition and emotional assessment): A clinical neuropsychological tool for early diagnosis of frontal variant of frontotemporal lobar degeneration. *Neuropsychology, 26*(1), 81–90. doi:10.1037/a0025318

Genova, H. M., Cagna, C. J., Chiaravalloti, N. D., DeLuca, J., & Lengenfelder, J. (2016). Dynamic assessment of social cognition in individuals with multiple sclerosis: A pilot study. *Journal of the International Neuropsychological Society: JINS, 22*(1), 83–88. doi:10.1017/S1355617715001137

Godfrey, H. P., Partridge, F. M., Knight, R. G., & Bishara, S. N. (1993, July). Course of insight disorder and emotional dysfunction following closed head injury: A controlled cross-sectional follow-up study. *Journal of Clinical and Experimental Neuropsychology, 15*(4), 503–515.

Godfrey, H. P., & Shum, D. (2000). Executive functioning and the application of social skills following traumatic brain injury. *Aphasiology, 14*(4), 433–444. doi:10.1080/026870300401441. http://search.ebscohost.com/login.aspx?direct=true&db=ufh&AN=3824904&site=ehost-live

Goodman, J. K., & Paolacci, G. (2017). Crowdsourcing consumer research. *Journal of Consumer Research, 44*(1), 196–210.

Grace, J., Grace, J., & Malloy, P. (2001). *FrSBe, Frontal Systems Behavior Scale: Professional Manual*. Lutz, FL: Psychological Assessment Resources.

Green, M. F., Bearden, C. E., Cannon, T. D., Fiske, A. P., Hellemann, G. S., Horan, W. P., Kee, K., Kern, R. S., Lee, J., Sergi, M. J., Subotnik, K. L., Sugar, C. A., Ventura, J., Yee, C. M., & Nuechterlein, K. H. (2011). Social cognition in schizophrenia, part 1: Performance across phase of illness. *Schizophrenia Bulletin, 38*(4), 854–864. doi:10.1093/schbul/sbq171

Green, M. F., Lee, J., & Ochsner, K. N. (2013). Adapting social neuroscience measures for schizophrenia clinical trials, part 1: Ferrying paradigms across perilous waters. *Schizophrenia Bulletin, 39*(6), 1192–1200.

Greene, J. D., & Hodges, J. R. (1996). Identification of famous faces and famous names in early Alzheimer's disease. Relationship to anterograde episodic and general semantic memory. *Brain, 119*(Pt 1), 111–128. www.ncbi.nlm.nih.gov/pubmed/8624675

Gregory, C., Lough, S., Stone, V., Erzinclioglu, S., Martin, L., Baron-Cohen, S., & Hodges, J. R. (2002). Theory of mind in patients with frontal variant frontotemporal dementia and Alzheimer's disease: Theoretical and practical implications. *Brain, 125*(Pt 4), 752–764. www.ncbi.nlm.nih.gov/pubmed/11912109

Griffin, J. W., Bauer, R., & Scherf, K. S. (2020). A quantitative meta-analysis of face recognition deficits in autism: 40 years of research. *Psychological Bulletin, 147*(3), 268–292.

Happe, F. G. (1994). An advanced test of theory of mind: Understanding of story characters' thoughts and feelings by able autistic, mentally handicapped, and normal children and adults. *Journal of Autism and Developmental Disorders, 24*(2), 129–154.

Healey, K. M., Combs, D. R., Gibson, C. M., Keefe, R. S., Roberts, D. L., & Penn, D. L. (2015). Observable social cognition – a rating scale: An interview-based assessment for schizophrenia. *Cognitive Neuropsychiatry, 20*(3), 198–221.

Herrmann, L. K., Welter, E., Leverenz, J. B., Lerner, A. J., Udelson, N., Kanetsky, C., & Sajatovic, M. (2018). A systematic review of dementia-related stigma research: Can we move the stigma dial? *The American Journal of Geriatric Psychiatry, 26*(3), 316–331. doi:10.1016/j.jagp.2017.09.006

Honan, C. A., Allen, S. K., Fisher, A., Osborne-Crowley, K., & McDonald, S. (2017). Social disinhibition: Piloting a new clinical measure in individuals with traumatic brain injury. *Brain Impairment, 18*(1). doi:10.1017/BrImp.2016.27

Honan, C. A., McDonald, S., Sufani, C., Hine, D. W., & Kumfor, F. (2016). The awareness of social inference test: Development of a shortened version for use in adults with acquired brain injury. *The Clinical Neuropsychologist, 30*(2), 243–264. doi:10.1080/13854 046.2015.1136691

Honan, C. A., McDonald, S., Tate, R., Ownsworth, T., Togher, L., Fleming, J., Anderson, V., Morgan, A., Catroppa, C., Douglas, J., Francis, H., Wearne, T., Sigmundsdottir, L., & Ponsford, J. (2017). Outcome instruments in moderate-to-severe adult traumatic brain injury: Recommendations for use in psychosocial research. *Neuropsychological Rehabilitation*, 1–21. doi:10.1080/09602011.2017.1339616

Horan, W. P., Nuechterlein, K., Wynn, J., Lee, J., Castelli, F., & Green, M. (2009). Disturbances in the spontaneous attribution of social meaning in schizophrenia. *Psychological Medicine, 39*(4), 635–643.

Horan, W. P., Reise, S. P., Kern, R. S., Lee, J., Penn, D. L., & Green, M. F. (2015). Structure and correlates of self-reported empathy in schizophrenia. *Journal of Psychiatric Research, 66–67*, 60–66. doi:10.1016/j.jpsychires.2015.04.016

Hsieh, S., Irish, M., Daveson, N., Hodges, J. R., & Piguet, O. (2013). When one loses empathy: Its effect on carers of patients with dementia. *Journal of Geriatric Psychiatry and Neurology, 26*(3), 174–184. doi:10.1177/0891988713495448

Johnson, S. K., Lange, G., DeLuca, J., Korn, L. R., & Natelson, B. (1997). The effects of fatigue on neuropsychological performance in patients with chronic fatigue syndrome, multiple sclerosis, and depression. *Applied Neuropsychology, 4*(3), 145–153.

Kelly, G., Todd, J., Simpson, G., Kremer, P., & Martin, C. (2006). The overt behaviour scale (OBS): A tool for measuring challenging behaviours following ABI in community settings. *Brain Injury, 20*(3), 307–319.

Kelly, M., & McDonald, S. (2020). Assessing social cognition in people with a diagnosis of dementia: Development of a novel screening test, the brief assessment of social skills

(BASS-D). *Journal of Clinical and Experimental Neuropsychology, 42*(2), 185–198. doi:10.10 80/13803395.2019.1700925

Kelly, M., McDonald, S., & Frith, M. H. J. (2017a). Assessment and rehabilitation of social cognition impairment after brain injury: Surveying practices of clinicians in Australia. *Brain Impairment, 18*(1), 11–35.

Kelly, M., McDonald, S., & Frith, M. H. J. (2017b). A survey of clinicians working in brain injury rehabilitation: Are social cognition impairments on the radar? *Journal of Head Trauma Rehabilitation, 32*(4), E55–e65. doi:10.1097/htr.0000000000000269

Kelly, M., McDonald, S., & Kellett, D. (2014). Development of a novel task for investigating decision making in a social context following traumatic brain injury. *Journal of Clinical and Experimental Neuropsychology, 36*(9), 897–913. doi:10.1080/13803395.2014.955784

Kelly, M., McDonald, S., & Wallis, K. (under review). *Empathy Across the Ages: "I May Be Older but I'm Still Feeling It"*.

Kelly, M., Mierndorff, S., Voeste, J., & Wales, K. (in prep). *Telehealth-based assessment of cognition, social cognition, mood and functional independence in older adults*.

Kern, R. S., Penn, D. L., Lee, J., Horan, W. P., Reise, S. P., Ochsner, K. N., Marder, S. R., & Green, M. F. (2013). Adapting social neuroscience measures for schizophrenia clinical trials, part 2: Trolling the depths of psychometric properties. *Schizophrenia Bulletin, 39*(6), 1201–1210.

Kertesz, A., Nadkarni, N., Davidson, W., & Thomas, A. W. (2000). The Frontal Behavioral Inventory in the differential diagnosis of frontotemporal dementia. *Journal of the International Neuropsychological Society, 6*(4), 460–468.

Kessels, R. P. C., Gerritsen, L., Montagne, B., Ackl, N., Diehl, J., & Danek, A. (2007). Recognition of facial expressions of different emotional intensities in patients with frontotemporal lobar degeneration. *Behavioural Neurology, 18*(1), 31–36.

Kessels, R. P. C., Montagne, B., Hendriks, A. W., Perrett, D. I., & de Haan, E. H. (2014). Assessment of perception of morphed facial expressions using the emotion recognition task: Normative data from healthy participants aged 8–75. *Journal of Neuropsychology, 8*(1), 75–93.

Kipps, C. M., Nestor, P. J., Acosta-Cabronero, J., Arnold, R., & Hodges, J. R. (2009). Understanding social dysfunction in the behavioural variant of frontotemporal dementia: The role of emotion and sarcasm processing [research support, non-U.S. Gov't]. *Brain: A Journal of Neurology, 132*(Pt 3), 592–603. doi:10.1093/brain/awn314

Kiser, K., Jonas, D., Warner, Z., Scanlon, K., Bryant Shilliday, B., & DeWalt, D. A. (2012). A randomized controlled trial of a literacy-sensitive self-management intervention for chronic obstructive pulmonary disease patients. *Journal of General Internal Medicine, 27*(2), 190–195. doi:10.1007/s11606-011-1867-6

Klin, A. (2000). Attributing social meaning to ambiguous visual stimuli in higher-functioning autism and Asperger syndrome: The social attribution task. *Journal of Child Psychology and Psychiatry, 41*(7), 831–846.

Klin, A., & Jones, W. (2006). Attributing social and physical meaning to ambiguous visual displays in individuals with higher-functioning autism spectrum disorders. *Brain and Cognition, 61*(1), 40–53.

Kohler, C. G., Turner, T. H., Bilker, W. B., Brensinger, C. M., Siegel, S. J., Kanes, S. J., Gur, R. E., & Gur, R. C. (2003). Facial emotion recognition in schizophrenia: Intensity effects and error pattern. *American Journal of Psychiatry, 160*(10), 1768–1774.

Konrath, S. H., O'Brien, E. H., & Hsing, C. (2010). Changes in dispositional empathy in American college students over time: A meta-analysis. *Personality and Social Psychology Review, 15*(2), 180–198. doi:10.1177/1088868310377395

Kumfor, F., Honan, C., McDonald, S., Hazelton, J., Hodges, J. R., & Piguet, O. (2017). Assessing the "social brain" in dementia: Applying TASIT-S. *Cortex*, *93*, 166–177. doi:http://dx.doi.org/10.1016/j.cortex.2017.05.022

Larsen, J. K., Brand, N., Bermond, B., & Hijman, R. (2003). Cognitive and emotional characteristics of alexithymia: A review of neurobiological studies. *J Psychosom Res*, *54*(6), 533–541.

Lawrence, E. J., Shaw, P., Baker, D., Baron-Cohen, S., & David, A. S. (2004). Measuring empathy: Reliability and validity of the empathy quotient. *Psychological Medicine*, *34*(5), 911.

Loukusa, S., & Moilanen, I. (2009). Pragmatic inference abilities in individuals with Asperger syndrome or high-functioning autism. A review. *Research in Autism Spectrum Disorders*, *3*(4), 890–904.

Ludwig, K. A., Pinkham, A. E., Harvey, P. D., Kelsven, S., & Penn, D. L. (2017). Social cognition psychometric evaluation (SCOPE) in people with early psychosis: A preliminary study. *Schizophrenia Research*, *190*, 136–143.

Luzzi, S., Baldinelli, S., Ranaldi, V., Fiori, C., Plutino, A., Fringuelli, F. M., Silvestrini, M., Baggio, G., & Reverberi, C. (2020). The neural bases of discourse semantic and pragmatic deficits in patients with frontotemporal dementia and Alzheimer's disease. *Cortex*, *128*, 174–191.

Mah, L., Arnold, M. C., & Grafman, J. (2004). Impairment of social perception associated with lesions of the prefrontal cortex. *American Journal of Psychiatry*, *161*(7), 1247–1255.

Malec, J. F., & Thompson, J. M. (1994). Relationship of the Mayo-Portland adaptability inventory to functional outcome and cognitive performance measures. *The Journal of Head Trauma Rehabilitation*, *9*(4), 1–15. https://journals.lww.com/headtraumarehab/Fulltext/1994/12000/Relationship_of_the_Mayo_Portland_Adaptability.3.aspx

Martinez, G., Alexandre, C., Mam-Lam-Fook, C., Bendjemaa, N., Gaillard, R., Garel, P., Dziobek, I., Amado, I., & Krebs, M.-O. (2017). Phenotypic continuum between autism and schizophrenia: Evidence from the movie for the assessment of social cognition (MASC). *Schizophrenia Research*, *185*, 161–166. doi:10.1016/j.schres.2017.01.012

Martin-Rodriguez, J. F., & Leon-Carrion, J. (2010). Theory of mind deficits in patients with acquired brain injury: A quantitative review. *Neuropsychologia*, *48*(5), 1181–1191. doi:10.1016/j.neuropsychologia.2010.02.009

Martins, M. J., Moura, B. L., Martins, I. P., Figueira, M. L., & Prkachin, K. M. (2011). Sensitivity to expressions of pain in schizophrenia patients. *Psychiatry Research*, *189*(2), 180–184.

Martyr, A., & Clare, L. (2018). Awareness of functional ability in people with early-stage dementia. *International Journal of Geriatric Psychiatry*, *33*(1), 31–38. doi:10.1002/gps.4664

Martyr, A., Nelis, S. M., Quinn, C., Rusted, J. M., Morris, R. G., Clare, L., & team, I. p. (2019). The relationship between perceived functional difficulties and the ability to live well with mild-to-moderate dementia: Findings from the IDEAL programme. *International Journal of Geriatric Psychiatry*, *34*(8), 1251–1261. doi:10.1002/gps.5128

Mathersul, D., McDonald, S., & Rushby, J. A. (2013a). Automatic facial responses to briefly presented emotional stimuli in autism spectrum disorder. *Biological Psychology*, *94*(2), 397–407. doi:10.1016/j.biopsycho.2013.08.004

Mathersul, D., McDonald, S., & Rushby, J. A. (2013b). Psychophysiological correlates of social judgement in high-functioning adults with autism spectrum disorder. *International Journal of Psychophysiology*, *87*(1), 88–94. doi:10.1016/j.ijpsycho.2012.11.005

Mathersul, D., McDonald, S., & Rushby, J. A. (2013c). Understanding advanced theory of mind and empathy in high-functioning adults with autism spectrum disorder. *Journal of Clinical and Experimental Neuropsychology, 35*(6), 655–668. doi:10.1080/13803395.2013.809700

Matsumoto, D., LeRoux, J., Wilson-Cohn, C., Raroque, J., Kooken, K., Ekman, P., Yrizarry, N., Loewinger, S., Uchida, H., Yee, A., Amo, L., & Goh, A. (2000). A new test to measure emotion recognition ability: Matsumoto and Ekman's Japanese and Caucasian brief affect recognition test (JACBERT). *Journal of Nonverbal Behavior, 24*(3), 179–209.

McDonald, S., Bornhofen, C., Shum, D., Long, E., Saunders, C. J., & Neulinger, K. (2006). Reliability and validity of the awareness of social inference test (TASIT): A clinical test of social perception. *Disability and Rehabilitation: An International, Multidisciplinary Journal, 28*(24), 1529–1542. doi:10.1080/09638280600646185

McDonald, S., & Flanagan, S. (2004). Social perception deficits after traumatic brain injury: Interaction between emotion recognition, mentalizing ability, and social communication. *Neuropsychology, 18*(3), 572–579. doi:10.1037/0894-4105.18.3.572

McDonald, S., Flanagan, S., Martin, I., & Saunders, J. C. (2004). The ecological validity of TASIT: A test of social perception. *Neuropsychological Rehabilitation, 14*, 285–302.

McDonald, S., Flanagan, S., & Rollins, J. (2011). *The Awareness of Social Inference Test Revised (TASIT-R).* Sydney, Australia: Pearson Assessment.

McDonald, S., Flanagan, S., & Rollins, J. (2017a). *The Awareness of Social Inference Test.* Sydney, Australia: ASSBI Resources.

McDonald, S., Flanagan, S., & Rollins, R. (2017b). *The Awareness of Social Inference Test* (3rd ed.). Sydney, Australia: ASSBI Resources.

McDonald, S., Flanagan, S., Rollins, J., & Kinch, J. (2003). TASIT: A new clinical tool for assessing social perception after traumatic brain injury. *The Journal of Head Trauma Rehabilitation, 18*(3), 219–238. www.ncbi.nlm.nih.gov/pubmed/12802165

McDonald, S., Honan, C. A., Allen, S. K., El-Helou, R., Kelly, M., Kumfor, F., Piguet, O., Hazelton, J. L., Padgett, C., & Keage, H. A. D. (2017). Normal adult and adolescent performance on TASIT-S, a short version of the assessment of social inference test. *The Clinical Neuropsychologist*, 1–20. doi:10.1080/13854046.2017.1400106

McDonald, S., Li, S., De Sousa, A., Rushby, J., Dimoska, A., James, C., & Tate, R. L. (2011). Impaired mimicry response to angry faces following severe traumatic brain injury. *Journal of Clinical and Experimental Neuropsychology, 33*(1), 17–29. doi:10.1080/13803391003761967

McKown, C., Allen, A. M., Russo-Ponsaran, N. M., & Johnson, J. K. (2013). Direct assessment of children's social-emotional comprehension. *Psychological Assessment, 25*(4), 1154.

Mecacci, L., & Righi, S. (2006). Cognitive failures, metacognitive beliefs and aging. *Personality and Individual Differences, 40*(7), 1453–1459. doi:10.1016/j.paid.2005.11.022

Mehrabian, A. (2000). *Manual for the Balanced Emotional Empathy Scale (BEES).* Monterey, CA: Albert Mehrabian.

Mendez, M. F., Anderson, E., & Shapira, J. S. (2005). An investigation of moral judgement in frontotemporal dementia. *Cognitive and Behavioral Neurology, 18*, 193–197.

Montagne, B., Kessels, R. P., Kammers, M. P., Kingma, E., de Haan, E. H., Roos, R. A., & Middelkoop, H. A. (2006). Perception of emotional facial expressions at different intensities in early-symptomatic Huntington's disease. *European Neurology, 55*(3), 151–154.

Montagne, B., Nys, G. M. S., Van Zandvoort, M. J. E., Kappelle, L. J., De Haan, E. H. F., & Kessels, R. P. C. (2007). The perception of emotional facial expressions in stroke patients with and without depression. *Acta Neuropsychiatrica, 19*(5), 279–283. doi:10.1111/j.1601-5215.2007.00235.x

Morrison, K. E., Pinkham, A. E., Kelsven, S., Ludwig, K., Penn, D. L., & Sasson, N. J. (2019). Psychometric evaluation of social cognitive measures for adults with autism. *Autism Research*, *12*(5), 766–778. doi:10.1002/aur.2084

Muller, F., Simion, A., Reviriego, E., Galera, C., Mazaux, J.-M., Barat, M., & Joseph, P.-A. (2010). Exploring theory of mind after severe traumatic brain injury. *Cortex*, *46*(9), 1088–1099.

Murphy, B. A., & Lilienfeld, S. O. (2019). Are self-report cognitive empathy ratings valid proxies for cognitive empathy ability? Negligible meta-analytic relations with behavioral task performance. *Psychological Assessment*, *31*(8), 1062–1072. doi:10.1037/pas0000732

Neumann, D. L., Sander, A. M., Perkins, S. M., Bhamidipalli, S. S., Witwer, N., Combs, D., & Hammond, F. M. (2020). Assessing negative attributions after brain injury with the ambiguous intentions hostility questionnaire. *The Journal of head trauma rehabilitation*, *35*(5), E450–E457. doi:10.1097/htr.0000000000000581

Neumann, D. L., & Westbury, H. R. (2011). The psychophysiological measurement of empathy. In Scapaletti, D. (Ed.), *Psychology of Empathy* (pp. 119–142). New York: Nova Science Publishers Inc.

Nunnally, J. C., & Bernstein, I. H. (1994). *Psychometric Theory* (3rd ed.). New York: McGraw Hill.

O'Brien, E., Konrath, S. H., Gruhn, D., & Hagen, A. L. (2013). Empathic concern and perspective taking: Linear and quadratic effects of age across the adult life span. *Journals of Gerontology Series B: Psychological Sciences and Social Sciences*, *68*(2), 168–175. doi:10.1093/geronb/gbs055

Olbert, C. M., Penn, D. L., Kern, R. S., Lee, J., Horan, W. P., Reise, S. P., Ochsner, K. N., Marder, S. R., & Green, M. F. (2013). Adapting social neuroscience measures for schizophrenia clinical trials, part 3: Fathoming external validity. *Schizophrenia Bulletin*, *39*(6), 1211–1218.

Olderbak, S., Wilhelm, O., Olaru, G., Geiger, M., Brenneman, M. W., & Roberts, R. D. (2015). A psychometric analysis of the reading the mind in the eyes test: Toward a brief form for research and applied settings. *Frontiers in Psychology*, *6*, 1503.

Osborne-Crowley, K., McDonald, S., & Francis, H. (2016). Development of an observational measure of social disinhibition after traumatic brain injury. *Journal of Clinical and Experimental Neuropsychology*, *38*(3), 341–353. doi:10.1080/13803395.2015.1115824

Ownsworth, T., Fleming, J., Doig, E., Shum, D. H. K., & Swan, S. (2019). Concordance between the awareness questionnaire and self-awareness of deficits interview for identifying impaired self-awareness in individuals with traumatic brain injury in the community. *Journal of Rehabilitation Medicine*, *51*(5), 376–379. doi:10.2340/16501977-2537

Palermo, R., O'Connor, K. B., Davis, J. M., Irons, J., & McKone, E. (2013). New tests to measure individual differences in matching and labelling facial expressions of emotion, and their association with ability to recognise vocal emotions and facial identity. *PLoS One*, *8*(6), e68126.

Pell, M. D., Monetta, L., Rothermich, K., Kotz, S. A., Cheang, H. S., & McDonald, S. (2014). Social perception in adults with Parkinson's disease. *Neuropsychology*, *28*(6), 905.

Pijnenborg, G., Spikman, J., Jeronimus, B., & Aleman, A. (2013). Insight in schizophrenia: Associations with empathy. *European Archives of Psychiatry and Clinical Neuroscience*, *263*(4), 299–307.

Pinkham, A. E., Harvey, P. D., & Penn, D. L. (2017). Social cognition psychometric evaluation: Results of the final validation study. *Schizophrenia Bulletin*, *44*(4), 737–748. doi:10.1093/schbul/sbx117

Pinkham, A. E., Harvey, P. D., & Penn, D. L. (2018). Social cognition psychometric evaluation: Results of the final validation study [article]. *Schizophrenia Bulletin, 44*(4), 737–748. doi:10.1093/schbul/sbx117

Pinkham, A. E., Hopfinger, J. B., Pelphrey, K. A., Piven, J., & Penn, D. L. (2008). Neural bases for impaired social cognition in schizophrenia and autism spectrum disorders. *Schizophrenia Research, 99*(1–3), 164–175.

Pinkham, A. E., Penn, D. L., Green, M. F., Buck, B., Healey, K., & Harvey, P. D. (2014). The social cognition psychometric evaluation study: Results of the expert survey and RAND panel. *Schizophrenia Bulletin, 40*(4), 813–823. doi:10.1093/schbul/sbt081

Pinkham, A. E., Penn, D. L., Green, M. F., & Harvey, P. D. (2016). Social cognition psychometric evaluation: Results of the initial psychometric study. *Schizophrenia Bulletin, 42*(2), 494–504.

Pinkham, A. E., Penn, D. L., Perkins, D. O., & Lieberman, J. (2003). Implications for the neural basis of social cognition for the study of schizophrenia. *American Journal of Psychiatry, 160*(5), 815–824.

Powell, P. A. (2018). Individual differences in emotion regulation moderate the associations between empathy and affective distress. *Motivation and Emotion, 42*(4), 602–613. doi:10.1007/s11031-018-9684-4

Prevost, M., Carrier, M. E., Chowne, G., Zelkowitz, P., Joseph, L., & Gold, I. (2014). The reading the mind in the eyes test: Validation of a French version and exploration of cultural variations in a multi-ethnic city. *Cognitive Neuropsychiatry, 19*(3), 189–204. doi:10.1080/13546805.2013.823859

Prigatano, G. P., & Altman, I. W. (1990). Impaired awareness of behavioural limitations after traumatic brain injury. *Archives of Physical Medication and Rehabilitation, 71*, 1058–1064.

Quinn, C., Jones, I., Martyr, A., Nelis, S. M., Morris, R. G., & Clare, L. (2019). Caregivers' beliefs about dementia: Findings from the IDEAL study. *Psychology & Health, 34*(10), 1214–1230.

Rabinowitz, A. R., & Levin, H. S. (2014). Cognitive sequelae of traumatic brain injury. *The Psychiatric Clinics of North America, 37*(1), 1.

Rapp, A. M., & Wild, B. (2011). Nonliteral language in Alzheimer dementia: A review. *Journal of the International Neuropsychological Society, 17*(2), 207–218.

Reniers, R. L. E. P., Corcoran, R., Drake, R., Shryane, N. M., & Völlm, B. A. (2011). The QCAE: A questionnaire of cognitive and affective empathy. *Journal of Personality Assessment, 93*(1), 84–95. doi:10.1080/00223891.2010.528484

Rosenberg, H., Dethier, M., Kessels, R. P., Westbrook, R. F., & McDonald, S. (2015). Emotion perception after moderate – severe traumatic brain injury: The valence effect and the role of working memory, processing speed, and nonverbal reasoning. *Neuropsychology, 29*(4), 509.

Rosset, E. (2008). It's no accident: Our bias for intentional explanations. *Cognition, 108*(3), 771–780. doi:10.1016/j.cognition.2008.07.001

Rossion, B., & Michel, C. (2018). Normative accuracy and response time data for the computerized Benton facial recognition test (BFRT-c). *Behavior Research Methods, 50*(6), 2442–2460. doi:10.3758/s13428-018-1023-x

Roth, R. M., Isquith, P., & Gioia, G. (2005). *BRIEF-A: Behavior Rating Inventory of Executive Function – Adult Version: Professional Manual*: Lutz, FL: Psychological Assessment Resources.

Samson, D., Apperly, I. A., Kathirgamanathan, U., & Humphreys, G. W. (2005). Seeing it my way: A case of a selective deficit in inhibiting self-perspective. *Brain, 128*(Pt 5), 1102–1111. doi:10.1093/brain/awh464

Schaffer, S. G., Wisniewski, A., Dahdah, M., & Froming, K. B. (2009). The comprehensive affect testing system – abbreviated: Effects of age on performance. *Archives of Clinical Neuropsychology*, *24*(1), 89–104.

Schieman, S., & Van Gundy, K. (2000). The personal and social links between age and self-reported empathy. *Social Psychology Quarterly*, *63*(2), 152–174. doi:10.2307/2695889

Schneider, D., Lam, R., Bayliss, A. P., & Dux, P. E. (2012). Cognitive load disrupts implicit theory-of-mind processing. *Psychological Science*, *23*(8), 842–847. doi:10.1177/0956797612439070

Scholten, M. R., Aleman, A., Montagne, B., & Kahn, R. S. (2005). Schizophrenia and processing of facial emotions: Sex matters. *Schizophrenia Research*, *78*(1), 61–67.

Schultz, I. Z., Sepehry, A. A., & Greer, S. C. (2018). Cognitive impact of fatigue in forensic neuropsychology context. *Psychological Injury and Law*, *11*(2), 108–119.

Sepeta, L., Tsuchiya, N., Davies, M. S., Sigman, M., Bookheimer, S. Y., & Dapretto, M. (2012). Abnormal social reward processing in autism as indexed by pupillary responses to happy faces. *Journal of Neurodevelopmental Disorders*, *4*(1), 17.

Sergi, M. J., Fiske, A. P., Horan, W. P., Kern, R. S., Kee, K. S., Subotnik, K. L., Nuechterlein, K. H., & Green, M. F. (2009). Development of a measure of relationship perception in schizophrenia. *Psychiatry Research*, *166*(1), 54–62. doi:10.1016/j.psychres.2008.03.010

Shamay-Tsoory, S. G., & Aharon-Peretz, J. (2007). Dissociable prefrontal networks for cognitive and affective theory of mind: A lesion study. *Neuropsychologia*, *45*(13), 3054–3067. doi:10.1016/j.neuropsychologia.2007.05.021

Shamay-Tsoory, S. G., Aharon-Peretz, J., & Levkovitz, Y. (2007). The neuroanatomical basis of affective mentalizing in schizophrenia: Comparison of patients with schizophrenia and patients with localized prefrontal lesions. *Schizophrenia Research*, *90*(1–3), 274–283.

Sherer, M., Bergloff, P., Boake, C., High, W. M., & Levin, E. (1998). The awareness questionnaire: Factor analysis structre and internal consistency. *Brain Injury*, *12*, 63–68.

Shimokawa, A., Yatomi, N., Anamizu, S., Ashikari, I., Kohno, M., Maki, Y., Torii, S., Isono, H., Sugai, Y., Koyama, N., & Matsuno, Y. (2000). Comprehension of emotions: Comparison between Alzheimer type and vascular type dementias. *Dementia and Geriatric Cognitive Disorders*, *11*(5), 268–274. doi:17249

Shinan-Altman, S., & Werner, P. (2017). Is there an association between help-seeking for early detection of Alzheimer's disease and illness representations of this disease among the lay public? *International Journal of Geriatric Psychiatry*, *32*(12), e100–e106.

Silberstein, J. M., Pinkham, A. E., Penn, D. L., & Harvey, P. D. (2018). Self-assessment of social cognitive ability in schizophrenia: Association with social cognitive test performance, informant assessments of social cognitive ability, and everyday outcomes. *Schizophrenia Research*, *199*, 75–82.

Snowden, J. S., Thompson, J. C., & Neary, D. (2004). Knowledge of famous faces and names in semantic dementia. *Brain*, *127*(Pt 4), 860–872. doi:10.1093/brain/awh099

Sollberger, M., Rosen, H. J., Shany-Ur, T., Ullah, J., Stanley, C. M., Laluz, V., Weiner, M. W., Wilson, S. M., Miller, B. L., & Rankin, K. P. (2014). Neural substrates of socioemotional self-awareness in neurodegenerative disease. *Brain and Behavior*, *4*(2), 201–214.

Sommerlad, A., Singleton, D., Jones, R., Banerjee, S., & Livingston, G. (2017). Development of an instrument to assess social functioning in dementia: The social functioning in dementia scale (SF-DEM). *Alzheimers and Dementia (Amst)*, *7*, 88–98. doi:10.1016/j.dadm.2017.02.001

Spek, A. A., Scholte, E. M., & Van Berckelaer-Onnes, I. A. (2010). Theory of mind in adults with high-functioning autism and Asperger syndrome. *Journal of Autism and Developmental Disorders*, *40*, 280–289.

Spikman, J. M., Timmerman, M. E., Milders, M. V., Veenstra, W. S., & van der Naalt, J. (2012). Social cognition impairments in relation to general cognitive deficits, injury severity, and prefrontal lesions in traumatic brain injury patients. *Journal of Neurotrauma*, *29*(1), 101–111. doi:10.1089/neu.2011.2084

Starkstein, S. E., Mayberg, H. S., Preziosi, T. J., Andrezejewski, P., Leiguarda, R., & Robinson, R. G. (1992). Reliability, validity, and clinical correlates of apathy in Parkinson's disease. *The Journal of Neuropsychiatry and Clinical Neurosciences*, *4*(2), 134–139. doi:10.1176/jnp.4.2.134

Stone, V. E., Baron-Cohen, S., & Knight, R. T. (1998). Frontal lobe contributions to theory of mind. *Journal of Cognitive Neuroscience*, *10*(5), 640–656. doi:10.1162/089892998562942. www.ncbi.nlm.nih.gov/pubmed/9802997

Tate, R. L. (2010). *A Compendium of Tests, Scales and Questionnaires: The Practitioner's Guide to Measuring Outcomes after Acquired Brain Impairment*. London: Psychology Press.

Tate, R. L., Broe, G. A., & Lulham, J. M. (1989). Impairment after severe blunt head injury: The results from a consecutive series of 100 patients. *Acta Neurologica Scandinavia*, *79*(97–107).

Taylor, G. J., Bagby, R. M., & Parker, J. D. A. (2003). The 20-item Toronto alexithymia scale-IV. Reliability and factorial validity in different languages and cultures. *Journal of Psychosomatic Research*, *55*, 277–283. doi:10.1016/s0022-3999(02)00601-3

Taylor, S. F., Kang, J., Brege, I. S., Tso, I. F., Hosanagar, A., & Johnson, T. D. (2012). Meta-analysis of functional neuroimaging studies of emotion perception and experience in schizophrenia. *Biological Psychiatry*, *71*(2), 136–145.

Torralva, T., Gleichgerrcht, E., Roca, M., Ibanez, A., Marenco, V., Rattazzi, A., & Manes, F. (2013). Impaired theory of mind but intact decision-making in Asperger syndrome: Implications for the relationship between these cognitive domains. *Psychiatry Research*, *205*(3), 282–284. doi:10.1016/j.psychres.2012.08.023

Torralva, T., Kipps, C. M., Hodges, J. R., Clark, L. A., Bekinschtein, T., Roca, M., Calcagno, M., & Manes, F. (2007). The relationship between affective decision-making and theory of mind in the frontal variant of fronto-temporal dementia. *Neuropsychologia*, *45*(2), 342–349. www.sciencedirect.com/science/article/B6T0D-4KKNJ8W-2/2/69a3b0dcf653cbf64b328b9a8953769c

Toussaint, L., & Webb, J. R. (2005). Gender differences in the relationship between empathy and forgiveness. *The Journal of Social Psychology*, *145*(6), 673–685.

Voracek, M., & Dressler, S. G. (2006). Lack of correlation between digit ratio (2D:4D) and Baron-Cohen's "reading the mind in the eyes" test, empathy, systemising, and autism-spectrum quotients in a general population sample. *Personality and Individual Differences*, *41*(8), 1481–1491. doi:10.1016/j.paid.2006.06.009

Wallis, K., Kelly, M., McRae, S., McDonald, S., & Campbell, L. (in press). *Scoping Review of Domains and Measures of Social Cognition in Acquired Brain Injury Neuropsychological Rehabilitation*.

Watson, P. J., & Morris, R. J. (1991). Narcissism, empathy and social desirability. *Personality and Individual Differences*, *12*(6), 575–579. doi:10.1016/0191-8869(91)90253-8

Wechsler, D. (1997). *Wechsler Memory Scale* (3rd ed.). San Antonio, TX: Psychological Corporation: Harcourt Assessment.

Wilmer, J. B., Germine, L., Chabris, C. F., Chatterjee, G., Williams, M., Loken, E., Nakayama, K., & Duchaine, B. (2010). Human face recognition ability is specific and highly heritable. *Proceedings of the National Academy of Sciences of the United States of America*, *107*(11), 5238–5241. doi:10.1073/pnas.0913053107

Wilson, B. A., Greenfield, E., Clare, L., Baddeley, A., Cockburn, J., Watson, P., Tate, R. L., Sopena, S., & Nannery, R. (2008). *The Rivermead Behavioural Memory Test* (3rd ed.). London: Pearson Assessment.

Wimmer, H., & Perner, J. (1983). Beliefs about beliefs: Representation and constraining function of wrong beliefs in young children's understanding of deception. *Cognition*, *13*(1), 103–128.

Young, A. P., Perret, D. I., Calder, A., Sprengelmeyer, R., Ekman, P., Young, A. W., & Calder, A. J. (2002). *Facial Expression of Emotion-Stimuli and Tests (FEEST)*. Thames Valley: Thames Valley Test Company.

Zalla, T., Sav, A.-M., Stopin, A., Ahade, S., & Leboyer, M. (2009). Faux pas detection and intentional action in Asperger syndrome. A replication on a French sample. *Journal of Autism and Developmental Disorders*, *39*(2), 373–382.

Zupan, B., Neumann, D., Babbage, D., & Willer, B. (2018). Sex-based differences in affective and cognitive empathy following severe traumatic brain injury. *Neuropsychology*, *32*(5), 554.

Chapter 10

Assessing social cognition in children

Louise Crowe, Simone Darling and Jennifer Chow

Social function encompasses social cognition as well as socio-behavioural manifestations (i.e. social skills and interactions as well as the social behaviours displayed by the individual) (Beauchamp & Anderson, 2010). Social cognition skills, or "social information processing" underpin socio-behavioural functioning or "social interaction", and involves social-affective processes that are specialised for the processing of social stimuli including encoding and interpreting a range of social cues, such as language, intonation, and non-verbal cues (i.e., facial expression, body language and gesture and eye contact) (McDonald, 2013; Beauchamp & Anderson, 2010). There are strong links to executive function (e.g., inhibitory control), which are the cognitive processes required for goal directed behaviour (Anderson, 2002) and social problem-solving which involves the integration of these two processes in responding to social stimuli (refer to Figure 10.1).

Social cognitive skills emerge throughout childhood and follow a developmental trajectory with maturation occurring throughout adolescence into early adulthood (Choudhury, Blakemore, & Charman, 2006; Tonks, Williams, Frampton, & Yates, 2007). Development of socio-cognitive skills begins with more basic skills such as facial emotion recognition and processing speed, which then form the foundation for more complex social cognition skills such as moral reasoning and theory of mind (Beaudoin & Beauchamp, 2020). Social cognition skills (refer to Figure 10.1) are influenced by external environmental factors (e.g., parenting style, family functioning), brain insult or disease related factors (e.g., type of insult, severity of insult) and internal child factors (e.g., temperament) (Beauchamp & Anderson, 2010; Yeates et al., 2007).

Social competence comprises a highly complex and intertwined amalgamation of social behavioural skills, social cognition and contextual factors (Beauchamp & Anderson, 2010). Measures of social cognition are therefore crucial to facilitate the disentanglement of social competence to illuminate the specific underlying socio-cognitive processes that may be contributing to a child's social difficulty (Beauchamp, 2017; Crowe, Beauchamp, Catroppa, & Anderson, 2011). Social cognition measures help distil specific socio-cognitive processes and allow the objective quantification of these processes (Bierman &

DOI: 10.4324/9781003027034-10

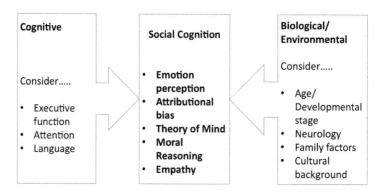

Figure 10.1 Assessment of social cognition

Welsh, 2000). This quantification allows the detection of specific areas of possible impairment which provides useful direction for the effective management and application of interventions to address social difficulty (Bierman & Welsh, 2000). Social cognition measures can also be used to identify changes in socio-cognitive processing over time due to developmental growth or clinical intervention (Beauchamp, 2017).

Social cognitive assessments

Clinical psychologists, neuropsychologists and educational psychologists working within paediatrics conduct psychological assessment for a variety of referral questions (see Box 10.1: Case Study: Christian in this chapter for an example). The *Diagnostic and Statistical Manual of Mental Disorders, 5th Edition* (DSM-5) highlights the importance of assessing social function or the 'social domain' for neurodevelopmental disorders (American Psychiatric Association, 2013). The social domain in the DSM-5 for intellectual disability and autism spectrum disorder (ASD) includes social cognitive skills, such as perceiving the social cues of others, and atypical responses to the social overtures of others (see Table 4.1) (APA, 2013). While some psychological disorders diagnosed in childhood such as ASD have social cognitive deficits as a core feature, the role of social cognition in both psychological and neurological disorders common in childhood is not always clear. For other referral questions and presentations, the presence of social cognitive problems may not be immediately apparent; however, research has shown that social cognitive deficits have a common morbidity with learning difficulties (Kavale & Forness, 1996), attention deficit hyperactivity disorder (ADHD) (Uekermann et al., 2010), conduct disorder (Happe & Frith, 1996) and behavioural problems (Toblin, Schwartz, Gorman, & Abou-ezzeddine, 2005). For neurological disorders, social cognitive problems have been associated with stroke (Lo et al., 2020), traumatic brain injury (McDonald, 2013), prematurity (Marleau, Vona, Gagner, Luu, & Beauchamp, 2020) and epilepsy (Operto et al., 2020).

Major areas to consider when developing a social cognition assessment protocol include emotion perception, attributional bias, theory of mind, moral reasoning and empathy, with most assessment tools focused in these areas (McDonald, 2017). Assessment methods include observation of the child in the school or home environment, child-based performance measures and questionnaires for children, parents and/or educators. Refer to Table 10.1 for information on the assessment tools mentioned in this chapter and published since 2000.

Emotion perception

Understanding the emotions of others using cues from facial expression, body language and speech are fundamental skills of social function. Gauging the emotions of others from facial expressions develops in the first year of life, with babies adjusting behaviour in accordance with parent facial expression (Walker-Andrews, 1998). Refining and understanding of more complex emotions continues into adolescence (Tonks, Williams, Frampton, & Yates, 2007). Many tasks have been developed to assess emotion recognition with some focused specifically on this including the *Minnesota Tests of Affective Processing* (Shaprio, Hughes, August, & Bloomquist, 1993), *Diagnostic Analysis of Nonverbal Accuracy-Second Edition (DANVA-2*: Nowicki & Duke, 1994; Nowicki & Duke, 2001), *Emotion Expression Scale for Children* (Penza-Clyve & Zeman, 2002), and the *Emotion Recognition Scales* (Dyck, Ferguson & Shocet, 2001). Others contain a subtest of emotion recognition and also assess other areas of social cognition including *Schedules for the Assessment of Social Intelligence* (Skuse, Lawrence & Tang, 2005), the *Paediatric Evaluation of Emotions Relationships and Socialisation* (PEERS, Thompson et al., 2018) and *The Awareness of Social Inference Test (TASIT)* for adolescents (McDonald, Fisher, Togher & Tate, 2015).

One of the most common ways these tools assess emotion recognition involves asking the child or adolescent to interpret an emotion from a facial expression of a person in a photograph. Perhaps the earliest example of this type of assessment is *Pictures of Facial Affect* published in the 1970s (Ekman & Friesen, 1976). This has evolved to similar methods including the Affect Recognition subtest on the *NEPSY-II* (Korkman, Kirk, & Kemp, 2007) and the Child Facial Expressions on the *DANVA-2* (Nowicki & Duke, 1994, 2001).

While speech and tone are also important factors in understanding emotion, there are few instruments available to measure this. The *DANVA-2* (Nowicki & Duke, 1994, 2001) has been highly cited (Crowe et al., 2011) and includes the Child Receptive Paralanguage test, which involves a child actor reading a sentence in high or low intensity, and children are asked to define if a

Table 10.1 Child based measures of social cognition and skills

Test	Verbal demands	Control	Time Mins	Simple to score	Internal reliability	Test-Retest	Convergent validity	Ecological validity	Clinical Sensitivity	Norms
TESTS OF EMOTION RECOGNTION										
Affect Recognition	Listen and point to answer	✗	10m	✓	✓	✓	✓	✗	✓	3–16 yrs
NEPSY-II DANVA (child subtests)	Listen and verbal responses	✗	20m	✓	✓	✓	✗	✗	✗	6–10 yrs
EE-C	Listen/Read questions and use likert scale	✗	<10m	✓	✓	✓	✓	✗	✓	6–10 yrs
RMFT	Listen and verbal responses	✗	20m	✓	✗	✗	✓	✗	✓	8–11 yrs
TESTS OF THEORY OF MIND										
IT	Listening and verbal responses	✗	20m	✗	✗	✗	✓	✗	✗	5–9 yrs
ToM-NEPSY-II	Listen and verbal responses	✗	<10m	✓	✓	✓	✓	✗	✓	3–16 yrs
TESTS OF EMPATHY										
ERS	Pictures and written questions with written responses	✗	30m	✗	✗ Comprehension <.70	✗	✓	✗	✓	9–16 yrs
TESTS OF ATTRIBUTIONAL BIAS										
SCAP-R	Listen and verbal responses to vignettes	✗	20m	✗	✗ Attributions <.70	✓	✓	✓	✓	Grade 2–4

TESTS OF SOCIAL COMMUNICATION²

Test	Mode of response		Time						Age
SLDT	Listen and verbal responses	✗	45m	✓	✓	✓	✓	✓	6–17 yrs

OVERALL TESTS OF SOCIAL COGNITION AND SOCIAL SKILLS

Test	Mode of response		Time						Age
SASI	Reading responses	✗	30m	✗ (Training required for TOM task)	✗	✗	✗	✓	6–60 yrs
PEERS	Listening/ Read questions and response	✓	1–10 mins per subtest	✓	✗	✓	✓	✓	4–18 yrs
SSIS Student	Read questions and responses	✗	10m	✓	+	✓	✓	✓	8–18 years

Control = a control condition is included which does not require social cognition. ✓ adequate, ✗ inadequate/not provided: Information taken from the associated reference except for ecological validity where ✓ refers to subsequent publication/s attest to ecological validity. Time estimated from test description when not specified.

DANVA = Diagnostic Analysis of Nonverbal Accuracy- Second Edition (DANVA-2: Nowicki & Duke, 2001)
EE-C = Emotion Expression Scale for Children (Penza-Clyve & Zeman, 2002)
ERS = Emotion Recognition Scales (Dyck, Ferguson, & Shocet, 2001)
SASI = Schedules for the Assessment of Social Intelligence (Skuse, Lawrence, & Tang, 2005)
PEERS = Paediatric Evaluation of Emotions, Relationships and Socialisation (PEERS, Thompson et al., 2018)
AR – NEPSY-II = Affect Recognition subtest on the NEPSY-II (Korkman, Kirk, & Kemp, 2007)
ToM-NEPSY-II = ToM subtest on the NEPSY-II (Korkman, Kirk, & Kemp, 2007)
RMFT = Reading the Mind in the Films Test (Golan, Baron-Cohen, & Golan, 2008)
IT = Irony Task (Filippova & Astington, 2008)
SLDT = Social Language Development Test (Bowers, Huisingh, & LoGiudice, 2010)
SCAP-R = Social Cognitive Assessment Profile- Revised (Hughes, Webster-Stratton, & Cavell, 2004)
SSIS = Social Skills Improvement System (Gresham & Elliott, 2008)

child is 'happy, sad, angry or fearful'. The *Reading the Mind in the Films Test* built on this idea using short films rather than static pictures, and interpretation of affect recognition uses visual, auditory and context cues to distinguish emotions (Golan et al., 2008). The ability to distinguish the emotions of others is a distinct skill to theory of mind.

Theory of mind

Theory of mind (ToM) first develops in early childhood (Cutting & Dunn, 1999). In its simplest form, it is the understanding that other's emotions, feelings or thoughts can be different to your own. It increases in complexity from understanding first-order beliefs that one person might have a different thought/emotion/belief to you up to third-order beliefs which involve a third-person perspective (Liddle & Nattle, 2006). Tasks that measure ToM include false-belief tasks which require the understanding that another child may hold a thought or belief that differs from themselves. Other measures that tap ToM include the ToM subtest on the *NEPSY-II* (Korkman, Kirk, & Kemp, 2007), *Reading the Mind in the Films Test* (Golan et al., 2008), *Strange Stories* test (Happe, 1994), *Irony task* (Filippova & Astington, 2008) and *Social Language Development Test* (Bowers, Huisingh, & LoGiudice, 2010).

Attributional bias

Attributional bias or intent attribution refers to the 'filter' or lenses that other's behaviour is interpreted through (McDonald, 2017). It is often referred to in studies of aggressive behaviour in children where children can interpret ambiguous situations as hostile. Measures to assess attributional bias involve the presentation of a scenario followed by questions that involve some elements of social problem-solving. For example, children would be shown/read a vignette describing a social situation where another person may provoke them or cause a problem. Children are then asked to describe the intentions of the other person. The intent can sometimes be interpreted as negative or ambiguous. As a result, children vary in the degree to which they interpret the person's intentions as benign or hostile. Measures of attributional bias typically incorporate a combination of executive (inhibition, cognitive flexibility) and social cognitive skills (emotion recognition, empathy, theory of mind, intent attribution) as they focus on making appropriate decisions in daily social situations that may require consideration of subtle or ambiguous social cues. Examples of these assessments include the *Social Cognitive Assessment Profile - Revised* (Hughes et al., 2004) and the *Social Information Processing Interview* (Quiggle, Garber, Panak, & Dodge, 1992), both of which use a verbal scenario, and the Social Intent subtest on the *PEERS* measure (Thompson et al., 2018; Dooley, Anderson, & Ohan, 2006), which uses video vignettes.

Moral reasoning

Moral reasoning is a complex skill that relies on early maturing social cognition skills including emotion recognition, ToM and empathy. It involves making moral judgements of right and wrong and is linked to social function and interpersonal relationship success (Moll et al., 2005). Moral reasoning develops over time from early concepts concerned with harm to others and to more complex understandings of justice and equality (Vera-Estay, Seni, Champagne & Beauchamp, 2016).

Traditional measures of moral reasoning have been adapted from adult tools. A well-known dilemma is the trolley dilemma, where the participant must make a decision on harming people in the vignette. More current research, however, has found that the original story in which the participant is a bystander retrieves different responses compared to one in which the participant has greater personal involvement (Dooley, Beauchamp, & Anderson, 2010). Likewise, different brain regions are activated when the participant is personally involved in the outcome as compared to a bystander (Greene, Somerville, Nystrom, Darley, & Cohen, 2001). This has led to new measures of moral reasoning such as the Multiple Morals task of the *PEERS* battery (Dooley et al., 2010). Other assessment tools focused in this area include the *Sociomoral Reflection Measure* (Gibbs, Basinger, & Fuller, 1992) and the *Prosocial Moral Reasoning Objective Measure* (Carlo, Eisenberg, & Knight, 1992).

Empathy

Empathy is closely related to ToM and is the ability to imagine another person's perspective, emotions and thoughts. There are two types of empathy: affective and cognitive. Affective empathy is being able to share others' feelings and can include mirroring others' emotions. Cognitive empathy is the capacity to identify and understand other people's emotions. Empathy for others is often measured through questionnaires and is an element of many broad social function questionnaires including the *Social Skills Improvement System* (Gresham & Elliott, 2008) and the *Walker McConnell Scales of Social Competence and School Adjustment* (Walker & McConnell, 1988). Measures focused specifically on empathy in children include the parent questionnaire, the *Griffith Empathy Measure* (Dadds et al., 2008).

Parent and teacher questionnaires

Questionnaires on behaviour and functional abilities commonly used in psychological assessment include the *Child Behavior Checklist (CBCL*; Achenbach & Rescorla, 2001), *Behavior Assessment Scale for Children (BASC*; Reynolds & Kamphaus, 2004), *Strengths and Difficulties Questionnaire (SDQ*;

Goodman, 1997, 2001) or the *Adaptive Behavior Assessment Scale (ABAS*; Harrison & Oakland, 2015), which all contain a social domain. These measures are quite generic in nature. However, delving deeper into some of the questions rated by parents or teachers may give some clue of social cognitive dysfunction. For example, the *CBCL* Social Problems scale contains an item that assesses children's attribution: [my child] "feels others are out to get him/her". The *ABAS* Social domain also contains items that could be interpreted as measuring social cognition. Items reference emotion recognition and empathy, e.g., [my child] "states when others seem happy, sad, scared, or angry", "shows sympathy for others when they are sad or upset", as well as understanding of jokes and irony, e.g., "laughs in response to funny comments or jokes", and others mental states, e.g., "refrains from saying something that might embarrass or hurt others". The *BASC* and the *SDQ* are more concerned with behaviours such as sharing, helping and encouraging others, and items tapping social cognitive processes are less apparent.

Highly cited questionnaires of social function include the *Social Skills Improvement System* (Gresham & Elliott, 2008), which is the new edition of the *Social Skills Rating Scale* (Gresham & Elliott, 1990). It is perhaps the most popular survey of social skills (Crowe et al., 2011), and although focused on social skills, it contains a few items that could be interpreted as measuring social cognition. Items that could tap social cognition and be of use to clinicians interested in this area include understanding the emotions of others, e.g., [my child] "tries to understand how you feel" and "tries to understand how others feel" and empathy, e.g., "tries to make others feel better", "tries to comfort others" and "shows concern for others". Examining the responses to certain items may lead the clinician to look at incorporating an assessment tool focused on a specific area of cognition, for example, facial emotion recognition or theory of mind.

Biological and environmental factors to consider

Both biological and environmental factors influence children's social cognitive skills. Biological variables include age and developmental stage as well as neurological factors. In terms of age and developmental stage, social cognitive skills develop throughout childhood, and therefore clinicians should have some expectations of expected skill level. It also highlights the importance of using assessment with age normative data. The presence of a neurological disorder or acquired brain injury should also be considered. Difficulties with social cognition have been identified in children with traumatic brain injuries (Dooley et al., 2010; McDonald, 2013), stroke (Lo et al., 2020), prematurity (Marleau, Vona, Gagner, Luu, & Beauchamp, 2020) and epilepsy (Operto et al., 2020). Social cognition has been linked to several brain structures, and therefore brain integrity and insults must be considered (Frith & Frith, 2007).

Environmental and family factors related to social cognition include maternal education and socioeconomic status, which have been found to influence moral reasoning (Hinnant, Nelson, O'Brien, Keane, & Calkins, 2013) and theory of mind (Cutting & Dunn, 1999). The role of culture is also seldom considered in social cognition assessment. It is now widely understood that culture plays a significant role in shaping an individual's beliefs, cognitions and behaviours, yet this notion is rarely reflected in the language and stimuli used in common social cognition measures (Wang, 2016). For example, in the *NEPSY-II* ToM subtest, the phrase "like two peas in a pod" is used (Korkman et al., 2007). This phrase is pervasive in many Western English-speaking cultures yet would be poorly understood by children who may not necessarily speak English as their first language. Additionally, performance on measures such as *Reading Mind in the Eyes* which present ethnically homogenous Caucasian faces have been found to vary across racial and ethnic groups, with Caucasian respondents more likely to demonstrate higher performance than non-White ethnic groups (Dodell-Feder et al., 2020). This lack of cultural sensitivity is a significant issue that plagues many measures of social cognition and highlights the need for future iterations of assessment to seriously incorporate important cultural considerations.

Cognitive considerations

There is a clear link between social cognition and cognitive skills including executive function, attention and language abilities. When assessing social cognition, the role of attention, memory, language and executive function should be considered and included in the assessment process. In terms of executive function, research has shown that social cognition is associated with conceptual reasoning, cognitive flexibility and verbal fluency (Vera et al., 2016; Hinnant et al., 2013). Attention abilities closely linked to executive function are also associated with social cognition. One example of how social cognition is impacted by these skills is in children with ADHD. Social cognitive impairments in children with ADHD are likely, in part, to reflect inattention as well as executive function difficulties in areas such as inhibitory control (Uekermann et al., 2010). See Case 1 (Box 10.1) for an example of a child with ADHD.

A child's language ability, including expressive and receptive language, has been linked to social cognition (Cutting & Dunn, 1999). This is especially true for some measures of social cognition that have high language requirements, for example, *The Irony task* (Filippova & Astington, 2008). Given these findings, an assessment of language is of importance when investigating social cognition to investigate whether it is at age-expected levels.

Issues with the assessment of social cognition in children

Given the rapid development and increasing focus on the assessment of social cognition in children, many social cognition assessment tools are being continually developed and made available (Bruneau-Bhérer et al., 2012). However, despite increased attention towards this area, measurement of social cognition in children is plagued with significant issues that limit the ecological validity, developmental suitability and clinical utility of assessments which, in turn, impede understanding social cognitive functioning in children.

Naturalistic observation, such as observing children in the school classroom or playground, is commonly employed in clinic assessment and provides valuable information on a child's functioning. While this method has been praised by some and referred to as the "gold standard" of social assessment (Merrell, 2001), there are significant disadvantages. For example, it is time and labour intensive with no guarantee of observing the behaviours of interest. Additionally, if children realise they are being watched, there is the possibility of behaving or reacting differently, i.e., the Hawthorne Effect (Oswald, Sherratt, Smith, 2014). Objectivity can be an issue with few formal methods of observation recording used (Crowe et al., 2011). Generally. observation is best combined with more formal or normed assessments of social cognition. Further, while a child may behave socially appropriately, such as showing behaviours of caring, it is hard to judge whether this may represent a high level of empathy or a drive to behave in a socially desirable manner while being observed.

Many performance-based measures of social cognition have been used in lab settings which aim to capture different processes such as ToM, emotion perception and recognition, or attributional bias. While many of these measures are designed to provide a direct assessment of social cognition and greater clarity for social dysfunction than global questionnaires may, many current performance-based measures are yet to demonstrate psychometric standards in terms of reliability (internal reliability, test-retest, inter-rater, etc.), sensitivity to change and/or validity (see Chapter 9 for further discussion of these issues). In particular, most social cognition tests used with children are limited by their lack of external validity, both in their stimuli selection and the generalisability of performance to everyday functioning (Bruneau-Bhérer et al., 2012). Many performance-based measures of social cognition, such as Ekman's Faces (Ekman & Friesen, 1976), Affect Recognition subtest on the NEPSY-II (Korkman, Kirk, & Kemp, 2007) and the Child Facial Expressions on the DANVA-2 (Nowicki, 2001), rely on photographs of faces that omit important subtle social cues present in dynamic real-life social situations (McDonald, 2017) but are also questionable whether they are developmentally appropriate (Crowe et al., 2011). For example, previous research has suggested that children have greater difficulty recognising emotions in photographs compared to drawings, and also have poorer facial recognition for adult faces compared to faces of their own age (Brechet, 2017; Rhodes & Anastasi, 2012).

Similarly, many measures are developed with adults, and simply modified or generalised for use with children (Crowe et al., 2011). For example, the commonly used trolley dilemma paradigm was initially applied to understand moral judgement and reasoning in adults but has now been widely used with children despite the cognitive confounds this paradigm places on a child's language comprehension and memory. Consequently, many measures lack an appropriate developmental framework, confounding the possibility of a universally accepted understanding of social cognition in children (Cordier et al., 2015).

A popular approach to assessing social cognition or social functioning more generally is through the use of pen-and-paper questionnaires which rely on child self-report, or parent and teacher secondary report. Such measures are thought to be able to capture social functioning in an ecologically valid fashion by assessing a child's functional social skills e.g., relationship with peers and social adaptability in different social contexts (Cordier et al., 2015). Whilst this approach is perhaps one of the more ecologically valid approaches to assessing social functioning as it captures a child's performance in real-life settings, pen-and-paper questionnaires are blunt instruments which do not reveal the complex and more nuanced socio-cognitive functions which underlie social performance. They are also afflicted with reporter bias effects (Crowe et al., 2011). For example, whilst widely used questionnaires such as the *Social Skills Improvement System* (Gresham & Elliott, 2008) include subscales such as communication and empathy and include specific questions which pertain to social cognition, these items provide a strictly preliminary and surface evaluation of these processes due to the small number of items and are better used as a starting point for further comprehensive assessment. Whether children can accurately rate their own skills is debated, with low correlations with others' ratings of their social competence (Frankel & Feinberg, 2002).

Parents are often used as raters; however, they are not always privy to their children's social abilities or what is 'typical'. Teachers can provide valuable information on how children interact with their peers at school and have a good knowledge of the social function of other children of the same age. However, the use of parent or teacher report poorly captures social functioning in different contexts and can be influenced by the subjective views of the rater (Cordier et al., 2015). The single reliance on pen-and-paper questionnaires is, therefore, insufficient, and child direct performance measures should also be used in order to garner a more comprehensive assessment of a child's social cognition ability.

Perhaps one of the greatest issues troubling the assessment of social cognition in children is the lack of appropriate age-based norms, with many measures only boasting modest, if any population norms (Henry et al., 2016). Several experimental tasks have been developed and used in studies, but they lack the normative data and psychometrics to be useful in clinical settings (Crowe et al., 2011). The lack of such standardised assessments with appropriate population and clinical norms significantly hampers the clinical utility of social cognition assessments (Beauchamp, 2017). This presents a significant area for future development in this growing field to lend greater utility to the wealth of social cognition assessments currently available.

The rapid growth and development of the social cognition field has meant that new measures of social cognition are continually evolving. As previously discussed, innovations in technology have meant that social cognition measures that feature dynamic and ecologically valid stimuli are becoming increasingly simple to administer via computerised or tablet-based tasks (Beauchamp, 2017; Crowe et al., 2011). These new technological advantages provide great optimism for the future development of social cognition measures that boast higher external validity and clinical utility.

Box 10.1   Case 1: Christian: Young person with suspected ADHD

History:

Christian is an 8-year-old boy referred with suspected ADHD as well as behaviour difficulties in the classroom and playground.

Neuropsychological and social cognitive evaluation:

A formal assessment of IQ revealed a score in the average range and assessment of attention skills demonstrated deficits in sustained attention. As part of the assessment battery, the clinician requested his parents complete the Child Behavior Checklist (CBCL) and the Adaptive Behavior Assessment Scale (ABAS). On the CBCL Parent report, Christian scored in the clinical range for aggressive behaviour. On the ABAS Parent report, Christian scored in the low range for self-care and the social domain. Further examination of their responses on the ABAS revealed that his parents have marked him as a "never" for "laughs in response to funny comments or jokes" and "refrains from saying something that might embarrass or hurt others". On the CBCL, the clinician also noted that his parents have marked "very often true" for "feels others are out to get him/her". This suggested to the clinician that Christian is having difficulty understanding the intentions of others in the form of what might embarrass them, understanding jokes and possibly sarcasm and allocates hostile attributes to others. Following up the suggestion of a social cognitive difficulty, the clinician utilised the NEPSY-II Affect Recognition and Theory of Mind subtests. Christian scored below average on both subtests. Understanding the contribution of other cognitive skills to social cognition, the assessment is tailored to examine memory and executive function. Christian is found to have difficulties inhibiting responses. A phone interview with this teacher found that Christian would become upset and aggressive if he got hit with a ball while playing or if other children were laughing in a group, assuming that children were making fun of him.

Opinion and recommendations:

Combining the results of the formal assessments, questionnaires and teacher interview, the clinician formulated that Christian fits the diagnosis of ADHD. Additionally, the clinician explained to the parents and his teacher that Christian also has some difficulties with social cognition. In particular, he has trouble understanding the intent of others with a tendency to feel that other children are excluding him or picking on him. He also has difficulty picking up on social cues, leading to misunderstandings. Recommendations were made about Christian working with the school counsellor on emotion recognition and trying to understand the perspective of others. At home and in the classroom, the clinician encouraged discussion of emotions and taking time before reacting.

Innovative measures of social cognition

The limitations of social cognition measures have been well established: adult measures inappropriately generalised to the paediatric context, a lack of ecological validity, use of static stimuli and often lacking breadth by only assessing a single component of social competence. In an attempt to address some of these limitations, and in parallel with the increased access to digital software and hardware (e.g., laptops, phones, tablets, internet, virtual reality, cloud-based data storage), digital approaches have been explored to provide more practical measures of social cognition. Digital technologies, such as touchscreens or wearables, facilitate the capturing of millions of pieces of real-time data, providing platforms to facilitate a more nuanced exploration of social cognition, and the engaging nature of "gamified" assessments is particularly attractive in the paediatric context (Shute & Ke, 2012). Technology has greatly reduced the burden of scoring assessments and preparing and sharing a clinical report with other healthcare providers. Digitisation of existing, validated tools such as the *NEPSY*, have minimised the administration burden for clinicians. Platforms such as Pearson's Q-Global are simple to use, web-based platforms for test administration, reporting and scoring. By using a web-based platform to perform these tasks, a clinician is able to save time and money on the administrative tasks associated with the assessment of social cognition.

Best practice advocates that social assessments should be 'ecologically sensitive and valid', that is, as close as possible to real life experience (Dooley, Anderson, Hemphill, & Ohan, 2008; Elliot, Malecki, & Demaray, 2001; John,

2001; van Overwalle, 2009). Virtual reality applications and well-produced videos have been used to depict real-life social situations and enhance emotional engagement in the task by enabling the 'testee' to become a part of the social situation. For example, *The Awareness of Social Inference Test (TASIT,* McDonald, Flanagan, Rollins, & Kinch, 2003) uses video vignettes to convey thoughts, intentions, feelings and meaning through facial emotional expression and tone. In a similar approach, virtual reality is an immersive experience, where the participant enters an alternative three-dimensional situation that has been contrived by the assessor. These innovative approaches to dynamic stimuli and immersive social situations address the limitations of using static stimuli (e.g., The Ekman faces) in the assessment of social cognition, which fails to accurately represent real-world social interactions. Furthermore, they allow the assessor to control and manipulate all elements in the social situation, including social cues (Parsons, Gaggioli, & Riva, 2017).

Digital products with automated 'stop rules' or machine learning algorithms have also been used to modify assessments to be personalised for each participant's individual ability level, reducing the need for excessive testing and the confounding impact of testing fatigue. Through adaptive, personalised gameplay, *Zoo U*, which is a point and click social problem-solving computer game, assesses and provides intervention for social skills, targeting emotion regulation, impulse control, communication, empathy, cooperation and initiation (DeRosier, Craig, & Sanchez, 2012). *Zoo U*'s uniqueness lies in the adaptive personalised game play, which modifies the stimuli and complexity of the scenarios based on the participants' real-time performance data.

One of the most comprehensive digital assessment tools for social cognition is the *Paediatric Evaluation of Emotions, Relationships and socialisation (PEERS)* battery (Thompson et al., 2018), which is comprised of an iPad-delivered, child-direct assessment of social cognition (PEERS Clinical or the brief PEERS screener) and web-based proxy- and self-reported measures of social functioning (PEERS-Q parent, teacher and self-report questionnaires). The *PEERS* battery can be used as a comprehensive assessment of social skills providing an overall measure of a child's social competency, or in a more nuanced fashion, to explore particular areas of concern. *PEERS* represents an innovative shift in the way social function, and specifically, social cognition, are assessed. *PEERS* provides an immediate detailed, yet comprehensive and actionable, 'social profile' for young people.

The development of *PEERS* was based on the biopsychosocial theoretical framework of the SOCIAL model (Beauchamp & Anderson, 2010), which includes three underlying cognitive domains of social development: attention-executive, social communication and socio-emotional skills. *PEERS* aims to describe the social profiles of children identified as at-risk for social difficulties and who would benefit from referral for tailored interventions. *PEERS* Clinical comprises 12 basic and complex subtests, each of which focuses on one of the three cognitive domains detailed in the SOCIAL model (Beauchamp &

Anderson, 2010). All subtests are derived from experimental paradigms from social neuroscience and modified to reflect real-life situations and developmental expectations. Basic subtests are designed to capture fundamental social skills, such as emotion recognition or perception, while complex subtests tap higher-order social skills, such as moral reasoning and theory of mind.

PEERS can be administered in full (all subtests) to derive a global social composite (mean (M) =100, standard deviation (SD) = 15) and domain scores (M =100, SD =15), or where specific concerns arise, the examiner can administer select subtests (M =10, SD =3) to efficiently and directly test a clinical hypothesis. All scoring is done automatically, and children's individual responses to sub-test items can be reviewed in the results screen. Both internal consistency (α = 0.665) and composite reliability (CR = 0.754) for the PEERS total score is good (Anderson et al., 2020). PEERS-Q is a questionnaire-based measure of social competence, completed by the parent, teacher or child (12 years+). PEERS-Q can be scored to produce six age-based subscale scores (Relationships, Participation, Behaviour, Social Rules, Social Communication and Social Cognition) as well as a total score. PEERS-Q was validated in a large-scale standardisation study (Hearps et al., 2020) and has excellent reliability (internal consistency Cronbach's Alpha range = 0.78–0.89 for subscales and CA = 0.95 for total PEERS-Q score).

Despite the significant benefits of using digital platforms for the assessment of social cognition, there are challenges that must be overcome. Firstly, accessibility barriers, for example internet connectivity issues or poor access to hardware (iPads, computers), may exacerbate existing inequity in healthcare, particularly for families from lower socio-economic status (SES) backgrounds (Hardiker & Grant, 2011). Accessibility issues should also be considered for those patients with sensory deficits, as this may prove to be a major barrier to participating in digital assessments (Caldwell et al., 2008). Secondly, regularly changing hardware and software means that measures leveraging digital technologies must be vigilantly checked for reliability and validity. Without this constant monitoring, previously validated measures may become invalid over a relatively short period of time. Lastly, many users are particularly sensitive to online data collection and related data privacy and security risks (Bradway et al., 2017). These concerns will need to be managed if digital technologies are to provide benefits to clinicians and their patients.

It is clear that despite the challenges with implementing digital solutions in the client/patient journey, digital technologies will be central to assessment approaches in the future. By leveraging technological advances in information technology software and hardware, solutions being grounded in theoretical and empirical science and incorporating methods that are engaging and attractive to young people and simulating the real world, digital solutions will provide professionals with convenient, practical, easy-to-interpret assessment tools while maintaining high levels of scientific rigour and assessment best-practice. With further validation and extensive testing, digital assessment solutions will likely become essential tools for any clinician in the assessment of social cognition and subsequent intervention approaches.

References

Achenbach, T. M., & Rescorla, L. A. (2001). *Manual for the ASEBA School-Age Forms & Profiles*. Burlington, VT: University of Vermont, Research Center for Children, Youth, & Families.

American Psychiatric Association. (2013). *Diagnostic and Statistical Manual of Mental Disorders* (5th ed.). Washington, DC: Author.

Anderson, P. (2002). Assessment and development of executive function (EF) during childhood. *Child Neuropsychology, 8*(2), 71–82.

Anderson, V. A., Darling, S., Hearps, S., Dooley, J., McDonald, S., Darby, D., Turkstra, L., & Beauchamp, M. (2020). *The Paediatric Evaluation of Emotions Relationships and Socialisation (PEERS) Manual*. Unpublished manual.

Beauchamp, M. H. (2017). Neuropsychology's social landscape: Common ground with social neuroscience. *Neuropsychology, 31,* 981–1002.

Beauchamp, M. H., & Anderson, V. (2010). SOCIAL: An integrative framework for the development of social skills. *Psychological Bulletin, 136*(1), 39–64.

Beaudoin, C., & Beauchamp, M. H. (2020). Social cognition. In *Handbook of Clinical Neurology* (Vol. 173, pp. 255–264). New York: Elsevier.

Bierman, K. L., & Welsh, J. A. (2000). Assessing social dysfunction: The contributions of laboratory and performance-based measures. *Journal of Clinical Child Psychology, 29*(4), 526–539.

Bowers, L., Huisingh, R., & LoGiudice, C. (2010). *Social Language Development Test – Adolescent Manual*. East Moline, IL: LinguiSystems, Inc.

Bradway, M., Carrion, C., Vallespin, B., Saadatfard, O., Puigdomènech, E., Espallargues, M., & Kotzeva, A. (2017). mHealth assessment: Conceptualization of a global framework. *JMIR mHealth and uHealth, 5*(5), e60.

Brechet, C. (2017). Children's recognition of emotional facial expressions through photographs and drawings. *The Journal of Genetic Psychology, 178*(2), 139–146.

Bruneau-Bhérer, R., Achim, A. M., & Jackson, P. L. (2012). Measuring the different components of social cognition in children and adolescents. In V. Anderson & M. H. Beauchamp (Eds.), *Developmental Social Neuroscience and Childhood Brain Insult* (pp. 138–160). New York: Guilford Press.

Caldwell, B., Cooper, M., Reid, L. G., Vanderheiden, G., Chisholm, W., Slatin, J., & White, J. (2008). *Web content accessibility guidelines (WCAG) 2.0*. WWW Consortium (W3C).

Carlo, G., Eisenberg, N., & Knight, G. (1992). An objective measure of adolescents' prosocial moral reasoning. *Journal of Research on Adolescence, 3,* 331–349.

Choudhury, S., Blakemore, S.-J., and Charman, T. (2006). Social cognitive development during adolescence. *Social Cognitive and Affective Neuroscience 1,* 165–174.

Cordier, R., Speyer, R., Chen, Y. W., Wilkes-Gillan, S., Brown, T., Bourke-Taylor, H., . . . Leicht, A. (2015). Evaluating the psychometric quality of social skills measures: A systematic review. *PLoS One, 10*(7), 1–32.

Crowe, L. M., Beauchamp, M. H., Catroppa, C., & Anderson, V. (2011). Social function assessment tools for children and adolescents: A systematic review from 1988 to 2010. *Clinical Psychology Review, 31*(5), 767–785.

Cutting, A. L., & Dunn, J. (1999). Theory of Mind, emotion understanding, language, and family background: Individual differences and interrelations. *Child Development, 70*(4), 853–865.

Dadds, M., Hunter, K., Hawes, D., Frost, A., Vassallo, S., Bunn, P., . . . El Masry, Y. (2008). A measure of cognitive and affective empathy in children using parent ratings. *Child Psychiatry and Human Development, 39*, 111–122.

DeRosier, M. E., Craig, A. B., & Sanchez, R. P. (2012). Zoo U: A stealth approach to social skills assessment in schools. *Advances in Human-Computer Interaction, 2012*.

Dodell-Feder, D., Ressler, K. J., & Germine, L. T. (2020). Social cognition or social class and culture? On the interpretation of differences in social cognitive performance. *Psychological Medicine, 50*(1), 133–145.

Dooley, J., Anderson, V., Hemphill, S., & Ohan, J. (2008). Aggression after pediatric traumatic brain injury: A theoretical approach. *Brain Injury, 22*(1), 836–846.

Dooley, J., Anderson, V., & Ohan, J. (2006). Assessment of social cognitive functioning after traumatic brain injury: Can it benefit the treatment of social skills impairments? *Brain Impairment, 7*(1), 63.

Dooley, J., Beauchamp, M., & Anderson, V. (2010). The measurement of sociomoral reasoning in adolescents with traumatic brain injury: A pilot investigation. *Brain Impairment, 11*(2), 152–161.

Dyck, M. J., Ferguson, K., & Shocet, I. M. (2001). Do autism spectrum disorders differ from each other and from non-spectrum disorders on emotion recognition tests? *European Child & Adolescent Psychiatry, 10*, 105–116.

Ekman, P., & Friesen, W. V. (1976). *Pictures of Facial Affect*. Palo Alto, CA: Consulting Psychologists Press.

Elliot, S., Malecki, C., & Demaray, M. (2001). New directions in social skills assessment and intervention for elementary and middle school students. *Exceptionality, 9*, 19–32.

Filippova, E., & Astington, J. (2008). Further development in social reasoning revealed in discourse irony understanding. *Child Development, 79*, 126–138.

Frankel, F., & Feinberg, D. (2002). Social problems associated with ADHD vs ODD in children referred for friendship problems. *Child Psychiatry & Human Development, 33*(2), 125–146.

Frith, C., & Frith, U. (2007). Social cognition in humans. *Current Biology, 17*(6), R724–R732.

Gibbs, J., Basinger, K., & Fuller, D. (1992). *Moral Maturity: Measuring the Development of Sociomoral Reflection*. Hillsdale, NJ: Lawrence Erlbaum Associates.

Golan, O., Baron-Cohen, S., & Golan, Y. (2008). The 'reading the mind in the films' task (child version): Complex emotion and mental state recognition in children with and without autism spectrum conditions. *Journal of Autism and Developmental Disorders, 38*, 1534–1541.

Goodman, R. (1997). The strengths and difficulties questionnaire: A research note. *Journal of Child Psychology and Psychiatry, 38*, 581–586.

Goodman, R. (2001). Psychometric properties of the strengths and difficulties questionnaire. *Journal of the American Academy of Child & Adolescent Psychiatry, 40*(11), 1337–1345.

Greene, J., Somerville, R., Nystrom, L., Darley, J., & Cohen, J. (2001). An fMRI investigation of emotional engagement in moral judgment. *Science, 293*, 2105–2108.

Gresham, F. M., & Elliott, S. N. (1990). *Social Skills Rating Scale*. Circle Pines, MN: American Guidance Service.

Gresham, F. M., & Elliott, S. N. (2008). *Social Skills Improvement System: Rating scales*. Bloomington, MN: Pearson Assessments.

Happe, F. G. E. (1994). An advanced test of theory of mind: Understanding of story characters' thoughts and feelings by able autistic, mentally handicapped, and normal children and adults. *Journal of Autism and Developmental Disorders, 24*, 129–154.

Happe, F. G. E., & Frith, U. (1996). Theory of mind and social impairment in children with conduct disorder. *British Journal of Developmental Psychology, 14*(4), 385–398.

Hardiker, N. R., & Grant, M. J. (2011). Factors that influence public engagement with eHealth: A literature review. *International Journal of Medical Informatics, 80*(1), 1–12.

Harrison, P. L., & Oakland, T. (2015). *Adaptive Behavior Assessment System* (3nd ed.). Torrance, CA: Western Psychological Services.

Hearps, S., Darling., S., Catroppa, C., Payne, J., Haritou, F., Beauchamp, M., Muscara, F., & Anderson, V. (2020). *Development and Validation of a Parent-Report Questionnaire of Social Skills for Children: The PEERS-Q.* Manuscript submitted for publication.

Henry, J. D., Von Hippel, W., Molenberghs, P., Lee, T., & Sachdev, P. S. (2016). Clinical assessment of social cognitive function in neurological disorders. *Nature Reviews Neurology, 12*(1), 1–12.

Hinnant, J. B., Nelson, J., O'Brien, M., Keane, S., & Calkins, S. (2013). The interactive roles of parenting, emotion regulation and executive functioning in moral reasoning during middle childhood. *Cognition and Emotion.* doi:10.1080/02699931.2013.789792

Hughes, J. N., Webster-Stratton, B. T., & Cavell, T. A. (2004). Development and validation of a gender-balanced measure of aggression-relevant social cognition. *Journal of Clinical Child and Adolescent Psychology, 33,* 292–302.

John, K. (2001). Measuring children's social functioning. *Child Psychology and Psychiatry Review, 6*, 181–188.

Kavale, K. A., & Forness, S. R. (1996). Social skill deficits and learning disabilities: A meta-analysis. *Journal of Learning Disabilities, 29*(3), 226–237.

Korkman, M., Kirk, U., & Kemp, S. (2007). *NEPSY-II Second Edition, Administration Manual.* San Antonio, TX: Pearson.

Liddle, B., & Nattle, D. (2006). Higher-order theory of mind and social competence in school-age children. *Journal of Evolutionary Psychology, 43*(3), 1589–5254.

Lo, W., Li, X., Hoskinson, K., McNally, K., Chung, M., Lee, J., Wang, J., Lu, Z., & Yeates, K. (2020). Pediatric stroke impairs theory of mind performance. *Journal of Child Neurology, 35*(3), 228–234.

Marleau, I., Vona, M., Gagner, C., Luu, T., & Beauchamp, M. (2020, July 27). Social cognition, adaptive functioning, and behavior problems in preschoolers born extremely preterm. *Child Neuropsychology.*

Merrell, K. (2001). Assessment of children's social skills: Recent developments, best practices, and new directions. *Exceptionality, 9*, 3-18.

McDonald, S. (2013). Impairments in social cognition following severe traumatic brain injury. *Journal of the International Neuropsychological Society, 19*, 231–246.

McDonald, S. (2017). What's new in the clinical management of disorders of social cognition?. *Brain Impairment, 18*(1), 2–10.

McDonald, S., Fisher, A., Togher, L., & Tate, R. (2015). Adolescent performance on the awareness of social inference test: TASIT. *Brain Impairment, 16*(1), 3–18.

McDonald, S., Flanagan, S., Rollins, J., & Kinch, J. (2003). TASIT: A new clinical tool for assessing social perception after traumatic brain injury. *The Journal of Head Trauma Rehabilitation, 18*(3), 219–238.

Moll, J., Zahn, R., de Oliveria-Souza, R., Krueger, F., & Grafman, J. (2005). The neural basis of human moral cognition. *Nature Reviews Neuroscience, 6*, 799–809.

Nowicki, S., & Duke, M. (1994). Individual differences in the nonverbal communication of affect: The diagnostic analysis of nonverbal accuracy scale. *Journal of Nonverbal Behavior*, *18*, 9–35.

Nowicki, S., & Duke, M. (2001). Nonverbal receptivity: The diagnostic analysis of nonverbal accuracy (DANVA). *Interpersonal Sensitivity: Theory and Measurement*, 183–198.

Operto, F. F., Pastorino, G. M., Mazza, R., Bonaventura, C. D., Marotta, R., Pastorino, N., . . . Roccella, M. (2020). Social cognition and executive functions in children and adolescents with focal epilepsy. *European Journal of Paediatric Neurology*, *28*, 167–175.

Oswald, D., Sherratt, F., & Smith, S. (2014). Handling the Hawthorne effect: The challenges surrounding a participant observer. *Review of Social Studies*, *1*(1), 53–73.

Parsons, T. D., Gaggioli, A., & Riva, G. (2017). Virtual reality for research in social neuroscience. *Brain Sciences*, *7*(4), 42.

Penza-Clyve, S., & Zeman, J. (2002). Initial validation of the emotion expression scale for children. *Journal of Clinical Child and Adolescent Psychology*, *31*, 540–547.

Quiggle, N. L., Garber, J., Panak, W. F., & Dodge, K. A. (1992). Social information processing in aggressive and depressed children. *Child Development*, *63*, 1305–1320.

Reynolds, C., & Kamphaus, R. (2004). *Behavior Assessment System for Children*. Circle Pines, MN: American Guidance Service.

Rhodes, M. G., & Anastasi, J. S. (2012). The own-age bias in face recognition: A metaanalytic and theoretical review. *Psychological Bulletin*, *138*(1), 146–174.

Shaprio, E. G., Hughes, S., August, G., & Bloomquist, M. (1993). Processing of emotional information in children with attention-deficit hyperactivity disorder. *Developmental Neuropsychology*, *9*, 207–224.

Shute, V. J., & Ke, F. (2012). Games, learning, and assessment. In *Assessment in Game-Based Learning* (pp. 43–58). New York, NY: Springer.

Skuse, D., Lawrence, K., & Tang, J. (2005). Measuring social-cognitive functions in children with somatotrophic axis dysfunction. *Hormone Research*, *64*, 73–82.

Thompson, E. J., Beauchamp, M. H., Darling, S. J., Hearps, S. J., Brown, A., Charalambous, G., Crossley, L., Darby, D., Dooley, J. J., Greenham, M., Jaimangal, M., & Anderson, V. (2018). Protocol for a prospective, school-based standardisation study of a digital social skills assessment tool for children: The paediatric evaluation of emotions, relationships, and socialisation (Peers) study. *BMJ Open*, *8*(2), e016633.

Toblin, R. L., Schwartz, D., Gorman, A. H., & Abou-ezzeddine, T. (2005). Social–cognitive and behavioral attributes of aggressive victims of bullying. *Journal of Applied Developmental Psychology*, *26*(3), 329–346.

Tonks, J., Williams, H. W., Frampton, I., & Yates, P. (2007). Assessing emotion recognition in 9–15-years olds: Preliminary analysis of abilities in reading emotion from faces, voices and eyes. *Brain Injury*, *21*(6), 623–629.

Uekermann, J., Kraemer, M., Abdel-Hammid, M., Schimmelmann, B. G., Hebebrand, J., Daum, I., . . . Kis, B. (2010). Social cognition in attention-deficit hyperactivity disorder (ADHD). *Neuroscience and Biobehavioral Reviews*, *34*, 734–743.

Van Overwalle, F. (2009). Social cognition and the brain: A meta-analysis. *Human Brain Mapping*, *30*, 829–858.

Vera-Estay, E., Seni, A. G., Champagne, C., & Beauchamp, M. (2016). All for one: Contributions of age, socioeconomic factors, executive functioning, and social cognition to moral reasoning in childhood. *Frontiers in Psychology*, *7*, 1–13.

Walker, H., & McConnell, S. (1988). *The Walker–McConnell Scale of Social Competence and Social Adjustment: A Social Skills Rating Scale for Teachers*. Austin, TX: Pro-ED.

Walker-Andrews, A. (1998). Emotions and social development: Infants' recognition of emotions in others. *Pediatrics*, *102*(Supplement E1), 1268–1271.

Wang, Q. (2016). Why should we all be cultural psychologists? Lessons from the study of social cognition. *Perspectives on Psychological Science*, *11*(5), 583–596.

Yeates, K. O., Bigler, E. D., Dennis, M., Gerhardt, C. A., Rubin, K. H., Stancin, T., Taylor, H. G., & Vannatta, K. (2007). Social outcomes in childhood brain disorder: A heuristic integration of social neuroscience and developmental psychology. *Psychological Bulletin*, *133*(3), 535.

Chapter 11

Remediating impairments in social cognition

Jacoba M. Spikman, Herma J. Westerhof-Evers and Anneli Cassel

Brain damage resulting from acute neurological disorders, such as traumatic brain injury (TBI) or stroke; insidious neurological disorders, such as brain tumors or multiple sclerosis (MS); or neurodegenerative diseases, such as frontotemporal dementia (FTD), can result in changes in social behaviour. This is particularly the case when prefrontal areas, or the circuits associated with these areas, are affected. Similar social behavioural presentations have been observed in various neurodevelopmental disorders, such as autism spectrum disorders (ASD), and neuropsychiatric disorders, such as schizophrenia spectrum disorders (SSD).

In 1990, Neil Brooks, who extensively investigated sequelae of brain damage, remarked the following: "*Of all three areas of deficit (physical, cognitive, behavioural) it is the behavioural deficit that lasts longest, is most difficult to treat, and has the most negative consequences on successful social and vocational rehabilitation*" (p. 77). In this citation, he emphasised not only the disruptive nature of behavioural changes but also their immunity to treatment. Despite this, for a long time, clinical neuropsychology neglected social behavioural problems in brain disorders as a relevant domain. Proper assessment and treatment methods were sorely needed but yet to be developed. This changed with the emergence of the field of social neuroscience at the end of the previous century. Social neuroscientists acknowledged that humans have to survive in a complex social world; hence, brain anatomy and function have evolved in such a way so as to optimally facilitate social interactions (Brothers, 1990). We humans, thus, have a social brain with specialised areas dedicated to the processing of socially relevant information.

Social cognitive information processing involves a series of stages (Adolphs, 2001; Beer & Ochsner, 2006). First, socially relevant information, e.g. expressions of emotions on other peoples' faces or in their voices (prosody), has to be attended to and perceived. Secondly, this perceived information, combined with knowledge regarding social rules and conventions, has to be interpreted, leading to an understanding of another's thoughts, feelings, and beliefs. In other words, this processing allows individuals to form a theory of other peoples' minds, and to take their perspective (the mentalising system; Frith & Frith,

DOI: 10.4324/9781003027034-11

2012). The perception of these social cues, and how they are interpreted, can be influenced by cognitive and attributional biases, i.e. the causal interpretations a person makes in response to events that occur in their lives (Peterson, 1988, 1991). Further, such mentalising may be achieved through different routes: either occurring fast and automatically with cognitive efficiency or in a slow and controlled way with greater cognitive demand (Happé, Cook, & Bird, 2017).

Perception of socially relevant, emotional information may also lead to empathy: that is, the sharing of others' feelings. It is thought that feeling emotions with others may support subsequent social cognitive processing via a contagion process such as the mirror system (Frith & Frith, 2012). The ability to share others' feelings is closely related to the ability to have and recognize one's own emotional feelings. Problems in self-awareness of one's own emotional state is referred to as alexithymia. Finally, being able to understand others, both cognitively and emotionally, is crucial in order to display appropriate behaviour within a specific social context (social behaviour "output"). This involves adapting one's behaviour to the social situation via the application of adequate social communicative skills, which in turn feeds into further, iterative, social cognitive processing cycles.

It follows, therefore, that social problem behaviours arising from brain damage, as well as neuropsychiatric and developmental conditions, may result from impairments in these "input" stages involved in the perception and understanding of social information. Following this social cognitive framework, various instruments have been developed in the field of clinical neuropsychology in the last decade that aim to assess impairments in aspects of social cognition, such as emotion recognition and theory of mind (ToM; for further discussion see Chapters 9 and 10).

In 2013 social cognition was included as one of the six major neurocognitive domains in the DSM-5 that should be assessed in brain disorders. Accumulating evidence shows that social cognitive deficits are prevalent in many different neurological and neuropsychiatric disorders in which behavioural problems are also commonly observed (Henry, Von Hippel, Molenberghs, Lee, & Sachdev, 2016). Studies have, indeed, demonstrated that such impairments relate to specific social behavioural problems in everyday life. In our own research, we found that social cognitive impairments after acquired brain injury (TBI and stroke) are associated with a range of behavioural indices (Buunk et al., 2016; Nijsse, Spikman, Visser-Meily, de Kort, & van Heugten, 2019b; Spikman, Timmerman, Milders, Veenstra, & Van Der Naalt, 2012). Poor emotion recognition and ToM skills are associated with impaired self-awareness, emotional indifference, lack of empathy, and disinhibition, as rated by a proxy of the patient (Buunk et al., 2017; Jorna et al., 2021; Nijsse, Spikman, Visser-Meily, de Kort, & van Heugten, 2019a; Spikman, Milders et al., 2013). Further, they are related to a decreased ability to learn from treatment (Spikman, Boelen et al., 2013) and to lower levels of vocational and social participation

(Meulenbroek & Turkstra, 2016; Westerhof- Evers, Fasotti, van der Naalt, & Spikman, 2019). This knowledge about the importance of the early cognitive processing of social information and its relation to adaptive behaviour offers new leads to develop treatments for social cognitive and social behavioural problems.

In this chapter we will discuss what these new developments have brought the field to date. We will start with providing a general overview of neuropsychological rehabilitation methods and then proceed with a review of neuropsychological interventions aimed at improving aspects of social cognition and social behaviour in patients with brain disorders, both neurological and neuropsychiatric. We will focus, in particular, on patients with brain injury due to TBI, with additional references to two specific clinical populations: patients with ASD and patients with SSD.

Neuropsychological rehabilitation: objectives, targets and methods

Neuropsychological rehabilitation involves the remediation of the cognitive, emotional and behavioural consequences of brain disorders with the overall aim to improve patients' functioning at different levels. To understand this, it is helpful to use the International Classification of Functioning, Disability and Health (ICF) system of the World Health Organisation (2001) that classifies consequences of illnesses at three levels.

The first level is that of bodily functions, which includes mental and neuropsychological functions; the second level refers to activities, as components of one's actions; and the third level refers to societal participation, the extent to which one fulfils social roles. Improvement in functioning through treatment may not only apply to improvement in neuropsychological performance, as measured using neuropsychological tests, but can also refer to improvement in function at the level of activities and social roles in daily life.

In the case of brain injury, any functional improvement can be conceived of as recovery: recovery does not necessarily mean a full return to pre-injury functioning but includes any progress from the level of an individual's functioning at the time of their brain damage. Recovery may take place at two levels: neurological (cerebral) and psychological (behavioural or experiential). The notion of recovery in other clinical populations is not always appropriate: here, progress can be conceptualised as any movement towards an individual reaching their perceived optimal physical, psychological, or social functioning.

Treatment approaches

Two treatment approaches can be distinguished that are related to these different recovery levels. Traditionally, the *restorative model* assumes that, with treatment, loss of function can be reversed: that is, the damaged cognitive function and its underlying brain structure can be restored. Theoretically, this is accomplished via stimulation of the damaged cognitive functions using a focused, repeated, practice approach. Through frequent exercises designed to tap a specific cognitive function, e.g. playing memory games to stimulate memory, it is assumed that this brain function will improve, just as a muscle becomes stronger as a result of exercise. This type of training is also called *function training*: it is expected to result in recovery of the damaged function. If that is the case, generalisation of this improvement to a wide range of different situations in everyday life can be expected.

In contrast, the *compensatory model* assumes that brain damage is irreversible, and aims to compensate for the consequences of brain damage by the deployment and use of the patient's intact functions and abilities (Spikman & Fasotti, 2017). According to Barbara Wilson's (1997) definition, this includes, "*Any intervention strategy or technique that is intended to help patients with cognitive problems caused by brain injury, and their families, to cope with these problems, to learn to live with them, to overcome and/or to reduce them*". This implies that the *compensatory model* includes any method which leads to better functioning of patients. These do not focus on the impairment itself, but on a reduction of restrictions that the patient encounters in daily life. Hence, treatment goals do not have to be confined to the individual patient, but can also extend to their physical and social environment (Spikman & Fasotti, 2017).

Under the label of compensatory treatments, different approaches can be distinguished. *Skills training* is the term used for interventions that require patients to practice tasks by repeatedly performing them, just as in function training. However, in contrast to function training, the aim is not to stimulate an underlying neuropsychological function, but rather to learn a specific, situation-related behavioural routine without the expectation that this will transfer to other situations. If patients have sufficient executive skills, they may be able to profit from *strategy training*. In this type of training the use of a general, top-down approach, usually existing of a series of steps, is taught that aims to achieve improved functioning in a wide range of different situations. Since a strategy describes the actions to take in a rather abstract manner, it is up to the patient to tailor this approach to suit specific situations.

Learning

Whether treatment approaches aim to restore brain functions or to teach patients to apply behavioural routines or strategies, they all involve learning with the objective to achieve a change in the patient's behaviour. Learning can take place at many different levels of complexity: consistently coupling a specific response to a specific stimulus can lead to a strong connection through simple association learning; a complex motor skill, such as riding a bicycle, can be procedurally learned via repeated practice; and knowledge from academic textbooks can be stored in one's memory through rote learning. These examples all involve forms of non-social learning. However, since we are social beings, much of our learning can be described as social learning, i.e. learning that is facilitated by observation of, or interaction with, other individuals.

In young children, this starts with imitating the behaviour of close others. However, when growing up, it becomes increasingly clear that simply copying others' behaviour may not always be wise. Hence, to make good use of social learning, we need to learn the right behaviours from the right others; those who know better than we do, via social learning strategies (SLSs; Heyes, 2016). However, deciding whom to imitate in order to successfully learn adaptive social behaviours relies heavily on social cognitive processes and involves both the mirror as well as the mentalising system. Relatedly, for patients with a social cognitive deficit, it would understandably become more difficult to learn such skills in a social context.

This is, indeed, what we found in a mixed group of patients with a brain injury participating in a rehabilitation treatment for executive deficits. The patients with impaired emotion recognition were less able to profit from this treatment, despite the fact that their executive deficits were no more severe than the patients with intact emotion recognition skills (Spikman, Boelen et al., 2013). Apparently, problems in recognising others' emotions hampered learning. Given this, it is not difficult to imagine that social learning plays an even larger role in treatments aimed to improve social cognition and social behaviour, while at the same time these processes are seriously impaired. This poses extra challenges to the design of any intervention aiming to treat impairments in social cognition.

When giving an overview of available interventions in the field of social cognition, the following aspects are relevant. First: what were the treatment objectives? In other words, what exactly was the intervention targeting? We can distinguish approaches that aimed to improve single aspects of social cognition, such as emotion perception, ToM, empathy, or social behaviour, or approaches that were multifaceted. Second: how did the authors establish whether these treatment targets were achieved? This relates to the outcome measures used in any study conducted to test the effectiveness of an intervention. Even if treatments are primarily aimed at improving aspects of social cognition, outcomes will only be ecologically valid if gains translate to more appropriate social behaviour in everyday life. Hence, to establish effectiveness of a treatment, the study should not only include measures of any purported "near" effects, such as social cognitive test performance, but also measure potential "far" effects, i.e. the associated skills related to everyday social behaviours. Third: what is the methodological quality of the treatment study? In this, we follow the distinction applied by Cicerone and colleagues (Cicerone et al., 2000; Cicerone et al., 2019) regarding three levels of evidence. Class I consists of prospective randomised controlled trials (RCTs), Class II includes prospective cohort studies, retrospective case-control studies or controlled clinical series, and Class III consists of uncontrolled clinical series or single subject studies. Only evidence from Class I studies can be considered solid, but evidence from studies with lower methodological quality may be relevant because they can highlight new developments in the field.

Interventions

Single target approaches

Perception of social-emotional information

Emotional expressions (from faces, voice tone, or body language) are one of the most important sources of social information. Impaired emotion perception is prevalent across a range of neurological, neurodevelopmental, and neuropsychiatric populations: it has been shown to affect those with a TBI (Babbage et al., 2011; Bornhofen & McDonald, 2008b), stroke (Buunk et al., 2017; Nijsse et al., 2019b), multiple sclerosis (Cotter et al., 2016), brain tumour (Goebel, Mehdorn, & Wiesner, 2018), ASD (Velikonja, Fett, & Velthorst, 2019), and SSD (Barkl, Lah, Harris, & Williams, 2014). In a study comparing patients with SSD to patients with ASD, more severe impairments in emotion perception were found in the latter group (Fernandes et al., 2018). Overall, emotion perception can be considered a relevant target for treatment in all these groups.

Within the field of brain injury, the first studies that aimed to improve social cognition focused on facial emotion perception. Pioneering work was carried out by Guercio, Podolska-Schroeder, and Rehfeldt (2004) and by the groups of McDonald and colleagues in Australia and Neumann and colleagues in the USA. Based on their work, different approaches to improving emotion perception can be distinguished. One method can be understood as a form of function training that involves practicing recognising various emotions, via repeated exercise, without providing an external strategy. Materials used can be pictures of emotional expressions and videos of emotional interactions. Preferably, exercises are graded, starting easy and, if that is successful, gradually increasing in difficulty. First, there is work on simple cues to affect recognition, for instance, still pictures, which can be eventually incorporated into training perception of complex and dynamic emotions, using video and role play. These interventions usually involve an errorless learning approach. This implies minimising the chance of making mistakes by encouraging the patient to focus attention carefully on the stimuli that are provided, i.e. different expressions of emotions, and to respond only when certain, after which immediate feedback is provided.

In addition, methods have been applied which can be understood as a metacognitive strategy approach, either through affective or cognitive routes. For instance, reflecting on previously experienced emotional episodes may help one to better recognise others' emotions. An example would be to ask a patient if he/she remembers an event from the past which triggered them to feel fear, and if so, if he/she can relive this feeling and express the matching facial expression.

Consequently, this self-reflection is used to relate to and help understand others' emotional expressions, and the patient is encouraged to apply this strategy in other situations. While this strategy can be considered as using an affective route to training, cognitive strategies can also be applied. In the context of facial emotion recognition, a cognitive approach could involve teaching patients to focus attention to the position of eyes, eyebrows and mouth, in order to rationally analyse these facial features. By comparing this information to knowledge regarding the typical positions of these facial cues for specific emotions, it can be deduced which emotion the observed configuration fits best.

Employment of the mirror system to support emotion recognition has also been described. This involves using one's own emotional expressions to assist in the recognition of others' facial emotional expressions. The most direct route is to teach the patient to imitate the facial expression of the other, which may result in recognition of the feeling that is triggered. Sometimes, use of a mirror to see one's own mimicked expression may be helpful. Such mimicry has been found to actually lead to emotional changes in the observer (Moody, McIntosh, Mann, & Weisser, 2007).

Several studies with sufficient methodological quality have been carried out comparing different (elements) of treatments aimed at improving emotion recognition within patients with TBI. Bornhofen and McDonald (2008a) compared a repeated practice approach using errorless learning with a strategic approach involving self-instruction and found that both TBI groups showed improvement on tests for emotion recognition, but only the errorless learning approach resulted in improved social behaviours. McDonald, Bornhofen, and Hunt (2009) compared facial-feature processing with mimicking but did not find that either strategy resulted in improved facial emotion recognition. However, the overall conclusion based on various studies in patients with brain injury is that there is evidence for improved emotion perception after training, irrespective of the method applied (Bornhofen & McDonald, 2008a, 2008c; Guercio et al., 2004; Radice-Neumann, Zupan, Tomita, & Willer, 2009; Neumann, Babbage, Zupan, & Willer, 2015). Less research has been carried out aimed at interventions targeting prosody or understanding of body language. McDonald et al. (2013) investigated whether a repeated practice approach could be effective for recognition of prosody in a mixed group of patients with brain injury, but found that the intervention did not result in better recognition of emotional expression in voices.

Emotion perception training has also been evaluated in neurodevelopmental and neuropsychiatric populations. The most commonly used approaches have focused on attention and facial-feature processing. In both patients with SSD and ASD, such treatments have been found to be effective in improving facial affect recognition (Cassel, McDonald, Kelly, & Togher, 2019; Nijman, Veling, van der Stouwe, & Pijnenborg, 2020; Pallathra, Cordero, Wong, & Brodkin, 2019). Indeed, large intervention effects (moderate to large range) have been observed when examining targeted emotion perception training programs amongst these populations (Roelofs, Wingbermühle, Egger, & Kessels, 2017). However, transfer of treatment effects to social functioning appears less robust (Pallathra et al., 2019; Roelofs et al., 2017), with concerns noted that such interventions may be "training to the task" rather than supporting generalisation to social behaviour.

Emotional self-awareness and emotional empathy

Despite the importance of intact empathy for the maintenance of meaningful relationships, and evidence for impaired empathy in patients with brain damage, ASD, and SSD, few attempts have been made to explicitly remediate impairments in self-emotional processing and empathy (Cassel et al., 2019). In the brain injury field, Neumann, Malec, and Hammond (2017) were the first group to explicitly target alexithymia in a treatment protocol. Individuals completed eight computerised lessons with a facilitator covering psychoeducation about emotional self-awareness and skill-building their emotional understanding repertoire (vocabulary, differentiating emotions, physical sensation awareness). Their proof-of-principle case series found positive changes which were observed before and after treatment in regard to both emotional self-awareness and emotion regulation, although further research is necessary before conclusions about efficacy can be made.

Similarly, impairments in self-emotional processing have been targeted in neuropsychiatric populations to varying degrees, although most often in populations other than ASD or SSD (see Cameron, Ogrodniczuk, & Hadjipavlou, 2014, for a review).

Theory of mind (ToM)

The term 'theory of mind' is most closely associated with ASD, as the first studies on this subject identified that the inability to take another's perspective and understand their thoughts, knowledge, and feelings was a core characteristic of autism. These first studies were soon followed by a plethora of studies demonstrating mentalising deficits in various other patient groups, both patients with brain injury as well as patients with SSD. It is unsurprising that problems in understanding others will have a negative impact on interpersonal relationships and result in decreased social and vocational participation. However, to date, there is a scarcity in ToM treatments for patients with brain injury (Cassel et al., 2019). Gabbatore et al. (2015) developed a treatment program (Cognitive Pragmatic Treatment; CPT) that aimed to improve the communicative skills of TBI patients through training social communication and mentalising skills. This treatment involved teaching patients to recognise that others have mental states that differ from their own and, therefore, to notice and infer the potential non-literal meaning behind another's communicative intent before responding.

Indeed, within-group improvement in social-communicative skills was found and maintained over three months following treatment, but effectiveness was tested in a small case series of 15 patients without a control condition.

In contrast, a wide range of programs that aim to treat ToM deficits in patients with ASD have been developed and evaluated. Early attempts involved a more functional approach, in which participants had to repeatedly practice first-order belief tasks, such as the well-known Sally-Anne task (Baron-Cohen, Leslie, & Frith, 1985). Different approaches have been used to facilitate learning, such as giving feedback, creating thought bubbles to make the thoughts of the characters depicted explicit, or to visualise others' beliefs as mental pictures (Cassel et al., 2019). Although these studies often demonstrated improvement on the tasks administered, no "far" effects have been evidenced: gains have not led to better performance on novel tasks or to real-world perspective taking. Only one study incorporated the actual translation of the above-mentioned approach to a real world context in order to increase understanding of patients that real people can hold false beliefs, but this had only modest success (McGregor, Whiten, & Blackburn, 1998).

In the field of SSD, several treatments have also been developed to improve mentalising, in which different strategy-based approaches have been employed. For example, realistic social vignettes have been utilised to train ToM skills extensively through both first- and second-order mental state inferencing. Still, these have tended to rely on artificial task materials to depict social situations with multiple characters, such as sketches or comic strips, in which there is little uncertainty over the supposed thoughts and intentions of the characters (e.g. Bechi et al., 2013; Choi & Kwon, 2006).

Greater effectiveness has been found for studies that use more realistic materials to improve perspective taking skills, for instance discussing video vignettes or experiential learning through role plays. Techniques applied to enhance comprehension of others' perspectives include explicitly noticing concrete contextual factors of an interaction (e.g. physical features, place, time); Socratic questioning to discuss and elaborate on hypotheses one might have about others' mental states; and using a cognitive-behavioural treatment model to better distinguish between one's own thoughts and feelings and those of another person (e.g. Fernandez-Gonzalo et al., 2015; Hogarty et al., 2004; Marsh et al., 2013). Cognitive distortions and attributional biases have additionally been well documented amongst this population and are known to influence beliefs about another's intentions (Green et al., 2008). Interventions to remediate these biases have typically utilised cognitive-behavioural strategies to support cognitive restructuring of biased social inferences, e.g. metacognitive training (Moritz & Woodward, 2007). Overall, targeted ToM interventions have been found to result in large intervention effects (small to large range) (Roelofs et al., 2017), although again the extent to which such training generalises to social functioning is less clear (Cassel et al., 2019).

Social behaviour and social communication

Given that it has long been known that social behavioural changes, and thus impairments in social functioning, are common consequences of serious brain injury, it is not surprising that the first interventions designed for this population were directly aimed at improving this behaviour. Helffenstein and Wechsler (1982) conducted one of the first studies targeting social skills and, using an RCT design, compared a method called interpersonal process recall (IPR) training with non-therapeutic attention involving eight patients with brain injury in each arm. In the IPR training, patients practiced social skills through role-play, which were recorded and subsequently reviewed with feedback to support reflection and insight building. Some improvement was found on observer ratings of social skills; however, no evidence was found for generalisation to social behaviour and societal participation, nor were treatment gains maintained at follow up. Other studies have focused on training social communication skills, such as expressing needs, listening, and using nonverbal communication. Dahlberg et al. (2007) conducted an RCT in a group of 52 patients with chronic TBI and found evidence for improvement in communication skills, measured using rating scales for observed communicative behaviour, of which gains were maintained at follow up.

Despite this early work, further treatment developments have been limited: almost 30 years after this publication, Driscoll, Dal Monte, and Grafman (2011) reported only three Class I RCTs with a focus on social skills training in their literature review for individuals with brain injury. In line with their conclusions, there is still limited evidence for the effectiveness and generalisiblity of treatments that focus solely on social skills training in patients with brain injury.

With regard to ASD, social skills training seems to lead to limited effects. A meta-analysis by Gates, Kang, and Lerner (2017) showed that social skills training resulted in patients showing improvement on relevant tasks and being very satisfied themselves with the gains. However, again generalisation was not apparent, with learned skills not translating to behaviour in other settings, such as family or school environments (as parent and teacher reports did not indicate improvement in social functioning). It is worth noting that there is also potential harm associated with some attempts to improve social skills in neurodiverse populations, particularly when using didactic approaches that aim to "teach" arbitrary neurotypical social rules (Randall, 2020; Vance, 2020). With regard to SSD, a meta-analysis by Turner et al. (2018) showed that social skills training may be effective in improving psychosocial outcomes for patients, but only for negative symptoms such as apathy and lack of social interest, and not for positive symptoms such as hallucinations.

Multifaceted approaches

In the previous section, single target treatments for separate aspects of social cognition were reviewed. Below we will present treatment approaches that aimed to improve a broader range of social cognitive processes and which have often combined various methods: in other words, are multifaceted.

One of the first studies evaluating such a multifaceted approach for patients with (traumatic) brain injury was the study of McDonald et al. (2008). In their protocol, which they labeled a social skills treatment program, they combined three different types of intervention: group training of social perception, group training of social behaviours, and in addition, individual therapy sessions targeting emotional adjustment. Training consisted of 12 weekly sessions, with three hours of group training and one hour of individual treatment. The social perception treatment involved both practicing the decoding of emotional expressions (face, voice, and gesture) as well as learning to understand social inferences.

The methods used were graduated practice, starting with simple materials, such as drawings or photos, and progressing to more dynamic emotion presentations, such as video, complex role plays, and games from the social skills literature. Patients were taught to focus their attention on relevant features, as well as to rehearse different modes of expression through mirror practice. Social behaviour was trained using the same structure in every session: warm-up games, review of homework, introduction of target skill, discussion of potential issues and solutions, therapist modelling of appropriate and inappropriate behaviour, and role-playing to develop skills.

In each session, a different facet of social behaviour was targeted, such as: greetings, introducing oneself, listening, giving compliments, starting a conversation, topic selection, being assertive, and coping with disagreements. Within this broader framework, individual goals were identified for each client, in relation to the specific difficulties that they encountered due to their brain injury. In all sessions, an acronym, WSTC, was used to represent the metacognitive strategy that patients learned to assist planning and monitoring of their behaviour (**W**hat am I doing, What is the best **S**trategy, **T**ry it, **C**heck it out), but treatment also involved extensive repetition of skills. Central to enhancing learning were the provision of immediate feedback and social reinforcement.

McDonald et al. (2008) compared this treatment with two control conditions in an RCT: social activity alone, and a waitlist control; in 39 patients, 13 in each condition. The authors concluded that social skills training yielded only modest gains with regard to social behaviour and no treatment effects were found for social perception.

The T-ScEmo (Treatment of Social cognition and Emotion regulation) program, designed by Westerhof and colleagues (Westerhof-Evers et al., 2017; Westerhof-Evers, Visser-Keizer, Fasotti, & Spikman, 2019), is another multifaceted treatment for people with brain injury. This treatment combines many of the approaches that have been evaluated before as effective or promising, in a new set-up. The protocol consists of 20 one-hour individual sessions and incorporates three modules: (1) emotion perception, (2) perspective taking and ToM, and (3) regulation of social behaviour. Each module builds upon the previous one.

The overall treatment aim is to improve social cognition, regulate social behaviour, and increase participation in everyday life. Important elements are homework assignments and involvement of a significant other, in addition to practice in the therapy sessions and treatment given by experienced therapists. Before starting the treatment, patients are provided with information about social cognition and its relation to social behaviour in two psychoeducation sessions: individualised feedback is further provided in relation to how the patient's specific social cognitive impairments may be influencing their changed social behaviour, based on the results of their neuropsychological assessment.

In module one, the patient is taught different emotion recognition strategies, such as facial-feature processing, using mimicry and emotional experiences, all to understand facial emotions, prosody, and body language, leading to the best, working, personalised strategy for each patient.

In module two, it is explained that recognising emotional expressions is an important prerequisite for understanding others, but that this also depends on the ability to recognise that others may have different thoughts and feelings. To train perspective taking and ToM, principles from cognitive behavioural therapy (CBT) are used to introduce to patients a simplified thoughts-feelings-behaviour (T-F-B) triangle, which is filled out both from the self as well as another's perspective. This is used only to focus on explicit communication about thoughts and feelings of self and others, not for reframing attributions or cognitive distortions. The scheme is applied in many different practice situations: using role-play, involvement of a close other, and real-life video clips. One strategy that is taught is to ask questions to enhance perspective taking, empathy, and social communication: e.g. what are the other's feelings? What are the other's thoughts? How can I influence the other? How will the other react?

In module three, social behaviour is treated through specific goals to increase self-awareness, to inhibit inappropriate behaviour, and to display socially desirable behaviour. Several basic skills are taught: general skills such as learning communication rules (listening, turn-taking, giving compliments, dealing with criticism); respecting others' personal space; and specific skills as these relate to a patient's impairments, such as social problem-solving, recognising precursors of inappropriate behaviour, and anger management.

In an RCT of 60 patients with TBI and impaired social cognition, the T-ScEmo protocol was compared to a control treatment involving computerised cognitive function training (Cogniplus). T-ScEmo led to improvements at a functional level (emotion perception, ToM) and also generalised to everyday life behaviours, evidenced by higher levels of proxy-rated empathy and societal participation. Given the multifaceted nature of the treatment, the design did not provide the means to determine whether there were specific treatment ingredients that improved these aspects of social cognition and social behaviour, or whether effectiveness was the final result of combining these elements.

Box 11.1   Case 1: John: Adult with serious TBI who underwent the T-ScEmo treatment because of problems in daily life social functioning

History:

John is a 39-year-old male, who is married and has three young children. He worked as a consultant in human resources. Two years prior to enrolling in T-ScEmo, he was hit on his bicycle by a car and sustained a severe traumatic brain injury (Glasgow Coma Scale: 8, posttraumatic amnesia: 21 days), with visible lesions in the prefrontal cortices on MRI. After two weeks acute hospital care, he was transferred to rehabilitation care. He was discharged home from rehabilitation after three weeks. However, there it became clear that his behaviour had changed. Most prominent were his problems in social functioning. For that reason, he was referred to a specialized rehabilitation facility.

Presentation:

At intake, John and his wife were interviewed by the clinical neuropsychologist. John reported his main complaints were fatigue, impulsivity, and that he frequently had anger outbursts. His wife reported that they had daily conflicts because John had trouble controlling his emotions, which led to expressions of anger. She mentioned that his personality had substantially changed. Before the injury, she described John as thoughtful, social, and easy going. Now she reported he was insensitive to the emotions of others (including herself and their children), his affect was blunt, and he did not display spontaneous affection to her and his children anymore. He also exhibited behaviours which where impulsive, inappropriate for the situation (such as acting too jovial to strangers), and sometimes rather childish (such as playing hide and seek with his son while shopping).

Assessment:

The neuropsychological assessment revealed in addition to general cognitive impairments (attention and planning, with intact memory) social cognitive impairments in facial emotion recognition, poor perspective taking, poor empathy, and problems in controlling his emotions.

Intervention:

Based on these findings, John was thought to be a suitable candidate for the T-ScEmo treatment program. He was willing to start with this, although he did not have a good insight into his changes, but he accepted the desire from his wife that she really wanted him to change, very seriously.

Together with the therapist and his wife at the start of the treatment, John formulated three treatment goals: (1) I want to control my anger outbursts, (2) I want to respond to my wife's emotions (and support her), and (3) I want to adjust my behaviour accordingly to the situation. Guided by the T-ScEmo protocol, John and his wife first received psycho-education based on his neuropsychological assessment, with a particular focus on understanding how his social cognitive deficits affected his changed behaviours. They reported this proved helpful for him to better understand how his brain injury had resulted in difficulties with the processing of social information, the understanding of others, and his ability to adjust his behaviours to the social situation.

Subsequently, in the first module focusing on improving perception of social-emotional information, he was trained to attend to others' facial emotions. He was stimulated to carefully observe others' emotional signals in real-life. Further, he applied the mimicry technique in playing situations with his youngest daughter. By doing this, he was forced to attend to her emotional expressions more carefully and was consequently able to fine-tune his behaviour to her needs more appropriately. Furthermore, in a safe and non-confronting manner, examples of his inappropriate behaviours were used to reflect on how this might lead to others' embarrassment. To support John's emotional self-awareness, he was asked to recollect emotional situations from the past (before the accident). He was stimulated by the therapist to use these to re-enliven the feelings that were elicited by these situations and use them to interpret new emotional situations. At first, he found it very difficult and exhausting to apply these strategies. However, as the treatment proceeded, he felt that the effort paid off as he realized that his mindfulness to others' feelings had increased. He started to believe that he could still contribute to adequate communication and cooperation in his family.

In the second module, focusing on improvement of theory of mind and empathy, John became increasingly aware that he had difficulties in understanding the thoughts and feelings of close others, which was a source for mutual distress and conflicts. By means of the Thoughts-Feelings-Behaviour cycle, he learned about his tendency to assume others' expectations, feelings, and needs. His wife participated in role plays in which John practiced inquiring about her actual thoughts and feelings. John tried hard to support his wife but was still limited in his ability to understand her as well as he used to. To further improve their reciprocal communication, his wife learned to be more explicit about her emotions and expectations.

In the third module, aiming to improve social behaviour, showing empathy was addressed in role plays. As treatment proceeded, more complicated emotional issues were addressed, also together with his wife. This was a helpful way to reconnect with and understand one another and served to prevent John from expressing his anger through an explosive reaction caused by misinterpretation. Furthermore, John was asked to monitor both his fatigue and his temper flares. It became clear that his anger outbursts frequently appeared in the late afternoon when he was tired. John, therefore, learned to signal fatigue before he started an activity. He started to ask himself questions: "how do I feel?" "how do I look (pale, tired?)" "is it sensible to start this complex/stressful activity at this moment?". By these means he increased his self-awareness to avoid activities that could led to cognitive overload or frustration in the moment. Further, he learned to cope with his lowered frustration tolerance by taking a functional time-out as soon as he noticed that his anger feelings were starting to increase. He was supported in ways to practice this. The first step was to say it out loudly, "I need a time out", when he was taking a time out, and not to just walk out the door. Sometimes his wife suggested to John that he take a time out with a specific and complete feedback instruction "John, your voice is too loud, I think a time out is helpful". John had learned to accept this corrective feedback by practicing the feedback steps in role-play together with his wife. Also, they agreed that his wife could take a time out herself when she was getting irritated or angry. The couple learned that they could more effectively talk about earlier conflicts when they were both relaxed and had had enough rest. Sometimes they used the Thoughts-Feelings-Behaviour cycle in the moment to prevent a discussion from escalating. For his wife, she reported appreciating apologies that John had learned to offer in situations where his reactions had still been too angry. She felt that her emotions were taken seriously by John, and that having a good relationship did matter for him. At the end of the third module, showing appreciation and giving compliments to others was addressed as an important social skill.

During one of the sessions his wife expressed that she missed his hugs and physical signs of loving her. John was willing to address her needs, although he felt no clear need for intimacy himself anymore. He was supported to remind himself to give his wife a hug or kiss using an alarm in his mobile phone. At first, these attempts felt unnatural for his wife, but she appreciated that he was willing to work so hard to compensate for his deficits. Increasingly, she started to feel loved by John again and she reported a growing confidence in the future of their relationship. To conclude, these outcomes were supported by their scores on several scales at follow-up. The couple reported treatment satisfaction (treatment satisfaction scale, score 4, range 1–5), and relationship quality (score 8, range 1–10). Furthermore, both John and his wife agreed that John had achieved his personal goals, measured with the treatment goal attainment scale (1 = not all, 10 = entirely). John's scores increased from 4–1–5 at baseline to 7–8–8 at follow up.

Similar to the T-ScEmo protocol, Cassel, McDonald, and Kelly (2020) designed a CBT-based group treatment protocol, called SIFT IT. The protocol broadly targets the three processes of social cognition: (1) perception of social cognitive cues, (2) interpretation of perceived social cues, and (3) translation into socially adaptive behaviour. These targets are addressed in five modules: (1) introductions and social cognitive psychoeducation, (2) improving awareness and understanding of self and others' emotions, (3) improving awareness and flexibility in understanding self and others' thoughts and intentions (perspective taking), (4) choosing socially adaptive responses, and (5) endings (review and therapy blueprint). Social-values based goals are developed and rated weekly, following a review of participants' satisfaction with their social relationships.

A proof-of-principle study has been carried out with two patients with severe TBI who showed reliable improvements on social cognitive measures and self-reported gains in everyday social functioning. This indicates that this approach may also show promise as a group treatment, but the program has not yet been evaluated for efficacy.

With regard to patients with ASD, there are many multifaceted treatment programs that have been developed and evaluated. Bishop-Fitzpatrick, Minshew, and Eack (2013) and Pallathra et al. (2019) have comprehensively reviewed the literature and described several treatments that target both emotion recognition and ToM, as well as incorporate a focus on social skills. However, few studies have employed a strong methodological design. The majority of these were interventions that targeted specific aspects of social cognition.

Similarly, two recent meta-analyses have been published evaluating treatment programs for patients with SSD (d'Arma et al., 2021; Nijman et al., 2020). These have indicated that multifaceted treatment programs targeting several aspects of social cognition are more effective than those that just aim to improve a single element. This is particularly the case when treatments also incorporate active training to support the transfer of treatment gains to every-day life situations.

One of the most researched multifaceted social cognition treatment programs in SSD has been Social Cognition Interaction Training (SCIT): a group-based approach informed by CBT to (1) support understanding of emotions, (2) increase awareness and challenging of social cognitive biases, and (3) integrate to social behaviour (Penn et al., 2005). This program includes a focus on attri-butional style and biases in ToM interpretations with the use of attributional bias characters (e.g. "Blaming Bill" to exemplify when an individual has made an externalising-personalising attribution), which act as externalised scaffolds when generating alternative perspectives. Of at least 12 trials of SCIT, results show that emotion perception and ToM improve irrespective of clinical sever-ity and setting (Fiszdon & Davidson, 2019). Externalising attributional biases to support perspective taking has also been adapted for use in other clinical populations, such as ASD (Turner-Brown, Perry, Dichter, Bodfish, & Penn, 2008) and in the SIFT IT protocol for people with brain injury described above (Cassel et al., 2020).

An interesting new development, which may facilitate better functioning in realistic social situations, is the use of virtual reality (VR). VR platforms have been developed primarily for people with SSD (e.g. SocialVille: Nahum et al., 2014; Rose et al., 2015; DISCoVR: Nijman et al., 2019) and are in their early testing phases. These programs are multifaceted in that they include comput-erised exercises that aim to train core social cognitive processes (e.g. emotion perception, social cue perception, ToM, attributional style, and empathy) based on principles of neuroplasticity-based learning. Their ability to be delivered remotely without the pragmatic constraints of requiring therapist availability or face-to-face scheduling is appealing. However, whilst both platforms have shown preliminary evidence of feasibility, further studies are required before claims of efficacy can be made.

Conclusions

Social cognition has emerged as an important area in the neuropsychological field, for which there is a sore need for effective neuropsychological treatments. In particular, in the last decade, various interventions have been developed to remediate impairments in social cognition and have been evaluated using designs with varying degrees of methodological quality. The majority of these treatments have been developed for patients with brain injury, ASD, and SSD. Some interventions are targeted to single aspects of social cognition, such as emotion perception or ToM. Others are multifaceted, addressing a broader range of social cognitive deficits.

Targeted and comprehensive, multifaceted, interventions have generally shown similar sized intervention effects (e.g. moderate to large effect sizes on relevant social cognitive outcome measures, such as emotion perception or ToM). However, whilst targeted interventions typically only establish effectiveness for these "near" outcome measures, multifaceted approaches have shown greater evidence of further generalisation to improved everyday social behaviours as well. These generalisation effects to social functioning are generally modest, with effect sizes ranging from small to large (Roelofs et al., 2017). This greater generalisability effect is reflected across the different clinical populations and noted in other reviews in the field (e.g. Bishop-Fitzpatrick et al., 2013; Cassel et al., 2019; Pallathra et al., 2019).

Clearly, there is a serious need to remediate social cognitive deficits across the populations that present with these impairments. Whilst treatment developments to date are already very promising, more work needs to be done. Identifying treatment mediators and moderators, ensuring treatment gains relate to everyday social behaviours, and utilising new technologies to support access to remediation, all pose interesting avenues for future developments.

References

Adolphs, R. (2001). The neurobiology of social cognition. *Current Opinion in Neurobiology, 11*(2), 231–239. doi:10.1016/S0959-4388(00)00202-6

Babbage, D. R., Yim, J., Zupan, B., Neumann, D., Tomita, M. R., & Willer, B. (2011). Meta-analysis of facial affect recognition difficulties after traumatic brain injury. *Neuropsychology, 25*(3), 277–285. doi:10.1037/a0021908

Barkl, S. J., Lah, S., Harris, A. W. F., & Williams, L. M. (2014). Facial emotion identification in early-onset and first-episode psychosis: A systematic review with meta-analysis. *Schizophrenia Research, 159*(1), 62–69. doi:10.1016/j.schres.2014.07.049

Baron-Cohen, S., Leslie, A. M., & Frith, U. (1985). Does the autistic child have a "theory of mind"? *Cognition, 21*(1), 37–46. doi:10.1016/0010-0277(85)90022-8

Bechi, M., Spangaro, M., Bosia, M., Zanoletti, A., Fresi, F., Buonocore, M., . . . Cavallaro, R. (2013). Theory of mind intervention for outpatients with schizophrenia. *Neuropsychological Rehabilitation, 23*(3), 383–400. doi:10.1080/09602011.2012.762751

Beer, J. S., & Ochsner, K. N. (2006). Social cognition: A multi level analysis. *Brain Research, 1079*(1), 98–105. doi:10.1016/j.brainres.2006.01.002

Bishop-Fitzpatrick, L., Minshew, N. J., & Eack, S. M. (2013). A systematic review of psychosocial interventions for adults with autism spectrum disorders. *Journal of Autism and Developmental Disorders, 43*(3), 687–694. doi:10.1007/s10803-012-1615-8

Bornhofen, C., & McDonald, S. (2008a). Comparing strategies for treating emotion perception deficits in traumatic brain injury. *Journal of Head Trauma Rehabilitation, 23*(2), 103–115. doi:10.1097/01.HTR.0000314529.22777.43

Bornhofen, C., & McDonald, S. (2008b). Emotion perception deficits following traumatic brain injury: A review of the evidence and rationale for intervention. *Journal of the International Neuropsychological Society, 14*(4), 511–525. doi:10.1017/S1355617708080703

Bornhofen, C., & McDonald, S. (2008c). Treating deficits in emotion perception following traumatic brain injury. *Neuropsychological Rehabilitation, 18*(1), 22–44. doi:10.1080/09602010601061213

Brooks, N. (1990). Behavioural and social consequences of severe head injury. In B. G. Deelman, R. J. Saan, & A. H. van Zomeran (Eds.), *Traumatic Brain Injury: Clinical, Social and Rehabilitational Aspects* (pp. 77–88). Amsterdam: Swets & Zeitlinger.

Brothers, L. (1990). The social brain: A project for integrating primate behavior and neurophysiology in a new domain. *Concepts in Neuroscience, 1,* 27–51.

Buunk, A. M., Groen, R. J. M., Veenstra, W. S., Metzemaekers, J. D. M., van der Hoeven, J. H., van Dijk, J. M. C., & Spikman, J. M. (2016). Cognitive deficits after aneurysmal and angiographically negative subarachnoid hemorrhage: Memory, attention, executive functioning, and emotion recognition. *Neuropsychology, 30*(8), 961–969. doi:10.1037/neu0000296

Buunk, A. M., Spikman, J. M., Veenstra, W. S., van Laar, P. J., Metzemaekers, J. D. M., van Dijk, J. M. C., . . . Groen, R. J. M. (2017). Social cognition impairments after aneurysmal subarachnoid haemorrhage: Associations with deficits in interpersonal behaviour, apathy, and impaired self-awareness. *Neuropsychologia, 103,* 131–139. doi:10.1016/j.neuropsychologia.2017.07.015

Cameron, K., Ogrodniczuk, J., & Hadjipavlou, G. (2014). Changes in alexithymia following psychological intervention: A review. *Harvard Review of Psychiatry, 22*(3), 162–178. doi:10.1097/HRP.0000000000000036

Cassel, A., McDonald, S., & Kelly, M. (2020). Establishing 'proof of concept' for a social cognition group treatment program (SIFT IT) after traumatic brain injury: Two case studies. *Brain Injury, 34*(13–14), 1781–1793. doi:10.1080/02699052.2020.1831072

Cassel, A., McDonald, S., Kelly, M., & Togher, L. (2019). Learning from the minds of others: A review of social cognition treatments and their relevance to traumatic brain injury. *Neuropsychological Rehabilitation, 29*(1), 22–55. doi:10.1080/09602011.2016.1257435

Choi, K. H., & Kwon, J. H. (2006). Social cognition enhancement training for schizophrenia: A preliminary randomized controlled trial. *Community Mental Health Journal, 42*(2), 177–187. doi:10.1007/s10597-005-9023-6

Cicerone, K. D., Dahlberg, C., Kalmar, K., Langenbahn, D. M., Malec, J. F., Bergquist, T. F., . . . Morse, P. A. (2000). Evidence-based cognitive rehabilitation: Recommendations for clinical practice. *Archives of Physical Medicine and Rehabilitation, 81*(12), 1596–1615. doi:10.1053/apmr.2000.19240

Cicerone, K. D., Goldin, Y., Ganci, K., Rosenbaum, A., Wethe, J. V., Langenbahn, D. M., . . . Harley, J. P. (2019). Evidence-based cognitive rehabilitation: Systematic review of the literature from 2009 through 2014. *Archives of Physical Medicine and Rehabilitation, 100*(8), 1515–1533. doi:10.1016/j.apmr.2019.02.011

Cotter, J., Firth, J., Enzinger, C., Kontopantelis, E., Yung, A. R., Elliott, R., & Drake, R. J. (2016). Social cognition in multiple sclerosis: A systematic review and meta-analysis. *Neurology, 87*(16), 1727–1736. doi:10.1212/WNL.0000000000003236

Dahlberg, C. A., Cusick, C. P., Hawley, L. A., Newman, J. K., Morey, C. E., Harrison-Felix, C. L., & Whiteneck, G. G. (2007). Treatment efficacy of social communication skills training after traumatic brain injury: A randomized treatment and deferred treatment controlled trial. *Archives of Physical Medicine and Rehabilitation, 88*(12), 1561–1573. doi:10.1016/j.apmr.2007.07.033

d'Arma, A., Isernia, S., Di Tella, S., Rovaris, M., Valle, A., Baglio, F., & Marchetti, A. (2021). Social cognition training for enhancing affective and cognitive theory of mind in schizophrenia: A systematic review and a meta-analysis. *Journal of Psychology: Interdisciplinary and Applied, 155*(1), 26–58. doi:10.1080/00223980.2020.1818671

Driscoll, D. M., Dal Monte, O., & Grafman, J. (2011). A need for improved training interventions for the remediation of impairments in social functioning following brain injury. *Journal of Neurotrauma, 28*(2), 319–326. doi:10.1089/neu.2010.1523

Fernandes, J. M., Cajao, R., Lopes, R., Jeronimo, R., & Barahona-Correa, J. B. (2018). Social cognition in schizophrenia and autism spectrum disorders: A systematic review and meta-analysis of direct comparisons. *Frontiers Psychiatry, 9,* 504. doi:10.3389/fpsyt.2018.00504

Fernandez-Gonzalo, S., Turon, M., Jodar, M., Pousa, E., Hernandez Rambla, C., García, R., & Palao, D. (2015). A new computerized cognitive and social cognition training specifically designed for patients with schizophrenia/schizoaffective disorder in early stages of illness: A pilot study. *Psychiatry Research, 228*(3), 501–509. doi:10.1016/j.psychres.2015.06.007

Fiszdon, J. M., & Davidson, C. A. (2019). Social cognitive interventions. In Lewandowski, K., & Moustafa, A. (Eds.), *Social Cognition in Psychosis* (pp. 269–293). London: Academic Press.

Frith, C. D., & Frith, U. (2012) Mechanisms of social cognition. *Annual Review of Psychology, 63*(1), 287–313.

Gabbatore, I., Sacco, K., Angeleri, R., Zettin, M., Bara, B. G., & Bosco, F. M. (2015). Cognitive pragmatic treatment: A rehabilitative program for traumatic brain injury individuals. *Journal of Head Trauma Rehabilitation, 30*(5), E14–E28. doi:10.1097/HTR.0000000000000087

Gates, J. A., Kang, E., & Lerner, M. D. (2017). Efficacy of group social skills interventions for youth with autism spectrum disorder: A systematic review and meta-analysis. *Clinical Psychology Review, 52,* 164–181. doi:10.1016/j.cpr.2017.01.006

Goebel, S., Mehdorn, H. M., & Wiesner, C. D. (2018). Social cognition in patients with intracranial tumors: Do we forget something in the routine neuropsychological examination? *Journal of Neuro-Oncology, 140*(3), 687–696. doi:10.1007/s11060-018-3000-8

Green, M. F., Penn, D. L., Bentall, R., Carpenter, W. T., Gaebel, W., Gur, R. C., . . . Heinssen, R. (2008). Social cognition in schizophrenia: An NIMH workshop on definitions, assessment, and research opportunities. *Schizophrenia Bulletin, 34*(6), 1211–1220. doi:10.1093/schbul/sbm145

Guercio, J. M., Podolska-Schroeder, H., & Rehfeldt, R. A. (2004). Using stimulus equivalence technology to teach emotion recognition to adults with acquired brain injury. *Brain Injury, 18*(6), 593–601. doi:10.1080/02699050310001646116

Happé, F., Cook, J. L., & Bird, G. (2017). The structure of social cognition: In(ter)dependence of sociocognitive processes. *Annual Review of Psychology, 68,* 243–267.

Helffenstein, D. A., & Wechsler, F. S. (1982). The use of interpersonal process recall (IPR) in the remediation of interpersonal and communication skill deficits in the newly brain-injured. *Clinical Neuropsychology, 4*(3), 139–142.

Henry, J. D., Von Hippel, W., Molenberghs, P., Lee, T., & Sachdev, P. S. (2016). Clinical assessment of social cognitive function in neurological disorders. *Nature Reviews Neurology, 12*(1), 28–39. doi:10.1038/nrneurol.2015.229

Heyes, C. (2016). Who knows? Metacognitive social learning strategies. *Trends in Cognitive Sciences, 20*(3), 204–213. doi:10.1016/j.tics.2015.12.007

Hogarty, G. E., Flesher, S., Ulrich, R., Carter, M., Greenwald, D., Pogue-Geile, M., . . . Zoretich, R. (2004). Cognitive enhancement therapy for schizophrenia: Effects of a 2-year randomized trial on cognition and behavior. *Archives of General Psychiatry, 61*(9), 866–876. doi:10.1001/archpsyc.61.9.866

Jorna, L. S., Westerhof-Evers, H. J., Khosdelazad, S., Rakers, S. E., Van Der Naalt, J., Groen, R. J. M., . . . Spikman, J. M. (2021). Behaviors of concern after acquired brain injury: The role of negative emotion recognition and anger misattribution. *Journal of the International Neuropsychological Society*. doi:10.1017/S135561772000140X

Marsh, P. J., Langdon, R., McGuire, J., Harris, A., Polito, V., & Coltheart, M. (2013). An open clinical trial assessing a novel training program for social cognitive impairment in schizophrenia. *Australasian Psychiatry*, *21*(2), 122–126. doi:10.1177/1039856213475683

McDonald, S., Bornhofen, C., & Hunt, C. (2009). Addressing deficits in emotion recognition after severe traumatic brain injury: The role of focused attention and mimicry. *Neuropsychological Rehabilitation*, *19*(3), 321–339. doi:10.1080/09602010802193989

McDonald, S., Tate, R., Togher, L., Bornhofen, C., Long, E., Gertler, P., & Bowen, R. (2008). Social skills treatment for people with severe, chronic acquired brain injuries: A multicenter trial. *Archives of Physical Medicine and Rehabilitation*, *89*(9), 1648–1659. doi:10.1016/j.apmr.2008.02.029

McDonald, S., Togher, L., Tate, R., Randall, R., English, T., & Gowland, A. (2013). A randomised controlled trial evaluating a brief intervention for deficits in recognising emotional prosody following severe ABI. *Neuropsychological Rehabilitation*, *23*(2), 267–286. doi:10.1080/09602011.2012.751340

McGregor, E., Whiten, A., & Blackburn, P. (1998). Teaching theory of mind by highlighting intention and illustrating thoughts: A comparison of their effectiveness with 3-year-olds and autistic individuals. *British Journal of Developmental Psychology*, *16*(3), 281–300. www.scopus.com/inward/record.url?eid=2-s2.0-0032384936&partnerID=40&md5 = 7a6581a06f-5ca175854fa0dc297d3cea

Meulenbroek, P., & Turkstra, L. S. (2016). Job stability in skilled work and communication ability after moderate-severe traumatic brain injury. *Disability and Rehabilitation*, *38*(5), 452–461. doi:10.3109/09638288.2015.1044621

Moody, E. J., McIntosh, D. N., Mann, L. J., & Weisser, K. R. (2007). More than mere mimicry? The influence of emotion on rapid facial reactions to faces. *Emotion*, *7*(2), 447–457. doi:10.1037/1528-3542.7.2.447

Moritz, S., & Woodward, T. S. (2007). Metacognitive training for schizophrenia patients (MCT): A pilot study on feasibility, treatment adherence, and subjective efficacy. *German Journal of Psychiatry*, *10*(3), 69–78. www.scopus.com/inward/record.url?eid=2-s2.0-34548327193&partnerID=40&md5 = 86311f458086ee4fb1d48d38aaec69d6

Nahum, M., Fisher, M., Loewy, R., Poelke, G., Ventura, J., Nuechterlein, K. H., . . . Vinogradov, S. (2014). A novel, online social cognitive training program for young adults with schizophrenia: A pilot study. *Schizophrenia Research: Cognition*, *1*(1), e11–e19. doi:10.1016/j.scog.2014.01.003

Neumann, D., Babbage, B. R., Zupan, B., & Willer, B. (2015). A randomized controlled trial of emotion recognition training after traumatic brain injury. *Journal of Head Trauma Rehabilitation*, *30*(3), E12–E23.

Neumann, D., Malec, J. F., & Hammond, F. M. (2017). Reductions in alexithymia and emotion dysregulation after training emotional self-awareness following traumatic brain injury: A phase I trial. *Journal of Head Trauma Rehabilitation*, *32*(5), 286–295. doi:10.1097/HTR.0000000000000277

Nijman, S. A., Veling, W., Greaves-Lord, K., Vermeer, R. R., Vos, M., Zandee, C. E. R., . . . Pijnenborg, G. H. M. (2019). Dynamic interactive social cognition training in virtual reality (DiSCoVR) for social cognition and social functioning in people with a psychotic disorder: Study protocol for a multicenter randomized controlled trial. *BMC Psychiatry, 19*(1), 272. doi:10.1186/s12888-019-2250-0

Nijman, S. A., Veling, W., van der Stouwe, E. C. D., & Pijnenborg, G. H. M. (2020). Social cognition training for people with a psychotic disorder: A network meta-analysis. *Schizophrenia Bulletin, 46*(5), 1086–1103. doi:10.1093/schbul/sbaa023

Nijsse, B., Spikman, J. M., Visser-Meily, J. M., de Kort, P. L., & van Heugten, C. M. (2019a). Social cognition impairments are associated with behavioural changes in the long term after stroke. *PLoS One, 14*(3). doi:10.1371/journal.pone.0213725

Nijsse, B., Spikman, J. M., Visser-Meily, J. M., de Kort, P. L., & van Heugten, C. M. (2019b). Social cognition impairments in the long term post stroke. *Archives of Physical Medicine and Rehabilitation, 100*(7), 1300–1307. doi:10.1016/j.apmr.2019.01.023

Pallathra, A. A., Cordero, L., Wong, K., & Brodkin, E. S. (2019). Psychosocial interventions targeting social functioning in adults on the autism spectrum: A literature review. *Current Psychiatry Reports, 21*(1). doi:10.1007/s11920-019-0989-0

Penn, D. L., Roberts, D. L., Munt, E. D., Silverstein, E., Jones, N., & Sheitman, B. (2005). A pilot study of social cognition and interaction training (SCIT) for schizophrenia. *Schizophrenia Research, 80*(2–3), 357–359. doi:10.1016/j.schres.2005.07.011

Peterson, C. (1988). Explanatory style as a risk factor for illness. *Cognitive Therapy and Research, 12*(2), 119–132. doi:10.1007/BF01204926

Peterson, C. (1991). The meaning and measurement of explanatory style. *Psychological Inquiry, 2*(1), 1–10. doi:10.1207/s15327965pli0201_1

Radice-Neumann, D., Zupan, B., Tomita, M., & Willer, B. (2009). Training emotional processing in persons with brain injury. *Journal of Head Trauma Rehabilitation, 24*(5), 313–323. doi:10.1097/HTR.0b013e3181b09160

Randall, K. (2020). An autistic SLP's experiences with social communication. *Therapist Neurodiversity Collective.* https://therapistndc.org/an-autistic-slps-experiences-with-social-communication/

Roelofs, R. L., Wingbermühle, E., Egger, J. I. M., & Kessels, R. P. C. (2017). Social cognitive interventions in neuropsychiatric patients: A meta-analysis. *Brain Impairment, 18*(1), 138–173. doi:10.1017/BrImp.2016.31

Rose, A., Vinogradov, S., Fisher, M., Green, M. F., Ventura, J., Hooker, C., . . . Nahum, M. (2015). Randomized controlled trial of computer-based treatment of social cognition in schizophrenia: The TRuSST trial protocol. *BMC Psychiatry, 15*(1). doi:10.1186/s12888-015-0510-1

Spikman, J. M., Boelen, D. H. E., Pijnenborg, G. H. M., Timmerman, M. E., Van Der Naalt, J., & Fasotti, L. (2013). Who benefits from treatment for executive dysfunction after brain injury? Negative effects of emotion recognition deficits. *Neuropsychological Rehabilitation, 23*(6), 824–845. doi:10.1080/09602011.2013.826138

Spikman, J. M., & Fasotti, L. (2017). Recovery and treatment. In R. Kessels, P. Eling, R. Ponds, J. M. Spikman, & M. van Zandvoort (Eds.), *Clinical Neuropsychology* (pp. 113–133). Amsterdam: Boom Publishers.

Spikman, J. M., Milders, M. V., Visser-Keizer, A. C., Westerhof-Evers, H. J., Herben-Dekker, M., & van der Naalt, J. (2013). Deficits in facial emotion recognition indicate behavioral changes and impaired self-awareness after moderate to severe traumatic brain injury. *PLoS One, 8*(6). doi:10.1371/journal.pone.0065581

Spikman, J. M., Timmerman, M. E., Milders, M. V., Veenstra, W. S., & Van Der Naalt, J. (2012). Social cognition impairments in relation to general cognitive deficits, injury severity, and prefrontal lesions in traumatic brain injury patients. *Journal of Neurotrauma*, *29*(1), 101–111. doi:10.1089/neu.2011.2084

Turner, D. T., McGlanaghy, E., Cuijpers, P., Van Der Gaag, M., Karyotaki, E., & MacBeth, A. (2018). A meta-analysis of social skills training and related interventions for psychosis. *Schizophrenia Bulletin*, *44*(3), 475–491. doi:10.1093/schbul/sbx146

Turner-Brown, L. M., Perry, T. D., Dichter, G. S., Bodfish, J. W., & Penn, D. L. (2008). Brief report: Feasibility of social cognition and interaction training for adults with high functioning autism. *Journal of Autism and Developmental Disorders*, *38*(9), 1777–1784. doi:10.1007/s10803-008-0545-y

Vance, T. (2020, December 4). Social stories for autism and the harm they can cause. *Neuro-Clastic*. https://neuroclastic.com/2020/12/04/social-stories-for-autism/

Velikonja, T., Fett, A. K., & Velthorst, E. (2019). Patterns of nonsocial and social cognitive functioning in adults with autism spectrum disorder: A systematic review and meta-analysis. *JAMA Psychiatry*, *76*(2), 135–151. doi:10.1001/jamapsychiatry.2018.3645

Westerhof- Evers, H. J., Fasotti, L., van der Naalt, J., & Spikman, J. M. (2019). Participation after traumatic brain injury: The surplus value of social cognition tests beyond measures for executive functioning and dysexecutive behavior in a statistical prediction model. *Brain Injury*, *33*(1), 78–86. doi:10.1080/02699052.2018.1531303

Westerhof-Evers, H. J., Visser-Keizer, A. C., Fasotti, L., Schönherr, M. C., Vink, M., Van Der Naalt, J., & Spikman, J. M. (2017). Effectiveness of a treatment for impairments in social cognition and emotion regulation (T-ScEmo) after traumatic brain injury: A randomized controlled trial. *Journal of Head Trauma Rehabilitation*, *32*(5), 296–307. doi:10.1097/HTR.0000000000000332

Westerhof-Evers, H. J., Visser-Keizer, A. C., Fasotti, L., & Spikman, J. M. (2019). Social cognition and emotion regulation: A multifaceted treatment (T-ScEmo) for patients with traumatic brain injury. *Clinical Rehabilitation*, *33*(5), 820–833. doi:10.1177/0269215519829803

Wilson, B. A. (1997). Cognitive rehabilitation: How it is and how it might be. *Journal of the International Neuropsychological Society*, *3*(5), 487–496. www.scopus.com/inward/record.url?eid=2-s2.0-0030884313&partnerID=40&md5=adf9730ed0194faf03c94180c3e53cf6

World Health Organization. (2001). *International Classification of Functioning, Disability and Health: ICF*. Geneva: World Health Organization.

Appendix

Supplementary Table 1 Tests of Face Recognition

Test	Psychometrics	Clinical Sensitivity	Normative data	Advantages	Disadvantages
The Benton Facial Recognition Test (BFRT) [1] **Available through parinc.com** The examinee matches a target face to one of six (Part 1: six items) and to three or six of six presented which differ with respect to head orientation (eight items) or lighting (eight items) (Part 2). There is also a short form of 12 items [2]. **Time to administer: 9 minutes (long form)**	Internal reliability: Long form: α: 0.61 [3], 0.69 [4], 0.72 [5], Short form: α: 0.41–0.53 [3, 5]. Computerised version r_shc: 0.61 (accuracy), 0.88 (reaction time) [6]. Test-retest (one year): Long Form: 0.71 [5] Short Form: 0.60 [2]. Convergent validity: Correlates with the CFMT (0.49 [4] and emotion perception subtest of TASIT (0.45 [7]). Does not correlate with self-ratings of face memory ability in adults [4].	Performed poorly by many people with acquired prosopagnosia [8, 9] but not all [10, 11] although in these cases, response times are inordinately slow, suggesting reliance on other strategies. Sensitivity is improved using adjusted normative cut-offs to the original [3] or considering response times [12].	Original cut-off for impairment was 40 [1]. Albonica et al. (N = 272 19–31 y.o. students) suggest their cut-off is 41.71 (i.e. 2s.ds below the mean) is more appropriate and sensitive [13, 14]. Norms available for elderly (N = 349, 60–90+) [5]	Numerous studies and associated normative samples. Is widely used and reasonably suitable for examinees from different ethnic origins to the target faces [3].	Accuracy does not seem to be the best index for identifying prosopagnosia, response times need to be considered also. There is no control task.
Cambridge Face Recognition Tasks: [10]: **Available through www.testable. org/library. The Australian version and others are available from author Brad. Duchaine@gmail.com.** **Face Memory test (CFMT)** Part 1: Examinees exposed to different images of the same face then Part 1: select image from other identities; Part 2: select novel image of identity from distractors; Part 3: select identity amongst images with heavy visual noise. Administration time 10–15 minutes **Face Perception test (CFPT)** [15]: Examinee sorts six morphed images below in similarity to target above in (1) upright and (2) inverted presentations. **Time to administer: 8–12 minutes**	Internal consistency: **CFMT:** α: 0.89–0.92; **CFPT:** α: 0.74 for upright faces, 0.50 for inverted faces [3, 4, 16, 17]. Test-retest (six months): **CFMT:** 0.70; **CFPT:** N/A. Convergent validity: **CFMT** correlates with the **CFPT** (upright) r = -0.61 [17], r = 0.67 [18] and long-term face memory (r = 0.72 [18], r = 0.51 [16]. Divergent validity: No correlation between **CFMT** scores and abstract visual [16] or verbal memory [16, 17]. Ecological validity: **CFMT** correlates with self-reported problems with face recognition (r = 0.14) [4].	Discriminative validity: 25/32 people with suspected prosopagnosia performed below the cut-off on the **CFMT** vs only 6/32 on the **BFRT** [3]. **CFPT:** People with prosopagnosia were only mildly impaired on the **CFPT** relative to the **CFMT** [17].	Normative data: N = 3000+ collected via the internet [16], and for young adults from USA (N = 50), Israel (N = 49), Germany (N = 153) and Australia (N = 117, 241) [3, 4] [17] and older adults from 35 to 79 [17]. Similar data for young to older adults (65–88 y.o.s) is available for the **CFPT** (N = 125) [17].	**CFMT** is differentially sensitive to prosopagnosia. In well-educated samples, education did not influence scores [17], although women tend to out-perform men (approx. 3-point advantage [3].	Ethnicity similarity between target items and examinees influences scores [17] The **CFPT** has been found to correlate with verbal memory [17], suggesting intelligence may play a role in scores.

Note. HC = Healthy Controls; ASD = Autism Spectrum Disorders; SSD = Schizophrenia Spectrum Disorders; TLE = Temporal Lobe Epilepsy; FTD = Frontotemporal Dementia; TBI = Traumatic Brain Injury; OCD = Obsessive-Compulsive Disorder; PTSD = Post Traumatic Stress Disorder; AD = Alzheimer's Disease; MCI = Mild Cognitive Impairment; PSP = PR =; ICC = Intraclass Correlation; α = Cronbach's Alpha; r_{sh} = Split Half Reliability; r_{12} = Test-Retest Reliability; MC= Multiple Choice.

1 Benton, A.L., et al. (1983). Facial recognition: Stimulus and multiple choice pictures. In A.L. Benton, et al., Editors. *Contribution to Neuropsychological Assessment.*. Oxford University Press: New York. 30–40.

2 Levin, H.S., K.d.S. Hamsher, and A.L. Benton (1975). A short form of the test of facial recognition for clinical use. *The Journal of Psychology*, **91**, 223–228.

3 Albonico, A., M. Malaspina, and R. Daini. (2017). Italian normative data and validation of two neuropsychological tests of face recognition: Benton facial recognition test and Cambridge face memory test. *Neurological Sciences*, **38**(9), 1637–1643.

4 Palermo, R., et al. (2017). Do people have insight into their face recognition abilities? *The Quarterly Journal of Experimental Psychology*, **70**(2). 218–233.

5 Christensen, K.J., et al. (2002). Facial recognition test in the elderly: Norms, reliability and premorbid estimation. *The Clinical Neuropsychologist*, **16**(1), 51–56.

6 Rossion, B. and C. Michel. (2018). Normative accuracy and response time data for the computerized Benton facial recognition test (BFRT-c). *Behavior Research Methods*, **50**(6), 2442–2460.

7 McDonald, S., et al. (2006). Reliability and validity of the awareness of social inference test (TASIT): A clinical test of social perception. *Disability and Rehabilitation: An International, Multidisciplinary Journal*, **28**(24), 1529–1542.

8 Barton, J.J.S., J. Zhao, and J.P. Keenan. (2003). Perception of global facial geometry in the inversion effect and prosopagnosia. *Neuropsychologia*, **41**(12), 1703–1711.

9 Gauthier, I., M. Behrmann, and M.J. Tarr, (1999). Can face recognition really be dissociated from object recognition? *Journal of Cognitive Neuroscience*, **11**(4): 349–370.

10 Duchaine, B. and K. Nakayama. (2006). The Cambridge face memory test: Results for neurologically intact individuals and an investigation of its validity using inverted face stimuli and prosopagnosic participants. *Neuropsychologia*, **44**(4), 576–585.

11 Duchaine, B.C. and K. Nakayama. (2004). Developmental prosopagnosia and the Benton facial recognition test. *Neurology*, **62**(7), 1219–1220.

12 Busigny, T. and B. Rossion. (2010). Acquired prosopagnosia abolishes the face inversion effect. *Cortex*, **46**(8), 965–981.

13 Yerys, B.E., et al. (2018). Arterial spin labeling provides a reliable neurobiological marker of autism spectrum disorder. *Journal of Neurodevelopmental Disorders*, **10**(1),: 32.

14 Vettori, S., et al. (2019). Reduced neural sensitivity to rapid individual face discrimination in autism spectrum disorder. *NeuroImage: Clinical*, **21**, 101613.

15 Duchaine, B., L. Germine, and K. Nakayama. (2007). Family resemblance: Ten family members with prosopagnosia and within-class object agnosia. *Cognitive Neuropsychology*, **24**(4), 419–430.

16 Wilmer, J.B., et al. (2010). Human face recognition ability is specific and highly heritable. *Proceedings of the National Academy of Sciences of the United States of America*, **107**(11), 5238–5241.

17 Bowles, D.C., et al. (2009). Diagnosing prosopagnosia: Effects of ageing, sex, and participant-stimulus ethnic match on the Cambridge face memory test and Cambridge face perception test. *Cognitive Neuropsychology*, **26**(5), 423–455.

18 Russell, R., B. Duchaine, and K. Nakayama. (2009). Super-recognizers: People with extraordinary face recognition ability. *Psychonomic Bulletin & Review*, **16**(2), 252–257.

Supplementary Table 2 Tests of Theory of Mind (ToM)

Test	Psychometrics	Clinical Sensitivity	Normative data	Advantages	Disadvantages
Reading the Mind in the Eyes – Revised (RMET) [1, 2] **Available from www.autismresearchcentre.com/arc_tests** 36 photographs of the eye regions of faces (taken from magazines). Examinee chooses a mental state term, e.g. "nervous", "playful", "pensive", "pre-occupied", from four options that best matches the eyes. **Time to administer: 6.6 minutes**	Internal reliability: α: 0.37 [3], 0.53–0.77 [4], 0.58 [5]. 0.6–0.63 [6] 0.64 [7]. Average tetrachloric intercorrelation of 0.08 (acceptable range 0.15–0.5 [8]) [9]. Test-retest: ICC (one month) = 0.83 [10], (12 months) 0.63 [11]. Convergent validity: Evidence is weak. Two studies found RMET correlates with text-based ToM tasks [12, 13] but others did not [14–16]. Does not correlate with empathy [17, 18]. Correlates with vocabulary (e.g., r = 0.62) [19, 20].	Many clinical disorders perform poorly including people with ASD [17], SSD [21, 22], anorexia nervosa [23], TBI [12, 24–27], euthymia and bipolar disorder [28], and dementia [12, 27].	Numerous reports in the literature provide normative data including some relatively large samples (e.g. N = 320 healthy adults age M/SD = 40/12 [17]; N = 98 middle-aged adults [21]. There is also at least one study that reports child performance (N = 67 aged 9–15 years) [29].	Very widely used and has minimal motor or speech demands.	Evidence suggests that the RMET is neither internally reliable nor a valid test of ToM. It is strongly predictive of vocabulary skills.
Strange Stories Test (SST) [30]. **Available from the author** 24 short texts ending with a non-literal lie, joke, pre-tense, etc. plus control stories. Examinees answer whether the final statement is true or not and why. **Time to administer: 20–60 minutes**	The stories have acceptable internal consistency α: 0.74–0.75 and inter-rater and test-retest reliability [31]. Convergent validity: correlates with other measures of ToM [31–34].	The mentalising (but not control stories) are typically poorly performed by people with ASD from childhood through to adult. [30, 32, 33, 35–39]).	Varying numbers of ToM stories from 5 upwards and normative data for children and adults (usually fairly small samples of 30 or less) can be found in these.		

(Continued)

Supplementary Table 2 (Continued)

Test	Psychometrics	Clinical Sensitivity	Normative data	Advantages	Disadvantages
Faux Pas Recognition Test (FPT) [40]. **Available from www. autismresearchcentre.com/ arc_tests** A series of short stories (usually 10 or 20), approximately half of which describe a situation in which a person commits a faux pas unintentionally. The stories are read aloud and then a series of questions are asked to probe comprehension. **Time to administer: approx. 22 minutes**	Internal reliability: α: 0.91 [41] as cited in [7, 42]. Test-retest: (three months) r_{12} = 0.83 [43] (4 weeks) = 0.76 [42]. Inter-rater reliability: 0.76 [43] to 0.98 [27]. Convergent validity: Correlates with the RMET [7, 12] but not always [42]. Correlates with SST [32, 42] (r = 0.29, 0.36 respectively) and indirect language [26]. Concurrent validity: Is associated with social function in SSD [43] and behavioural problems in people with TBI [44].	The FPT is performed poorly by many kinds of clinical disorders including ASD [45], neuropsychiatric conditions [46–48], TBI [49] and dementia [12, 27].	Many clinical studies of the FPT, e.g. [44, 46, 48, 50, 51] provide data on normal healthy controls in middle adulthood (N 41, 36, 152, 33, 88 respectively) that can be useful to derive normative comparisons. There are also norms for children [52] N = 59 7, 9, and 11 year olds.	Quick and easy to administer. Freely available. Numerous translations (e.g. [7, 42, 45, 48, 53].	Requires reading/ listening and reliance on working memory/ memory.
The Hinting Task (HT) [54] **Available from the authors** 10 short stories describing an interaction between two characters, which end with one of the characters making a hint. At the end of each passage, the participant is asked what the hint meant. **Time to administer: 6 minutes**	Internal reliability: α: 0.56 [21], 0.57 [55] for HC 0.73 for SD [21]. Test-retest: r_{12} (2–4 weeks) = 0.42–0.51 (HC) and 0.64–0.70 (SSD) [19, 21]. Convergent validity: Correlates with other measures of ToM [56, 57]. Loads with other ToM tests (FPT [58] and TASIT [59]) on a single factor, separate to emotion perception and cognition. Concurrent validity: associated with in vivo social skills and functional outcomes in SSD [19, 21, 56] but not always [60].	The HT discriminates between people with SSD [19, 21, 61] and people with OCD [62] and healthy adults. It is also one of the most sensitive of a range of social cognitive measures for discriminating adults with ASD [59].	Normative data: There are a number of sources of normative data for middle-aged adults for the Hinting task including [59], N = 95; [19], N = 154; [21], N = 104; [54], N = 30; [63]; N = 30; [61], N = 32. There are also some normative data for children N = 20 10–15 years [64].	Simple and quick to administer. Freely available.	Does not have a control condition to determine what other non-social difficulties may be contributing.

Test description	Reliability/Validity	Sensitivity	Norms	Strengths	Limitations
TASIT [65] **& TASIT-S** [66]: **Part 2 (Social Inference -Minimal) and Part 3 (Social Inference Enriched). Available from www.assbi. com.au/TASIT-S-The-Awareness-of-Social-Inference-Test-Short** Videos of actors engaged in conversations that are sincere or sarcastic (Part 2) or sarcastic or lies (Part 3). Examinees answer four questions per item regarding thoughts, feelings, and intentions. **Time to administer: 40–50 minutes (long form) and 20 minutes (short form).**	_Reliability: Test-retest:_ Part 2: $r = 0.88$; Part 3: $r = 0.83$ (1 week); _Alternative form:_ Part 2: $r = 0.62$; Part 3: $r = 0.78$ (5–26 weeks); _Internal Consistency:_ Short version: Rasch item reliability estimates all > 0.89. _Validity: Convergent:_ Correlates with socially orientated tasks of new-learning and executive processing and experimental social tasks [67]. _Construct:_ TASIT-S correlated with original (all r's > 0.87) [68] _Concurrent:_ Correlates to poor social communication in vivo [69].	TASIT Parts 2 and/or 3 have proven sensitive to ToM impairments in SSD [70–73], major depression [74], multiple sclerosis [76, 77], Parkinson's disease [78], and FTD [73].	**TASIT**: 270 Australian adults aged 16–74 and 150 adolescents (aged 13–16) [65] **TASIT-S:** Normative data for 616 Australians including 226 adolescents (13–19) and 390 adults aged 20–75+ along with 180 U.S. residents (aged 20–74) [79].	Uses videos, everyday type conversations that mimic real world emotion processing than many tests. Has alternate forms.	TASIT correlates with measures of working memory and processing speed but not with non-social executive function and learning tasks [67]. Full version is lengthy.
Movie for the Assessment of Social Cognition (MASC) [34] **Available from the authors** 15-minute movie of four people interacting, regularly paused and a question is asked as to the thoughts/feelings or intentions of the relevant characters. Also MC format **Time to administer: 45 minutes**	_Internal Reliability:_ α: entire scale = 0.84–0.86 [34, 80]. Inter-rater: ICC = 0.99 [34] Test-retest (one year) $r_{12} = 0.67$ [81] Convergent validity: Correlates with the SST in ASD [34, 80] and with emotion recognition and RMET in healthy controls [34, 80, 82].	Differentiates b/w healthy adults and people with ASD [80], SSD [83, 84], and antisocial personality disorder [85]. This is true for most scores including under-mentalising errors but not over-mentalising [82–84].	Range of norms for young adults, e.g. N = 71 age: M/SD = 29.3/7.7 [84], N = 80, age: 39.1/10.7 [83], N = 42, age 37.5/15.9 [85], N = 71, age 29.3/7.7 [82], N = 26, 27.2/4.7 [80].	Ecologically valid assessment that combines verbal and non-verbal cues. Samples a range of mental state inferences.	Not all questions sample mental state terms. The over-mentalising errors seem to lack validity. Not yet consistent agreement about how scores/errors are categorized.

(Continued)

Supplementary Table 2 (Continued)

Test	Psychometrics	Clinical Sensitivity	Normative data	Advantages	Disadvantages
The Social Attribution Task (SAT) [86, 87] **Available from the authors** Adaption of Himmel and Siedler's 60-second cartoon of animated geometrical shapes. Explanations of the shapes' actions are rated for Pertinence, Salience, ToM, ToM affective, Animation, Person, and Problem Solving. There is also a multiple-choice format [88] and parallel versions [19]. **Time to administer: 10 minutes**	Internal reliability: α: 0.74 [19] and 0.83 [88] (MC version). Inter-rater reliability: ICCs (2 raters) 0.76–0.90 [86]. Test-retest (two weeks) 0.55 for parallel MC versions [19]. (ES = 0.49). Convergent validity: Correlates with the BLERT (r = 0.47) and the HT (r = 0.37) but not IQ [86, 87]. Is associated with neuropsychological test scores in SSD [88]. Concurrent validity: Correlated with financial, communication, and social skills in SSD but not another measure of real-world function [19].	The SAT discriminates between people with ASD, SSD, and HC [19, 86–88].	Norms for the MC version are provided for 154 adults [19] and 85 adults [88] in mid adulthood.	Requires minimal verbal comprehension. Has both free response and MC with detailed scoring procedures. High IRR is reported for both scoring systems.	Psychometrics are not well established. The free response scoring systems are detailed and complex.
The Yoni Task [89] **Available from the authors** Uses items with a central schematic face "Yoni" with changing eye gaze/mouth. In the corners around Yoni are objects (1st order ToM) or other faces with adjacent objects (2nd order ToM). Questions are of the form "Yoni is thinking of:." "Yoni loves . . ." (1st order) or "Yoni is thinking of/loves the fruit that – wants/loves" (2nd order). Control items tests physical judgements. **Time to administer: varies**	Internal consistency: N/A. Test-retest N/A. Adults with SSD improve on the test 18 months later, suggestive of practice effects: η2 = 0.193 [90]. Construct validity: Yoni scores are associated with cognition in some [91, 92] but not all studies [93]. Yoni task- 2nd order ToM is associated with comprehension of irony [89]. Concurrent validity: Correlated with Health-related Quality of Life in PD [93] and with positive and negative symptoms in SSD [94, 95], although not always [96] also psychopathy [97].	The 1st order tasks are poor at differentiating clinical groups [89, 91, 93–95, 97–99]. The 2nd order task is sensitive to brain lesions [89, 96–98], PD [93], MCI [100], OCD [91], HD [101], and SSD [90, 92, 95, 96, 99, 102], bipolar disorder [94], ASD [99], and psychopathy [97]. Affective vs cognitive tasks differentiate different disorders, e.g. affective task is difficult for people with psychopathy or ventromedial frontal lesions [89, 96, 97].	Normative data is limited and varies depending on the number of trials. Several studies using the original 64 items version [89, 90, 97, 99] provide percent accuracy estimates (and SDs) for small samples of adults (43, 44, 20, and 30 healthy adults respectively). One study using a 54 version, presents normative data (raw scores) for 316 normal adults age M/SD = 23.3/7.8 years [103].	Simple and has limited verbal demands. Has been used in a number of studies using healthy adults and is sensitive to clinical disorders. Provides the capacity to look at cognitive and affective ToM and there appears to be evidence that these dissociate in some clinical conditions.	Psychometrics are not established. Does correlate with cognitive abilities in some studies at least. The use of different numbers of (and possibly type of) trials across studies limits generalisability. Very little normative information.

Note. HC = Healthy Controls; ASD = Autism Spectrum Disorders; SSD = Schizophrenia Spectrum Disorders; TLE = Temporal Lobe Epilepsy; FTD = Frontotemporal Dementia; TBI = Traumatic Brain Injury; OCD = Obsessive-Compulsive Disorder; PTSD = Post Traumatic Stress Disorder; AD = Alzheimer's Disease; MCI = Mild Cognitive Impairment; PSP = PR =; ICC = Intraclass Correlation; α = Cronbach's Alpha; r_{sh} = Split Half Reliability; r_{t2} = Test-Retest Reliability; MC= Multiple Choice.

1   Baron-Cohen, S., et al. (1997). Another advanced test of theory of mind: Evidence from very high functioning adults with autism or Asperger syndrome. *Journal of Child Psychology & Psychiatry & Allied Disciplines*, **38**(7), 813–822.

2   Baron-Cohen, S., et al. (2001). The "reading the mind in the eyes" test revised version: A study with normal adults and adults with Asperger's syndrome or high functioning autism. *Journal of Child Psychology and Psychiatry*, **42**, 241–251.

3   Khorashad, B., et al. (2015). The "reading the mind in the eyes" test: Investigation of psychometric properties and test – retest reliability of the Persian version. *Journal of autism and developmental disorders*, **45**.

4   Prevost, M., et al. (2014). The reading the mind in the eyes test: Validation of a French version and exploration of cultural variations in a multi-ethnic city. *Cognitive Neuropsychiatry*, **19**(3), 189–204.

5   Harkness, K.L., et al. (2010). Mental state decoding in past major depression: Effect of sad versus happy mood induction. *Cognition and Emotion*, **24**(3), 497–513.

6   Voracek, M. and S.G. Dressler. (2006). Lack of correlation between digit ratio (2D:4D) and Baron-Cohen's "reading the mind in the eyes" test, empathy, systemising, and autism-spectrum quotients in a general population sample. *Personality and Individual Differences*, **41**(8), 1481–1491.

7   Soderstrand, P. and O. Almkvist. (2012). Psychometric data on the eyes test, the faux pas test, and the dewey social stories test in a population-based Swedish adult sample. *Nordic Psychology*, **64**(1), 30–43.

8   Clark, L.A. and D. Watson. (1995). Constructing validity: Basic issues in objective scale development. *Psychological Assessment*, **7**(3), 309–319.

9   Olderbak, S., et al. (2015). A psychometric analysis of the reading the mind in the eyes test: Toward a brief form for research and applied settings. *Frontiers in Psychology*, **6**, 1503–1503.

10   Vellante, M., et al. (2013). The "reading the mind in the eyes" test: Systematic review of psychometric properties and a validation study in Italy. *Cognitive Neuropsychiatry*, **18**(4), 326–354.

11   Fernández-Abascal, E.G., et al. (2013). Test-retest reliability of the 'reading the mind in the eyes' test: A one-year follow-up study. *Molecular Autism*, **4**(1), 33.

12   Torralva, T., et al. (2009). A neuropsychological battery to detect specific executive and social cognitive impairments in early frontotemporal dementia. *Brain*, **132**(Pt 5), 1299–1309.

13   Ferguson, F.J. and E.J. Austin. (2010). Associations of trait and ability emotional intelligence with performance on theory of mind tasks in an adult sample. *Personality and Individual Differences*, **49**(5), 414–418.

14   Ahmed, F.S. and L. Stephen Miller. (2011). Executive function mechanisms of theory of mind. *Journal of Autism and Developmental Disorders*, **41**(5), 667–678.

15   Duval, C., et al. (2011). Age effects on different components of theory of mind. *Consciousness and Cognition*, **20**(3), 627–642.

16   Gregory, C., et al. (2002). Theory of mind in patients with frontal variant frontotemporal dementia and Alzheimer's disease: Theoretical and practical implications. *Brain*, **125**(4), 752–764.

17   Baron-Cohen, S., et al. (August 2015). The "reading the mind in the eyes" test: Complete absence of typical sex difference in ~400 men and women with autism. *PLoS One*, **10**(8), ArtID e0136521.

18   Spreng, R.N., et al. (2009). The Toronto empathy questionnaire: Scale development and initial validation of a factor-analytic solution to multiple empathy measures. *Journal of Personality Assessment*, **91**(1), 62–71.

19   Pinkham, A.E., P.D. Harvey, and D.L. Penn. (2018). Social cognition psychometric evaluation: Results of the final validation study. *Schizophrenia Bulletin*, **44**(4), 737–748.

20   Peterson, E. and S. Miller. (2012). The eyes test as a measure of individual differences: How much of the variance reflects verbal IQ? *Frontiers in Psychology*, **3**(220).

21   Pinkham, A.E., et al. (2016). Social cognition psychometric evaluation: Results of the initial psychometric study. *Schizophrenia Bulletin*, **42**(2), 494–504.

22   Savla, G.N., et al. (2012). Deficits in domains of social cognition in schizophrenia: A meta-analysis of the empirical evidence. *Schizophrenia Bulletin*, **39**(5), 979–992.

23   Russell, T.A., et al. (2009). Aspects of social cognition in anorexia nervosa: Affective and cognitive theory of mind. *Psychiatry Research*, **168**(3), 181–185.

24   Geraci, A., et al. (2010). Theory of mind in patients with ventromedial or dorsolateral prefrontal lesions following traumatic brain injury. *Brain Injury*, **24**(7–8), 978–987.

25   Havet-Thomassin, V., et al. (2006). What about theory of mind after severe brain injury? *Brain Injury*, **20**(1), 83–91.

26   Muller, F., et al. (2010). Exploring theory of mind after severe traumatic brain injury. *Cortex: A Journal Devoted to the Study of the Nervous System and Behavior*, **46**(9), 1088–1099.

27   Gregory, C., et al. (2002). Theory of mind in patients with frontal variant frontotemporal dementia and Alzheimer's disease: Theoretical and practical implications. *Brain*, **125**(4), 752–764.

28 Bora, E., et al. (2005). Evidence for theory of mind deficits in euthymic patients with bipolar disorder. *Acta Psychiatrica Scandinavica*, **112**(2), 110–116.

29 Tonks, J., et al. (2007). Assessing emotion recognition in 9–15-years olds: Preliminary analysis of abilities in reading emotion from faces, voices and eyes. *Brain Injury*, **21**(6), 623–629.

30 Happe, F. (1994). An advanced test of theory of mind: Understanding of story characters' thoughts and feelings by able autistic, mentally handicapped, and normal children and adults. *Journal of Autism & Developmental Disorders*, **24**(2), 129–154.

31 McKown, C., et al. (2013). Direct assessment of children's social-emotional comprehension. *Psychological Assessment*, **25**(4), 1154–1166.

32 Spek, A.A., E.M. Scholte, and I.A. Van Berckelaer-Onnes. (2010). Theory of mind in adults with high-functioning autism and Asperger syndrome. *Journal of Autism and Developmental Disorders*, **40**, 280–289.

33 Lahera, G., et al. (2013). Social cognition and interaction training (SCIT) for outpatients with bipolar disorder. *Journal of Affective Disorders*, **146**(1), 132–136.

34 Dziobek, I., et al. (2006). Introducing MASC: a movie for the assessment of social cognition. *Journal of Autism and Developmental Disorders*, **36**(5), 623–636.

35 White, S., et al. (2009). Revealing Mentalizing Impairments in Autism. *Child Development*, **80**(4), 1097–1117.

36 Rogers, K., et al. (2007). Who cares? Revisiting empathy in Asperger syndrome. *Journal of Autism and Developmental Disorders*, **37**, 709–715.

37 Jolliffe, T. and S. Baron-Cohen. (1999). The strange stories test: A replication with high-functioning adults with autism or Asperger syndrome. *Journal of Autism and Developmental Disorders*, **29**(5), 395–406.

38 Kaland, N., et al. (2005). The strange stories test – a replication study of children and adolescents with Asperger syndrome. *European Child & Adolescent Psychiatry*, **14**(2), 73–82.

39 Baron-Cohen, S., S. Wheelwright, and T. Jolliffe. (1997). Is there a "language of the eyes"? Evidence from normal adults, and adults with autism or Asperger syndrome. *Visual Cognition*, **4**(3), 311–331.

40 Stone, V., S. Baron-Cohen, and R.T. Knight. (1998). Frontal lobe contributions to theory of mind. *Journal of Cognitive Neuroscience*, **10**(5), 640–656.

41 Yeh, Z., M. Hua, and S. Liu. (2009). Guess what I think? The reliability and validity of Chinese theory of mind tasks and performance in the elderly. *Chinese Journal of Psychology*, **51**, 375–395.

42 Chen, K.-W., et al. (2017). Psychometric properties of three measures assessing advanced theory of mind: Evidence from people with schizophrenia. *Psychiatry Research*, **257**, 490–496.

43 Zhu, C.-Y., et al. (2007). Impairments of social cues recognition and social functioning in Chinese people with schizophrenia. *Psychiatry and Clinical Neurosciences*, **61**(2), 149–158.

44 Milders, M., S. Fuchs, and J.R. Crawford. (2003). Neuropsychological impairments and changes in emotional and social behaviour following severe traumatic brain injury. *Journal of Clinical & Experimental Neuropsychology*, **25**(2), 157–172.

45 Zalla, T., et al. (2009). Faux pas detection and intentional action in Asperger syndrome. A replication on a French sample. *Journal of Autism and Developmental Disorders*, **39**, 373–382.

46 Ibáñez, A., et al. (2014). From neural signatures of emotional modulation to social cognition: Individual differences in healthy volunteers and psychiatric participants. *Social Cognitive and Affective Neuroscience*, **9**(7), 939–950.

47 Ibanez, A., et al. (2012). Neural processing of emotional facial and semantic expressions in euthymic bipolar disorder (BD) and its association with theory of mind (ToM). *PLoS One*, **7**(10), e46877.

48 Negrão, J., et al. (2016). Faux pas test in schizophrenic patients. *Jornal Brasileiro de Psiquiatria*, **65**, 17–21.

49 Martin-Rodriguez, J.F. and J. Leon-Carrion. (2010). Theory of mind deficits in patients with acquired brain injury: A quantitative review. *Neuropsychologia*, **48**, 1181–1191.

50 Spikman, J.M., et al. (2012). Social cognition impairments in relation to general cognitive deficits, injury severity, and prefrontal lesions in traumatic brain injury patients. *Journal of Neurotrauma*, **29**(1), 101–111.

51 Westerhof-Evers, H., et al. (2017). Effectiveness of a treatment for impairments in social cognition and emotion regulation (T-ScEmo) after traumatic brain injury: A randomized controlled trial. *Journal of Head Trauma Rehabilitation*, **32**(5), 296–307.

52 Baron-Cohen, S., et al. (1999). Recognition of faux pas by normally developing children with Asperger syndrome or high-functioning autism. *Journal of Autism & Developmental Disorders*, **29**(5), 407–418.

53 Altamura, A., et al. (2015). Correlation between neuropsychological and social cognition measures and symptom dimensions in schizophrenic patients. *Psychiatry Research*, **230**(2), 172–180.

54 Corcoran, R., G. Mercer, and C.D. Frith. (1995). Schizophrenia, symptomology and social inference: Investigating "theory of mind" in people with schizophrenia. *Schizophrenia Research,* **17,** 5–13.

55 Campos, D., et al. (2019). Exploring the role of meditation and dispositional mindfulness on social cognition domains: A controlled study. *Frontiers in Psychology,* **10,** 809.

56 Canty, A.L., et al. (2017). Evaluation of a newly developed measure of theory of mind: The virtual assessment of mentalising ability. *Neuropsychological Rehabilitation,* **27**(5), 834–870.

57 Wastler, H.M. and M.F. Lenzenweger. (2019). Self-referential hypermentalization in schizotypy. *Personality Disorders: Theory, Research, and Treatment,* **10**(6), 536–544.

58 Fernandez-Modamio, M., et al. (2019). Neurocognition functioning as a prerequisite to intact social cognition in schizophrenia. *Cognitive Neuropsychiatry,* No Pagination Specified.

59 Morrison, K.E., et al. (2019). Psychometric evaluation of social cognitive measures for adults with autism. *Autism Research,* **12**(5), 766–778.

60 Mallawaarachchi, S.R., et al. (2019). Exploring the use of the hinting task in first-episode psychosis. *Cognitive Neuropsychiatry,* **24**(1), 65–79.

61 Park, S. (2018). A study on the theory of mind deficits and delusions in schizophrenic patients. *Issues in Mental Health Nursing,* **39**(3), 269–274.

62 Tulaci, R.G., et al. (2018). The relationship between theory of mind and insight in obsessive-compulsive disorder. *Nordic Journal of Psychiatry,* **72**(4), 273–280.

63 Sanvicente-Vieira, B., et al. (2017). Theory of mind impairments in women with cocaine addiction. *Journal of Studies on Alcohol and Drugs,* **78,** 258–267.

64 Saban-Bezalel, R., et al. (2019). Irony comprehension and mentalizing ability in children with and without autism spectrum disorder. *Research in Autism Spectrum Disorders,* **58,** 30–38.

65 McDonald, S., S. Flanagan, and R. Rollins. (2017). *The Awareness of Social Inference Test 3rd ed.,* Sydney: ASSBI Resources.

66 McDonald, S., C. Honan, and S. Flanagan. (2017). *The Awareness of Social Inference Test-Short,* Sydney: ASSBI Resources.

67 McDonald, S., et al. (2006). Reliability and validity of the awareness of social inference test (TASIT): A clinical test of social perception. *Disability and Rehabilitation: An International, Multidisciplinary Journal,* **28**(24), 1529–1542.

68 Honan, C.A., et al. (2016). The awareness of social inference test: Development of a shortened version for use in adults with acquired brain injury. *Clinical Neuropsychologist,* **30**(2), 243–264.

69 McDonald, S., et al. (2004). The ecological validity of TASIT: A test of social perception. *Neuropsychological Rehabilitation,* **14**(3), 285–302.

70 Bliksted, V., et al. (2017). The effect of positive symptoms on social cognition in first-episode schizophrenia is modified by the presence of negative symptoms. *Neuropsychology,* **31**(2), 209–219.

71 Chung, Y.S., J.R. Mathews, and D.M. Barch. (2011). The effect of context processing on different aspects of social cognition in schizophrenia. *Schizophrenia Bulletin,* **37**(Suppl 5), 1048–1056.

72 Green, M.F., et al. (2012). Social cognition in schizophrenia, part 1: Performance across phase of illness. *Schizophrenia Bulletin,* **38**(4), 854–864.

73 Kern, R.S., et al. (2009). Theory of mind deficits for processing counterfactual information in persons with chronic schizophrenia. *Psychological Medicine,* **39,** 645–654.

74 Ladegaard, N., et al. (2014). Higher-order social cognition in first-episode major depression. *Psychiatry Research,* **216**(1), 37–43.

75 McDonald, S. and S. Flanagan. (2004). Social perception deficits after traumatic brain injury: interaction between emotion recognition, mentalizing ability, and social communication. *Neuropsychology,* **18**(3), 572–579.

76 Genova, H.M., et al. (2016). Dynamic assessment of social cognition in individuals with multiple sclerosis: A pilot study. *Journal of the International Neuropsychological Society,* **22**(1), 83–88.

77 Genova, H.M. and S. McDonald. (2019). Social cognition in individuals with progressive multiple sclerosis: A pilot study using TASIT-S. *Journal of the International Neuropsychological Society,* 1–6.

78 Pell, M.D., et al. (2014). Social perception in adults with Parkinson's disease. *Neuropsychology,* **28**(6), 905–916.

79 McDonald, S., et al. (2017). Normal adult and adolescent performance on TASIT-S, a short version of the assessment of social inference test. *The Clinical Neuropsychologist,* 1–20.

80 Lahera, G., et al. (2014). Movie for the assessment of social cognition (MASC): Spanish validation. *Journal of Autism and Developmental Disorders,* **44**(8), 1886–1896.

81 Vonmoos, M., et al. (2019). Improvement of emotional empathy and cluster B personality disorder symptoms associated with decreased cocaine use severity. *Frontiers in Psychiatry,* **10,** 213–213.

82 Vaskinn, A., et al. (2018). Emotion perception, non-social cognition and symptoms as predictors of theory of mind in schizophrenia. *Comprehensive Psychiatry,* **85,** 1–7.

83 Montag, C., et al. (2011). Different aspects of theory of mind in paranoid schizophrenia: evidence from a video-based assessment. *Psychiatry Research*, **186**(2–3), 203–209.

84 Engelstad, K.N., et al. (2019). Large social cognitive impairments characterize homicide offenders with schizophrenia. *Psychiatry Research*, **272**, 209–215.

85 Newbury-Helps, J., J. Feigenbaum, and P. Fonagy. (2016). Offenders with antisocial personality disorder display more impairments in mentalizing. *Journal of Personality Disorders*, **31**(2), 232–255.

86 Klin, A. (2000). Attributing social meaning to ambiguous visual stimuli in higher-functioning autism and Asperger syndrome: The social attribution task. *Journal of Child Psychology and Psychiatry*, **41**(7), 831–846.

87 Klin, A. and W. Jones. (2006). Attributing social and physical meaning to ambiguous visual displays in individuals with higher-functioning autism spectrum disorders. *Brain and Cognition*, **61**(1), 40–53.

88 Bell, M.D., et al. (2010). Social attribution test – multiple choice (SAT-MC) in schizophrenia: Comparison with community sample and relationship to neurocognitive, social cognitive and symptom measures. *Schizophrenia Research*, **122**(1–3), 164–171.

89 Shamay-Tsoory, S.G. and J. Aharon-Peretz. (2007). Dissociable prefrontal networks for cognitive and affective theory of mind: A lesion study. *Neuropsychologia*, **45**(13), 3054–3067.

90 Ho, K.K., et al. (2018). Theory of mind performances in first-episode schizophrenia patients: An 18-month follow-up study. *Psychiatry Research*, **261**, 357–360.

91 Liu, W., et al. (2017). Disassociation of cognitive and affective aspects of theory of mind in obsessive-compulsive disorder. *Psychiatry Research*, **255**, 367–372.

92 Li, D., et al. (2017). Comparing the ability of cognitive and affective theory of mind in adolescent onset schizophrenia. *Neuropsychiatric Disease and Treatment*, **13**, 937–945.

93 Bodden, M.E., et al. (2010). Affective and cognitive theory of mind in patients with Parkinson's disease. *Parkinsonism & Related Disorders*, **16**(7), 466–470.

94 Wang, Y.-y., et al. (2018). Theory of mind impairment and its clinical correlates in patients with schizophrenia, major depressive disorder and bipolar disorder. *Schizophrenia Research*, **197**, 349–356.

95 Zhang, Q., et al. (2016). Theory of mind correlates with clinical insight but not cognitive insight in patients with schizophrenia. *Psychiatry Research*, **237**, 188–195.

96 Shamay-Tsoory, S.G., J. Aharon-Peretz, and Y. Levkovitz. (2007). The neuroanatomical basis of affective mentalizing in schizophrenia: Comparison of patients with schizophrenia and patients with localized prefrontal lesions. *Schizophrenia Research*, **90**(1), 274–283.

97 Shamay-Tsoory, S.G., et al. (2010). The role of the orbitofrontal cortex in affective theory of mind deficits in criminal offenders with psychopathic tendencies. *Cortex*, **46**(5), 668–677.

98 Hu, Y., et al. (2016). Impaired social cognition in patients with interictal epileptiform discharges in the frontal lobe. *Epilepsy & Behavior*, **57**(Pt A), 46–54.

99 Tin, L., et al. (2018). High-functioning autism patients share similar but more severe impairments in verbal theory of mind than schizophrenia patients. *Psychological Medicine*, **48**(8), 1264–1273.

100 Rossetto, F., et al. (2018). Cognitive and affective theory of mind in mild cognitive impairment and Parkinson's disease: preliminary evidence from the Italian version of the Yoni task. *Developmental Neuropsychology*, **43**(8), 764–780.

101 Adjeroud, N., et al. (2016). Theory of mind and empathy in preclinical and clinical Huntington's disease. *Social Cognitive and Affective Neuroscience*, **11**(1), 89–99.

102 Ho, K.K., et al. (2015). Theory of mind impairments in patients with first-episode schizophrenia and their unaffected siblings. *Schizophrenia Research*, **166**(1–3), 1–8.

103 Terrien, S., et al. (2014). Theory of mind and hypomanic traits in general population. *Psychiatry Research*, **215**(3), 694–699.

Test	Psychometrics	Clinical Sensitivity	Normative data	Advantages	Disadvantages
Facial Expression of Emotion: Stimuli and Tests (FEEST) [1] Formerly available through Thames/ Pearson Assessment Two tests of emotion identification (1) *The Ekman 60 Faces Test* and (2) *The Emotion Hexagon Test*. **Time to administer: approx. 10 minutes**	Internal reliability [1]: 60 Faces: r_{sh} = 0.62 (total score); 0.21–0.66 (individual emotions): Hexagon test: r_{sh} = 0.92 (total score); 0.18–0.92 (individual emotions): Convergent validity: 60 faces correlates with TASIT (Part 1; 0.69) [2] vocal emotion (0.65), posture (0.70) and social judgements in people with ASD [3].	TLE reduces 60 Faces scores [4]. Fear is selectively poor with amygdala damage [5–7]. FTD also leads to impairment [8], while face recognition is preserved [9]. People with ASD and SSD do poorly on 60 Faces [10] but not necessarily face recognition [3].	Manual has data for *60 Faces Test* (N = 227, ages 20–70 years); *Emotion Hexagon Test* (N = 125, ages 20–75) [1]. Other studies with *60 Faces* provide normative data, e.g. [11] N = 33; [12]; N = 88; [13], N= 51; [14] N = 58.	The Ekman Faces are the most widely used images in emotion perception research.	The Ekman faces are outdated, black and white and posed.
The Comprehensive Affect Test System (CATS) [15]. Short form also available. **Manual currently inaccessible**[1] 13 subtests examining facial, prosodic and cross-modal affect **Time to administer: approx. 20 mins.**	Internal reliability: α – 0.15 to 0.76 [16] in children [17, 18] and adults [19]. Test-retest: Subtest 11 in children: r_{12} = 0.7 (12 months) [17]. Construct validity: Subtests 5 and 6 inter-correlate (r = 0.61) [19]. Subtest 11 correlates with DANVA, Strange stories, posture recognition in children, reflecting developmental trends [17].	SSD and BPD have poor face identification [20], naming and conflict judgements (prosody) and name/affect matching. [20–22]. FTD, AD, vascular dementia are poor at voice and face affect [23]. People with (left lateralised) PD have difficulty with prosody but not facial affect (CATS-A) [24].	Normative data for the CATS is reportedly in the manual for 20–79-year olds[1]. For the CATS-A the means and SDs for the individual subtests (N = 48, aged 18–60) are reported in [25] and for the composite scales (N = 60, aged 20–79) [26].	In adults, simple and complex emotions are not influenced by age but women outperform men. Allows testing of separate modalities.	Scores influenced by fluid reasoning (MR) and age [26]. Faces are outdated, black and white and posed.
The Emotion Recognition Task (ERT) [27] Freely available: Contact r.kessels@donders. ru.nl 96 videos of faces morphing into an emotional expression (40%, 60%, 80%, 100% intensities) **Time to administer: 20 minutes (long form) and 10 minutes (short form).**	Internal reliability: Based on N = 54 (TBI and healthy controls) [28], α for emotions range from 0.51 (happy) to 0.84 (anger) Construct validity: Reanalysing published data [28], ERT correlates with TASIT Part 1 (r = 0.78). Concurrent validity: The ERT correlates with informants' view of difficulties with communication after TBI [29].	The ERT is sensitive to TBI [28–31]; SSD [32], ASD [33, 34], OCD [35], BPD (Gray et al., 2006), PTSD [36], depersonalisation disorder [37], Korsakoff's amnesia [38], amygdalectomy [39], HD [40], FTD [41], social anxiety disorder [42] and Noonan syndrome [43] and stroke [44].	Regression-based norms are available from a sample of 373 healthy participants from Australia, Ireland and Europe, aged 8–75 [27] and also based on many clinical comparison studies, e.g. [29]. N = 42; [34]. N = 50; [43]. N = 40.	Translated into multiple languages.	Limited psychometric data to date.

(Continued)

Supplementary Table 3 (Continued)

Test	Psychometrics	Clinical Sensitivity	Normative data	Advantages	Disadvantages
The Awareness of Social Inference Test (TASIT) [45] & **TASIT-S** [46]. **Part 1: Emotion Evaluation Test** Available through **www.assbi.com.au/TASIT-S-The-Awareness-of-Social-Inference-Test-Short (short form)** 28 videos (nine in TASIT-S) of professional actors. Examinee classifies emotion. **Time to administer: 20 minutes (long form) and 10 minutes (short form)**	_Internal reliability:_ Short version: Rasch item reliability estimates all > 0.89 [47]. _Test-retest:_ r_{12} = 0.74 (1 week); _Alternative form:_ r_{AB} = 0.83 (5–26 weeks) [48]; _Construct validity:_ Correlates with socially orientated tasks of new-learning and executive processing and experimental social tasks [48]. Short version correlated with original (all r's > 0.87 [47]. _Concurrent:_ Correlates with poor social communication in vivo [49].	TASIT Part 1 has proven sensitive to emotion perception impairments in many clinical populations, including stroke [2], acquired brain injury [50], multiple sclerosis [51] and Alzheimer's disease [52].	**TASIT**: 270 Australian adults aged 16–74 and 150 adolescents (aged 13–16) [45] **TASIT-S**: Normative data for 616 Australians including 226 adolescents (13–19) and 390 adults aged 20–75+ along with 180 U.S. residents (aged 20–74) [53].	Uses videos everyday type conversations that mimic real-world emotion processing than many tests. Has alternate forms.	TASIT correlates with measures of working memory and processing speed but not with non-social executive function and learning tasks [48]. Full version is lengthy.
The Penn Emotion Recognition Test (ER-40) [54] Available from developers. See **https://penncnp.med.upenn.edu/request.pl** 40 colour photographs of four face emotions (i.e. happiness, sadness, anger or fear) at high and low intensity and neutral. **Time to administer = 3.5 minutes**	_Internal reliability:_ α = 0.56–0.65–(HC), 0.75–0.81 (SSD) [55, 56]. _Test-retest (2–4 weeks):_ r_{12}= 0.68–0.75 (patients and controls) [55, 56]. _Convergent validity:_ Correlates with the BLERT (r = 0.59) [55]. _Concurrent validity:_ Predicts functional and social outcomes in people with SSD. Confidence ratings/reaction times predict functional outcomes beyond neurocognitive measures [56].	ER-40 differentiates patients with SSD from health controls with medium to large effect size (d = 0.71) [55].	Normative data is available from Pinkham [55], N = 104; age 39.2 (13.70) and [56], N = 154: age = 41.95 (12.42).	The ER-40 is quick and simple to administer. Gender, age and ethnicity are varied and balanced across each emotional category.	

The Bell-Lysaker Emotion Recognition Test (BLERT) [57] Available from author morris.bell@yale.edu 21 x 10-second videos of a male actor expressing one of six emotions and neutral via face, voice and upper body movement. **Time to administer: 7 minutes.**	Internal reliability: α: 0.74–0.78 (SSD), 0.57–0.63 (HC) [55, 56]. Test-retest (2–4 weeks): r_{12} 0.70–0.81 (SSD) 0.63–0.68 (HC) [55, 56]. Convergent validity: Correlated with cognition measures [58]. Correlates with ER-40 (r = 0.59) [55]. Concurrent validity: Predicts functional and social outcomes in SD more strongly than TASIT, ER-40 or RMET [55].	The BLERT differentiates patients with SSD from healthy controls [59] with medium to large effect size (d = 0.76) [55, 60].	Normative data: Normative data is available for middle adulthood from Pinkham [55], N = .98 and [56], N = 148, [58]. N = 63.	Quick (7 minutes) and simple to administer and a good predictor of functional outcomes in people with schizophrenia, i.e. has good ecological validity.

Note. HC = Healthy controls; ASD = Autism Spectrum Disorders; SSD = Schizophrenia Spectrum Disorders; TLE = Temporal Lobe Epilepsy; FTD = Frontotemporal Dementia; TBI = Traumatic Brain Injury; OCD = Obsessive-Compulsive Disorder; PTSD = Post Traumatic Stress Disorder; AD = Alzheimer's Disease; MCI = Mild Cognitive Impairment; PSP = PR =; ICC = Intraclass Correlation; α = Cronbach's Alha; r_{sh} = Split Half Reliability; r_{12} = Test-Retest Reliability; MC= Multiple Choice; ^{1} The manual is advertised as online but according to the authors is no longer available.

1 Young, A., et al. (2002). *Facial Expression of Emotion-Stimuli and Tests (FEEST)*. Bury St Edmunds, England: Thames Valley Test Company.
2 Cooper, C.L., et al. (2014). Links between emotion perception and social participation restriction following stroke. *Brain Injury*, **28**(1), 122–126.
3 Philip, R.C., et al. (2010). Deficits in facial, body movement and vocal emotional processing in autism spectrum disorders. *Psychological Medicine*, **40**(11), 1919–1929.
4 Amlerova, J., et al. (2014). Emotion recognition and social cognition in temporal lobe epilepsy and the effect of epilepsy surgery. *Epilepsy & Behavior*, **36**, 86–89.
5 Broks, P., et al. (1998). Face processing impairments after encephalitis: Amygdala damage and recognition of fear. *Neuropsychologia*, **36**(1), 59–70.
6 Calder, A.J., et al. (1996). Facial emotion recognition after bilateral amygdala damage: Differentially severe impairment of fear. *Cognitive Neuropsychology*, **13**(5), 699–745.
7 Sprengelmeyer, R., et al. (1999). Knowing no fear. *Proceedings of the Royal Society of London. Series B: Biological Sciences*, **266**(1437), 2451–2456.
8 Kumfor, F., et al. (2011). Are you really angry? The effect of intensity on facial emotion recognition in frontotemporal dementia. *Social Neuroscience*, **6**(5–6), 502–514.
9 Keane, J., et al. (2002). Face and emotion processing in frontal variant frontotemporal dementia. *Neuropsychologia*, **40**(6), 655–665.
10 Sparks, A., et al. (2010). Social cognition, empathy and functional outcome in schizophrenia. *Schizophrenia Research*, **122**(1–3), 172–178.
11 Spikman, J.M., et al. (2012). Social cognition impairments in relation to general cognitive deficits, injury severity, and prefrontal lesions in traumatic brain injury patients. *Journal of Neurotrauma*, **29**(1), 101–111.
12 Westerhof-Evers, H., et al. (2017). Effectiveness of a treatment for impairments in social cognition and emotion regulation (T-ScEmo) after traumatic brain injury: A randomized controlled trial. *Journal of Head Trauma Rehabilitation*, **32**(5), 296–307.
13 Trepáčová, M., et al. (2019). Differences in facial affect recognition between non-offending and offending drivers. *Transportation Research Part F: Traffic Psychology and Behaviour*, **60**, 582–589.
14 Rowland, J.E., et al. (2013). Adaptive associations between social cognition and emotion regulation are absent in schizophrenia and bipolar disorder. *Frontiers in Psychology*, January 3.
15 Froming, K., et al. (2006). *The Comprehensive Affect Testing System*. Psychology Software, Inc.
16 Schaffer, S.G., et al. (2006). *Emotion Processing: The Comprehensive Affect Testing System User's Manual*. Psychology Software Inc.
17 McKown, C., et al. (2013). Direct assessment of children's social-emotional comprehension. *Psychological Assessment*, **25**(4), 1154–1166.
18 McKown, C., et al. (2009). Social-emotional learning skill, self-regulation, and social competence in typically developing and clinic-referred children. *Journal of Clinical Child and Adolescent Psychology*, **38**, 858–871.
19 Albuquerque, L., et al. (2014). STN-DBS does not change emotion recognition in advanced Parkinson's disease. *Parkinsonism & Related Disorders*, **20**(2), 166–169.

20 Martins, M.J., et al. (2011). Sensitivity to expressions of pain in schizophrenia patients. *Psychiatry Research*, **189**(2), 180–184.

21 Rossell, S.L., et al. (2013). Investigating affective prosody in psychosis: A study using the comprehensive affective testing system. *Psychiatry Research*, **210**(3), 896–900.

22 Rossell, S.L., et al. (2014). Investigating facial affect processing in psychosis: A study using the comprehensive affective testing system. *Schizophrenia Research*, **157**(1), 55–59.

23 Shany-Ur, T., et al. (2012). Comprehension of insincere communication in neurodegenerative disease: Lies, sarcasm, and theory of mind. *Cortex: A Journal Devoted to the Study of the Nervous System and Behavior*, **48**(10), 1329–1341.

24 Ventura, M.I., et al. (2012). Hemispheric asymmetries and prosodic emotion recognition deficits in Parkinson's disease. *Neuropsychologia*, **50**(8), 1936–1945.

25 Hulka, L., et al. (2013). Cocaine users manifest impaired prosodic and cross-modal emotion processing. *Frontiers in Psychiatry*, **4**, 98.

26 Schaffer, S.G., et al. (2009). The comprehensive affect testing system – abbreviated: Effects of age on performance. *Archives of Clinical Neuropsychology*, **24**(1), 89–104.

27 Kessels, R.P.C., et al. (2014). Assessment of perception of morphed facial expressions using the emotion recognition task: Normative data from healthy participants aged 8–75. *Journal of Neuropsychology*, **8**(1), 75–93.

28 Rosenberg, H., et al. (2015). Emotion perception after moderate-severe traumatic brain injury: The valence effect and the role of working memory, processing speed, and nonverbal reasoning. *Neuropsychology*, **29**(4), 509–521.

29 Rigon, A., et al. (2018). Facial-affect recognition deficit as a predictor of different aspects of social-communication impairment in traumatic brain injury. *Neuropsychology*, **32**(4), 476–483.

30 Rosenberg, H., et al. (2014). Facial emotion recognition deficits following moderate-severe traumatic brain injury (TBI): Re-examining the valence effect and the role of emotion intensity. *Journal of the International Neuropsychological Society*, **20**(10), 994–1003.

31 Byom, L., et al. (2019). Facial emotion recognition of older adults with traumatic brain injury. *Brain Injury*, **33**(3), 322–332.

32 Scholten, M.R.M. et al. (2005). Schizophrenia and processing of facial emotions: Sex matters. *Schizophrenia Research*, **78**(1), 61–67.

33 Law Smith, M.J., et al. (2010). Detecting subtle facial emotion recognition deficits in high-functioning Autism using dynamic stimuli of varying intensities. *Neuropsychologia*, **48**(9), 2777–2781.

34 Evers, K., et al. (2015). Reduced recognition of dynamic facial emotional expressions and emotion-specific response bias in children with an autism spectrum disorder. *Journal of Autism and Developmental Disorders*, **45**(6), 1774–1784.

35 Montagne, B., et al. (2008). Perception of facial expressions in obsessive-compulsive disorder: A dimensional approach. *European Psychiatry*, **23**(1), 26–28.

36 Poljac, E., B. Montagne, and E.H. de Haan. (2011). Reduced recognition of fear and sadness in post-traumatic stress disorder. *Cortex*, **47**(8), 974–980.

37 Montagne, B., et al. (2007). Emotional memory and perception of emotional faces in patients suffering from depersonalization disorder. *British Journal of Psychology*, **98**(3), 517–527.

38 Montagne, B., et al. (2006). Processing of emotional facial expressions in Korsakoff's syndrome. *Cortex*, **42**(5), 705–710.

39 Ammerlaan, E.J.G., et al. (2008). Emotion perception and interpersonal behavior in epilepsy patients after unilateral amygdalohippocampectomy. *Acta Neurobiologiae Experimentalis*, **68**(2), 214–218.

40 Montagne, B., et al. (2006). Perception of emotional facial expressions at different intensities in early-symptomatic Huntington's disease. *European Neurology*, **55**(3), 151–154.

41 Kessels, R.P.C., et al. (2007). Recognition of facial expressions of different emotional intensities in patients with frontotemporal lobar degeneration. *Behavioural Neurology*, **18**(1), 31–36.

42 Montagne, B., et al., Reduced sensitivity in the recognition of anger and disgust in social anxiety disorder. *Cognitive Neuropsychiatry*, **11**(4), 389–401.

43 Roelofs, R.L., et al. (2015). Alexithymia, emotion perception, and social assertiveness in adult women with Noonan and Turner syndromes. *American Journal of Medical Genetics, Part A*, **167**(4), 768–776.

44 Montagne, B., et al. (2007). The perception of emotional facial expressions in stroke patients with and without depression. *Acta Neuropsychiatrica*, **19**(5), 279–283.

45 McDonald, S., S. Flanagan, and R. Rollins. (2017). *The Awareness of Social Inference Test*. 3rd ed. Sydney: ASSBI Resources.

46 McDonald, S., C. Honan, and S. Flanagan. (2017). *The Awareness of Social Inference Test-Short*. Sydney: ASSBI Resources.

47 Honan, C.A., et al. (2016). The awareness of social inference test: Development of a shortened version for use in adults with acquired brain injury. *The Clinical Neuropsychologist*, **30**(2), 243–264.

48 McDonald, S., et al. (2006). Reliability and validity of the awareness of social inference test (TASIT): A clinical test of social perception. *Disability and Rehabilitation: An International, Multidisciplinary Journal*, **28**(24), 1529–1542.

49 McDonald, S., et al. (2004). The ecological validity of TASIT: A test of social perception. *Neuropsychological Rehabilitation*, **14**(3), 285–302.

50 McDonald, S. and S. Flanagan. (2004). Social perception deficits after traumatic brain injury: Interaction between emotion recognition, mentalizing ability, and social communication. *Neuropsychology*, **18**(3), 572–579.

51 Genova, H.M. and S. McDonald. (2019). Social cognition in individuals with progressive multiple sclerosis: A pilot study using TASIT-S. *Journal of the International Neuropsychological Society*, 1–6.

52 Kumfor, F., et al. (2014). Degradation of emotion processing ability in corticobasal syndrome and Alzheimer's disease. *Brain: A Journal of Neurology*, **137**(11), 3061–3072.

53 McDonald, S., et al. (2017). Normal adult and adolescent performance on TASIT-S, a short version of the assessment of social inference test. *The Clinical Neuropsychologist*, 1–20.

54 Kohler, C.G., et al. (2003). Facial emotion recognition in schizophrenia: Intensity effects and error pattern. *American Journal of Psychiatry*, **160**(10), 1768–1774.

55 Pinkham, A.E., et al. (2016). Social cognition psychometric evaluation: Results of the initial psychometric study. *Schizophrenia Bulletin*, **42**(2), 494–504.

56 Pinkham, A.E., P.D. Harvey, and D.L. Penn. (2018). Social cognition psychometric evaluation: Results of the final validation study. *Schizophrenia Bulletin*, **44**(4), 737–748.

57 Bryson, G., M. Bell, and P. Lysaker. (1997). Affect recognition in schizophrenia: A function of global impairment or a specific cognitive deficit. *Psychiatry Research*, **71**(2), 105–113.

58 Bryson, G., M. Bell, and P. Lysaker. (1997). Affect recognition in schizophrenia: A function of global impairment or a specific cognitive deficit. *Psychiatry Research*, **71**(2),: 105–113.

59 Cornacchio, D., et al. (2017). Self-assessment of social cognitive ability in individuals with schizophrenia: Appraising task difficulty and allocation of effort. *Schizophrenia Research*, **179**, 85–90.

60 Fiszdon, J.M. and J.K. Johannesen. (2010). Functional significance of preserved affect recognition in schizophrenia. *Psychiatry Research*, **176**(2–3), 120–125.

Test	Psychometrics	Clinical Sensitivity	Normative data	Advantages	Disadvantages
ATTRIBUTIONAL BIAS **The Ambiguous Intentions and Hostility Questionnaire (AIQ)** **Available from the authors** 15 vignettes (five in short version) representing accidental, ambiguous and intentional events. Examinee writes down reason for behaviour and how they would respond (both rated later, as the Hostility Bias (HB) and Aggression Bias (AB) index, 1–5). Three additional ratings derive the Blame Score (BS). **Time to administer: 5–7 minutes.**	*Internal consistency* BS (av 3 Likert scales): α: 0.84–0.86 [1] and 0.34–0.85 [2]. *Inter-rater:* ICCs 0.91–0.99 (HB), 0.93–0.99 (AB) [1]. *Test-retest:* r_{12} (2–4 weeks) 0.57 (HB), 0.70 (Aggression) and 0.76 (BS) [2]. *Convergent validity:* Scores higher for intentional vs ambiguous/ accidental vignettes. [1]. BS associated with SCID Paranoia subscale (esp. ambiguous scenarios (r = 0.25–0.26). [1]. *Concurrent validity* BS (but not others) correlated with real world function (the SLOF) in SSD. [2].	*Discriminant Validity:* SSD vs HCs perform poorly on HB and BS but not AB [2].	322 undergraduate students [1], 104 healthy community adults [2]. Based on Pinkham et al. (2016), *Healthy M (SD):* HB: 1.99 (0.60); AB: 1.83 (0.26); BS: 7.02 (2.31).	Discriminates people with SSD from HCs and is associated with other measures of paranoia	Does not predict functional outcomes in people with SSD.
SOCIAL COMMUNICATION **Latrobe Communication Questionnaire (LCQ)** [3] **Available from the authors** 30 items (six reverse scored) answered on a four-point scale from 1 (never) to 4 (always). Total score: 30 to 120, higher scores = greater impairment. Six sub scores: Conversational tone, Effectiveness, Flow, Engagement, Partner sensitivity and Conversational attention/focus. Self-completion and informant versions. **Time to administer: 15 minutes (informant): 30 minutes (interview).**	*Internal consistency:* α: 0.85–0.86 (healthy adult) α = 0.91–0.92 (TBI) *Test-retest:* Normative sample (eight weeks) r_{12} = 0.48 (Informant) 0.76 (self); ABI: (two weeks): r_{12} = 0.87 (informant) r_{12} = 0.81 (self). *Concurrent Validity:* Associated with exec deficits [4] and deficits in social perception [5].	*Discriminant validity:* Discriminates people with brain injury from healthy adults [4, 5].	147 young adults and 109 close others [6].	Good construct validity, high internal consistency and good stability in the ABI sample [7], freely available from the authors, easy to administer, simple language.	Lengthy, reverse scoring can be confusing and people with cognitive impairment need assistance to complete.

The Relationships Across Domains (RAD) [8]. **Available from the authors** The abbreviated version has 15 written vignettes involving male-female dyads representing one of four relational models (communal sharing, authority ranking, equality matching, and market pricing). Examinees read vignette and answer three yes/no questions about whether a future behaviour is likely to happen given the described relationship. Performance is scored as the total number of correct responses (ranging from 0 to 45). [8]. **Time to administer: 14–16 minutes.**	_Internal consistency:_ α: 0.72 (SSD), 0.81 (ASD); 0.63–0.70 (HCs) [2,9]. _Test-retest:_ (2–4 weeks) r_{12}= 0.751 (SSD), 0.756 (HCs) [2]. _Convergent validity:_ Loads on a "social appraisal" factor with TASIT and the HT in ASD, associated with TASIT in HCs [9]. _Concurrent Validity:_ In SSD RAD is correlated with real world function (SLOF; r = 0.202), financial/ communication skills (UPS A: r = 0.439) and social skills (SSPA: r = 0.243) [2].	_Discriminant Validity:_ Discriminates SSD from HCs (Cohen's d = 0.93) [2] and also ASD (Cohens d = 0.41) [9].	Discriminates SSD from HC. One of the only measures of social perception available.
		104 HCs from the community [2].	Has floor effects, where a high proportion of patients performed a t chance levels. It does not predict functional outcomes once neurocognitive performance is accounted for. It is also relatively long to administer. It was not recommended by Pinkham et al., 2016 for these reasons.
SELF-AWARENESS **Toronto Alexithymia Scale (TAS) [10]** **Available from the authors** 20-items with three subscales: Difficulty Describing Feelings (DDF): Difficulty Identifying Feeling (DIF): Externally-Oriented Thinking (EOT): All items are rated from 1 = strongly disagree to 5 = strongly agree. Five items are reverse scored. **Time to administer: 3–5 minutes.**	_Internal consistency:_ Total scores: α: 0.81–0.86; DDF and DDI Subscales (α: 0.71–0.78). [10,11]. Less support for EOT (0.66–0.80) [10–12]. _Test-retest: Depressed patients (5 years):_ 0.46 (Total), 0.35 (DDF), 0.49 (DDI), 0.57 (EOT) [13]; _People with psoriasis: (10 weeks)_ 0.69 (Total) [14]; _HC adolescents (4 years):_ 0.50–0.64 [15] _HC adults (11 years):_ r = 0.51–0.63 [16]. _Convergent Validity:_ Correlates with Bermond and Vorst Alexithymia Questionnaire [17] and the Observer Alexithymia Scale [12]. _Concurrent validity:_ High TAS-20 scores predict depression 4 and 11 years later [16], low social supports in adolescents [15] and alcohol use [12].	_Discriminant Validity:_ Discriminates many clinical disorders including traumatic brain injury [18–21], autism spectrum disorder [17], anxiety and depression [22–24] and eating disorders [25–27].	The subscale EOT less consistent than the other two.
		The TAS-20 uses cut-off scoring; equal to or less than 51 = non-alexithymia, equal to or greater than 61 = alexithymia. Scores of 52 to 60 = possible alexithymia.	Widely used (cited in over 3,000 research studies) to assess alexithymia. Remarkably consistent over time, consistent with personality variable.

(Continued)

Supplementary Table 4 (Continued)

Test	Psychometrics	Clinical Sensitivity	Normative data	Advantages	Disadvantages
Awareness Questionnaire (AQ) [28] **Available from the Combi site: The Awareness Questionnaire (tbims.org)** Seventeen-item scale uses clinician, informant and/or self-ratings to measure patient's awareness of functioning from 1 (much worse) to 5 (much better) in: Motor-sensory (four items), Cognition (seven items), and Behavioural/affective (six items) relative to pre-injury. Discrepancy between self- and informant = awareness. **Time to administer: 10 minutes.**	_Internal consistency:_ Self & Informant α = 0.88 (Total score). _Test-retest reliability:_ N/A. _Construct validity:_ Factor analysis supports 3 subscales: cognitive, behavioural/ affective and motor/ sensory. _Convergent validity:_ Higher correlation with similar ratings: Clinician vs Informant: r = 0.44 Clinicians vs DRS: r = -0.46, vs FIM r = 0.35.	_Sensitivity/ responsivity:_ Reduced discrepancy score after awareness intervention [29].	Norms not applicable.	Brevity (only 17 items). Strong psychometric properties. Well established use in TBI – inpatients, outpatients and community. AQ is in the public domain via the COMBI site.	Reliance on collateral ratings and the usual issues affecting their reliability (relative/clinician), no test-retest reliability.
Mayo-Portland Adaptability Inventory: 4 (MPAI-4) [30] **Available from the COMBI site** Mayo-Portland Adaptability Inventory (tbims.org) MPAI-4 is completed by clinician, informant or self with 29 core and six additional items. Core items: common sequelae of acquired brain injury in physical, cognitive, emotional, behavioural and social domains in three subscales: Ability (12 items), Adjustment (nine items), Participation (eight items). Pre-existing and associated conditions (six items: not scored). Responses on a five-point scale from 0 (mild problem without interference in activity) to 4 (severe problem interferes with activities > 75% of the time). (see [7] for full details).	_Internal consistency:_ α = 0.89; Inter-rater: N/A; Test-retest: N/A. Construct validity (MPAI-Version I only): Cognitive Index & RAVLT/ WCST, r = -0.55/0.56; Lower correlations with dissimilar constructs: Non-cognitive Index & RAVLT/WCST, r = -0.22/0.29; _Concurrent validity:_ Disability Rating Scale: r= 0.81; [30], admission MPAI-4 predicts discharge MPAI-4 participation [31] and living status at 1 yr. follow-up [32].	_Clinical sensitivity:_ Discriminates between two subgroups of the Ranchos Los Amigos Levels of Functioning Scale (Kruskall – Wallis = 22.07, p < 0.001[30]. Highly responsive to change (d = 1.71; [32] in response to treatment effort.	Norms not applicable.	MPAI-4 is a well-refined scale designed specifically for acquired brain injury. Subscales are reflective of key areas of global function. Clinician, informant and self-rated versions.	No inter-rater or test-retest reliability estimates.

Discrepancy between self and informant can be used to assess loss of awareness. **Time to administer: 8–10 minutes.** **The Patient Competency Rating Scale (PCRS) [33]** **Available from COMBI site** **www.tbims.org/combi/pcrs/pcrsref.html** Thirty-item scale with self, relative, clinician versions assesses current competency from 1 = Can't do, to 5 = Can do with ease. Subject's responses are compared to a significant other (a relative or therapist) who rates them on the identical items. Impaired self-awareness is inferred from discrepancies such that the subject overestimates his/her abilities compared to the informant. Various domains: activities of daily living, behavioural and emotional function, cognitive abilities, and physical function can be assessed separately. A short form of 13 items was developed for inpatient neurorehabilitation units, by excluding items not relevant to the inpatient context or which did not cohere with others in a factor analysis [34]. **Time to administer: 3–5 minutes.**	*Internal consistency:* α = 0.91 (patients), 0.93 (relatives) [35] and 0.82 (short form) [35]; *Test-retest reliability:* r_{12}= 0.92 (relatives), 0.97 (ABI) [33] ICC = 0.85 patients (one week) [35]. *Construct validity:* PCRS discrepancy scores correlate with indices of injury severity in some studies [36] but not others [33]. PCRS does not seem to correlate with neuropsychological findings [33,37] but does correlate negatively with depression or emotional distress [35,37], lending support to the idea that emotional reactions to disability follow the onset of deficit awareness. *Responsiveness:* Is used to measure changes in awareness for different domains over time [35] and response to intervention [38]. In the latter study, self and relative reports on the PCRS changes (indicating better functioning), whilst the discrepancy score did not significantly change.	Norms not applicable.	Brevity, available to the public (COMBI site), self, relative and clinician versions. Captures perceived current behavioural functioning across different domains – which is helpful separate to measuring awareness per se. Comparison with premorbid functioning is not required.	Usual concerns with discrepancy-based methods for awareness (does this reflect awareness deficits or relative's emotional state?) and the issue of interpreting change over time, which can arise from change in relative's score, not the shifting self-perceptions of the person with TBI.

(Continued)

Supplementary Table 4 (Continued)

Test	Psychometrics	Clinical Sensitivity	Normative data	Advantages	Disadvantages
Self-Awareness of Deficits Interview (SADI) [39] **Available from the authors** The SADI is a semi-structured interview that assesses the individual's awareness of changes in functioning, associated implications and the capacity to set realistic goals. Each section is scored on a 4-point scale: 0 (accurate knowledge, awareness of functional implications, and ability to set reasonably realistic goals) to 3 (no knowledge of deficits, acknowledgement of functional consequences, or realistic appraisal of the future level of functioning). The total score ranges from 0 to 9, with higher scores indicating greater unawareness. **Time to administer: 20–30 minutes.**	*Inter-rater reliability:* Total score: ICC = 0.82 [39]; *Test-retest reliability* (2–4 weeks) total score: ICC = 0.94 [40] *Convergent validity:* SADI correlates with AQ: r = 0.62 [41]; Discrepancy index on the DEX: r = 0.40 [42]; *Concurrent validity:* Predicts severity classification of Traumatic ABI (mild-moderate vs severe) with 75% sensitivity and 71% specificity [42].	The SADI Is sensitive to change, e.g. detected improved awareness pre vs post discharge [43].	Norms not applicable.	The interviewer can integrate information provided by the informant with their own observations to guide scoring. Unlike questionnaires, interviewer can rephrase questions and provide prompts to elicit self-perceptions.	The timeframe for administration is around = 30–40 mins, is not feasible for regular administration. Verbal skills and retrospective recall are likely to influence self-reported difficulties.
SOCIAL BEHAVIOUR **The Frontal Systems Behaviour Scale (FrSBe)** [44] **Available from PAR: www. parinc.com/Products/ Pkey/116#:~:text=The%20 FrSBe%20fills%20a%20 gap,may%20be%20targeted%20 for%20treatment.** The FrSBe is designed to measure changes in behavior as a consequence of frontal systems dysfunction.	*Internal consistency:* Family form – Total: α = 0.92 (Apathy: 0.78, Disinhibition: 0.80, Executive: 0.97), Self-Form – Total: α = 0.88 (Apathy: 0.72, Disinhibition: 0.75, Executive: 0.79); *Inter-rater reliability:* 0.83–0.89 for the total score and 0.79–0.92 for subscales [45]. *Test-retest* (three mns), r_{12} = 0.78 (Total score) *Construct validity:* Principal component analysis: 3 components account for 41% of the variance:	"After" functioning ratings on an earlier version (FLOP) revealed significant differences between patients with frontal lesions > patients with non-frontal lesions > controls [47].	Has some, but not extensive, normative data (n = 436) [44].	"Before" and "after" ratings, can be used in conjunction or separately. Subscales that are clinically meaningful and verified statistically. –	Needs to be purchased.

It is a 46-item scale, with three subscales: Apathy (14 items), Disinhibition (15 items) and Executive dysfunction (17 items). Self-rating and family forms have identical items, phrased as appropriate— can rate 'before' and 'after' injury.

Items are rated in a five-point scale: 1 (almost never), 2 (seldom), 3 (sometimes), 4 (frequently), 5 (almost always). Four scores are obtained: Total, Apathy, Disinhibition and Executive. Scores greater than T = 65 are considered clinically significant.

Time to administer: 5–10 minutes.

Frontal Behaviour Inventory (FBI) [48]
Available from the authors
The FBI in an informant rated scale with 24 items: 12 negative behaviours: apathy, aspontaneity, indifference, inflexibility, concreteness, personal neglect, disorganization, inattention, loss of insight, logopenia, verbal apraxia and alien hand, and 12 positive behaviours: perseveration, irritability, excessive or childish jocularity, irresponsibility, inappropriateness, impulsivity, restlessness, aggression, hyper orality, hyper sexuality, utilization behaviour and incontinence. Each item is scored on a four-point scale: none, mild, moderately, severe.

Time to administer: 5–10 minutes.

Executive dysfunction (14 items), Disinhibition (9 items) and Apathy (10 items) [46]. Higher correlations with similar constructs (FrSBe Apathy with Verbal Fluency (VF): r = -0.47, FrSBe Disinhibition with TMT-B errors: r = 0.42), and lower correlation with dissimilar constructs (FrSBe Apathy with TMT-B errors: r = 0.17; FrSBe Disinhibition with VF: r = -0.16) in a sample of 131 people SSD and 51 HC [45].

Internal consistency: α = 0.89 [49], 0.93 [50], 0.97 [51]; _Inter-rater reliability:_ Kappa = 0.89 [49], 0.92 [50], ICC: 0.91–0.92 [51]; _Test-retest_ (two weeks) r = 0.90 [50], (three weeks) 0.96– 0.97 [51]; _Convergent validity:_ Negative items correlate with the Madras Dementia Rating Scale and the MMSE [52]; _Concurrent Validity:_ The positive items correlate with the Zarit Burden Inventory (carers) [52].

Discriminant validity: The FBI differentiates patients with FTD from those with other dementias [50–58]. The FBI is also sensitive to deterioration over time [52,54] and is better able (98%) to differentiate patients with FTD from AD than cognitive tests (MMSE, WMS, WAIS, WAB: 78%).

Normative Data: As a measure of aberrant behaviours, most studies examine people with dementia classification. A cut-off score of 30 is recommended as useful for differentiating FLD from AD, vascular dementia and those with depression [49,55].

The FBI seems to have better sensitivity to deterioration over time than the NPI [52].

(Continued)

Supplementary Table 4 (Continued)

Test	Psychometrics	Clinical Sensitivity	Normative data	Advantages	Disadvantages
Overt Behaviour Scale (OBS) [59] **Available from COMBI site** OBS Rating Form (tbims.org) A clinician rating scale to measure challenging behaviors in people with ABI in the community. Contains nine categories, eight have three to six hierarchical levels (total of 34 levels across the scale): (1) Verbal Aggression (four levels), Aggression against objects (four levels), Aggression against self (four levels), Aggression against people (four levels), Inappropriate sexual behavior (six levels), Perseveration/repetition (three levels), Wandering/ absconding (three levels), Inappropriate social behavior (five levels). The final category, Lack of initiative has a single level. Hierarchical levels within the categories = increasing severity. Scoring uses three indices: **Cluster score**, which refers to the number of categories where the behavior occurs (range 0–9). **Total Levels** score, which refers to the number of levels that are endorsed (range 0–34), and **Total Clinical Weighted Severity** score, which is a summation of severity scores assigned to each of the levels – severity scores vary among the	*Inter-rater reliability* (two raters) r= 0.97 *Test-retest* (one week): r_{12} (Total score) = 0.77 [59]. *Construct validity*: Convergent validity: moderate-to-strong coefficients (range 0.37–0.66) between the OBS and MPAI, Current Behaviour Scale, Neurobehavioural Rating Scale-Revised). Divergent validity: No correlation between the OBS and the sub-scales of these tools that do not measure challenging behavior [59].	Responsiveness: Significant improvement in OBS scores after four months of treatment (Weighs: Time 1 Median = 11.0 vs Time 2 Median = 7.5; z = -2.24, p = 0.025) [59].	Norms not applicable.	Provides comprehensive understanding of nature, frequency and severity of challenging behavior. Quite good psychometric properties. Becoming increasingly widely used. Available free of charge.	Only includes 1 item on deficiencies in behavior (initiation), and other instruments will provide a more comprehensive analysis of that component of behavior (e.g. Apathy Evaluation Scale; FrSBe apathy subscale). OBS is quite a complex scale with a range of indices, and the user needs to be prepared to spend time and practice on administration and scoring.

categories and range from 1 to a maximum of 5. The Total Clinical Weighted Severity score ranges from 0 to 84).

Time to administer: 10–20 minutes.

DysExecutive Questionnaire (DEX) [60]

Available from Pearson Assessment www. pearsonclinical.com.au/ products/view/32 for purchase

The DEX is a rating scale that samples everyday problems commonly associated with frontal systems dysfunction. It can be used as a measure of awareness, by calculating a discrepancy score between self and informant responses.

Comprises 20 items sampling four domains: emotional, motivational, behavioural and cognitive with two forms, Self and Informant, same items, phrased as appropriate. All items are rated for frequency on a five-point scale: 0 (never) to 4 (very often). Scores are summed and the total scores range from 0 to 80, with higher scores indicating greater problems with executive functioning. The discrepancy score to measure awareness ranges from -80 to +80; scores in the positive direction indicate that the informant endorses greater frequency of problem than the patient, suggestive of the patient having problems with awareness.

Time to administer: generally brief.

Internal Consistency: $\alpha > 0.90$ in four different types of raters [61]. *Inter-rater reliability*: Neuropsychologist and OT ratings correlated 0.79 [61]. Family ratings correlate less. *Test-retest reliability*: N/A. *Construct validity*: The factor structure of the DEX contains either three or five factors: (1) Behaviour, Cognition & Emotion [62]; (2) Inhibition, Intentionality, Executive Memory, Positive Affect and Negative Affect [63]. The DEX has higher correlations with similar constructs: DEX-Inhibition vs TMT-B, r = 0.43; (2) DEX-Intentionality vs SET, r = 0.46 [63] than dissimilar constructs: Inhibition/Intentionality vs RBMT, both r = 0.06 [63].

A brief measure of self-reported and other-reported EF difficulties. Covers several domains of executive dysfunction.

Factor analyses suggest the DEX measures a series of constructs, not one [63–67]. However, it is unclear how separate subscales should be decided, as factor analyses were conflicting, with three-, four- and five-factor structures reported. The questionnaire must be purchased in conjunction with the BADS. Other measures such as the FrSBe and the BRIEF-A have superior psychometric properties and are available for purchase individually.

(Continued)

Supplementary Table 4 (Continued)

Test	Psychometrics	Clinical Sensitivity	Normative data	Advantages	Disadvantages
The Behavior Rating Inventory of Executive Function- Adult Version (BRIEF-A) [68] **Available from https://paa.com.au/product/brief-a/ for purchase** The BRIEF-A is a standardised measure of an adult's executive functions or self-regulation in his or her everyday environment. Two formats are used: a Self-report and an Informant report each with 75 items within nine clinical scales that measure various aspects of executive functioning: Inhibit, Self-Monitor, Plan/Organise, Shift, Initiate, Task Monitor, Emotional Control, Working Memory and Organisation of Materials. The clinical scales form two broader indexes: Behavioral Regulation (BRI) and Metacognition (MI), and these indexes form the overall summary score, the Global Executive Composite (GEC). The BRIEF-A also includes three validity scales (Negativity, Inconsistency and Infrequency). All 75 items are rated in terms of frequency on a three-point scale: 0 (never), 1 (sometimes), 2 (often). Raw scores for each scale are summed and T scores (M = 50, SD = 10) are used to interpret the individual's level of executive functioning. **Time to administer: 10-15 minutes.**	*Internal consistency:* α (self-report) 0.73–0.90 for clinical scales, 0.93–0.96 for the indexes and overall score. α (informant) 0.80–0.98 for the clinical scales, indexes and overall score [68]. *Inter-rater reliability:* Correlations between self- and informant report were moderate (0.44–.68). 50–70% of individuals and their informants reported T scores within one standard deviation of each other. A number of individuals rated themselves as having more difficulties than their informant (22.2% were between 1–2 SD higher, 6.7% were >2 SD higher), whereas only approximately 7% of individuals reported lower T scores on the overall scale than their informants. [68] *Test-retest reliability:* r$_{12}$ (four wks: self-report) 0.82–0.94 for the clinical scales, indexes and overall score: r$_{12}$ (four weeks: informant) 0.91–0.94 for the clinical scales and 0.96 for the indexes and overall score were 0.96. *Construct validity:* Moderate to strong correlations with the FrSBe for the majority of scales and indexes. BRIEF-A indexes correlated significantly with the executive dysfunction scale of the FrSBe for both self-report form (0.63–0.67) and informant-report form (0.68–0.74). Also, Total score on the DEX correlated with BRI (0.84), MI (0.73) and GEC (0.84) [68].	*Discriminant validity:* BRIEF-A Self-Report forms for 23 patients with TBI (60% mild, 10% moderate, 30% severe) were compared to 23 healthy individuals. Significant group differences were found for the GEC (η^2 = 0.19), BRI (η^2 = 0.23) and MI (η^2 = 0.08), as well as the individual scales Shift (η^2 = 0.14), Initiate (η^2 = 0.17), Working Memory (η^2 = 0.26), Plan/Organise (η^2 = 0.22), and Task Monitor (η^2 = 0.22) [68].		It is a reasonably brief measure of self-reported and informant-reported EF difficulties. Covers various aspects of EF and provides T scores for each scale. Strong psychometric properties for each scale, as well as indexes and GEC. Reasonably well priced. Can be administered and scored by individuals who do not have formal training.	

| Social Functioning in Dementia Scale (SF-Dem) [69]
Available from the authors
Uses self and informant ratings to evaluate social activities (10 items, e.g. "seen friends or family in own home") and Personal relationships (seven items: e.g. "asked other people about their feelings or concerns") each rated on a four-point scale (0: Never, to 3: Very often) Max score = 51. Higher scores = better function.
Time to administer: 13 minutes.
(people with dementia), 11 minutes (caregivers) | *Internal consistency:* α = 0.62 (patient rated) and 0.64 (carer rated) [69]
Inter-rater reliability: Two raters: ICC = 0.99 (patient), 0.99 (carer); *Test-retest:* (29 days) ICC = 0.80 (patient) and 0.89 (carer).
Convergent validity: Moderate correlation (r = 0.59) between overall scores from patient rated and caregiver-rated *Baseline:* No correlation with social domain of Health Status Questionnaire -12 (r = -0.26) (patients) or QOL-AD (r = 0.33) (carers); 6–8 months: sig correlation with QOL-AD (r = 0.47) (patients) 0.49 (carers). | *Discriminant validity:* No comparisons yet made with normative groups or different kinds of dementia. | None yet available. | One of very few measures that look at specific interpersonal behaviours in dementia.

Very little research to date. |
| Social Skills Questionnaire-TBI (SSQ-TBI) [70]
Available from the authors
The SSQ-TBI has 41 items that are completed by self or informant, rated on a five-point Likert scale, from 1 = Not at all to 5 = Very often.

Items reflect behaviours that are important for normal social interactions, as well as those impaired following ABI including emotion recognition, empathy, egocentrism and language skills. The SSQ-TBI taps 16 positive behaviours (e.g. "Shows interest in what another is saying (e.g. "with appropriate facial movements, comments and questions") and 24 negative behaviours (e.g. "Talks about a limited number of things"), | *Internal Consistency:* α = 0.90; *Convergent Validity:* The SSQ-TBI (family report) correlates with the FrSBe (Total Score and subscales: Apathy, Disinhibition and Executive Function (r = 0.84, 0.64, 0.84 0.75 respectively). The SSQ-TBI (Self report) correlated with FrSBe Disinhibition and Executive Dysfunction but not Apathy or Total Scores. The SSQ-TBI was associated with Disinhibited behaviour on the Neuropsychiatric Inventory (r = 0.5–0.63). It is only marginally correlated with TASIT Part 3 (r = 0.32, p = 0.053) but not Parts 1 or 2. *Concurrent validity:* SSQ-TBI (family report) predicts psychosocial outcomes (the Sydney Psychosocial Reintegration Scale) in Occupational, Interpersonal and Leisure domains (r = -0.38–0.69) [70]. | *Discriminant Validity:* The SSQ-TBI has only been used in a TBI sample to date so performance in normal healthy adults is not available. | Not available. | One of few questionnaires designed to examine specific social behaviours after TBI. It is the only questionnaire for clinical disorders that asks for both positive behaviours (strengths) and negative behaviours (weaknesses).

Not widely used. |

(Continued)

Supplementary Table 4 (Continued)

Test	Psychometrics	Clinical Sensitivity	Normative data	Advantages	Disadvantages
which can yield negative and positive subscales respectively. A final item provides an overall impression of social functioning. Positive items are reverse scored to produce a Total score (41 to 205) with higher scores suggesting greater difficulties. **Time to administer: 5–10 minutes.**					
OMNIBUS TESTS **The Social and Emotional Assessment (SEA)** [71] **Available from the authors** The SEA is designed to provide an overview of social cognitive abilities in FTD. It comprises five subtests. Emotion Perception (label 35 emotional expressions from Ekman and Freisen (max score = 15). Reward sensitivity/emotional reversal learning (Learn simple visual rule which then reverses: Max score = 5); Behavioural control: learn three rules for selecting visual squares (Max score = 5); Faux Pas test (Max score = 15) (10 stories: five of which contain a Faux Pas). (Total score max = 15) Apathy Scale (Carer version) (Max score = 15, transformed from total of 42) Scale taken from Starkstein et al., 1992) 14 items answered on three-point scale. For Items 1–8: 3 = "not at all." to 0 = "a lot.". For items 9–12 scale was reversed.	*Internal consistency:* N/A; *Test-retest reliability:* N/A; *Divergent validity:* None of the SEA subtests correlate with measure from the Frontal Assessment Battery within an FTD sample. Within an AD sample, only a word recall list was associated with the SEA, specifically higher apathy scores [71]. *Concurrent Validity:* N/A	**Discriminative validity:** All subtests of the SEA discriminate people with FTD from HCs [71,72]. Subtests, other than Reward sensitivity and behavioural control discriminate FTD from AD [71]. People with AD < HCs on Emotion perception, Apathy and SEA total scores [71].	Normative data: N/A However, based on their initial study (22 AD, 22 FTD and 30 HCs), Funkiewiez et al. recommended a cut-off of 39.4 as indicative of pathology. In a comparison between 19 people with MDD and 17 patients with FTD, cut-offs for differentiating between these conditions are recommended at 35.28 and 22.05, respectively for the SEA and the miniSEA.	Provides a comprehensive assessment of social cognition and inhibition in people with dementia filling a current gap.	Needs further research to establish psychometric properties and normative data. Requires computer program to administer several subtests.

A MiniSEA comprises Subtests 1 and 4 only [72]. **Time to administer: SEA – one hour; mini SEA – 30 minutes.**		People with MDD < HCs on Total scores SEA, miniSea and Apathy ratings [72]. Both the SEA and miniSea discriminate people with depression from people with FTD [72].	
Brief Assessment of Social Skills in Dementia (BASS-D) Available from the authors The BASS-D [73] is a test designed to assess social skills in dementia comprising five subtests (1) Face Emotion Perception Task (54 photos: max = 54); (2) Facial Identification Task (16 photos of famous faces: max = 48); (3) Empathy/ Theory of Mind Task (19 images of social scenes and participants asked questions about events and associated feelings: max = 133); (4) Social Disinhibition: Part I: (10 items: participants asked to inhibit comments about socially undesirable behaviour in images: max = 5). Part II: modified Stroop naming task where participants have to inhibit responses to their own name. Scores were calculated as the difference between the inhibition and reading conditions for both completion time and errors; (5) Social Reasoning Task	_Internal consistency:_ N/A; _Test-retest reliability:_ N/A; _Convergent validity:_ In a mixed sample of people with dementia and HCs, BASS subtests correlated with similar measures e.g. BASS Emotion perception correlated with TASIT EET (r = 0.81), BASS Face identity correlated with NUFFACE (HCs only: r = 0.604), BASS Empathy correlated with BEES (self-report) (r = 0.37), BASS Social Disinhibition Part II correlated with WMS-IV, Brief Cognitive Examination -Inhibition subtest (time r = 0.56, errors [HC only]: r = 0.43; BASS Social reasoning correlated with TASIT Part 3 (r = 0.320). However, BASS Face Memory did not correlate with a similar measure (WMSIII Face Memory) [74]; _Concurrent Validity:_ BASS Total score is correlated with a general cognitive measure (ACE-III) especially	_Discriminative validity:_ All subtests of BASS, except for the Face memory subtests discriminated people with dementia from healthy controls [74]. _Normative data:_ N/A.	Provides a comprehensive assessment of social cognition and inhibition in people with dementia filling a current gap. Needs further research to establish psychometric properties and normative data.

(Continued)

Supplementary Table 4 (Continued)

Test	Psychometrics	Clinical Sensitivity	Normative data	Advantages	Disadvantages
(five images of awkward social situations and participants need to answer questions about why they are award: max score = 5); (6) Memory for Familiar Faces (four photos, two of which were shown earlier: maximum score = 4); **Time to administer: 30–40 minutes.**	attention, memory and language domains of the ACE-III. The BASS is also associated with years since diagnosis, a proxy for dementia severity [74].				

HC = Healthy Controls; ASD = Autism Spectrum Disorders; SSD = Schizophrenia Spectrum Disorders; TLE = Temporal Lobe Epilepsy; FTD = Frontotemporal Dementia; ABI = Acquired Brain Injury; OCD = Obsessive-Compulsive Disorder; PTSD = Post Traumatic Stress Disorder; AD = Alzheimer's Disease; MCI = Mild Cognitive Impairment; ICC = Intraclass Correlation; a = Cronbach's Alpha; r_{sh} = Split Half Reliability; r_{t2} = Test-Retest Reliability; MC= Multiple Choice; RAVLT = Rey Auditory Verbal Learning Test; WCST = Wisconsin Card Sorting Test; TMT = Trail Making Test; MMSE= Mini Mental State Exam; WAIS= Wechsler Adult Intelligence Scale; WAB= Western Aphasia Battery.

1 Combs, D.R., Penn, D.L., Wicher, M., et al. (2007, March), The ambiguous intentions hostility questionnaire (AIHQ): A new measure for evaluating hostile social-cognitive biases in paranoia. *Cognitive Neuropsychiatr*, 12(2), 128–143.

2 Pinkham, A.E., Penn, D.L., Green, M.F., et al. (2016, March). Social cognition psychometric evaluation: Results of the initial psychometric study. *Schizophrenia Bulletin*, 42(2), 494–504.

3 Douglas, J., Bracy, C., Snow, P. (2000), *La Trobe Communication Questionnaire*. Bundoora, Victoria: Victoria School of Human Communication Sciences, La Trobe University.

4 Douglas, J.M. (2010, April). Relation of executive functioning to pragmatic outcome following severe traumatic brain injury. *Journal of Speech, Language, and Hearing Research*, 53(2), 365–382.

5 Watts, A.J., Douglas, J.M. (2006). Interpreting facial expression and communication competence following severe traumatic brain injury. *Aphasiology*. 20(8), 707–722.

6 Douglas, J.M., Bracy, C.A., Snow, P.C. (January–February, 2007), Measuring perceived communicative ability after traumatic brain injury: Reliability and validity of the La Trobe communication questionnaire. *Journal of Head Trauma Rehabilitation*, 22(1), 31–38.

7 Tate, R.L. (2010). *A Compendium of Tests, Scales and Questionnaires: The Practitioner's Guide to Measuring Outcomes after Acquired Brain Impairment*. Hove, UK: Psychology Press.

8 Sergi, M.J., Fiske, A.P., Horan, W.P., et al. (2009). Development of a measure of relationship perception in schizophrenia. *Psychiatry Research*, 166(1), 54–62.

9 Morrison, K.E., Pinkham, A.E., Kelsven, S., et al. (2019). Psychometric evaluation of social cognitive measures for adults with autism. *Autism Research*, 12(5), 766–778.

10 Bagby, R.M., Parker, J.D.A., Taylor, G.J. (1994). The 20-item Toronto alexithymia scale. 1. Item selection and cross validation of the item structure. *Journal of Psychosomatic Research*, 38, 23–32.

11 Taylor, G.J., Bagby, R.M., Parker, J.D.A. (2003), The 20-item Toronto alexithymia scale-IV. Reliability and factorial validity in different languages and cultures. *Journal of Psychosomatic Research*, 55, 277–283.

12 Thorberg, F.A., Young, R.M. Sullivan, K.A., et al. (July, 2010), A psychometric comparison of the Toronto alexithymia scale (TAS-20) and the observer alexithymia scale (OAS) in an alcohol-dependent sample. *Personality and Individual Differences*, 49(2), 119–123.

13 Saarijärvi, S., Salminen, J.K., Toikka, T. (2006). Temporal stability of alexithymia over a five-year period in outpatients with major depression. *Psychotherapy and Psychosomatics*, 75(2), 107–112.

14 Richards, H.L., Fortune, D.G., Griffiths, C.E., et al. (January, 2005). Alexithymia in patients with psoriasis: Clinical correlates and psychometric properties of the Toronto alexithymia scale-20. *Journal of Psychosomatic Research*, 58(1), 89–96.

15 Karukivi, M., Polonen, T., Vahlberg, T., et al. (October, 2014). Stability of alexithymia in late adolescence: Results of a 4-year follow-up study. *Psychiatry Research*, 219(2), 386–390.

16 Tolmunen, T., Heliste, M., Lehto, S.M., et al. (September–October, 2011). Stability of alexithymia in the general population: An 11-year follow-up. *Comprehensive Psychiatry*, 52(5), 536–541.

17 Berthoz, S., Hill, E.L. (May, 2005). The validity of using self-reports to assess emotion regulation abilities in adults with autism spectrum disorder. *European Psychiatry*, 20(3), 291–298.

18 Allerdings, M.D., Alfano, D.P. (2001). Alexithymia and impaired affective behavior following traumatic brain injury. *Brain and Cognition*, 47, 304–306.

19 Henry, J.D., Phillips, L.H., Crawford, J.R., et al. (2006). Cognitive and psychosocial correlates of alexithymia following traumatic brain injury. *Neuropsychologia*, 44, 62–72.

20 Neumann, D., Zupan, B., Malec, J.F., et al. (2013). Relationships between alexithymia, affect recognition, and empathy after traumatic brain injury. *Journal of Head Trauma Rehabilitation*, 29(1), E18–E27.

21 Williams, C., Wood, R.L. (March, 2010). Alexithymia and emotional empathy following traumatic brain injury. *Journal of Clinical and Experimental Neuropsychology*, 32(3), 259–267.

22 Hintikka, J., Honkalampi, K., Lehtonen, J., et al. (2001). Are alexithymia and depression distinct or overlapping constructs?: A study in a general population. *Comprehensive Psychiatry*, 42(3), 234–239.

23 Honkalampi, K., Hintikka, J., Antikainen, R., et al. (2001). Alexithymia in patients with major depressive disorder and comorbid cluster c personality disorders: A 6-month follow-up study. *Journal of Personality Disorders*, 15(3), 245–254.

24 Monson, C.M., Price, J.L., Rodriguez, B.F., et al. (2004). Emotional deficits in military-related PTSD: An investigation of content and process disturbances. *Journal of Traumatic Stress*, 17(3), 275–279.

25 Gramaglia, C., Ressico, F., Gambaro, E., et al. (August, 2016). Alexithymia, empathy, emotion identification and social inference in anorexia nervosa: A case-control study. *Eating Behaviors*, 22, 46–50.

26 Råstam, M., Gillberg, C., Gillberg, I.C., et al. (May, 1997). Alexithymia in anorexia nervosa: A controlled study using the 20-item Toronto Alexithymia Scale. *Acta Psychiatrica Scandinavica*, 95(5), 385–388.

27 Taylor, G.J., Parker, J.D.A., Bagby, R.M.I., et al. (December, 1996). Relationships between alexithymia and psychological characteristics associated with eating disorders. *Journal of Psychosomatic Research*, 41(6), 561–568.

28 Sherer, M., Bergloff, P., Boake, C., et al. (1998). The awareness questionnaire: Factor analysis structure and internal consistency. *Brain Injury*, 12, 63–68.

29 Schmidt, J., Fleming, J., Ownsworth, T., et al. (2013). Video-feedback on functional task performance improves self-awareness after traumatic brain injury: A randomised controlled trial. *NeuroRehabilitation and Neural Repair*, 27, 316–324.

30 Malec, J.F., Thompson, J.M. (1994). Relationship of the Mayo-Portland adaptability inventory to functional outcome and cognitive performance measures. *The Journal of Head Trauma Rehabilitation*, 9(4), 1–15.

31 Malec, J.F., Parrot, D., Altman, I.M., et al. (September 3, 2015). Outcome prediction in home- and community-based brain injury rehabilitation using the Mayo-Portland adaptability inventory. *Neuropsychological Rehabilitation*, 25(5), 663–676.

32 Malec, J.F. (2001). Impact of comprehensive day treatment on societal participation for persons with acquired brain injury. *Archives of Physical Medicine and Rehabilitation*, 82(7), 885–895.

33 Prigatano, G.P., Altman, I.M. (December, 1990). Impaired awareness of behavioral limitations after traumatic brain injury. *Archives of Physical Medicine and Rehabilitation*, 71(13), 1058–1064.

34 Borgaro, S.R., Prigatano, G.P. (October, 2003). Modification of the patient competency rating scale for use on an acute neurorehabilitation unit: The PCRS-NR. *Brain Injury: [BJ]*, 17(10), 847–853.

35 Fleming, J.M., Strong, J., Ashton, R. (1998). Cluster analysis of self-awareness levels in adults with traumatic brain injury and relationship to outcome. *Journal of Head Trauma Rehabilitation*, 13, 39–51.

36 Prigatano, G.P., Bruna, O., Mataro, M., et al. (October, 1998). Initial disturbances of consciousness and resultant impaired awareness in Spanish patients with traumatic brain injury. *Journal of Head Trauma Rehabilitation*, 13(5), 29–38.

37 Ranseen, J.D., Bohaska, L.A., Schmitt, F.A. (1990). An investigation of anosognosia following traumatic head injury. *International Journal of Clinical Neuropsychology*, 12(1), 29–36.

38 Ownsworth, T., Fleming, J., Shum, D., et al. (2008). Comparison of individual, group and combined intervention formats in a randomized controlled trial for facilitating goal attainment and improving psychosocial function following acquired brain injury [article]. *Journal of Rehabilitation Medicine*, 40(2), 81–88.

39 Fleming, J.M., Strong, J., Ashton, R. (1996). Self-awareness of deficits in adults with traumatic brain injury: How best to measure? *Brain Injury*, 10, 1–15.

40 Simmond, M., Fleming, J. (April, 2003). Reliability of the self-awareness of deficits interview for adults with traumatic brain injury. *Brain Injury: [BJ]*, 17(4), 325–337.

41 Wise, K., Ownsworth, T., Fleming, J. (September, 2005). Convergent validity of self-awareness measures and their association with employment outcome in adults following acquired brain injury. *Brain Injury: [BJ]*, 19(10), 765–775.

42 Bogod, N.M., Mateer, C.A., MacDonald, S.W. (March, 2003). Self-awareness after traumatic brain injury: A comparison of measures and their relationship to executive functions. *Journal of the International Neuropsychological Society*, 9(3), 450–458.

43 Fleming, J.M., Winnington, H.T., McGillivray, A.J., et al. (2006). The development of self-awareness and emotional distress during early community re-integration after traumatic brain injury. *Brain Impairment*, 7, 83–94.

44 Grace, J., Malloy, P.F. (2001). *FrSBe, Frontal Systems Behavior Scale: Professional Manual*. Lutz: FL: Psychological Assessment Resources, Inc.

45 Velligan, D.I., Ritch, J.L., Sui, D., et al. (2002). Frontal systems behavior scale in schizophrenia: Relationships with psychiatric symptomatology, cognition and adaptive function. *Psychiatry Research*, 113(3), 227–236.

46 Stout, J.C., Ready, R.E., Grace, J., et al. (March, 2003). Factor analysis of the frontal systems behavior scale (FrSBe). *Assessment*, 10(1), 79–85.

47 Grace, J., Stout, J.C., Malloy, P.F. (1999). Assessing frontal lobe behavioral syndromes with the frontal lobe personality scale. *Assessment*, 6(3), 269–284.

48 Kertesz, A., Davidson, W., Fox, H. (1997). Frontal behavioral inventory: Diagnostic criteria for frontal lobe dementia. *Canadian Journal of Neurological Sciences*, 24(1), 29–36.

49 Kertesz, A., Nadkarni, N., Davidson, W., et al. (2000). The frontal behavioral inventory in the differential diagnosis of frontotemporal dementia. *Journal of the International Neuropsychological Society*, 6(4), 460–468.

50 Milan, G., Lamenza, F., Iavarone, A., et al. (April, 2008). Frontal behavioural inventory in the differential diagnosis of dementia. *Acta Neurologica Scandinavica*, 117(4), 260–265.

51 Alberici, A., Geroldi, C., Cotelli, M., et al. (April, 2007). The frontal behavioural inventory (Italian version) differentiates frontotemporal lobar degeneration variants from Alzheimer's disease. *Neurological Sciences*, 28(2), 80–86.

52 Boutoleau-Bretonnière, C., Lebouvier, T., Volteau, C., et al. (2012). Prospective evaluation of behavioral scales in the behavioral variant of frontotemporal dementia. *Dementia and Geriatric Cognitive Disorders*, 34(2), 75–82.

53 Kertesz, A., Davidson, W., McCabe, P., et al. (October–December, 2003). Behavioral quantitation is more sensitive than cognitive testing in frontotemporal dementia. *Alzheimer Disease and Associated Disorders*, 17(4), 223–229.

54 Marczinski, C.A., Davidson, W., Kertesz, A. (December, 2004). A longitudinal study of behavior in frontotemporal dementia and primary progressive aphasia. *Cognitive and Behavioral Neurology: Official Journal of the Society for Behavioral and Cognitive Neurology*, 17(4), 185–190.

55 Kertesz, A., Davidson, W., Fox, H. (February, 1997). Frontal behavioral inventory: Diagnostic criteria for frontal lobe dementia. *Canadian Journal of Neurological Sciences*, 24(1), 29–36.

56 Milan, G., Iavarone, A., Lorè, E., et al. (March 1, 2007). When behavioral assessment detects frontotemporal dementia and cognitive testing does not: Data from the frontal behavioral inventory. *International Journal of Geriatric Psychiatry*, 22, 266–267.

57 Blair, M., Kertesz, A., Davis-Faroque, N., et al. (2007). Behavioural measures in frontotemporal lobar dementia and other dementias: The utility of the frontal behavioural inventory and the neuropsychiatric inventory in a national cohort study. *Dementia and Geriatric Cognitive Disorders*, 23(6), 406–415.

58 Konstantinopoulou, E., Aretouli, E., Ioannidis, P., et al. (2013). Behavioral disturbances differentiate frontotemporal lobar degeneration subtypes and Alzheimer's disease: Evidence from the Frontal Behavioral Inventory. *International Journal of Geriatric Psychiatry*, 28(9), 939–946.

59 Kelly, G., Todd, J., Simpson, G., et al. (January 1, 2006). The overt behaviour scale (OBS): A tool for measuring challenging behaviours following ABI in community settings. *Brain Injury*, 20(3), 307–319.

60 Burgess, P., Alderman, N., Wilson, B., et al. (1996). The dysexecutive questionnaire. In: *Behavioural Assessment of the Dysexecutive Syndrome*. Bury St Edmunds, UK: Thames Valley Test Company.

61 Bennett, P.C., Ong, B., Ponsford, J. (2005). Measuring executive dysfunction in an acute rehabilitation setting: Using the dysexecutive questionnaire (DEX). *Journal of the International Neuropsychological Society*, 11(4), 376–385.

62 Wilson, B.A., Alderman, N., Burgess, P.W., et al. (1996). *The Behavioural Assessment of the Dysexecutive Syndrome*. London: Thames Valley Test Company/Harcourt Assessment/Psychological Corporation.

63 Burgess, P.W., Alderman, N., Evans, J., et al. (1998). The ecological validity of tests of executive function. *Journal of the International Neuropsychological Society*, 4(6), 547–558.

64 Burgess, P.W., Alderman, N., Wilson, B.A., et al. (1996). Validity of the battery: Relationship between performance on the BADS and ratings of executive problems. In: Wilson BA, editor. *Bads: Behavioural Assessment of the Dysexecutive Syndrome Manual*. Bury St Edmunds, UK: Thames Valley Test Company.

65 Chaytor, N., Schmitter-Edgecombe, M., Burr, R. (April, 2006). Improving the ecological validity of executive functioning assessment. *Archives of Clinical Neuropsychology*, 21(3), 217–227.

66 Bodenburg, S., Dopslaff, N. (January, 2008). The dysexecutive questionnaire advanced-item and test score characteristics, 4-factor solution, and severity classification. *Journal of Nervous and Mental Disease*, 196(1), 75–78.

67 Simblett, S.K., Bateman, A. (2011). Dimensions of the dysexecutive questionnaire (DEX) examined using Rasch analysis. *Neuropsychological Rehabilitation*, 21(1), 1–25.

68 Roth, R.M., Isquith, P.K., Gioia, G.A. (2005). *BRIEF-A: Behavior Rating Inventory of Executive Function – Adult Version: Professional Manual*. Lutz, FL: Psychological Assessment Resources; 2005.

69 Sommerlad, A., Singleton, D., Jones, R., et al. (2017). Development of an instrument to assess social functioning in dementia: The social functioning in dementia scale (SF-DEM). *Alzheimers Dement (Amst)*, 7, 88–98.

70 Francis, H.M., Osborne-Crowley, K., McDonald, S. (2017). Validity and reliability of a questionnaire to assess social skills in traumatic brain injury: A preliminary study. *Brain Injury*, 1–8.

71 Funkiewiez, A., Bertoux, M., Cruz de Souza, L., et al. (2012). The SEA (social cognition and emotion assessment): A clinical neuropsychological tool for early diagnosis of frontal variant to frontotemporal lobar degeneration. *Neuropsychology*, 26(1), 81–90.

72 Bertoux, M., Delavest, M., de Souza, L.C., et al. (April, 2012). Social cognition and emotional assessment differentiates frontotemporal dementia from depression. *Journal of Neurology, Neurosurgery, and Psychiatry*, 83(4), 411–416.

73 Kelly, M., McDonald, S. (2020). Assessing social cognition in people with a diagnosis of dementia: Development of a novel screening test, the brief assessment of social skills (BASS-D). *Journal of Clinical and Experimental Neuropsychology*, 42(2), 185–198.

74 Kelly, M., McDonald, S. (2020). Assessing social cognition in people with a diagnosis of dementia: Development of a novel screening test, the brief assessment of social skills (BASS-D). *Journal of Clinical and Experimental Neuropsychology*, 42(2), 185–198.

Index

Note: Page numbers in *italics* indicate a figure and page numbers in **bold** indicate a table on the corresponding page.

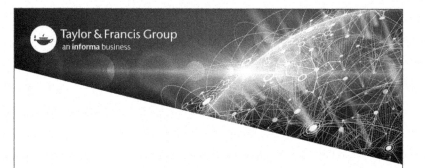

For Product Safety Concerns and Information please contact our EU
representative GPSR@taylorandfrancis.com
Taylor & Francis Verlag GmbH, Kaufingerstraße 24, 80331 München, Germany

www.ingramcontent.com/pod-product-compliance
Ingram Content Group UK Ltd.
Pitfield, Milton Keynes, MK11 3LW, UK
UKHW021450080625
459435UK00012B/443